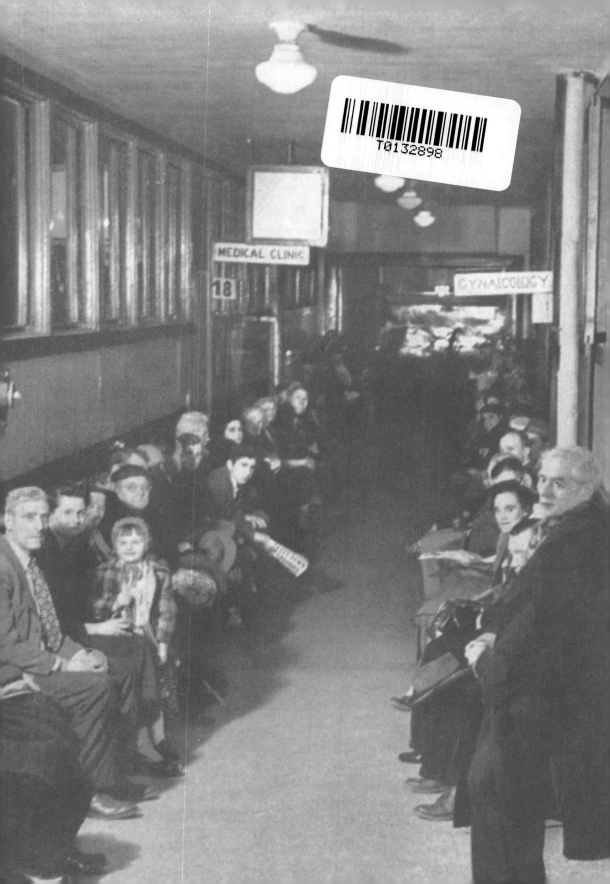

The General

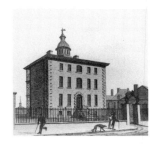

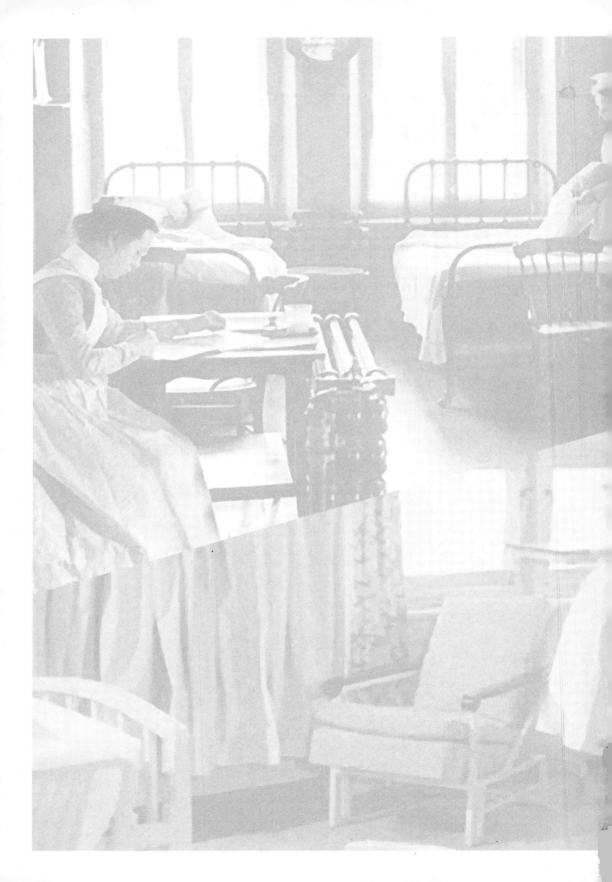

The General

A History of the Montreal General Hospital

EDITED BY JOSEPH HANAWAY AND JOHN H. BURGESS

Published for the Montreal General Hospital Foundation
by
McGill-Queen's University Press
Montreal & Kingston • London • Chicago

ISBN 978-0-7735-4685-1 (cloth)
ISBN 978-0-7735-9864-5 (ePDF)

Legal deposit third quarter 2016
Bibliothèque nationale du Québec

Printed in Canada on acid-free paper

McGill-Queen's University Press acknowledges the support of the Canada
Council for the Arts for our publishing program. We also acknowledge the
financial support of the Government of Canada through the Canada Book
Fund for our publishing activities.

Library and Archives Canada Cataloguing in Publication

General (Montréal, Québec)
The General : a history of the Montreal General Hospital, 1819–1997
/ edited by Joseph Hanaway and John H. Burgess.

Includes bibliographical references and index.
Issued in print and electronic formats.
ISBN 978-0-7735-4685-1 (cloth).–ISBN 978-0-7735-9864-5 (ePDF)

1. Montreal General Hospital–History. 2. Hospitals–Québec
(Province)–Montréal–History. I. Hanaway, Joseph, 1933–, author, editor
II. Burgess, John H., 1933–, author, editor III. Title.

RA983.M652M65 2016   362.1109714'28   C2016-901545-9
                                            C2016-901546-7

Front endsheets: 1892 MGH OR scene from Hugh Ernest McDermott, *A
History of the Montreal General Hospital, 1888–1983* (Montreal: Montreal
General Hospital, 1950), 60. Photographer unknown. MGH clinic waiting
room circa 1920 from "The Montreal General Hospital, 1821–1956: A Picto-
rial Review," special issue, *Montreal General Hospital Bulletin* 2, no. 8, 21.
Photographer unknown.

Rear endsheets: Top: MGH nurses attending beds, 1920s. Bottom: Nurses
making a bed, 1955. Photos courtesy of Robert Derval and the MGH photo
archives. Photographer unknown.

To the Molson Family

We dedicate this volume on the history of the Montreal General Hospital to the Molson family, whose members have been involved in its management and development for 190 years. Starting with John Molson the elder, who was the third president of the hospital from 1831 to 1835, throughout the decades, members of the family have been presidents and members of the Board of Directors. Whenever improvements in facilities to strengthen patient care were being considered, the Molsons could be relied on to help. This dedication was and is from a sincere interest in the hospital's mission.

The Molsons and the MGH have grown up together. In many ways, the hospital would not be the great clinical and research centre it is today without the friendship of this extraordinary family.

Contents

Abbreviations

AAMGHSN Alumnae Association of the Montreal General Hospital School of Nursing

AAOG American Association of Obstetrics and Gynecology

AAOOL American Association of Ophthalmologists and Otolaryngologists

AAOS American Academy of Orthopedic Surgeons

AAST American Association of the Surgery of Trauma

AC Audit Committee

ACOG American College of Gynecologists

ACS American College of Surgeons

ACTH adrenocortic trophic hormone

AGA American Gynelogical Association

AIDS acquired immune deficiency syndrome

ALA American Laryngology Association

AMI Allen Memorial Institute

ANPQ Association of Nurses of the Province of Quebec

ARNPQ Association of Registered Nurses of the Province of Quebec

ATLS advanced trauma life support

B of D Board of Directors

B of G Board of Governors

B of M Board of Management

Bill 65 Quebec Medical Insurance Act, 1970

BIPP Bismuth Iodoform Paraffin Paste

BSc(N) bachelor of nursing

BUN blood urea nitrogen

CAMC Canadian Army Medical Corps

CAR Canadian Association of Radiologists

CARO Canadian Association of Radiation Oncologists

CBE Companion of the British Empire

CBH Catherine Booth Hospital

CCCN Canadian Coronary Care Nurses Association

CCPM Canadian College of Physicists in Medicine

CDC Centers for Disease Control

CEA carcinoembryonic antigen

CEGEP Colleges d'Enseignment Generale et Practiques

CEO chief operating officer

CGH#3 Canadian General
    Hospital No. 3, McGill
MCHI Montreal Chest Institute
    (old Royal Edward Laurentien
    Hospital)
CHA Canada Health Act
CHUM Centre hospitalier
    universitaire de Montréal
CIDA Canadian Infectious Disease
    Agency
CLSCs Centre Local Santé
    Communitaire
CMA Canadian Medical
    Association
CME continuing medical
    education
CMG Companion of the Order of
    St Michael and St George
CNA Canadian Nurses Association
CNS clinical nurse specialist
CN Council of Nurses
COA Canadian Orthopaedic
    Association
COG Children's Oncology Group
COQAR Committee of Quality
    and Risk Management
COTOLS Canadian Otolaryngo-
    logical Society
COS Canadian Ophthalmological
    Society
CPC Clinical Pathological
    Conference
CPDP Council of Physicians,
    Dentists and Pharmacists
CPR Canadian Pacific Railway
CPR cardio-pulmonary
    resuscitation

CQRS Quebec Council on Social
    Research
CRC Canadian Red Cross
CRCP Certificate of Royal College
    of Physicians
CRN Centre for Research in
    Neuroscience
CT computed tomography
CTU clinical teaching unit
CUSM Centre Universitaire Santé
    McGill
CVS cardiovascular surgery
CVT cardiovascular thoracic
    surgery
DG director general
DH Douglas Hospital (old Verdun
    Protestant Hospital)
DN director of nursing
DPS director of professional
    services
DSC Départements de santé
    communautaire
*DSM Diagnostic and Statistical
    Manual*
DVM doctor of veterinary
    medicine
ECT electroconvulsive therapy
ED Emergency Department
ED executive director
EEG Electroencephalogram
EM emergency medicine
EMG Electromyogram
ENT ear, nose, and throat
ER emergency room
ERG/VER electroretinogram/
    visual-evoked response

FACOG Fellow of the American College of Gynecology

FLQ Front du Libération de Québec

FMSQ Federation of Medical Specialists of Quebec

FRCPC Fellow of the Royal College of Physicians of Canada

FRCSC Fellow of the Royal College of Surgeons of Canada

FRSQ les Fonds de la Recherche en Santé du Québec

GEC Governing and Ethics Committee

GERD gastrointestinal reflux disease

GFT geographic full time

GI Gastroenterology

GISM Groupe Immobilier Santé McGill (MUHC PPP)

Glen site Notre-Dame-de-Grâce (NDG) site of MUHC, old railway marshalling yard

GP general practitioner

GYN gynaecology

HSSA Health and Social Service Agency

HSSS Health Services and Social Services Act

HIDS Hospital Insurance and Diagnostic Services Act

IBM International Business Machines

ICD-9 International Classification of Disease-9

ICN International Council of Nursing

ICO International Congress of Ophthalmology

ICU Intensive Care Unit

ID infectious disease

IDRC International Development Research Centre

ISRS International Stereotactic Radiosurgery Society

JGH Jewish General Hospital

kVP kilovoltage peak

LH Lachine Hospital (of the MUHC)

MBE Member of the British Empire

MCH Montreal Children's Hospital

MGH Montreal General Hospital

MH minister of health

MMH Montreal Maternity Hospital

MMI Montreal Medical Institute

MNH Montreal Neurological Hospital

MNI Montreal Neurological Institute

MNQ Module du Nord Québécois

MQUP McGill-Queen's University Press

MR magnetic resonance

MRC Medical Research Council

MRI magnetic resonance imaging

MSN master of science in nursing

MSSS Ministère de la Santé et des Services Sociaux

MUHC McGill University Health Centre

MUA McGill University Archives

NASET National Symptomatic
   Enarterectomy Trail
NCEs nurse clinician educators
NDG Notre Dame De Grasse
NDH Notre Dame Hospital
NHRDP National Health Research
   and Development Program
NHRP National Health and
   Research Program
NICU Neurointensive Care Unit
OBE Order of the British Empire
OBS/GYN Obstetrics and
   Gynaecology
OC Order of Canada
OHQ L'Order des Infirmiers et
   Infirmieres du Québec
OPD Outpatient Department
OQ Order of Quebec
OTL Otolaryngology
PhD doctor of philosophy
PPP public/private partnership
PROS Paediatric Radiation
   Oncology Society
PTU Pregnancy Termination Unit
QA quality assurance
QC Commander of the Order
   of Quebec
QCPS Quebec College of
   Physicians and Surgeons
QHIS Quebec Hospital Insurance
   Services
QMA Quebec Medical Association
QMVH Queen Mary Veterans
   Hospital
RCPC Royal College of Physicians
   of Canada

RCPSC Royal College of Physicians
   and Surgeons of Canada
REI Royal Edinburgh Infirmary
RMC Risk Management
   Committee
RMH Reddy Memorial Hospital
RN registered nurse
RRC Royal Red Cross
RTOG Radiotherapy Oncology
   Group
RVH Royal Victoria Hospital
RVHMMH Royal Victoria
   Montreal Maternity Hospital
SOGC Society of Gynaecologists
   of Canada
SSHRC Social Sciences and
   Humanities Research Council
StJH St Justine Hospital
TAU Health Technology
   Assessment Unit
TBc tuberculosis
TC-99m Technetium-99 m isotope
TDC Tropical Diseases Centre
TQM total quality management
UBC University of British
   Columbia
UMF unmyelinated fibers
VFR visiting friends and relatives
VON Victorian Order of Nurses
VPH Verdun Protestant Hospital
Western Western General Hospital/
   University of Western Ontario
WHO World Health Organization

Preface

Following the decision to group most of the McGill University hospitals under the single banner of the McGill University Health Centre (MUHC) in 1997 it was thought that the Montreal General Hospital would cease to exist. Joseph Hanaway felt this was the right time to write a history of the General. He began drumming up interest in the project among MGH staff and the idea was well received. He then asked John Burgess to be a co-editor and onsite coordinator to help recruit authors for individual chapters.

Burgess and Hanaway trained at McGill University Medical School in Montreal. Burgess graduated in 1958 and trained in cardiology, and Hanaway graduated two years later and trained in neurology. Both have extensive research and writing experience. Hanaway is the co-author of *McGill Medicine*, a two-volume history of the McGill Medical School (1996, 2006), and Burgess is the author of *Doctor to the North* (2008), which chronicles his career and the history of healthcare and heart disease among Canadian Inuit.

We planned this book to be an authoritative and documented record of the MGH from 1819 to 2012. We did not consider it a memoir or a coffee-table book. We organized it according to (1) subspecialties in medicine and surgery, (2) other non-specific specialties related to medicine and surgery (social service, pathology, etc.), and (3) nursing, and we asked others to contribute chapters. This proved more difficult than we had anticipated due to many factors, including finding people who had the knowledge and time to devote to the project. We had to write several chapters ourselves as manuscripts failed to materialize. The majority of the chapter authors, however, had a stake in the department they wrote about and endeavoured to trace important developments and to highlight changes in treatment and infrastructure.

The chapters that present the history of the hospital's many departments differ in perspective and style. Some of the authors were personally involved in the development of divisions and departments and had excellent records; others had to rely on memory alone as no minutes or other historical documents existed to supply references.

From the historical perspective, we considered four main periods of the MGH that influenced its policies. The first period, the early years (1819–85), consisted of a struggling institution run by businesspeople with no experience managing a hospital (learning-while-doing) and staffed by dedicated family practitioners who practised the medicine of the day and had no specialty medical training and limited surgical training, which offered little help to their patients.

The second period, the rise of specialization (1885–1957), coincided with scientific developments in Europe, the appearance of anaesthesia, and antisepsis and the global hunt for microbes. Add to these the appointment of a brilliant group of academic leaders to the MGH (Craik, Campbell, Howard, Ross, Roddick, and Osler, to name a few) who took advantage of these advances to lead the General into an era of unparalleled accomplishment.

The third period consists of the government takeover of healthcare in Quebec (1961–97). We review the various federal and provincial medical care bills and discuss how they affected the administration of the MGH. Because of their impact on the operation of the hospital, we also discuss the language bills, Bill 22 (1974) and Bill 101 (1977).

The fourth period concerns the emergence of the concept of a united hospital centre for all McGill's' hospitals (the McGill University Health Centre, or the MUHC/CUSM). Driven by financial pressures to keep McGill's half-filled hospitals open, the MUHC was created in 1997. All the individual hospitals were to close and move to a single site at an abandoned railway switching yard in Notre-Dame-de-Grâce (NDG). The plan, however, proved financially impossible and the idea was reconsidered in 2003. The decision has since been made to have the MGH remain on Cedar Avenue and to be renovated over the coming years.

The authors were sent a statement of the goals of the MGH history, a tentative table of contents, and a model chapter written by Burgess that set the standard for chapter organization, style, and documentation. They were to confine their chapters to their specialties and to restrict accounts of the origin of the MGH, about which there is an entire chapter (chapter 2). The page limit for each chapter was to be forty-five pages more or less, and authors were to conform to MQUP guidelines for citations and endnotes, which are to be located at the end of each chapter. The editors accept that variations in writing style and intensity are going to be found with fifty-five or so authors, but we edited to keep a certain standard throughout. A short introductory paragraph at the beginning of each chapter tells the reader what the author emphasizes.

The pictures posed a problem in many cases. We searched through the audio-visual files, conference rooms, hallways, and photos from friends for all that we could find, and we even appealed in EN BREF (a publication of the MUHC/CUSM) for pictures. We also looked at the Notman Collection and the McGill University Archives (MUA). We could not find pictures for two departments and are lacking important ones for a number of others, for which we apologize. We are disappointed that we could not find everything we wanted.

Joseph Hanaway
John H. Burgess

Acknowledgments

The acknowledgment pages of any book are important because they cite the unsung members of the team of experts in many fields who work to get a history like this published. We thank the Molson family and, more recently, the Molson Foundation for supporting the MGH for almost 196 years as well as our project to write and compile a history of the institution that owes them so much.

Phil Cercone, the director of McGill-Queen's University Press (MQUP), listened to our proposal ten years ago and agreed to take us on, never realizing how long it would take. Phil, a friend for more than two decades, has seen MQUP thrive and move to its present headquarters.

Time has imposed more and more rules and regulations on university presses, requiring an increasing need for editorial specialists to deal with various policies and still get books published. We are happy to have Kyla Madden as our editor. She has helped us to focus, style, and organize the book, and this has strengthened it. Helen Hajnoczky has given us the guidelines for choosing the many photographs that appear in this book – a daunting task given that they come from a plethora of sources, are of different quality, and some have never before been published. Joanne Richardson made a major contribution as copy editor. It is these people that give MQUP its integrity.

Finding and organizing our many illustrations was another story. Without the enthusiastic help of Robert Derval, director of the audio-visual department of the MGH, who has hundreds of pictures filed on the computer, we could never have found what we needed. Robert took extra photos in halls and conference rooms for us, always with a positive and helpful approach. Unfortunately, we were unable to find photographs in offices, halls, and conference rooms of some of the divisions and departments, despite considerable searching.

Herb Bercovitz, a personality well known at the MGH for decades, collected and filed hundreds of pictures about the institution and staff and collected memorabilia that have been turned over to the MUHC Archives group. Herb found an original ambulance sign used by Jos. Wray, the funeral director who supplied the first MGH ambulances in the 1880s.

Enough cannot be said about the behind-the-scenes reference work conducted at the Osler Library, the McGill University Archives (MUA), and the Notman Photographic Archives owned by McGill (approximately 400,000 photographs). Pam Miller, director of the Osler Library (r. 2011); Chris Lyons, the present director; and the intrepid Lily Szczygiel have found obituaries, dates, and other information for us over the years. Gordon Burr, director of the MUA and a friend for two decades, has never failed to find a time-worn minute books and other ancient volumes from the MGH. Nora Hague, keeper and curator of the fabulous Notman Archives, was always able to come up with pictures we had never seen before.

Near the beginning of the project, Nan Carlin, known to many at the MGH, helped find early records and articles in the *MGH News*. The appearance of Kelly Ann McCulloch-Glover has been quite an experience. Her enthusiasm and expertise in organizing and editing the manuscript and for the project has been a delight.

It is said, in football, that "the team makes the coach," and so the team above has made our book, and we thank you all.

Last, we co-dedicate our book to our friends and fellow authors who have died since we started this project: Joseph Stratford, neurosurgeon; J. Dick McLean, tropical medicine; Don Baxter, neurology; Alan Mann, psychiatry; R. Roy Forsey, dermatology; David Hawkins, rheumatology; Michael Laplante, urology; and Shirley Woods, Molson historian.

Foreword by Abe Fuks

Abe Fuks is a former dean of medicine at McGill University and a member of the attending staff of the Montreal General Hospital (MGH) in the Division of Allergy and Immunology.

This wonderful volume, prepared by the department and division heads of the MGH under the inspired leadership and persistence of Joseph Hanaway, a loyal alumnus of our Faculty of Medicine and erstwhile trainee of the MGH; and John H. Burgess, a former director of cardiology; is a special tribute to an extraordinary institution that has served, taught, and inspired multiple generations of Montrealers and their families. The book and the institution it describes offer many lessons in the richness of the partnership between a community and the institutions it initiates and nurtures and that, in turn, serve the members of that community over a span of centuries. From the outset, the impetus for the creation of the hospital was the need to care for the burgeoning influx of immigrants, primarily from Ireland, Scotland, and England, who left their native lands to seek better fortunes in the New World. Hence, the General was created as a charitable institution and its attending physicians were barred from charging fees to their indigent patients. The hospital was founded by Montreal's Protestant community, including leaders from the Scots-Canadian community whose Presbyterian faith instilled in them a strong sense of service (particularly to their less fortunate brethren) and whose vision as Freemasons encompassed the construction of lasting institutions whose design and support merged both physical and spiritual values. The line of one founder and immigrant from Lincolnshire, John Molson (the elder), can be traced to seventh-generation offspring who live in Montreal and who use the General as "their" hospital. This sense of family among staff and patients is a feature of the institution's corporate ethos, and it is cited by all who work within it as characteristic of the quality of its healing environment. It is noteworthy that the original institution was first called the House of Charity and then the House of Recovery, a name that would befit the aspirations of a modern hospital.

It is emblematic of the cultural rootedness of a great institution such as the General that it still serves its two original communities – (1) the hardworking offspring of the indigent newcomers who populated the parts of the Island of Montreal known as Verdun, St Henri, and Point St Charles and (2) the offspring of the founding families whose stately homes are higher up the mountain in Westmount. A final noteworthy feature of the original mindset behind the founding of the General is that it, unlike its sister Catholic institutions, was neither supported nor run by the Church but, rather, was the first of many institutions of its kind in Montreal funded directly by members of the community, both in terms of capital needs and operating costs. This pattern is replicated in all the partners of the McGill University Health Centre, including the university itself, all of whom depended and depend on community philanthropy to propel them beyond the quotidian to the levels of excellence that characterize their current missions as they continue to plan for a new and exciting future. It is also of note that, although the General was set up to serve patients of a particular community, it served Catholic patients from the outset and now caters to the great multicultural diversity of Montreal.

Another highlight of the volume is the early association between the General and the then nascent Faculty of Medicine at McGill, the first medical school in Canada and the founding faculty of the university. Indeed, this early and significant connection between the faculty and its first teaching hospital led to the quality of teaching that garnered kudos for McGill from Abraham Flexner in his famed 1910 report. Though separate institutions, McGill University and the Montreal General Hospital owe their existence to the same Montreal community of philanthropists and visionary entrepreneurs who gave not only money and land but also managerial and political leadership to their community institutions – a two-vector symbiosis between faculty and hospital and between institutions and community. The founding professors at the medical school were the early attending physicians at the hospital, namely, Holmes, Stephenson, Caldwell, and Robertson, who themselves provided a link to the General's sister medical school in Edinburgh, a model for McGill well into the twentieth century. The physician William Osler, whose skills and fame helped spread the reputation of the faculty throughout the English-speaking world, began his clinical career as a pathologist at the MGH, where his painstaking autopsies laid the groundwork for his seminal textbook, *The Principles and Practice of Medicine*. The MGH has many other firsts, for example, Thomas Cotton's introduction of the electrocardiograph in 1914 and Phil Gold and Samuel Freedman's discovery of a tumour marker for malignancy in 1965.

The reader will find a clear example of how many teaching hospitals in North America evolved, beginning as charitable hospices for the indigent. The physicians who attended these people would then utilize them as teaching cases and volunteer at the medical school, having honorary appointments in both establishments and seeing both the provision of care and teaching as communal obligations – a sort of medical "tithe" through service. With the increasing complexity of both university and hospital work, the university developed part-time faculty positions with some remuneration followed by the later innovation of geographic full-time hospital physicians, who generally held university appointments. The two institutions grew in tandem with an ease of cooperation that made possible the seminal development of the McGill model of the academic physician.

This particular model of the birth and development of the modern academic health centre is evident in the pages of this history. The first complement to clinical care has generally been the teaching mission. Once that is in place, it generates a demand for clinicians who are not only role models for their junior colleagues and students but who also provide the highest levels of clinical care, eventually offering locally all that is innovative in other centres of excellence throughout the world. With that comes the imperative to recruit clinical leaders with international perspectives and widespread collegial links. This, in turn, averts too high a degree of inbreeding that could undermine the level of quality. Over time, the teaching hospital becomes a referral centre and provider of tertiary and quaternary care. All outstanding examples, at least in North America, have also developed a strong and complementary research mission.

At McGill, the initial research facilities developed on the university campus, followed by a dramatic increase in the breadth and depth of basic and clinical research at the hospital in the second half of the twentieth century. By the end of the century, the hospital had a very robust and well developed research institute with a wide range of investigators using and developing leading-edge technologies in work designed to elucidate the mechanisms of significant human diseases. In addition to molecular biologists and geneticists with their analytic approaches, these researchers included clinical scientists and epidemiologists developing clinical trials and contributing to the new(er) world of evidence-based medicine.

The General contributed to teaching in a great many domains. It had its own nursing school until the late 1960s, while also training radiology technicians, dieticians, and a host of other health care professionals. One of the General's major contribution was the hierarchical teaching structure of its clinical teaching units, encompassing teams of clinical fellows, residents at various levels, clinical clerks, and junior medical students learning physical diagnosis. Wards were the crossroads of a constant stream of specialist consultants who represented the growing list of medical and surgical specialties, starting with the cardiac clinic inaugurated in the mid-1920s by Harold Segall. This expansion of services eventually led to the construction of new facilities at the Western Division and then the current site on Cedar Avenue. It, in turn, will become one of the physical venues of the new MUHC, formally created among the teaching hospital partnership in 1997.

It is not at all coincidental that many of the chapters of this retrospective were written by those who were responsible for the development of the divisions, departments, and units they describe. The General's sense of mission and its deep engagement with its founding and supportive communities led to its being pervaded by a strong ethos of family and belonging. Hence, the majority of its clinical staff arrived as young recruits and served until retirement. True enough, some were called to leadership positions elsewhere. Nonetheless, the corporate ethos was founded on close relationships over long spans of time. This was true of mentors and recruits; physicians and surgeons (and other caregivers) and their patients; the members of the board; philanthropic leadership; and the ladies auxiliary, the successor to the Montreal Ladies Benevolent Society of 1815, which spurred the founding of the small forerunner hospital. This pervasive fraternity and mutual collegial respect enhanced the quality of care, permitting many to engage in the care of each patient, and was a powerful magnet for new recruits.

Just as the library doors of the current General were the main doors of the old hospital, so all those involved in this volume – a true labour of love – will wish to present this ethos, this collective mission of service to the patient within a teaching-research environment, as a heritage gift to those who will lead the newly minted MUHC.

SECTION 1

The Beginnings

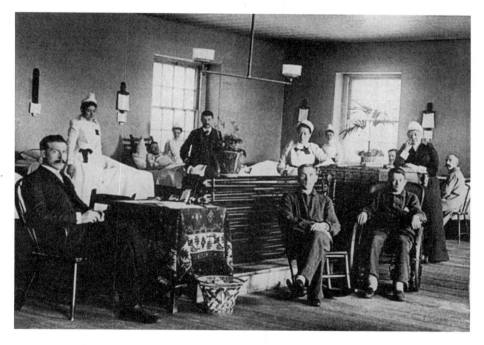

S.1 1892 Ward rounds with Robert Kirkpatrick (far left), C.F. Martin (standing behind table), and Nora Livingston (in back, far right).

The Molson Story

Shirley E. Woods, Jr

Shirley Woods, an author of children's books, wrote *The Molson Saga*, the definitive history of the Molson family.[1] He traces the relationship of the Molson family to the MGH, starting with John Molson, the elder, and the early problems of getting a general hospital built in Montreal in the 1820s. He leads the reader through six or seven generations of Molsons who have been presidents and board members of the MGH and have donated, bequeathed, and granted on request large sums of money over almost two centuries – money that the hospital could not have reached its present status without. Through the government health and language issues, the 1970 October Crisis, and other external pressures, the Molson family has continued to run the brewery and other interests and, up to the present, has never failed the MGH. This chapter has been reviewed and approved by members of the Molson family.

The Molson family has supported the MGH for two centuries. No family in Canada, and few, if any, on the North American continent can match this bond with a medical institution. In January of 1819, John Molson – the founder of the brewing dynasty – petitioned the legislature of Lower Canada for a grant to build a public hospital in Montreal. At that time, medical care was largely in the hands of religious orders, a situation that restricted public access to treatment. The need for a second hospital – Montreal's population was over sixteen thousand – was made clear in his petition, which reads, in part:

> THAT the present hospital for the sick attached to the Hotel Dieu in this Town is capable of containing only thirty patients, and the inconvenience arising to the nuns from their constant attendance on the sick, and the inadequacy of their funds for that purpose, renders some remedy for this evil absolutely necessary; and by an order of the superintendent of 1817, which excluded all cases of fever of whatever denomination from

being admitted, the advantages resulting from the Institution are necessarily extremely limited.

THAT the rapid increase of population in this District (it being at
least doubled within the last ten years), the strong tide of emigration
that has extended itself to Canada, and the increased number of sick
naturally attendant on such causes, imperiously call for some asylum
where they may receive that aid and relief their impoverished and un-
sheltered condition urgently demand.

THAT of those emigrants who have lately arrived in this District
there are at present upwards of two hundred sick, destitute of every
comfort and almost of every necessity of life, who are solely dependent for medical assistance on the humanity of the Medical Gentlemen
of the town, whose professional aid must be in a great measure rendered nugatory, from the destitute and helpless condition these poor
people are at present in. Besides, from their being scattered in miser-
able hamlets about the town, exposed to every inclemency of weather
they cannot receive that attention they otherwise would, were they collected in an establishment for their purpose.

As expected, John Molson's petition was referred to a committee for further study. The committee, which included three respected doctors, recommended that ten thousand pounds be appropriated for a public hospital in
Montreal. This proposal was then debated on the floor of the Legislative Assembly and would likely have passed, had it not been denounced by Michael
O'Sullivan, the member for Huntingdon.

O'Sullivan's opposition illustrates yet another source of friction between
the Canadians who emigrated from the Old World: the enmity between Irish
Roman Catholics and English Protestants. On language questions the Irish
usually sided with the English, but on religious matters the Irish Roman
Catholics and the French were united by the Mother Church. O'Sullivan,
born in Ireland, was a fervent Roman Catholic. Because the petition for a
public hospital – open to all – had been sponsored in the main by Protestants, O'Sullivan fought the proposal.

O'Sullivan's speech, fuelled by prejudice, ignored the facts. After lauding
the nuns and denouncing the medical sorority as "mercenary hirelings" he
dismissed the problem of destitute emigrants as a temporary inconvenience
caused by "a few birds of passage" (though emigration was increasing, and

most were from Ireland). He also defended the nuns' decision *not* to treat infectious diseases in the Hotel Dieu, knowing that many of the emigrants suffered from cholera or typhus. And he mocked the doctors on the committee for stating that a public hospital would "promote the perfection of medical science." Distorting the phrase, he told the assembly that a teaching hospital would "promote the *fatal* perfection of medical science." When Molson's petition was put to a vote, the French majority in the House sided with O'Sullivan to defeat the motion.[3]

On 1 May 1819, fewer than three weeks after the duel, the committee rented a stone house on Craig Street with space for twenty-four beds. This temporary arrangement was the beginning of the Montreal General Hospital. From the outset, the hospital was a haven for sick immigrants. Many of these immigrants were in such a wretched state that a section of the stable had to be partitioned off "for the purpose of purifying those parts of the wearing apparel of the patients unfit to be cleaned in the hospital on account of vermin and contagious matter."[4]

Two years later, on 5 June 1821, there was general rejoicing in Montreal when the cornerstone was laid for a permanent hospital on Dorchester Street (see chapter 2 for a description of the laying of this cornerstone). The original structure on Dorchester was three stories high, measured 23.2 by 12.7 metres and could accommodate up to eighty patients. Wooden galleries were attached to the rear of the stone building so that patients could convalesce in the fresh air. An ornamental cupola on the roof acted as a source of light for the operating room. The land and building were paid for by personal subscription, the main benefactor being John Richardson, a public-spirited citizen of great wealth. John Molson, Sr, also gave generously to the building fund, and, when construction was completed, he donated a stout iron fence to enclose the premises. Shortly after the new hospital opened its doors on 3 May 1822, the rented facility on Craig Street was phased out of existence.

The Montreal General Hospital received its Royal Charter in 1823. John Molson and his three sons – John, Jr, Thomas, and William – were among the founding governors. Taken individually or together (they were all partners in John Molson & Sons), these men represented a powerhouse of influence and ability. Since their time, the Molson name has kept recurring on the board and in volunteer activities connected with the hospital. For the family, supporting the MGH means more than simply writing cheques: it also means giving one's time. This tradition dates back to the earliest days, when John Molson's duties as a governor required him to make regular inspections of the hospital and to record his findings. One of his reports reads:

> I have visited all the occupied wards, kitchen etc., and found every part in the most perfect good order except Ward No. 5, and there is a very disagreeable smell which the Matron suspects is a rat or some dead animal between the floor and the ceiling underneath.
>
> I was under the necessity of enforcing the regulations by hurrying out a woman who refused leaving the Hospital when desired, that had called to see a man that had undergone amputation.[5]

In 1823, the year that the hospital received its Royal Charter, it also established the Montreal Medical Institution, Canada's first medical school. Six years later, the medical school was transferred to McGill University to provide the college with a fully staffed medical faculty. Until 1843, the medical school was the only functioning faculty at McGill. The symbiotic relationship between the hospital and the university was a contributing factor in the Molson family's decision to make a long-term commitment to McGill as well as to the MGH. Over the years, the brewery line has made timely financial donations, endowed chairs of learning, and given academic prizes, buildings, and a sports stadium.

John Molson, Sr, died on 7 January 1836. In addition to a fulsome obituary in the *Montreal Gazette*, he received a tribute from *Le Canadien*, a staunch supporter of his political opponent, Louis-Joseph Papineau:

> We hasten to associate ourselves with the regrets which have been expressed by our Montreal contemporaries, on the occasion of the loss experienced by Canadian industry through the death of the Hon. John Molson, to whom Lower Canada owes the introduction of steam in inland navigation, and who was at all times a zealous supporter of every important commercial and industrial enterprise. Few men have rendered better service to their country in connection with its material development.[6]

John Molson Jr, the eldest of the founder's three sons, died in 1860. His biography, which appears in Henry J. Morgan's *Sketches of Celebrated Canadians*, published in London in 1862, concludes with this paragraph:

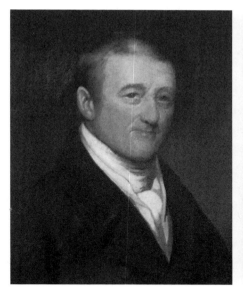 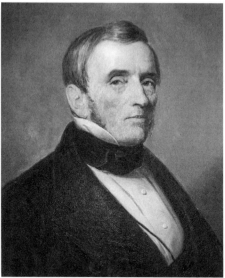

Fig. 1.1 John Molson, Sr, MGH president, 1831–35
Fig. 1.2 John Molson, Jr, MGH president, 1857–59

As a private citizen, Mr. Molson was highly esteemed. The cause of education and philanthropy ever found him a friend, and there is scarcely an important educational or charitable institution in Montreal with which his name has not been connected. The Molson Chair in the McGill college; endowed by the liberality of the three brothers, may especially be mentioned as an instance of munificence and public spirit. As a governor for many years of the MGH, from the presidency of which he retired about a year previous to his death, owing to his failing health, his zeal will be long remembered, which considering the magnitude of his business engagement, often surprised his coadjutors, in the management of that benevolent institution.[7]

The second of the founder's sons, Thomas Molson, died in 1863. Montreal's leading French newspaper, *La Minerve*, made the appalling mistake of publishing his obituary the day *before* he died. This faux pas was noted with glee by the English press, who printed very brief tributes. The obituary in the *Montreal Gazette* was typical:

We regret to learn that Thos. Molson, an old and wealthy citizen of Montreal, died yesterday at the age of seventy-one years. He enjoyed vigorous health up to his last illness. He was noted for some eccentricities in his later years; but in the prime of life he was remarkable for great business energy, to which he owed the accumulation of his fortune. He was connected, we believe, with the early establishment of steamboat communication between Quebec and Montreal.[8]

Thomas Molson's obituary failed to mention his most notable achievements: as a brewer and distiller. It was Thomas – not the founder – who established the tradition of technical excellence in the family trade. And it is Thomas Molson's descendants who comprise the brewery line.

William Molson, the last member of the second generation, died on 18 February 1875. He was the founding president of Molson's Bank. Chartered in 1855, Molson's Bank had 125 branches when it was taken over by the Bank of Montreal seventy years later. At his death William was president of the Montreal General Hospital and a governor of McGill University as well as a member of the boards of many other commercial and charitable enterprises.

Control of the brewery had already been transferred to John Henry Robinson Molson, Thomas Molson's eldest son. John H.R. was a successful businessman and philanthropist who also supported the MGH and McGill University (and had declined the chancellorship of the latter). At his death in 1897, John H.R. left the brewery to his brother, John Thomas Molson.

The fact that Thomas Molson had two sons whose first name was "John" deserves an explanation. John Molson, Sr, had wanted to leave the brewery to Thomas – the brewer and distiller in the family – but he was afraid to do so because Thomas didn't have a marriage contract. If Thomas predeceased his wife, the brewery could then "pass into the hands of strangers." The old man solved the problem by entailing the brewery to the third generation in this manner: "I give and bequeath to my Grandson John Molson, son of Thomas Molson, the whole of those extensive buildings comprising brewery, houses, Stores (old & new) with the lot of ground whereon the same erected." The will then went on to stipulate:

If my Grandson should not survive to the age of twenty-one years, or that he shall not be brought up to follow the brewing business – then I do give and bequeath the same to my next Grandson called John Molson, and should he die before the age of twenty-one years, or not be brought up to follow the brewing business, then I direct that the said last mentioned premises shall go into & form part of the residue of my Estate.[9]

Thomas was pleased that his son had been left the brewery, but he was gnawed by anxiety. Nine-year-old John H.R. was a sickly child, and Thomas wasn't sure he would live to maturity. If John H.R. died before he reached twenty-one, John Molson, Jr, had a son named John who would qualify to inherit the brewery.

Thomas weighed the risk and decided upon a pragmatic solution. When his next son was born in October 1837, he named him John Thomas Molson. This improved the actuarial odds considerably as the founder had bequeathed his brewery to "my Grandson, John Molson, son of Thomas Molson." The will did not stipulate *which* John Molson, son of Thomas Molson.

John Thomas Molson died after a long illness in October 1910. He was married twice and had eight children. His eldest son, Herbert, inherited the brewery. The MGH and McGill were among the charitable institutions that received substantial bequests.

Harry Markland Molson, a nephew of John Thomas, went down with the *Titanic* in April 1912. Just before his death, *Moody's Magazine* had rated Harry as one of the most influential businessmen in Canada. During his active life he had supported many charities, but only two were remembered in his will: the Canadian Society for the Prevention of Cruelty to Animals, of which he had been president, and the MGH.

Doctor William Alexander Molson, a grandson of the founder, died in January 1920. After obtaining his degree from McGill, he completed his medical studies in London, Edinburgh, and Vienna. He began his general practice in Montreal in 1877 and was later appointed senior physician at the MGH. He was also examining surgeon of the Montreal Garrison Artillery during the North West Rebellion in 1885. As well as a highly qualified physician, William Alexander Molson was a deeply caring person. Alton Goldbloom, former chief of paediatrics at the Montreal Children's Hospital, wrote in his memoir *Small Patients* (Lippincott, Philadelphia, 1959):

During my first-year of life I fell ill with pneumonia and it apparently looked as if I, too, were to follow the path of the other three. For several days I lay close to death. The doctor was William Alexander Molson, a member of the famous brewing family, who was a physician at the

MGH. He was the physician to the poor Jews of Montreal whom he attended without fee. He came often and willingly. He lived on his wealth and gave freely of himself. My mother never tired of recounting the critical night of that illness – how Dr Molson sat at the cribside in the hovel on St Antoine Street, waiting. She would vividly describe Dr Molson's uncertainty at the outcome; her fears, indeed her terror, of the fourth child going the way of the other three; her fervent prayers; the first discernible sign of impending improvement as the critical night wore on, and the great change for the better by dawn. She never tired of talking of Dr Molson and hoped that I too, when I became a doctor, would treat the poor as he treated us.[10]

Frederick William Molson, Harry Molson's brother, died suddenly in 1929. He had been a governor of the MGH and a prominent businessman. In its obituary, the *Financial Post* described Fred Molson (who was also Herbert Molson's partner and managing director of the brewery) as "one of a small group of Montreal financiers who have for a number of years been the most important financial group in Canada." His only charitable bequest was to the MGH, observing in his will: "Having contributed liberally during my lifetime to charitable and other like purposes I have not made other contributions for such purposes."[11]

Fllowing Fred Molson's death in 1929, Herbert Molson returned to the brewery as president and CEO. He had been semi-retired since the end of the First World War, in which he was decorated and seriously wounded. Now, with the economy collapsing, Herbert was faced with numerous challenges. He continued as president of the MGH – which he still visited every day – but found it increasingly difficult to maintain the hospital's services on a shrinking budget. He also chaired a special survey committee that produced the rescue plan that enabled McGill University to survive the Depression.

Colonel Herbert Molson underwent surgery for cancer in 1936. The operation appeared to be a success, but the following year he suffered a relapse. This time his doctors told him the malignancy was inoperable. At the beginning of March 1938, he indicated that his end was near when he resigned as president of the MGH. Herbert Molson was the fourth member of the family to hold this position, and his portrait hangs on the east wall of the hospital's boardroom. He died on 21 March 1938. Hundreds of people sent the family letters of condolence. Among the letters that his wife Bessie Molson received was one from John Buchan, first Baron Tweedsmuir, who was governor general of Canada. His letter was written from Government House in Ottawa:

> Dear Mrs. Molson,
> I heard in Montreal yesterday that Colonel Molson was sinking and now I get the melancholy news of his death. We cannot regret that he is now free from pain. With him goes one of the great figures of Canadian life, for Canada has no finer citizen. There was no good cause to which he did not lend a hand. It is a hard fate for Canada that in the last year she has lost so many of her leading men. But the chief loss is your own. I want you to know how deeply my wife and I sympathize with you in your great sorrow.
>
> Yours Very Sincerely,
> Tweedsmuir [12]

Colonel Molson's controlling block of brewery stock was left to his two sons, Thomas Henry Pentland and Hartland de Montarville. Tom, the eldest, received the majority of shares. The MGH and McGill University were each endowed with one-quarter of a million dollars.

Tom and Hartland were active members of the board of the MGH for many decades. In 1950, Hartland took time off from the brewery to chair a joint fundraising drive for the MGH, the Children's Memorial Hospital, and the Royal Edward Laurentian Hospital. It was the first time such a drive was held in Montreal, and, because of the huge amount being sought – $8 million – many were sceptical that it could be done. The objective was reached within three months at a cost of less than 1 percent of the donations. This enabled the three hospitals to expand their facilities.

Tom Molson, who had been a governor since 1934, chaired the General's building committee. It was a project dear to his heart and one that he was eminently suited to lead, having recently completed a six-year overhaul of the brewery. Tom used the same architects and consulting engineers for the General that he had used for Molson's expansion in Montreal and its new brewery in Toronto. It wasn't a coincidence that the sterile operating rooms in the hospital had the same tiles, the same quality valves and pipes, and the same temperature control systems as Molson's yeast rooms. Similarities between the hospital and the brewery were everywhere – the elevators, stairwells, railings, windows, even the exterior bricks.

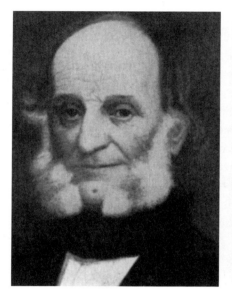 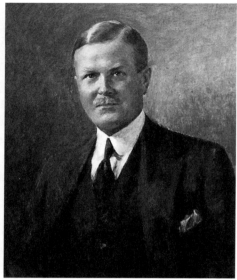

Fig. 1.3 William Molson, president, 1868–74
Fig. 1.4 Herbert Molson, president, 1923–38

Tom's interest in the General began years before the planned expansion and continued long after the Cedar Avenue building was completed in May 1955. A stickler for detail, his inspection tours – which could occur at any time of the night or day – were dreaded by the maintenance staff. As well as keeping a vigilant eye on the operations, he also cared for the welfare of the patients. On Christmas day, he would often leave his family for a few hours to visit the public wards.

Herbert William "Bert" Molson – the eldest son of Fred Molson – died in the spring of 1955. Bert was president of the brewery from 1938 to 1953. Among his many bequests he left both an outright amount and an endowment to the MGH.

The Molson Foundation was established by federal charter in November 1958. The original capital for the foundation was donated by Tom and Hartland Molson, who wanted a formal structure for their personal philanthropy and that of future generations. Tom and Hartland were especially interested in giving money to "innovative projects in the fields of health and welfare, education and social development, and the humanities.[13] As well as endowing the Molson Prizes (administered by the Canada Council), the Molson

Foundation has supported the MGH for the past half century and disbursed millions of dollars to an eclectic mix of charitable organizations.

In 1971, Tom Molson was presented with a special Award of Merit medal for his dedication and exceptional service to the MGH. Only three of these medals were struck to mark the institution's sesquicentennial anniversary. Tom Molson died in April 1978, at the age of seventy-six. In addition to his outstanding career at the brewery, Tom had been vice-president of the MGH and had served on its Board of Management for thirty-three years. He also left a substantial bequest to the MGH. At the time of his death, Tom was the largest individual shareholder of the brewery. Control of the firm passed to his eldest son, Eric Herbert Molson. Eric was forty years old and executive vice-president of the company's brewing division. A director of the Montreal General since 1968, he was the sixth generation of the Molson family to serve on the hospital's board.

Senator Hartland Molson died in September 2002. The last of the fifth generation, he had a long and distinguished career that included many honours. In his will he left significant sums to McGill University and the MGH. When Eric Molson became a director of the MGH it was administered by a single board. Later, the MGH was split into a number of boards: one was responsible for operations, another for property, a third for the Research Centre, and a fourth for the Hospital Foundation. Eric has served on all these boards. Eric Molson is proud of every facet of the hospital, but he's most enthusiastic about its world-class performance in sports medicine. For decades, specialists from the General have looked after the Montreal Canadiens and their families. Eric, a self-described rink rat (as well as chancellor emeritus of Concordia University and chairman emeritus of Molson-Coors), has rooted for the Habs since he was tall enough to see over the boards.

In November 2004, the MGH presented Eric Molson with a special Award of Merit – the same medal that his father, Tom Molson, had received thirty-five years earlier. In his acceptance speech Eric shared some amusing anecdotes and reflected on the family's enduring commitment to the hospital. Looking to the future, he mentioned that his three sons – Andrew, Geoffrey, and Justin – were introduced to the MGH at an early age, having been born on the seventh floor.

Eric's three sons are known collectively by the media as the Molson brothers. In partnership, they now own a majority interest in the Montreal Canadiens, the Bell Centre, and related assets. Geoff Molson is the general partner and chair of the syndicate. In a recent interview, Geoff acknowledged the benefit of the MGH's sports medicine to the hockey team, and then confirmed his family's long-standing relationship to the hospital: "The MGH has played an integral role in our community since 1821, and the Molson family has supported it from the outset. We, the seventh generation, remain committed to this great institution."[13]

NOTES

1 Shirley E. Woods, *The Molson Saga, 1763–1985* (Toronto: Doubleday, 1983).
2 Ibid., 65–6. John Molson's letter to the governor general in 1819 requesting public funds for a hospital in Montreal.
3 Ibid., 67 The resulting duel between Caldwell from the MGH and O'Sullivan (who opposed the Protestant plan for a hospital) is found in chapter 2 of this book, under "The Caldwell-O'Sullivan Duel.
4 Ibid., 69.
5 Ibid., 70.
6 Ibid., 102.
7 Ibid. 164.
8 Ibid., 167.
9 Ibid., 103–4.
10 Alton Goldbloom, *Small Patients* (Toronto: Longman Green and Co., 1959), 19.
11 Woods, *Molson*, 253.
12 Ibid. 266
13 Karen Molson, *The Molsons: Their Lives and Times, 1780–2000* (Buffalo: Firefly Books, 2001), 394.

Early History, 1819–85

Joseph Hanaway

The practice of medicine is an art, based on science.[1]

Introduction

The idea of having a general hospital in Montreal in 1818 came from an organized group of benevolent women, known as the Female Benevolent Society, who wanted to provide health care for the hundreds of neglected, poor, and homeless immigrants who were on the streets of the city. They raised money to rent a house (the first house, built in 1818, was too small) on Craig Street in 1819 as a temporary arrangement until they could raise enough money to build a dedicated general hospital. Preparing for this eventuality, while on Craig Street, an administration was formed (with a board of governors), rules and regulations were decided upon, and regular meetings were held and recorded in an MGM minute book between 1 May 1819 and 3 May 1821.

There is no official founding date for the MGH on Dorchester Street. Since 1821 is on the wall in the lobby on Cedar Avenue, it is likely that this date was chosen because, on 26 January 1821, enough money had been raised to begin construction on Dorchester Street. This date applies only to the Dorchester Street building, not to the MGH that had been founded and opened two years before, in May 1819, on Craig Street.

To further confuse founding dates, the Massachusetts General Hospital (Boston MGH) in Boston and the Montreal General Hospital (Montreal MGH) had bronze plaques near their lobbies citing 1821 as their founding dates, implying a common bond between the hospitals. However, it appears that the Boston MGH was actually founded in 1811 (when a charter was granted by the state) and the Montreal MGH in 1819. The cornerstone was laid for the Boston MGH in 1818 and for the Montreal MGH on 6 June 1821. The opening dates were September 1821 in Boston and 3 May 1822 in Montreal. Eighteen twenty-one was a busy year for both hospitals, but since neither the Boston MGH nor the Montreal MGH were founded in 1821, it appears we have a small international historic error, which is part of MGH legend.

This is the story of the Montreal General Hospital. Founded by benevolent citizens for the care of the indigent poor in 1819, it mitigated a major problem of health care for mainly homeless immigrants even if its rude beginnings included only a few rooms and straw mattresses. As the ethos of Montreal changed with the acquisition of an increasingly diverse and increasingly wealthy population, so the medical profession changed as it increased in number and experience, and the MGH expanded to provide more space, beds, surgical facilities, and clinics. It is about the men and women at the MGH who cared for the sick and taught students as well as many generations of young doctors and nurses that I write.

Immigrant Health in Montreal in the Early 1800s

The origins of the MGH can be traced back to about 1815,[2] when the war between England and the United States ended (i.e., the War of 1812). Travel on the Atlantic was hazardous in an unarmed vessel during the war, so few ships docked in Montreal between 1812 and 1815. Records reveal that the number of ships docking in 1813 was nine and in 1814 thirteen.[3] After the war, when the British again dominated the Atlantic, sixty-two ships docked in Montreal in 1816 and more in subsequent years. Emigration of the disenfranchised and poor from England, Ireland, and Scotland resumed and increased, hundreds crossing the ocean for a chance of a new life in colonial Canada. Most of the poor that came had no idea how hard the winters were, that Quebec was a French and Roman Catholic province where English was not spoken much outside Montreal, and that there was no industry to employ them. The trip across the Atlantic crammed in small sailing vessels was arduous. Many arrived in Quebec City or Montreal sick and desperate. After eight to ten weeks at sea with poor facilities, bad food, and no medical care, most had to rest and recover in cities before moving to other locations. With experience mostly in poor farming situations in Ireland, these immigrants had few prospects of similar jobs in Lower Canada, where fur trading, shipping, and more prosperous farming were the main occupations. Those who arrived late in the season during cold weather were even worse off because travel and jobs in the country were non-existent. So with no place to go these people remained in Montreal, essentially homeless and dependent on local citizens for help. In 1817, the population of Montreal was nearly twenty thousand, and an estimated fifteen hundred immigrants were destitute and living in the suburbs.[4]

Montreal was a thriving small city on the St Lawrence River, headquarters of the North West Company, a centre for river trade with Upper Canada – a trade that stretched into western Canada and the northern United States to the Pacific Ocean. By 1818, the old walled city had expanded east, north, and west – way beyond the original walls. Self-sufficient to a degree, Montreal survived without major economic problems until the postwar emigration from Europe. A local depression and a crop failure in 1816–17 occurred, threatening the population and requiring the government to acquire grain subsidies from outside Lower Canada.

A Plan for Immigrant Health Care, 1816

The dismal plight of the immigrants did not go unnoticed. Local citizens and the Protestant clergy raised money for the poor, but there was no guiding organization. Help came from a spirited group of women who formed the Female Benevolent Society (also called the Montreal Ladies Benevolent Society) announced in the *Montreal Gazette* February 1816.[5] The members called for volunteers to raise money to provide food for the poor and education for their children. This extraordinary group of women was well organized and had regular meetings as well as a charter. It soon began to coordinate the churches' fundraising efforts. A soup kitchen was opened in 1818 and the children were schooled in the basics wherever room could be found to hold classes. The need was so great that another society, called the Society for the Relief of Immigrants, was formed in 1818 and the two organizations worked together.

The health of the homeless population, which had not been addressed, became a priority in 1818 when it became apparent that there was no provision for the treatment of the sick poor. A few doctors made charitable calls, but this was not sufficient to meet the demands. The Female Benevolent

Society decided to do something to provide the needed care, and a few doctors agreed to treat the poor if a facility could be made available.

The First Hospital in a Rented House, 1818

To this end, in 1818, the Female Benevolent Society rented a four-room house in the Recollect suburb (west of the old walls) to be used as a small hospital and school. Furnishings, bedding (straw mattresses), used clothing, and stoves were obtained from government stores by Isaac Winslow-Clarke, a United Empire Loyalist who came from Boston at the time of the American Revolution. He became deputy commissar general in charge of military stores and had access to used items in storage. He provided these essential items with the permission of the governor general of Canada, the Duke of Richmond.[6]

This meagre beginning was named the House of Recovery in 1818.[7] There is some confusion about the name, which was initially the House of Charity: this was an unsuitable name and it was changed. One room of the house was used as a schoolroom and probably for any surgery that was performed. Should any surgery have occurred (and, again, this is only supposition), only a table and sheets would have been required. The enterprise was considered a success after one year, with thirty-nine admissions. This small step was the first of many in the establishment of the MGH. There were other limited hospital facilities in Montreal. The Hotel Dieu, which was founded in 1640, was a thirty-bed Catholic facility, would not take fever patients, and favoured Catholics. (The present Hotel Dieu was built in 1861.) The Grey Nuns convent would take mental patients for custodial purposes but had no capacity to care for people with other illnesses. The city needed a general hospital big enough to take patients of all denominations with any diagnosis, including fever.

A Proposal for Government Funding of a General Hospital in Montreal, 1818

The Female Benevolent Society, with the help of other citizens' groups, determined what it would cost to build a proper hospital big enough for the area, but it had no funds except for church donations. It was decided to approach the legislature of Quebec and on 13 October 1818. James Andrew Smyth wrote a letter to the Duke of Richmond outlining a proposal for provincial support of a general hospital in Montreal. Nothing was heard from the duke for two months, so John Molson resubmitted the proposal in January 1819. This time MP Michael O'Sullivan, a Catholic who took exception to the Protestant proposal, actively opposed it in the legislature. He proposed expanding the Hotel Dieu instead, but he didn't stop there. In a long diatribe, some of which made sense, he criticized the Protestant plan and suggested that the nursing in such a facility would be unprofessional compared to that provided by the nuns (here he is referring to the nuns' devotion to duty, not to any special training).

O'Sullivan also suggested that medical students who would have access to the hospital in the future would subject patients to experiments.[8] This was all that William Caldwell, MD, one of the founding doctors of the hospital, could take. He wrote an unsigned rebuttal to O'Sullivan's remarks in the Canadian Current in April 1819 and, in a veiled manner, called O'Sullivan a coward. The latter demanded the name of the author of the letter and, when Caldwell's name was revealed, challenged him to a duel.

The Caldwell-O'Sullivan Duel over the French Rejection of the Montreal Proposal, 1819

The famous duel was fought on Windmill Point in Point Claire, a 0.81-hectare spit of land that projects out into the St Lawrence River and in the centre of which sits an ancient windmill.[9] This windswept point of land, now the site of a Catholic retirement facility, was a remote and ideal spot for duels. The two met with seconds at sunrise on Saturday 11 April 1819. It appears they came fully intending to do harm to each other. The duelling custom of the day was for the combatants to stand 18.3 metres (twenty long paces) apart with loaded pistols held high and, at a signal, fire. This sure-death situation was mitigated by the terrible aim of the parties. After exchanging four shots of twenty-eight-gram lead balls and missing, which would have ended most duels, O'Sullivan, the offended party, insisted on continuing (a bad decision). Apparently one of Caldwell's coat collars was torn, indicating a near miss. The parties took aim a fifth time, and both were wounded. Caldwell was shot in the right forearm, which shattered one of the bones, and he lived with a stiff arm for the rest of his life. O'Sullivan was shot in the right side of the chest, just missing the heart. Miraculously, both survived what may have been the longest duel in local history.[10]

Caldwell died fourteen years later (1833) of typhus fever, and O'Sullivan lived another thirty years with a lead ball against his spine (discovered at autopsy), which was not life-threatening but gave him a lot of grief. Quite obviously this ended any further attempts to obtain financial support from the government. Caldwell was a hero, but the project still needed funding.

The Second Hospital in a Rented House on Craig Street, 1819

In the meantime, the Female Benevolent Society and the Society for Relief of Immigrants raised enough money to rent a bigger house on Craig Street, two doors east of Bluery. It had room for twenty-four beds and a dispensary. Again, Isaac Clarke, who had been involved in organizing the facility, provided the extra furnishings in addition to what was brought from the House of Recovery. It opened on 1 May 1819 and was ambitiously called the Montreal General Hospital, with a board of directors and a list of rules and regulations for all the officers, committees, staff, and so on. Regular quarterly meetings were held. It has to be said, therefore, that 1819 was the first year of the MGH, not 1822, when the building on Dorchester Street was opened (which, over the years, many have believed to be the real opening date of the hospital).

Not forgetting the ultimate goal to build a new hospital, a meeting of the subscribers was held on 25 April 1820 at the courthouse, with the Honourable John Richardson called to the chair. The following were elected officers (and others present at the meeting): Samuel Gerard (treasurer), and John Christie (secretary), Isaac Winslow Clarke, Frederick Ermatinger, James Leslie, George Garden, Thomas McCord, Robert Gillespie, David Ross, Thomas Blackwood, Horatio Gates, John Frothingham, J.T. Barrett, John Try, Thomas Phillips, John Fisher Robert Armour, James Miller, George Moffat, Jacob Dewitt, Jab Dewitt, James Woolrich, Thomas Turner, Henry Driscoll, John Molson, Sr, Steven Sewell, W.M. Porter, Thomas Torrence, John Torrence, George Auldjo, B. Gibb, William Grey, Alex Skakel, and Andrew Porteous. The original attending physicians were William Robertson, William Caldwell, Thomas Blackwood, and Ferrenden and Christie. The latter resigned and were replaced by Andrew Fernando Holmes, Henry Loedel, and, eventually, John Stephenson. Blackwood resigned, so the final five were Robertson, Caldwell, Stephenson, Holmes, and Loedel, men who were willing to devote many hours per week, with no compensation and at considerable inconvenience, to treat the indigent (also eventually to teach students).

Henry Loedel resigned soon after this because of illness and died of typhus in 1825.[11] In a 1 November 1820 meeting of the board, the statistics of the first year and six months were: 138 admitted, 106 discharged, 15 dead, and 17 remaining in the hospital. At the same meeting it was decided to retain Mr and Mrs Jamieson as managers and Mrs Patons as matron to take care of patients.

Although the house was bigger, the care was basic and primitive. Rats and roaches were a problem with which everyone had to live. The question is: Why did so many recover? The doctors didn't make much difference except to support the patients. A relatively clean environment, regular food, and bed rest together with hardy host resistance probably saved most patients with serious illnesses.

There were no nurses and no available training until Florence Nightingale (1820–1910) founded her Nightingale School for Nurses in London in 1860,[12] which resulted in the beginning of professional training for nurses. There were no records or charts except for the medical and surgical ledgers that were kept by the apothecary.

Freemasons in Quebec and Their Involvement with the MGH

Freemasonry was well established in Lower Canada at the time, and many of the leading businesspeople and supporters of the MGH project were Freemasons. It was a secret fraternal order of Protestant men started by stonemasons in England who built castles, cathedrals, and large country homes in medieval times. The attraction of the society was its founding principles of the brotherhood of God and of man. Freemasonry teaches man's duty to God, his neighbours, and himself; in other words, service to humanity was the guiding policy. The organization grew through the centuries, becoming an elaborate society of Protestants claiming many in the military in Ireland, England, and Scotland.[13]

Freemasons appeared in Quebec in about 1720, originally as army officers from England. Eventually, civilians were involved. Many provincial premiers, Canadian prime ministers, and most of the presidents of the United States were Freemasons (including George Washington). Locally the organization became a prestigious society by the 1800s, with many Masonic lodges in Montreal. Most of the city's prominent businessmen were members. Thus, the planning and construction of the MGH, which involved many Freemasons, became the most important Masonic event in the area, with many men devoting their time and money to the project for the public good.

Plans for the Dorchester Street MGH, 1820

As long as the Craig Street facility was open, the indigent and sick were cared for while plans were being made for a new building. The first step was to purchase the land, which was acquired by the Honourable John Richardson, the Honourable William McGillivray, and the Honourable Samuel Gerard on their joint credit. It was deeded in trust, the purpose being to erect a hospital on the property, and announced to the managers on 30 November 1820. In a St Lawrence suburb they purchased thirty-six-by-fifty-five metres owned by a gardener who was using it for a nursery on the corner of Dorchester and St Dominique streets. It had been the site of a house that had been fortified to defend against Aboriginal attacks in the mid-1600s. A building committee was appointed to make arrangements for the construction. The men chosen for this daunting task had no idea how to design or build a hospital, and there were no architects, builders, masons, and so on with any experience. At least the architects sought hospital plans from firms in England to get started.

The proposed twenty-three-by-twelve-metre building was to face north, with a central entrance on Dorchester Street.[14] There were two stories for wards, an attic and basement, and room for all the services (kitchen, laundry, boiler room, storage, autopsy room, and rooms for the attendants). Together with the furniture, double windows (with the shutters on the outside), outhouses, and cupola, the estimated cost was twenty-two hundred pounds. In a short time, this amount was raised by subscription letters and church appeals. The architect Thomas Phillips (1777–1842), an MGH founder and a general contractor, designed the building with help of senior members of the board. Phillips was a wealthy professional who had supervised many major projects but had never designed or built a hospital. The masonry contractors were John Redpath and William Reilly; the carpenters were Edward Bennett and Gordon Forbes.

The lack of experience caused the costs to rise to almost double the original estimate. The people were waiting for the hospital to open, so John Richardson secretly paid for the cost overruns in order to keep the building on schedule. He can be considered the father of the original hospital because of the money and time he devoted to its completion. The total cost of construction was £5,856.8s.

Laying the Cornerstone of the Dorchester Street MGH, 1821

Little happened in Montreal in the first quarter of the nineteenth century that brought the city together more than the laying of the cornerstone and the opening of the MGH. The Craig Street facility had been a success, and although this was the real origin of the MGH (in 1819), neither the Masonic orders nor the city in general had been aroused to civic action by its existence.

The Female Benevolent Society and a group of community businesspeople brought the urgent need for a general hospital to the public's attention. Most of the directors and other influential men of the city were Freemasons, so when serious plans to build a hospital were being considered, the brethren saw this as a worthy endeavour. Considering that the laying of the cornerstone would be a grand Masonic event, a parade route was chosen, building decorations were encouraged, and ships in the harbour agreed to fly their flags and to fire their guns. Stands were erected at the building site for dignitaries, ladies, and a band. Not to be outdone, the Montreal Horticultural Society constructed a huge floral arch at the entrance of the MGH property, and all who went to the building site passed under it.

The Masonic brethren gathered in their meeting rooms at the City Tavern on St Paul Street before noon on 6 June 1821 in preparation for the parade to the building site. The MGH directors, the Masonic hierarchy, a military band, and an honour guard of the 60th Montreal Regiment left the tavern about 11:00 AM. Approximately two hundred strong marched through the residential city to be seen by crowds along the parade route. According to an 1839[15] map and the newspaper accounts, the van marched east on St Paul Street, north to McGill, east on Notre Dame Street, through Place D'Arms to St Gabriel Street. From here it went north to the Scottish church, which all entered for a service. The van, on leaving the church, walked east on St James Street to the main street of the St Lawrence suburb and to Dorchester Street, where it turned west to the MGH building site. The Masons, dressed in their ceremonial hats, sashes, and aprons, together with the regimental band and honour guard made a grand procession that passed under the floral arch and arranged themselves in the stands at the building site in preparation for the ceremony. Full Masonic protocol and tradition was observed for the solemn laying of the cornerstone. Surrounded by brethren, the top of the cornerstone was lifted exposing a cavity in the lower stone into which a crystal cylinder was placed containing parchments listing the names of the contributors to the hospital, a brief history, and eleven different gold and silver coins of the time. Sealed with lead, the cavity was closed and the top stone lowered and cemented in place. The band played "Rule Britannia" and "God Save the King" to three rousing cheers from the assembled. The Masonic brethren, according to tradition, spread corn, wine, and oil around the cornerstone, and this was followed by a speech from the grand master and a cannon salute. When the ceremonies were finished, all retired to the City Tavern for a sumptuous dinner to celebrate the event.[16]

The Opening of the Dorchester Street MGH, 1822

The newly constructed MGH, as we know it today, officially opened on 3 May 1822 (fig. 2.1) when eight patients were transferred there from the Craig Street building. Isaac Clarke came forward, again supplying beds, straw mattresses, stoves, and chairs for the new building. As the first president, 1819–21, he also arranged for the official Royal Charter, which unfortunately was not granted until January 1823 after he had died. The second president, John Richardson, was a contemporary of James McGill, whose name was given to a college and a street in Montreal. Richardson, in comparison, preferred to keep a low profile in Montreal history.

This worthy man helped found the prosperous North West Company, which was based in Montreal and competed with the London-based Hudson's Bay Company as well as a leading business and financial institution, Forsythe-Richardson and Company. John Richardson, like James McGill, became an MP from Lower Canada. He was instrumental in the construction of the Lachine Canal, which allowed shipping on the St Lawrence to bypass the Lachine Rapids. Between 1822 and 1831, when he died, he supported the hospital with anonymous donations that kept it open.

The Original Staff of the Dorchester Street MGH

The original medical staff was a dedicated, Edinburgh-educated group of doctors. Henry Loedel resigned in 1823 because of illness. The other four men[17] – William Caldwell (1782–1833), William Robertson (1784–1844), John Stephenson (1794–1842), and Andrew Fernando Holmes (1797–1860) – agreed to serve without compensation and were interested in founding a medical school associated with the MGH. These men, well educated for the

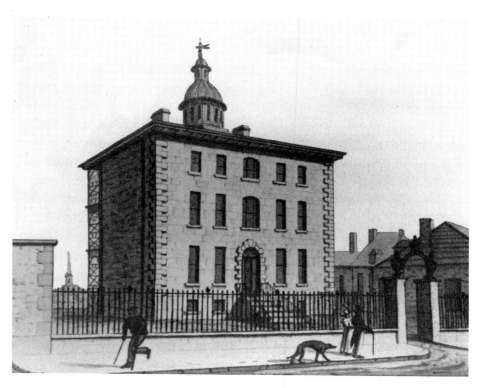

Fig. 2.1 The original MGH central building, 1822. Drawing by John Paod Drake, 1826

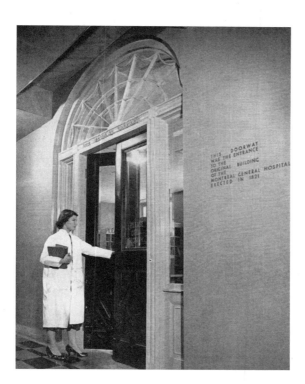

Fig. 2.2 The original front doors of the MGH on Dorchester Street, which now are the doors to the medical library on Cedar Avenue. Note the window above the doors. MGH photographer unknown, taken from the *MGH Bulletin* 1955

time, nevertheless practised the medicine of the era, which involved using many useless symptomatic treatments, observing the patients, making them comfortable and feeding them, and hoping for the best. The physicians knew that there was little they could do, but they cared and gave hope to many, and this made the difference. The majority of admitted patients were discharged so the doctors could take credit for Mother Nature's bountifulness.

William Robertson (1784–1844) was born in the Scottish highlands and, as was the custom of the day, enrolled in a highland regiment at age thirteen. He showed leadership qualities beyond his age, which was concealed from the troops. He studied medicine at Edinburgh University from 1802 to 1805, with no record of graduation (in 1832 he received a degree, "Honoris Causa," from the University of Vermont, which was willing to grant a degree for a fee with proof of education elsewhere). His timing was right because as a faculty leader he had to have a degree before the first graduation ceremony in 1833. His only degree was from the University of Vermont, which, like McGill, was a school founded by Edinburgh graduates.

Robertson continued in the military as a physician (without a degree) and was stationed in Canada on Cape Breton Island, where he met the sixteen-year-old daughter of the governor in 1805 and was married in 1806. He was a military surgeon to the regiment that fought in the Niagara campaign in 1815 and eventually retired in Montreal to practise medicine. In addition to being one of the founding physicians of the MGH, he co-founded the Montreal Medical Institution (MMI), which opened in 1823, where he was a lecturer in obstetrics and diseases of women and children.

Described as a good lecturer in an account of the time, Robertson was a mostly private person. However, in 1832, as a magistrate, he was involved in a riot in Place D'Arms in which three people were killed after he read the riot act and troops fired on the crowd. He was accused of murder and ordering the use of arms (never proven), and he was so insulted by Louis Papineau, who defended the victims, that he challenged him to a duel. Papineau wisely rejected the challenge. If Robertson had shot or killed Papineau, the French response might have ended the fledgling medical school.

As senior member of the staff, Robertson substituted for the absent principal in awarding McGill's first degree in 1833 to William Leslie Logie, a medical graduate. Robertson died at age sixty in Montreal, and a copy of his portrait hangs in the office of the dean of medicine at McGill, the original having been burned in the fire of 1907.

The most controversial person is *William Caldwell* (1782–1833), who was born in Scotland and, like Robertson, went to medical school at Edinburgh University in the early 1800s and did not graduate. Nevertheless, he joined the military as a surgeon, working his way up in a Scottish regiment and was sent to Canada during the War of 1812. Deciding to remain in Canada, he retired from the military in 1815 (all this time without a medical degree) and ended up in Montreal, where there were a number of Edinburgh-trained physicians.

He became friends with Robertson, Stephenson, and Holmes, and, in 1817, he applied, with his Edinburgh record, to the Marischal Medical College of Aberdeen University for an MD, which was granted by attestation (meaning he paid a fee) and, with his Edinburgh record, was given the degree. This was a common practice in Scotland at the time. With the others, he helped found the MGH and the MMI. Not one to avoid controversy, he challenged and shot a critic of the MGH proposal for government funding and later was involved in a riot outside St Gabriel church over the choice of a new minister.

He taught a course entitled Principles and Practices of Medicine. Later he became terrified of cholera, which was epidemic in 1830, to the point where he wouldn't go to the cholera isolation sheds but would send students instead. Tragically, he developed typhus (a flea-borne infection) in 1833 and died before McGill's Faculty of Medicine was four years old and before its historic first graduation. His students so respected Caldwell that they replaced the horses in the funeral train and personally pulled his hearse to his burial place.

John Stephenson (1794–1842), the leader of the staff, had an extraordinary personal history. He was born in Montreal with a cleft soft palate and a significant speech defect, which he overcame through his academic ability. He was a Protestant educated in a Catholic school in Montreal (College de Montreal), where the director who recognized his ability understood him despite his significant speech disability. The director's brother was an anatomist in Paris who later helped Stephenson get a position. Stephenson apprenticed with William Robertson after graduating from the College de Montreal and went to Edinburgh in 1817 to attend medical school. It was common for students in these medical schools to come and go because they paid by the course. In 1819, Stephenson decided to get some lab experience and went to Paris to work in the clinic of Philibert Joseph Roux, a surgeon (1780–1854) who took on students and who did not meet Stephenson for months. Finally they met and, hearing Stephenson's nasal speech, Roux became interested in his problem. After examining Stephenson's oral cavity, Roux told him that the defect could be closed if he was willing to take the risk and if he agreed to say nothing in case of failure. Stephenson, never dreaming that it could be possible, accepted the terms and, without anaesthesia or antisepsis, had his soft palate sutured closed on 28 September 1819. Done in a sitting position, crude forceps were used to reach the back of the oral cavity, reflected light and long sutures were placed with needles, one of which broke during the procedure, which, according to Stephenson's own account, took approximately one hour. The operation was such a success that it launched a career for Roux and, fourteen or twenty days later (he mentions two dates in his thesis), Stephenson returned to Edinburgh to recover and continue his studies. Approximately a year after his surgery he read his thesis, "De Velosynthesis," which was based on his own operation, in the Fall of 1820 and graduated with his MD. A copy of this thesis is in the Osler Library, and W.W. Francis and Lloyd Stephenson wrote a short paper on it in 1963.[18] This was thought to be the first successful closing of a soft palate defect, but prior claim goes to Carl Ferdinand Graefe (1787–1849) who performed the operation in 1816.[19]

Stephenson returned to Montreal after Edinburgh and became involved in the MGH organization as one of the original staff. His speech improved to a degree, but he was still hard to understand at times. His intelligence and executive abilities made him a leader in the formation of the medical school the four friends had planned. He led the effort to obtain the bequest from James McGill, which his wife's family contested until 1829 (see below). In 1832, to speed up the process, he hand-carried to Quebec City the statutes, rules, and ordinances of the Faculty of Medicine of McGill College, which the province required of any institution before degrees could be granted. Of the four founders, Stephenson played the most important role in the establishment of McGill and probably would have been its first dean had he not died at age forty-eight in 1842.

The last of the founders, and the one who served the longest, is *Andrew Fernando Holmes* (1797–1860). His parents were shipwrecked on their way to Canada in 1897, captured by a French warship, and put ashore in Spain. He was born in Cadiz, and, at age four, his parents took him to Canada, their ultimate destination. He was educated in Montreal and was apprenticed to a well known local physician, Daniel Arnoldi. He eventually went to Edinburgh for formal training, graduating in 1821. He returned to Montreal and became associated with Robertson, Caldwell, and Stephenson in the founding of the MGH and the MMI. These Edinburgh-educated physicians had a great respect for higher education, thus their interest in forming a medical school after the MGH opened in 1822. Stephenson placed an ad in a local paper offering to teach basic and clinical medical subjects, and the response was so good that the Edinburgh four decided to go ahead with their plans to start a medical school in 1823. At the Montreal Medical Institution (MMI) Holmes taught chemistry, pharmacy, and material medica. He introduced chloroform to Montreal in 1848,[20] and the stethoscope in 1850.[21] He was the first dean of the Faculty of Medicine (1854–60), and his name is perpetuated in the Holmes Gold Medal (established by George Campbell, MD, the second dean of medicine, in 1865), which is given to the student with the highest grade-point average for four years. What made these men so respected in the community was not their medical practices but their willingness to devote many hours, without compensation, to teach others what was known about medicine and to start a tradition that developed beyond their wildest dreams.

Early Diagnoses and Early Surgical and Medical Treatments

Many diagnoses in the first half of the nineteenth century were noted in archaic Latin terms found in the MGH case books. This a list of the most common diagnoses: Ambustio was a burn or scald, contusio a bruise, cynanche a sore throat, fractura a fracture, gelato was frostbite, psora any skin disease, synochus a continued fever, uter.gest was gestation, vulnus was a gunshot, and white swelling was tuberculosis (Tbc) of the knee joint. Typhus, typhoid fever, cholera, smallpox, edema, dropsy, jaundice, stupor, dyspepsia, pneumonia, tonsillitis, quinsy, fever of unknown origin, trauma with various fractures, pregnancy, syphilis, anasarca, asthma, abscesses, ulcers amenorrhea, Tbc, dislocations, pleurisy, and hysteria were also recorded.

Early surgery was seriously restricted because of constant threat of fatal infection. Operations, other than for superficial problems, were uncommon. Maybe twenty-five per year were approved by the Medical Board. The most common necessary operation was amputation for a compound fracture, which had up to 80 percent mortality. The first operation recorded at the MGH was for a compound fracture of the femur on 14 May 1823. This resulted in amputation of the leg, and the patient survived. The first tonsillectomy, which was performed on 29 November 1838, also survived and was discharged. Otherwise, without anaesthesia until 1847 and antisepsis in 1877, surgery was limited, and both the physician and patient were heroic to undergo procedures without these benefits (see chapter 19).

Medical therapy was untested, symptomatic, frequently toxic, and often made the patients worse. There were a few items, such as digitalis (Withering 1785),[22] for heart failure and edema; cinchona (extract from a tree bark, Barba 1642),[23] used to treat malaria; morphine (narcotic principle of opium), used for pain; and citrus fruit (Vitamin C), used to treat and prevent scurvy in the British navy (Lind, 1758).[24] Limes were more available, thus the nickname "limey" for British sailors.

Most of the other medical treatments were nostrums that everyone used for want of other choices – Silver nitrate (a tonic and antispasmotic) and Dover's Powders (ipecac and opium). Thomas Dover was a physician/buccaneer and ship-owner who discovered Alexander Selkirk on San Fernando Island in the Pacific Ocean in 1710. He had been marooned for four and one-half years and gladly joined the pirates. Dover later practised medicine after making a fortune on the high seas (his story was written in a novel by Daniel Defoe entitled *Robinson Crusoe* and published in 1719). Other compounds were Castor oil (cathartic), Fowler's Solution (arsinite of potassium), magnesia (magnesium carbonate), James' Powder (antimonial powder), blistering compounds (skin irritants like mustard), ipecac, calomel, and tarter. Bleeding, an ancient treatment based on the idea of bad "humours" in the blood, was used up until 1870, when it was recognized as useless. Throughout the nineteenth century, leeches were used to debride tissue. "Cupping" (heated, wet brass cups, applied along the spine – used to treat pneumonia and as counter-pain) was last seen at the MGH in 1872.[25] Electrical treatments became popular in the mid-nineteenth century but were pure quackery. Ice, in the form of ice packs, was used as a treatment at the MGH starting in the 1850s. Wine, beer, and whisky were used to calm the patients. For obstetrical practices, see chapter 27.

Examples of Hospital Expenses in the 1820s

A list of expenses in a minute book of the Committee of Management, 1 August 1822, in the MUA gives the reader a glimpse of the annual cost of what had to be supplied to keep the MGH open.

Fuel	£ 54.8.1
Groceries	£ 42.9.5
Oats, flour & pork	£ 15.0.0
Baker	£ 9.16.3
Butcher	£ 7.15.3
Apothecary	£ 27.15.0
Sundry	£ 25.4.0
Salaries: matron,	
Two nurses, steward	£ 19.15.0

Seven years later, on 1 May 1829, the following were recorded:

Drugs	£ 29.14.0
Meat	£ 60.9
Sugar	£ 36.8
Butter	£ 25.8
Fish	£ 2.16.3
Eggs	£ 3.4.8
Beer	£ 4.13./11
Rum	£ 2.14.6
Wine	£ 10.9.6.
Vegetables	£ 14.1.11
Fuel	£ 61.15.4
Water	£ 30.19.8
Icehouse	£ 2.5

Missing are the costs of bread and poultry. Two cows were purchased in 1825 to defray to cost of milk, and two more were acquired about ten years later. Many more items were needed to keep the hospital running and to provide health care. A lot of butter, sugar, bread, meat, and beer were used by the employees, who had strict allotments of these items. The treasurer was responsible for checking these expenses and inquiries into any irregularities (which did occur at times).

During 1829, the patient population was broken down by religion and nationality. During the year 556 Irish, 103 English, 103 Scots, 134 Canadians, and 12 Americans were admitted. Catholics out-numbered Protestants 3–4:1. In 1832–33, 1,210 patients were admitted and 1,148 were seen in the clinic. One thousand and ninety-two of those admitted were fever patients, 546 of these having been diagnosed with typhus.

Beginning Organization of the Dorchester Street MGH, 1822

After the Craig Street facility opened on 1 May 1819, plans were being made to build a permanent hospital, and the governors began to organize in preparation for this. The minute books of the Board of Directors of the Craig Street MGH reveal a budding professional organization as the members learned how to manage a hospital for the public – an enterprise foreign to all involved. The Montreal General Hospital Corporation owned the property and was legally responsible for it. It annually elected a board of directors as its governing body.

The Board of Directors officially established itself and elected officers in April 1820.[26] Twenty-six governors were elected, mainly the original contributors to the project and twenty-six life governors as well as a resident physician who was appointed and who was to be in daily attendance. The board would meet quarterly. Admission policy allowed for recommendations from the clergy, governors, and members of the medical staff. Laypersons could admit people to the hospital to be cared for by the medical staff. However, if someone from out of town was admitted, the recommending person was held responsible for hospital and mortuary costs if the patient could not pay.

The first meeting of the Board of Directors in the new hospital occurred on 7 May 1822, four days after the MGH opened its doors. The Craig Street facility was closed and eight patients transferred. The all-important Committee of Management was appointed by the Board of Governors in May: it was to be responsible for running the hospital and it met weekly. This committee was the major supervising force at the MGH. It kept the hospital running by carefully managing all its business – finances, food supplies, the domestic staff, the medical staff, buildings and grounds, and the cows. Not enough praise can be given to these men who, under serious financial stress, every week for decades, devoted hours of free time and received little thanks for a job well done.

The Medical Board also appointed in May 1822, consisted of all the attending staff, who credentialed staff and house surgeon appointments, disciplined staff, and directed patient diets. The long-awaited charter for incorporation applied for in 1821 finally arrived in 1823, signed by the Right Honourable George Ramsay, 9th earl of Dalhousie, and governor general of Lower Canada.

Rules and Regulations of the MGH[27]

The original rules and regulations of the MGH, which Quebec required to grant a charter, were extensively revised in the charter of 1823 on twenty folio pages in the minute book of the governors, and it clearly establishes the guidelines for establishing the Montreal General Hospital Corporation and who was eligible for the boards and committees, the election of officers and their terms and responsibilities, and the behaviour of the medical attending staff and students. It lists the qualification for stewards, matrons, nurses, and apothecaries as well as rules for in- and outpatient behaviour. It also describes penalties for patient misbehaviour, for receiving fees, and for altering the rules and regulations. This extraordinary document is a sophisticated manual for the organization of this enterprise, and it is a tribute to the men who created it. It served MGH's guideline for decades.

Student Access to the MGH and Their Responsibilities

Students were there to learn to take histories and to perform physical exams, and they were not to discuss any medical course of patient treatment except with the staff. This failure to involve students in the management of the patients, which is what they would have to do when practising medicine, weakened the clinical training at the MGH and McGill for a century. This was not unique to McGill; rather, it was a failure of the senior physicians to see beyond tradition. It was not challenged until William Osler, chief of medicine at Johns Hopkins Medical School in the 1890s, insisted on a real clinical clerkship whereby students with house officers cared for patients supervised by the attending staff. Students at the MGH had to keep their own notes on patients. These were taken from the casebooks that were kept in the apothecary's office in the lobby. Only the house officers wrote in these casebooks, and what they wrote was frequently dictated by the attendings on rounds.

A unique feature of the MGH was that it offered fairly liberal access to patients during visiting hours and at other specified times without staff being present. The doors were definitely not open at any time, but what was allowed was better than what was available at most university hospitals in North America. The MGH Board of Governors was comprised of Montreal businessmen who took their jobs seriously and who tended to make decisions for the hospital and not for the medical school.

In 1825, twenty-three diagnoses were recorded (see above); 447 patients were seen in the hospital and the clinic. The majority of these were Catholics and Irish immigrants, reflecting the number of Irish coming to Canada looking for a better life.

The MGH, the Montreal Medical Institution, and McGill College (opened in 1829)

When the MGH finally opened in 1822, the founders intended to use the hospital as a base for a medical school. Called the Montreal Medical Institution (MMI), its first advertisement appeared in the *Montreal Herald*, 11 October 1823. It opened shortly thereafter. By 1828, both the MMI and McGill faced serious legal challenges. The response to the MMI's 1826 request for the right to grant degrees (answered in 1828) was that it could not do so until formally associated with a higher institution of learning. This decision affected students in the MMI who, knowing that they couldn't get a degree, dropped out and went to the University of Vermont or the University of Edinburgh for a degree. By 1829, the situation at the MMI was desperate, and it was losing students.

At that time the only seminary of higher education was McGill College, which was looking for a way to start teaching. McGill College (the University of McGill College up until 1885, thereafter McGill University) had a charter (1821), and a principal and faculty (1824), but this was all on paper The college faced pressure as, according to James McGill's will, it was to start teaching within ten years after his death in 1813. This was extended by the repeated appeals launched by his wife's relatives, who contested the will.

James McGill's Burnside property was initially awarded to McGill on 7 June 1820. Further prolonged litigation over the property didn't stop in 1820, and it prevented the college from opening on the McGill estate. A final Privy Council (London) decision was handed down in favour of McGill on 31 March 1829. Now McGill College could start functioning because it had the property, and that part of the bequest litigation was finally finished.

In order to start teaching as soon as possible, it was necessary to conduct a search for professors. When the staff of the MMI heard about the court decision and McGill's quandary, they approached the governors of the Royal Institution for the Advancement of Learning, which represented McGill, and offered to be its first faculty. Considering the good standing of the MMI and the reputation of its founders it was an offer McGill couldn't refuse. Therefore, on 29 June 1829, with a bit of fanfare, there was a gathering of prominent Protestant clergy and other invited guests at James McGill's Burnside Estate (an 1829 version of a press conference).[28]

The Reverend George Jehosaphat Mountain, the Anglican archbishop of Quebec and McGill's principal, presided over the first meeting of the governors of McGill College and formally announced to the assembled guests the opening of the college as a medical school. Later, as prearranged, he met separately with the four members of the MMI. They were formally asked to accept being "engrafted" onto McGill as its first teaching faculty, which they accepted and, in so doing, stepped into Canadian history as the founding faculty of the country's first university and first medical school. The MGH, not to be left out, sponsored student teaching as far back as 1822 and can be said to be the oldest teaching hospital in Canada.

Although perhaps a little out of context, it is appropriate here to mention the front doors of the old Dorchester MGH (fig. 2.2). The doors in figure 2.2 are the original front doors of the 1822 central building of the MGH. Apparently, when the move to the new MGH on Cedar took place in 1955, MGH neurosurgeon Harold Elliott visited the original Dorchester site of the hospital, which was being vacated. Elliott saved the original doors, and they were installed as the sixth-floor library entrance, where they are still serving the hospital and are 193 years old.

Richardson died in 1831. The father of the MGH, he left money for a statue, but better sense prevailed and it was used to build a badly needed wing on the east side called the Richardson Wing, which the Board felt was a more appropriate way to spend the money. It is perpendicular to the central building on its east side and had beds for fifty to sixty patients, almost doubling MGH's capacity in 1832 (fig. 2.3).

John Molson, Sr, was elected president of the hospital in 1831. The new wing was to be constructed like the original building of 1822, and the cornerstone laying was seen as another Masonic opportunity for pageantry and tradition. The event is depicted in an almost life-sized painting in the main hall of the Masonic Temple on Sherbrooke Street. The masons are dressed in their traditional bibs, aprons, and hats and are standing next to the

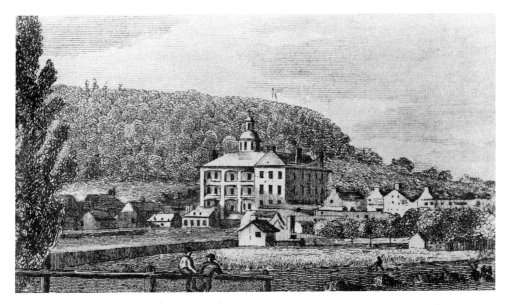

Fig. 2.3 The MGH from the southeast, showing the back of the central building (1822) and the Richardson (1832) Wing. Drawn in 1839. Artist unknown.

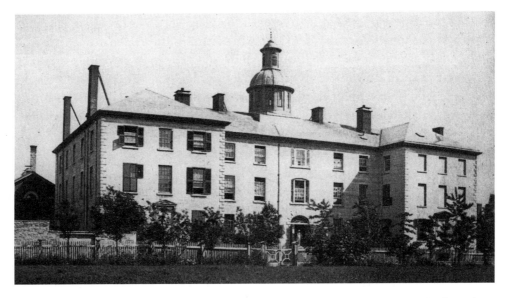

Fig. 2.4 The earliest photograph of the MGH (1849). The Reid Wing (1848) on the far right has boarded windows and has not been completed. Photographer unknown.

cornerstone. The wing was a shell and was finished in 1832, when it was dedicated. It was completed approximately one year later.

In February 1832, the year's statistics included thirty-eight diagnoses, the majority being fever patients with infectious diseases.

Annual Recurring Problems from the Committee of Management Minutes, 1822–85

The daily affairs of the MGH, of the Committee of Management, and of the Medical Board are generally routine and uninteresting. Recurring problems, however, give a better picture of how the volunteer management and medical staff tried to cope with running a public institution.

Hospital Finances

The major problem of the Committee of Management was finances. The hospital ran on a meagre income for decades, and, for years, shortfalls were made up by John Richardson, Sam Gerard, and John Molson (Richardson died in 1831). The MGH was an English institution supported by the Montreal public.

As early as 1823, the government gave the MGH £250 per year. This was raised in 1857 to five thousand pounds, which was a considerable increase but still not enough. Money from volunteer collectors remained a major source of hospital income. Other income came from the monthly campaigns of the Protestant churches, occasional gifts from grateful patients, gifts from the Board of Governors, the sale of student tickets, the two-dollar-per-day patient charge, and the annual amount contributed by Richardson to make up the deficit.

The accounting was conducted by professional bookkeepers, who made detailed monthly, quarterly, and annual reports of the MGH's income and expenses. The money went to pay the staff, to buy provisions for patients and staff, medicines, and a hundred other items. Repairs were made only if essential, and things were so bad at times that plumbing and carpentry work had to be postponed for lack of funds. Other gifts, such as of barrels of oats, cornmeal, and used clothing, were received. At times, the Committee of Management had to close wards and restrict admissions in order to save expenses. A few large gifts and bequests were given over the years by Richardson (i.e., the Richardson Wing), the family of Justice Reid (i.e., the Reid Wing [fig. 2.4]), friends of Thomas Moreland (i.e., the Moreland Wing [fig. 2.5]), and David Greenshields and George Stevens (Greenshields and Campbell Pavilion) for capitol expansions.

Eighteen seventy-two was an anomalous year because the MGH had a surplus of $6,358.55 thanks to good collections and reduced expenditures (not explained). In 1869, however, the deficit was so serious that the attending physicians reduced admissions by one hundred patients. The Committee of Management saved the day again.

MacDermot details a number of expenses in 1872 that are worth mentioning:

Employees	$2,848.49
Wine, beer, etc.	$813.88
Medicines	$1,802.12
Chloroform	$40.83
Batting	$66.70
Bandages	$60.07
Leather and oilskins	$20.78
Linseed meal	$152.80
Lard and mustard	$69.75
Gutta percha	$59.80
Surgical instruments	$97.27
Alcohol for treatments	$160.75
Lime juice, cider	$19.09

These are desultory, but they give the reader a little insight into the sorts of things the hospital needed.

In the twenty-first century, the MGH was caring for many thousands of patients, and the expenses in 1922, one hundred years after opening in 1822, were:

Total income from all sources	$486,482.83
Total expenditures	$608,092.89
Operating deficit	$121,610.06

This gives the reader some idea of the annual hospital deficit,[29] which, in 1996, was about $1 million. The major source of support now is from the Province of Quebec. Under the 1966 Canada Medicare Act, Ottawa supplies the money for the individual provincial programs to spend on their own

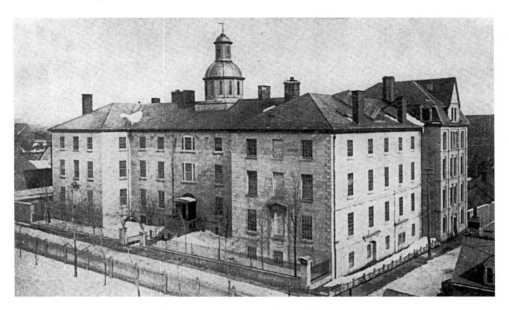

Fig. 2.5 The MGH in 1881, looking east down St Dominique Street. The Moreland Wing (1875) is east of the Reid Wing (1848) on the right. Note the separate entrance for the basement clinics on St Dominique Street. Photographer unknown.

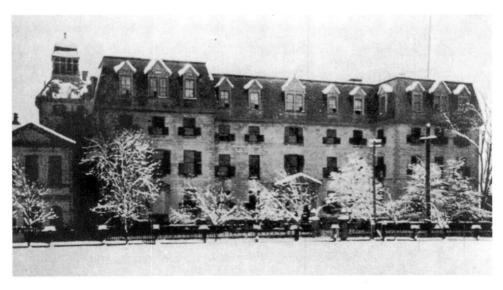

Fig. 2.6 The MGH in 1895. The Mansard Nurses quarters on the roof of the central building (1889–90) made nursing at the MGH more attractive. Note the separate pathology building (1894) to the left of the Richardson Wing and the smallpox isolation tower behind the Richardson Wing (1868). Fred Tees, pioneer orthopaedic surgeon, 1895, was the photographer.

medical care. Quebec passed its version in 1970, the Quebec Medical Care Act, which supplies the money for all medical care (including hospitalization) in the province.

Domestic Staff

Once the MGH opened, a small domestic staff had to be hired by the Committee of Management (should have been the Medical Board): a matron (who had to be able to read and write) and two nurses (untrained women who attended the sick and who did not have to know how to read and write to get the job). "Nurse" is a term that was used as far back as 1590 for women who cared for the sick (no level of training is implied). A housemaid, a cook, and a male steward (who also did not have to know how to read or write to get the job) were also hired. The salaries were five dollars a month for the women and seven dollars a month for the men (not much has changed). The salaries were low even for the 1820s–40s, but in addition there was a Spartan food and drink allowance for each employee. The matron was responsible for the staff and had the committee's approval to hire and fire when deemed necessary (the committee, of course, had to be notified). The turnover was high, as can be imagined, and people were dismissed mainly for bad behaviour, insolence, incompetence (frequent), ignorance, stealing food, and drunkenness. The training was poor, as were the incentives. Matrons were not excluded from dismissal, and the Committee of Management fired them for drunkenness, stealing food, housing family members who irritated everyone (matrons had the option to live in the MGH), disorderly conduct, using bad language, and not doing the job.

The number of "nurses" who took care of the patients gradually increased, and, by 1832, with the Richardson Wing, there were more than one hundred beds to attend. There were six day and two night nurses, which meant that each nurse had about twenty patients during the day. Considering the nurses' level of expertise, many treatments that were ordered by the attendings were never administered, and this led to complaints from patients and doctors. Nevertheless, the number of nurses was gradually increased as new wings were added in 1848, 1868, and 1874, bringing another one hundred beds to the MGH. Housework on the wards was taken care of by the nurses and the housemaid, and, by the mid-1830s, a laundress was hired. For more information, see Section 5 (Nursing).

The cook was busy preparing all the meals, and the steward functioned as an orderly when a man was needed throughout the hospital. The steward also had to help bury out-of-town patients and help the church sexton once a deceased patient's church had been identified. The matron had to pitch in but was, in the main, a supervisor. This was all the MGH could afford, so it is easy to imagine how hard these people had to work and why turn-over was common.

By 1859, staff problems had to be resolved by trying to get a higher class of employee;[30] consequently, the base wage was raised to six dollars per month, with an annual bonus for good performance. In 1862, the wage was raised to seven dollars per a month, and the incentive worked. This did not, however, eliminate the basic problem of poor supervision on the part of the medical staff, who were ultimately responsible. Eventually, the Committee of Management (remember that this was comprised of Montreal business-men) handed the domestic staff problem over to the Medical Board, which should have been responsible for them from the beginning. It was the med-ical attendings who had daily contact with the domestic staff, and it made sense that they should be in charge.

Lack of training led to many complaints from patients that treatments ordered, such as hot packs, were never administered. Mistakes pertaining to medicines were made because of poor record keeping. In 1847, laudanum (opium), when ordered, was provided in marked wine bottles that were kept at the patient's bedside. On one occasion, a partially blind patient gave his bottle to another patient without knowing its contents. The other patient, thinking it was wine, took an overdose and died. The investigation revealed that the bottles were frequently not labelled, and it was a miracle that this sort of thin had not happened before. There were many other, albeit less dra-matic, stories of missed treatments and medications, and this did not change until professional nurses came on the scene in the 1880s and 1890s.

Fever Patients

A divisive and perennial problem concerned the admission of fever patients, who constituted the largest group of medical diagnoses. In 1842, and for decades, the list of admissions averaged 70 percent fever patients. Smallpox, typhus, typhoid fever, cholera, tuberculosis, pneumonia, abscesses, pleurisy, diarrhoea, urinary tract infections, scrofula (Tbc gland infection), erysipelas, and fever of unknown origin were typical diagnoses.

Smallpox, typhus, typhoid fever, and cholera were the most common dis-eases seen at the MGH during its first seventy-five years. Epidemic typhus (a rickettsial disease) was spread by lice from rats to humans and then from human to human. In 1832–33, 526 patients were admitted with the diagnosis of typhus (clinical diagnosis only). Typhus tended to come in good weather as immigrants disembarked from rat-infested ships, and then it spread from person to person. In 1847, 3,140 patients died in a great Montreal epidemic. The cause of this epidemic was not known, but it was guessed to be due to overcrowding and poor hygiene (resulting in body lice). It killed Caldwell and Blackwood and a medical student, all of whom died treating patients.[31]

Typhoid fever (a salmonella infection spread by fecal contamination of water and food) has GI symptoms (Identified by Eberth in 1880).[32] Cholera, another epidemic enteric disease (a vibrio), is also spread by fecal contamination of water and food (it was identified by Koch in 1884).[33] Epidemics occurred in 1831 (four thousand deaths in Montreal), 1834 (one thousand deaths), and again in 1866–67. Patients with these diagnoses often had other medical conditions as well, and this created a serious problem as some patients entered the MGH with one diagnosis and left with two, having contracted something else while admitted.

Smallpox, in contrast, was a very dangerous, highly contagious disease known for centuries to have killed hundreds of thousands in epidemics in Europe. It was seen regularly at the MGH, which built a smallpox isolation ward in 1868, consisting of forty beds with no bathroom or kitchen, southeast of the Richardson Wing (fig. 2.6). Everyone feared smallpox, despite vaccination, which was reported by Jenner in 1789.[34] The smallpox ward was important for the MGH because it allowed the patients to be isolated. In the great epidemic of 1885–86, an estimated fifty-seven hundred patients died in the greater Montreal area.[35]

Vaccination for smallpox, probably one of the most far-reaching discoveries in the annals of medical history, had been generally accepted by this time (Osler had been vaccinated). Despite almost guaranteed immunity with vaccination, in Montreal in 1885 the French population resisted due to ignorance, lake of exposure to the procedure, a vigorous anti-vaccination campaign, and their fatalistic attitude. The MGH lobbied the province to establish a smallpox hospital in the city so that patients could be admitted there instead of the general hospitals. Such a hospital was opened in 1876 and was supposed to help the City of Montreal and the MGH, which stopped admitting smallpox patients. In practice, the smallpox hospital was too small, and didn't solve the problem because people were afraid to go there. The reason so many died of smallpox in 1885–86 had to do with widespread ignorance and suspicion among the French population and weak public health officials who did not demand compulsory vaccination. Instead, these officials kowtowed to a suspicious and angry French public, and fifty-seven hundred people died. It was after this that McGill began to take a greater interest in public health, and, in 1894, Lord Strathcona endowed the Strathcona Chair of Public Health, which was given to the very talented Robert Craik.

The idea that invisible organisms could cause so many diseases led to a massive hunt for microbes between 1870 and 1890. This hunt became so important that it subverted interest in pathology, which was still the foundation of understanding human disease. Pasteur (1822–95) and Koch (1843–1916) may be considered the founders of the bacteriological movement in the late 1880s. A few others who made major contributions are: leprosy, Hansen (1875); typhoid fever, Eberth (1880); lobar pneumonia, Pasteur and many others (1880); Tbc, Koch (1882); diphtheria, Klebs (1883); erysipalis, Fehleison (1883); tetanus, Nicolaier (1884); cholera, Koch (1884); Malta fever, Bruce (1887); scarlet fever, Klein (1887); and diphtheria antitoxin, Behring and Kitasato (1890).[37] Diagnoses could now be made, but there was still no specific treatment except diphtheria antitoxin and, with regard to prevention, smallpox vaccination.

The objection to fever patients was that they dominated the hospital to the degree that they excluded other diagnoses, spent weeks and months recovering, and often spread their infection. Economics prevailed in the 1870s, when, for a short time, fever patients were refused admission.

Parallel events that helped control infectious disease included the development of antisepsis, which was introduced to the MGH in 1869 by Craik, who did not follow Lister's procedure to the letter and was not impressed with its benefits. In 1877, Roddick, who *did* follow Lister's antiseptic procedure to the letter, had excellent results in dramatically reducing post-operative infections. Many of his colleagues adopted his procedure with the same results. Something else that helped with the control of infectious disease was the 1891 forty-thousand-dollar bequest by David Greenshields (matched by George Stevens) in the name of George Campbell to build, in 1892, a separate surgical building south of the Moreland Wing (fig. 2.7) to isolate surgical patients.

Finally, the appearance of professionally trained nurses, who, in the 1880s and 1899s, insisted on cleaner hospital conditions, controlled hospital infections. In 1887, these women included the first operating room nurse, Alicia Dunn,[38] who was old-fashioned but who took over the OR and demanded antisepsis, civility, and conformity. No one crossed swords with this dedicated, short-tempered woman who had no time for anyone who didn't understand her way of doing things.

Length of Stay in the Hospital

The prolonged length of stay on the part of many patients, usually three to four months, posed an ongoing problem for which there seemed no solution. It is hard for contemporary physicians to conceive of such long admissions as, today, routine infectious diseases cost eighth-hundred dollars per day and there are squads of people roaming around the hospital telling the doctors to get the patients moving. Since in the mid- to late nineteenth century there were no laboratories to help with progress and prognosis, the attending physician had to stand passively by and watch the natural history of a disease run its course.

Once recovered, the patients, who were kept in bed most of the time, had to be mobilized (there were no therapists) by the nurses or steward. It took time for the patient to regain strength before she or he could be discharged. There were no referral facilities, nursing homes, or half-way houses, so the patient had to remain in the MGH until he or she convinced the medical staff that he or she could manage at home. It took half a century and two world wars to realize that early mobilization hastened recovery from literally all illnesses.

Fire Hazard

There was constant concern about fire at the MGH and, indeed, in the City of Montreal, where fires were common. The water supply was uncertain. Water had to be pumped from the river, which was a problem for the MGH, which needed it for hospital use as well as for fire prevention. Water pipes were laid down in Montreal in the 1820s, and the water was pumped from the St Lawrence up to the city. It was a significant help when the reservoir below the Royal Victoria Hospital (RVH) was finally completed in the 1840s.

Lighting in the early hospital was provided by oil lamps, which were a constant hazard. Matrons had to watch patients carefully when they used the lamps, and smoking was absolutely forbidden and was grounds for expulsion. When gas was finally installed in the wards, the stopcocks were mounted high on the walls out of reach of the patients, and everyone breathed easier when the lamps were discarded.

Heat provided by coal stoves was of equal concern, and this hazard was finally eliminated by central steam heating. Despite the constant risk, it is a tribute to the vigilance of the staff that there was never a major fire at the MGH.

Stimulants on the Wards

The use of stimulants (i.e., wine, beer, brandy, and whisky) on the wards was a common practice as it helped to relax the patients. On admission, each patient was given a choice of a four- to eight-ounce bottle of whisky or brandy, or a bottle of port or ale. There were complaints, even though the patients were told to drink only a little each day and were cautioned that abuse was not tolerated and would be seen as grounds for expulsion. The problem of staff abuse, however, was not really addressed, and it is believed that the staff drank much of the patients' allotment. But it must be said that, with individual exceptions, this was never proven.

Every now and then staff, and even matrons, were fired for drunkenness. A complaint was brought to the attention of the Committee of Management that the patients used too much alcohol and that this needed to be investigated. In the 1880s, it was determined to everyone' surprise that, over a twenty-year period, there was no increase in expenditure on either alcohol or alcohol abuse. I cannot determine when the custom of providing patients with alcohol came to an end, but it is suspected that Nora Livingston had something to do with it.

The Outpatient Clinic

The original clinic, or dispensary, consisted of two rooms off the lobby for years and was initially staffed by house officers before attending staff were appointed in 1840s. More and more doctors wanted positions at the MGH because of the prestige that was now being associated with the hospital and McGill. The number of outpatient physicians started at two and was steadily increased to four and then to eight in the 1880s, while the number of inpatient physicians was fixed at eight, all of whom worked as volunteers.

Clinic expansion, which was badly needed, was finally provided when the Moreland Wing was constructed in 1875. The basements of the Moreland and Reid wings were divided into a number of rooms to meet the increasing patient load, and the clinic remained there for many years until a new building was constructed after 1910. A separate entrance on St Domimique Street made the clinic more accessible.

The hospital hierarchy was typical of the British Empire at the time – that is, a small number of devoted physicians had inpatient positions, which they kept until death or retirement. This number was kept fixed as a reward for long service. However, this reward came at a considerable sacrifice for these physicians received no compensation for their time. The authors of this volume do not know what days or for how many hours a day the clinic was open. What we do know is that physician advancement from clinic service to inpatient service only occurred when a senior died or retired, which might happen every ten or twelve years.

In Europe, the full-time clinical staff were paid by the state to see patients, teach students, and conduct research, quite a contrast when compared to McGill, where the medical staff had to make their livings in private practice in offices outside the hospital. Because of the infection problem, surgery in the clinic was strictly minor. And, because of the lack of training in surgical procedures, it took years for the staff to fully utilize Roddick's technique.

After 1875, the clinic was a dark set of rooms with dark wooden benches in the halls, where the patients sat and waited to be called. They signed in in a book on a first-come, first-served basis, and a doctor called out their names before seeing them in alcoves behind curtains. Almost all doctors wore head mirrors to focus the poor lighting from the gas lights onto the patients (see below). Electricity was installed in the MGH in 1892, but the hospital remained dark and dismal.

The clinic was poorly run because there was no money to staff it properly. Record keeping, which was stipulated in the rules and regulations, was not up to date because the house officer who was in the clinic did not have enough time to keep it up. He not only had to assist the medical staff in seeing the patients and in performing small procedures but also had to pick up and clean up. There were no nurses or secretaries to help, so things just didn't get done.

Instruments and rooms were not properly cleaned, and the staff had to make it on their own. Still, everyone got used to it and lived with it as there was no other free medical service offered in Montreal. In 1880, the number of house officers was increased by four, with one assigned to the clinic. This was an improvement, but this person was still too busy to keep things in order. None of this changed substantially until professionally trained nurses came to the MGH in the 1890s.

Another ongoing problem in the clinic was created by Frank Buller (1844–1905), the first eye doctor at the MGH, who arrived in 1877. Being the first trained eye specialist in Montreal, Buller rapidly had a huge clientele and flooded the clinic with patients. He saw too many patients, took too much time, and encroached on the time of the other clinics. He was well trained in his work and was given the first Chair of Ophthalmology and Otology at McGill in 1883, with no salary. In 1894, he moved to the RVH, where he directed its eye, ear, nose and throat department.

The Ambulance and Emergency Services, 1883

In 1883, the undertaker for the MGH, Joseph Wray, agreed to supply an ambulance service for the hospital, initially using his hearses to carry patients. Business was so good that Wray constructed wagons to be used specifically as ambulances (fig. 2.8). They were on four wheels, were about 2.1 metre high and 3.7 metres long, and were pulled by one or two horses depending on the weather. They could accommodate two stretchers. The house officer and driver, like stage coach drivers, sat in front on a bench seat exposed to the elements. The hospital did supply a worn, heavy coat for winter and a Macintosh for rainy weather. In winter, skis replaced the wheels, and, frequently, two or more horses were needed. Joseph Wray had his sheds and stables downtown near the MGH on St Dominique Street to be nearby when needed. When called, the driver would hitch up the hoses, get the bell ringing at the MGH, and drive to the front entrance, expecting the house officer to be outside waiting. Any delay would result in a chastising from the driver, who wanted to get to the patient first.

The house officers who were on call would answer the bell rung in the lobby and race to the front door to answer the call and pick up a hat and coat, which would be hanging on a hook. Speed was important because there were two ambulance services in Montreal in 1894, one for the MGH and one for the RVH, and Joseph Wray supplied the wagons for both. Later, Notre Dame Hospital got a service, and, by 1900, frequently all three hospitals were called by patients and raced to the scene, with bells ringing, on a first-come, first-to-get-the-patient basis.

Arguments would result when they all arrived together, but the first to touch the patient had priority. The house officer could administer first aid, bandage a wound, splint a fracture, and give morphine for pain, but otherwise he had to bundle the patient in blankets and race back to the MGH. One can imagine what the patient had to endure in an unheated wagon in freezing weather.[39]

All medical emergencies went through the front doors, where the ambulance patients were delivered and admitted. The clinic had no capacity to deal with emergencies, and the concept of an emergency service or room (ER) was decades away.

The Early Appearance of Specialization at the MGH

In the second half of the nineteenth century, specialization – was inevitable. It was impossible for a well educated MD, while travelling in Germany, France, and Austria after graduating from medical school, to turn a blind eye to the advances in science and medicine apparent in these countries. The return of these students with their new ideas, the proliferation of medical journals, the increasing number of medical societies and meetings, better communication with European centres – all contributed to an awareness of the need to specialize. Doctors travelling to centres in the west (e.g., the British Medical Association meeting in Montreal in 1897), the telephone, the appearance of new medical equipment, and the anticipation of change also contributed to a rising interest in specialization and a waning interest in generalization. The medical profession had to accept that knowing a lot about one subject was ultimately better for the patient than knowing a little about a lot of subjects. Both had a place in the diagnostic and treatment hierarchy.

Into this world stepped the remarkable William Osler, who went to Europe after graduating from McGill in 1872. With an incredibly open mind, he started slowly, and it was Rudolph Virchow, the German pathologist, who opened his eyes. Osler grasped Virchow's message immediately: through careful pathologic studies, both gross and microscopic, the causes of human disease could be found. Virchow was very thorough, very careful with tissues, and observed everything, most of which he reported. And he had a profound effect on Osler.

After also having experience in Vienna with Karl Rokitansky, the great Austrian pathologist, Osler returned to Montreal in 1874, primed to introduce real pathology to McGill and the MGH. He had been hired by McGill because of his blood cell research in England, but it was through pathology that he made his lasting influence on the university. He was appointed pathologist to the MGH in 1877 and was to conduct all the autopsies. He quickly made pathology the most interesting subject in the medical school. While at McGill (1874–84) he gave demonstrations to both students and staff, delivered talks, and wrote hundreds of publications that rendered pathology more relevant to students than any other subject. Indeed, pathology and its findings became an obsession in the medical world in the second half of the 1800s, only rivalled by the hunt for microbes between 1870 and 1900. William Osler performed 780 autopsies during his ten years at the MGH, and he set the stage for clinical specialists to come to McGill.

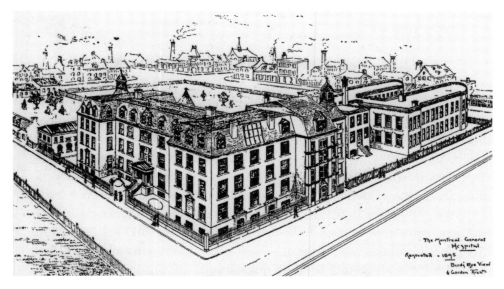

Fig. 2.7 An architectural overview of the MGH campus in 1895, showing the new Greenfield and Campbell Surgical Pavilions (1892) (U-shaped). Drawn by Gordon Trents, architect, 1895.

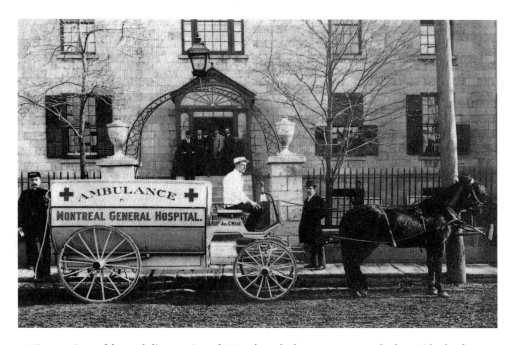

Fig. 2.8 One of funeral director Joseph Wray's ambulance wagons parked outside the front entrance of the MGH in the early 1900s. Originally he used hearses with reversible signs, but business was so good that Wray built dedicated ambulance wagons for the MGH. All emergencies came through the front entrance. The concept of an emergency service would not appear for many decades. Photographer unknown.

Prominent Medical Staff up to 1885

As the original founding staff died (Caldwell, 1832; Stephenson, 1842; Robertson, 1844; and Holmes 1860), each was replaced by able, well trained younger physicians. These I now list.

George Campbell (1810–82) replaced Caldwell in 1835. He was an outstanding student and practitioner who was appointed professor of surgery in 1842 and dean of medicine from 1860 to 1880. He was one of the great leaders in the early years. In 1861, Campbell, as dean of medicine, convinced the McGill Corporation to change the medical degree from MD to MD, CM in order to acknowledge the surgical as well as the medical training acquired in medical school. Following the University of Edinburgh's 1858 decision to add the "CM" to its medical degree,[40] the McGill Corporation agreed to Campbell's proposal. Starting in 1862, the twenty graduates in medicine of that year were awarded the degree of doctoris medicinae et chirurgiae magristri (MD, CM) for the first time.[41] This degree is still offered. In 1865, he also created the Holmes Gold Medal.

Michael McCullough (1795–1854) took Stephenson's place in 1842 as professor of obstetrics and gynaecology and diseases of women and children. He was the first director of the University Lying-In Hospital in 1843.

On Robertson's death in 1844, Andrew F. Holmes became professor of medicine in 1845 and the first dean of medicine, 1854–60. Of the four founders, Holmes is the only one whose name is remembered in the Holmes Gold Medal, which is awarded annually to the graduate with the highest grade-point average in the four years of medical school. It was first awarded in 1865.

James Crawford was appointed in 1845 as the first professor of clinical medicine and surgery, and he took over the teaching at the MGH, relieving the other professors who taught students at the medical school. It soon became too much for Crawford to teach both medicine and surgery, so in 1849 he relinquished the medical teaching to Robert McDonnell (1812–78), who was then professor of clinical medicine. Crawford was killed in a carriage accident in 1854.

Crawford was replaced by William Scott (1823–82), a physician-surgeon and the professor of anatomy until his death in 1883. He was a traditional anatomist with no special training, and he never insisted on dissection of the chest, abdomen, pelvis, or nervous system because these were never viewed by the surgeons of the time. Thinking that students ought to learn anatomy in the same manner as he had, he neither illustrated his lectures nor went to the dissecting room

Frank Shepherd, a young anatomist who started in 1875, brought a modern view to anatomy. He lavishly illustrated his lectures and, after Roddick introduced antiseptic surgery, thus allowing head, neck, chest, abdomen, pelvis, joints, and bones to be operated on, he pushed for the total dissection of the cadaver. Until his death, Shepherd was in conflict with Scott (It should be noted that William Scott is our present-day Harry Scott's great-grandfather.)

After 1855, a dramatic change in the MGH's milieu occurred with of series of appointments of exceptional physicians who, together, formed a team that exceeded their individual reputations.

Robert Palmer Howard (1823–89), an outstanding McGill graduate of 1848 was appointed professor of clinical medicine in 1856 and professor of medicine in 1860. He was dean of medicine from 1882 to 1889. He was McGill's first great academic figure trained in pathology and its correlation with human disease. Having a large personal library, he influenced many students (William Osler in particular).

George Fenwick (1825–94), a surgeon ahead of his time, was professor of clinical surgery in 1867 and professor of surgery in from 1875 to 1890. He was a fast operator and didn't meddle with post-op patients, who generally did well. He edited two medical journals and was vice-president of the Canadian Medical Association (CMA) from 1881 to 1882. He quickly adopted Lister's antiseptic techniques. He was professor of surgery when Roddick introduced antisepsis to the MGH, and he was particularly interested in Tbc of the knee joint with excision, publishing a few cases. His biggest contribution to McGill was convincing young Tom Roddick, who was on his way to Edinburgh to medical school, to apply to McGill in 1864. Fenwick recognized a teenage prodigy in Roddick, and few knew how much this was going to mean to McGill's future.

Robert Craik (1829–1906) graduated first in his class of 1854. He was appointed professor of clinical surgery in 1861, of chemistry in 1867, and dean of medicine in 1889 on Howard's death. He practised medicine at the MGH and was a brilliant philosopher of medicine who influenced improvements in the medical school (1889–1901), was involved in the creation of RVH, and saw many other changes during his fifty-two years at McGill.

Thomas George Roddick (1843–1923), a prodigious genius and Holmes medalist on graduation in 1868, was appointed professor of surgery 1890 and was dean of medicine from 1901 to 1908. He was knighted in 1914. He was the most important surgical figure in Canada in the latter 15 years of the century for promoting antiseptic surgery and establishing the Dominion Medical Council, whose examinations allow a Canadian physician to practise anywhere in the country. He was a born politician and charmed everyone he met.

Francis Shepherd (1851–1929), a winner of the Primary Examination prize on graduation in 1873, was appointed professor of anatomy in 1883 and dean of medicine in 1914. His academic career as a surgeon was hampered somewhat by his being a professor of anatomy but only a lecturer in surgery (McGill would allow only one professorship per person). He insisted on total dissection of the cadaver. He became the leading surgeon at the MGH, performed the first nephrectomy in Lower Canada in 1885, had a large series of successful thyroidectomies, and was one of the first dermatologists in Canada. He should have been knighted for his thyroid work but did not have the political abilities that Roddick had. Still, he was a giant in the history of surgery at McGill.

William Osler (1834–1919), a prize winner on graduation in 1872, started his academic career in basic physiology, histology, and pathology (at the Institutes of Medicine). The latter formed the background for his subsequent career in medicine. By the time he left McGill in 1884 he had performed hundreds of autopsies over ten years and demonstrated, discussed, and published his findings. He went on to become the most influential figure in American and Canadian medicine between 1893 and 1919, when he died. His textbook of medicine, *The Principles and Practice of Medicine*, published in 1893, was the world's authority for at least forty years.

George Ross (1842–92), Holmes Gold Medalist on graduation in 1866, was an exacting and brilliant teacher who intimidated students in his attempts to get them to do better. Punctual, methodical, short tempered, up to date, intolerant of inferior performance, he was one of those teachers any dean would love to appoint a professor. He edited the *Montreal Medical Journal* from 1879 to 1893, was president of the Canadian Medical Association, and, unfortunately, died at age forty-seven due to complications of hypertension.

Alexander Dougall Blackader (1847–1932), an outstanding student, had multiple careers, all which made him famous. He trained in diseases of children, became a lecturer in paediatrics at McGill in 1883, and went on to become one of the founding members of the American Pediatric Society in 1889. He was professor of the diseases of children (1896–1921), chair of paediatrics (1921–32), and acting dean of medicine (1915–19). He was also professor of materia medica and therapeutics (1892–94) and of therapeutics and pharmacology (1895–1921). He was president of virtually every major medical and paediatric association in North America. To cap his brilliant career, he was editor-in-chief of the *Canadian Medical Association Journal* from 1921 until his death. He was responsible for this journal's international credibility when he was already over seventy-two years old.

Francis Buller (1844–1905), a graduate of the Toronto School of Medicine (the medical branch of Victoria College) in 1869, had advanced training in ophthalmology in Germany and London before coming to the MGH in 1877 as McGill's first surgical subspecialist and ophthalmologist. He was appointed the first chair of ophthalmology and otology at McGill in 1883 and chair of ophthalmology at the RVH in 1994. He introduced the ophthalmoscope to McGill in 1877 and published articles on gonorrhoea of the eye and its prevention, operative techniques, and methyl alcohol blindness. (His great-grandson, Sean Murphy, MD, CM, became chair of ophthalmology at McGill and has Buller's original ophthalmoscope.)

James Chalmers Cameron (1852–1912), winner of the Final Examination Prize on graduation in 1874, received extensive training in obstetrics and gynaecology in Dublin, Berlin, Paris, and Vienna before returning to Montreal. He was appointed professor of obstetrics and diseases of children and brought modern concepts of obstetrics to McGill at the Montreal Maternity Hospital (obstetrics and gynaecology were separate specialties until Cameron's death in 1912, when they were recombined)

William Gardner (1842–1926), winner of the Final Examination Prize on graduation in 1866, was appointed the first professor of gynaecology at McGill in 1883 with no surgical training or privileges. Apparently he could teach the subject to McGill's satisfaction. In 1884, he arranged to spend six months as a surgical assistant to a famous British gynaecologist during the winter of 1885. He kept his professorship in gynaecology and became gynaecologist-in-chief at the new RVH in 1895. He was not an academician but was highly qualified and was the first specially trained gynaecologist in Montreal.

Ross and Howard in medicine; Roddick, Shepherd, and Fenwick in surgery; Cameron in obstetrics; Gardner in gynaecology; Blackader in paediatrics (who was better trained than Cameron, who insisted on controlling paediatrics); Buller in ophthalmology; Craik in chemistry and as dean of medicine; and Osler in pathology – almost all prize winners on graduation from medical school – formed an extraordinary faculty of unrivalled academic ability.

The State of the MGH in 1885

The condition of the MGH in the 1880s was not good. The lobby walls were papered with pages from the *London Illustrated News*, and the woodwork was dark and dingy. The heater in the lobby stood on one leg, the others propped up by bricks. The walls were unpainted and stained from the gas lights. The men's ward was overcrowded, and many had to be moved to tents on the grounds during warm weather. As mentioned, the heating was provided by stoves in the open wards until steam pipes and radiators were installed in 1892.[42]

Plumbing on the men's side consisted of one bath with a WC, bathtub, and wash basin, which was grossly inadequate for sixty people (the capacity of two open wards at the MGH). When drains were blocked it was not a sure thing that the plumbers would be called: it depended on the funds available.[43] The basement clinics were dark and dingy and poorly lit with gas light. Patients sat on benches in the waiting room. There was still no Emergency Room (ER) at the MGH.

Most doctors wore head mirrors to focus light on the patients – light reflected from the gas lights that were located behind the patients and that could be quite bright when turned up. The food service was primitive. With the kitchen in the basement, food had to be brought up by dumb waiters on trays and served by the staff and by ambulatory patients who volunteered to help. This became a real drill because all the staff had to pass the food around on the wards three times a day and then had to clean up. The "nurses" were employees who did everything from cleaning the wards, making beds, performing various housekeeping tasks, to attending to the patients.

The mattresses were straw-filled and rested on metal-framed beds, which created a mess on the floor around the beds. The laundry under one of the first-floor wards sent odours upwards. There was no drying area, so wet or drying sheets and bedding were hung wherever there was room. The urinals and bedpans were made of china and were not warmed in the cold weather. The floors were not just worn but, in some places, worn through. There was a major problem with rats on the wards and in the MGH in general, and roaches flourished in the warm weather. Both had to be accepted as part of the scene at the hospital.[44]

A provocative and literate description of the condition of the MGH, provided by an outsider and taken from an 1877 newspaper, is quoted in Hugh MacDermot's *History of the School of Nursing of the Montreal General Hospital*:

> There is only one bathroom for all the wards on the male side of the hospital. It is more inconveniently located and, in short is entirely inadequate for the purpose for which it was designed. The water closets are in the immediate vicinity, and as if some malevolent genius of unfitness had taken charge of the arrangements, the shaft by which the meals are hoisted from the lower regions, is only separated from both by a wooden partition. Meals are prepared for distribution on the landing in full sight of this trinity of incompatibilities …
>
> The smallness of the wards allowing an insufficiency of cubic inches to each bed; the poverty of window room; the scanty means for natural and the absurd attempts at artificial ventilation throughout a large proportion of the wards; the total absence of anything that deserves the name of light in some of the passages; the impossibility of admitting many essential conveniences from want of space; the unavoidably unwholesome condition of the walls from age and porosity of materials, allowing them to become impregnated with various miasmatae; the shocking accommodations for violent weak-minded patients in the basement, more like provocatives to insanity than prophylactic agencies; the situation of the laundry immediately under the wards, aggravated by the case with which noxious vapours there from can ascend to the first floor, imparting in their passage quaint unwelcome flavours to flesh, fish , and fowl; the wholly uncalled for little nests of pestilence which obtrude themselves with disagreeable familiarity at almost every turn and corner in this no-mans-land; may be included in the bill of objections which we would bring against our otherwise admirable MGH.[45]

Although the Nightingale School for Nurses was opened in London in 1860, few nurses had made it to Canada, where there was no formal training for them. The women hired as "nurses" had no experience in hospital care but learned to take care of patients with the help of the doctors. The nursing directors that were hired by the MGH in the 1870 and 1880s not only had to deal with intolerant doctors, very poor living conditions, and poor salaries but were also expected to initiate nurses training (which didn't happen).

In 1890, Nora Livingston, seeing the problems others had had at the MGH, demanded more respect for her nurses – better pay, better living conditions, and relief from housekeeping duties – or she wouldn't consider the challenge. She also promised to start a school for nurses as a priority, all of which MGH authorities accepted in order to have her come to Montreal.

The nurses' quarters were cubicles built into an old ward and had thin walls and leaky ceilings. They had no sitting rooms or lounge. There is little wonder that young women were not attracted to nursing when they had to live under those conditions.[46] This improved in 1890, when a Mansard addition was built on the top of the MGH as a nurses' quarters. There was not a lot of room, but at last nurses had their own quarters. Nora Livingston would not have come to the MGH in 1890 without them. There were no offices in the hospital for the senior staff, all of whom were McGill professors. Also, there were no chiefs of the clinical departments at the RVH and MGH – only senior professors at McGill – until about 1918, when McGill insisted on chairs in all the clinical departments, just as there had been in the pre-clinical departments for decades.[47]

The autopsy room was a small, dingy room in the basement, with a wooden autopsy table, a wooden instrument table, and a chair. It was in this dismally lit room that Osler performed his autopsies by the light of an oil lamp or two and taught himself the pathological bases of human disease.[48] There were complaints from patients that the odours from the post-mortem room could, at times, be smelled on the wards above.

Members of the board were supposed to visit the hospital weekly on rotation and write a critique of what they saw in a ledger that existed just for these comments. Most did a superficial inspection and wrote useless notes praising the hospital's condition. Occasionally, visitors took their time and wrote detailed and critical notes about the true condition of the MGH, which was poor.[49]

Once the RVH opened in 1893, it was clear to the Montreal General Hospital Corporation and Board of Governors that the old buildings needed serious renovations and additions. The surgical pavilions, finished in 1892 (fig. 2.7), and the major renovations of the other buildings in 1894 were enough of a facelift to appeal to students and house surgeons.

Presidents of the MGH 1820–87

Isaac Winslow Clarke	1820
John Richardson	1821–31
John Molson, the elder	1831–35
Samuel Gerard	1835–57
John Molson, the younger	1857–59
John Redpath	1859–68
William Molson	1868–74
Peter Redpath	1871–81
Andrew Robertson	1881–87

MGH Buildings and Extensions, 1821–94

Main Central Building	1821
Richardson Wing (east side)	1832
Reid Wing (west side)	1848
Fever and Smallpox Wing	1868
Morland Wing (west side)	1875
Extension to Morland Wing	1884
Mansard story above all wings as a nurses' residence	1889–90
Campbell and Greenshields Surgical Wing	1891
Major internal remodeling of wings	1894
Pathological Building (east of Richardson Wing)	1894

NOTES

1 W. Osler, *Aequanimitas and Other Addresses* (Philadelphia: Blaikston Son and Co., 1905), 36.

2 Maude Abbott, "Historical Sketch of the Medical Faculty of McGill University," *Montreal Medical Journal* 31, 8 (1902): 603–6.

3 Kathleen Jenkins, *Montreal, Island City in the St. Lawrence* (New York: Doubleday, 1966), 221; Abbott, "Historical Sketch," 626.

4 Abbott, "Historical Sketch," 564–6.

5 A Committee for the Society, History of the Montreal Ladies Benevolent

Society, 1815–1920 , Montreal: Ladies Benevolent Society, 1920), 9 (located in Osler Library); Abbott, "Historical Sketch," 626–8. This is the actual notice from the *Montreal Gazette*, 26 February 1816.

6 The Quebec Act, 1774, established a lieutenant-governor of Upper Canada and Lower Canada. A governor general of Canada was apparently appointed by 1776 and reconfirmed by a change in the Constitution in 1791.

7 Abbott, "Historical Sketch," 567–8, 606–7.

8 Ibid., 631–3. This is O'Sullivan's speech and response to John Molson's letter of January 1819, which led to the famous duel.

9 I visited Windmill Point in Point Claire. The ancient windmill still stands on the windswept 0.8-hectare point jutting out into the St Lawrence River. A remote and forbidding spot that would have been ideal for duelling.

10 E.H. Bensley and B.R. Tunis, "The Caldwell-O'Sullivan Duel," *Canadian Medical Association Journal* 100 (1969): 1092–5.

11 H.E. MacDermott, *History of the Montreal General Hospital* (Montreal: Montreal General Hospital, 1950), 4.

12 M.S.E. Abbott, "Florence Nightingale as Seen in Her Portraits," *Boston Medical and Surgical Journal* September (1916): 14, 21, 28. Reprinted in book form for the Canadian Red Cross in 1916. See M.S.E. Abbott, *Florence Nightingale as Seen in Her Portraits* (Boston: privately published, 1916), 51–2.

13 Agaib Milborne, *Freemasonry in the Province of Quebec, 1759–1959* (Montreal: Free-masons of Quebec, 1960), chap. 1. This is the history of Freemasonry in Quebec published by the Order. It is authoritative and is available at the Grand Lodge in Montreal.

14 Abbott, "Historical Sketch," 610–11; MacDermott, *History of the Montreal General Hospital*, 7–11.

15 Bosworth Newton, *Hochelaga Deptica: The Early History and Present State of the City and Island of Montreal* (Montreal: William Craig, 1839). An 1839 map of Montreal, which shows all the streets of the parade route, is inserted in the back of the book.

16 Abbott, "Historical Sketch," 611–19; *Montreal Herald*, 9 June1821; *Montreal Gazette*, 13 June 1821.

17 J. Hanaway and R. Cruess, *McGill Medicine: The First Half Century* (Montreal-Kingston: McGill-Queen's University Press, 1996), 1:143–9.

18 John Stephenson, "De Velosynthesis," a graduation thesis submitted to the University of Edinburgh, 1 August 1820, for the degree of MD. Stephenson describes the operation and post-op period. A copy of the thesis is in the Osler Library. See also, W. Francis, "Repair of a Cleft Palate by Philibert Roux in 1819:

A Translation of John Stephenson's 'De Velosynthesis,'" *Journal of the History of Medicine and Allied Sciences* 18, 3 (1963): 209–19.

19 C. Von Graefe, "Die Gaoumenath, ein neuentdeckts Mittel gegen angborne Fehler der Sprache," *J. Chir. Augenhelk* 1 (1820) 1–54. This is the only reported operation on a congenital cleft palate before Stephenson's.

20 A.F. Holmes, "Employment of Chloroform," *British American Journal of Medical and Physical Science* 3 (1848): 263–4.

21 A.F. Holmes, "Valedictory address read to students, the Faculty of Medicine, McGill College, 1850," *British American Journal of Medical and Physical Science* 6 (1850): 53 (mentions the stethoscope)

22 W. Withering, *An Account of Foxglove and Some of Its Medicinal Uses* (London: G.J. and J, Robinson, 1785).

23 Pedro Barba, *Vera Praxis ad Curationem Tertianae* (Hispali, 1642).

24 J. Lind, *A Treatise on Scurvy* (Edinburgh: Sands, Murray & Cochran, 1753). Lind was not the first to find that citrus fruit could cure and/or prevent scurvy. It was reported at least one hundred years before but not widely known. Lind gets the credit for getting the story of scurvy and citrus fruit to the public.

25 MacDermot, *History of the Montreal General Hospital*, 43; R. Dunglison, *Dictionary of Medical Sciences*, 2nd ed. (Philadelphia: Blanchard and Lea, 1858).

26 The Board of Governors was first established at Craig Street A., 1820.

27 Minutes of the Board of Governors, rules and regulations for the Montreal General Hospital, 8 April 1823, MUA. It takes twenty folio-sized, handwritten pages to cover these rules and regulations.

28 Abbott, "Historical Sketch," 665–9.These are the actual minutes of this historic meeting, which was held on 29 June 1829.

29 MacDermot, *History of the Montreal General Hospital*, 59, 89.

30 Ibid., 29–33.

31 Ibid., 45–50.

32 C.J. Eberth, "Die Organismen in den Orgaren bei Typhus Abdominalis," *Virchow Arch. Path. Anat.* 81 (1880): 58–74; R. Koch, "Uber die Cholerabakterien," *Dtsch, Med. Wschr.* 10 (1884): 725–28.

33 Hanaway and Cruess, *McGill Medicine*, 1:143–49.

34 E. Jenner, *An Inquiry into the Causes and Effects of Variolae Vaccinae* (London: S. Low, 1798). Although Jenner was not the first to vaccinate for smallpox, he deserves the credit for his careful study, for his book and for introducing the concept of vaccination to the world.

35 M. Bliss., *The Making of Modern Medicine* (Toronto: University of Toronto Press, 2011), 18–21. This book is a gem written by Canada's premier medical

historian. I owe the description of the smallpox problem in Montreal to Bliss's account.

36 Ibid., 22–9.

37 E.A, Behring and S. Kitasato, "Uber das Zustandekommen der Diptherie-Immunitat und der Tetnus-Immunitat bei Thierin," *Dtsch. med. Wschr.* 16 (1890):1113–14, 1145–8. The eleven references given above are found in F.H. Garrison and L.T. Morton, *A Medical Bibliography*, 3rd ed. (London: Andre Deutsch Ltd., 1970), 5020–5546.4

38 H.E. MacDermot, *A History of the School of Nursing of the Montreal General Hospital* (Montreal: Alumnae Association, 1940), 49. Alicia Dunne was trained by Roddick and Fenwick as an OR nurse or technician. She quickly took over the management of the OR and ruled staff and physicians for ten years from 1887 to 1897.

39 F.J. Shepherd, *Origin and History of the Montreal General Hospital* (Montreal: published by the author, n.d.), 29–30; S. Lewis, *Royal Victoria Hospital, 1887–1947* (Montreal and Kingston: McGill-Queen's University Press, 1969), 112–15; N. Terry, *The Royal Vic* (Montreal and Kingston: McGill-Queen's University Press, 1994), 133–6. There is not much written about the ambulance service or the emergency facility at the MGH.

40 J.D. Comrie, *History of Scottish Medicine* (London: Baillere, Tindall and Cox, 1932), 11:586, 789.

41 Minute Book of the Corporation of McGill University, 24 April 1861 (1861–62) and 6 May 1862 (1862–63), MUV.

42 MacDermot, *History of the School of Nursing*, 39–40.

43 *MacDermot, History of the Montreal General Hospital*, 78.

44 Ibid.

45 MacDermott, *History of the School*, 29–35.

46 Ibid., 34.

47 M. Entin, J. Hanaway, and T. Nimeh, "The Principal and The Dean," *Canadian Bulletin of the History of Medicine* 20, 1 (2003): 154, 160.

48 C.F. Martin, *The Montreal General Hospital in Osler's Time* (Montreal: MGH publication, 1955), 13–14.

49 MacDermot, *History of the Montreal General Hospital*, 41–2. Visiting Governors' Book started by Stephenson, 10 October 1822. The governors, on a rotation, had to visit the hospital and write their opinions in the book. If someone didn't show up on his assigned date, Stephenson would note his absence in

the book for all to see. There is a fair amount of information about the MGH in general and the clinic in: W.B. Howell, F.J. Shepherd, *Surgeon: His Life and Times* (London: J.M. Dent, 1935); H.E. MacDermott, *Sir Thomas Roddick: His Work in Medicine and Public Life* (Toronto: Macmillan, 1938); F.J. Shepherd, *Reminiscences of Student Days and Dissecting Room* (Montreal: self-published, 1919); F.N. Gurd, *The Gurds, the Montreal General and McGill: A Family Saga* (Burnstown, ON: General Store Publishing House, 1986); R.W. Pound, *Rocke Robertson: Surgeon and Shepherd of Change* (Montreal and Kingston: McGill-Queen's University Press, 2008).

SECTION 2

Department of Medicine
and Its Divisions

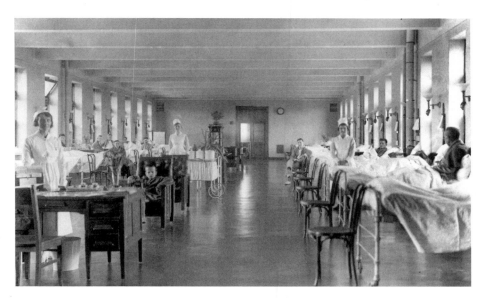

S.2 Old medical ward in MGH on Dorchester, 1900

General Medicine

James H. Darragh

Jim Darragh was a senior physician at the Montreal General Hospital during the Doug Cameron era and was subsequent CEO of the Royal College of Physicians and Surgeons of Canada. He was an author of the second volume of the history of the McGill Faculty of Medicine.

In the 1890s, with additions to the hospital and new appointments to the hospital staff, the Board of Management developed a more formal organization plan. In 1896, the board passed a resolution creating the Department of Medicine, which occupied the rebuilt and remodelled Reid, Richardson, and Moreland wings, providing four wards of forty-seven metres, arranged for 150 beds. There was a new and commodious outpatient department on the ground floor of the Richardson Wing. This resolution resulted from changes that had occurred gradually over the previous fourteen years.

From the opening of the hospital in 1822 until 1882, the MGH attending staff were general practitioners. Their practices included medicine, surgery, and obstetrics. Occasionally they or the housemen conducted post-mortem examinations. In 1871–72, MGH attending physicians were divided into two services:

	Howard Service	Ross Service
1st quarter	William Fraser	John Reddy
2nd quarter	William E. Scott	William Wright
3rd quarter	Duncan C. McCallum	George Fenwick
4th quarter	Robert Palmer Howard	Joseph Morley Drake

Seven of the eight attending physicians were senior members of the medical faculty. Howard, born in Montreal in 1823, graduated MD, CM from McGill in 1848. After several other faculty appointments, he was professor of medicine from 1860. Fenwick was professor of surgery; McCallum was professor of midwifery and diseases of children; Scott was professor of anatomy; Fraser taught the principles of medicine; and Wright taught materia medica. The attending physicians supervised the house officers: George Ross, house surgeon; Thomas. G. Roddick, assistant house surgeon; and T.A. Roger, apothecary.

In 1877, the first specialists were appointed to the MGH staff – Francis Buller in ophthalmology and William Osler as pathologist to the hospital. Osler had been teaching at the Institutes of Medicine since 1874.

George Ross was born in Quebec in 1845, attended McGill in arts and medicine. and graduated MD, CM with the Holmes Medal in 1866. As well as being a brilliant student, he was recognized as an outstanding teacher. After six years as a house officer, in 1872 he was appointed to the attending staff as professor of clinical medicine. In 1882, he took an important decision – to limit his practice to medical cases.[1]

In 1882, the eight attending doctors were divided into two teams – four physicians and four surgeons. Howard and Ross were two of the four physicians. There were two medical services for the indoor patients, with two physicians on each service. At first, the physicians took three-month shifts on ward duty. Later this was changed to six months. After 1882, an appointment to the indoor staff was either as a physician or as a surgeon. For instance, in 1883, when W.E. Scott died, F.J. Shepherd was appointed attending surgeon. Prior to 1882, there was no system for assigning hospital beds according to patients' illnesses. In the next fourteen years, separate wards were developed for medical and surgical patients.

In the 1870s and 1880s, Palmer Howard and George Ross played a part in the development of medicine at McGill and the MGH. Howard gave the lecture course in medicine and Ross supervised the teaching of medical students on the MGH wards. After Palmer Howard died in 1888, Ross was professor of medicine from 1888 to 1892, and Richard MacDonnell was professor of clinical medicine 1888 to 1891. When Ross died in 1892, James Stewart was appointed professor of medicine.

Fred Finley and Henri Lafleur Era, 1894–1924

In 1894, Stewart left MGH to be physician-in-chief at the new RVH, where he continued as McGill's professor of medicine. The position of professor of clinical medicine was discontinued. This presented a problem for Robert

Craik, who had succeeded to the deanship when Palmer Howard died in 1889. Who would teach the medical students at MGH? Two of the indoor physicians, Alexander Blackader and William Molson, were not candidates. Blackader was interested in therapeutics, pharmacology, and diseases of children; Molson was not interested in teaching medical students. Craik found a solution in two young physicians, Fred Finley and Henri Lafleur.

Frederick Gault Finley was born in Melbourne, Australia, in 1861.[2] His family moved to Montreal in 1865. He attended High School of Montreal, graduated MB from the University of London, and MD, CM from McGill in 1885. After his internship at MGH, he was outdoor assistant physician and demonstrator of anatomy at McGill. Soon he was recognized as an outstanding teacher and was promoted to lecturer in 1893, assistant professor in 1894, and associate professor in 1897.

Henri Amedee Lafleur was born in Longueil, Quebec, in 1862 into a family of scholars.[3] At the High School of Montreal and McGill, he was an exceptional student, graduating MD, CM in 1886, and was appointed a house officer at MGH. Osler invited him to come to Johns Hopkins Hospital to be his first medical resident. On returning to Montreal, he was appointed lecturer in medicine at McGill in 1894, assistant professor in 1895, and associate professor in 1897.

Finley and Lafleur were physicians at MGH for many years, each directing a medical service. In 1907, when James Stewart died, they were promoted to professors of medicine and held that rank until they retired in 1924. Finley served overseas with the Royal Canadian Army Medical Corps (RCAMC) in the First World War. He was the first chair of the McGill Department of Medicine, 1920–21, and was dean of medicine from 1921 to 1922. Due to the work of Finley and Lafleur, aided by C.A. Peters and A.H. Gordon, MGH dominated the McGill Department of Medicine from 1907 to 1924.

Campbell Howard Era, 1924–36

Nineteen twenty-four was a "watershed year" in Montreal medicine. C.F. Martin was appointed the first full-time dean of medicine in 1923. In the summer of 1924, J.C. Meakins returned from Edinburgh to be professor of medicine, chair of the McGill Department of Medicine, physician-in-chief at Royal Victoria Hospital, and, most important, director of the Rockefeller-funded, RVH University Medical Clinic, the first research department in an academic hospital in Canada. Campbell Howard returned to Montreal from

Iowa as a professor of medicine, physician at MGH, chair of the MGH Department of Medicine, and director of one of the two medical services.[4] Unlike Meakins, Howard wanted to be in private practice as chairman of the MGH medical department (one suspects Osler's hand in this decision), and the MGH staff rejected an offer by Martin to include them in the request for funds for a research centre from the Rockefeller Foundation. They did not want the Faculty of Medicine to have anything to do with the way medicine was practised at the MGH. A.H. Gordon was associate professor and director of the second medical service and frankly competed with Howard. There being no office space in the MGH, Howard had his office for private patients at 1487 Mackay Street.

Campbell Palmer Howard, youngest son of Robert Palmer Howard, was born in Montreal in 1877. He graduated MD, CM from McGill in 1901. He was a house officer at MGH for four years and then at Johns Hopkins with William Osler for a second four years. After studying in Europe, he returned to Montreal with appointments as junior assistant physician at MGH and demonstrator of clinical medicine and clinical chemistry at McGill. In 1910, he accepted an appointment as professor and chair of the Department of Medicine at the University of Iowa.

Under his leadership, Iowa became one of the leading departments of medicine in the United States. During his postgraduate training, and his years at MGH, Baltimore, and Iowa, Howard investigated a variety of subjects, with particular emphasis on cirrhosis of the liver and the relationship of liver function to various types of anaemia. He was a member of the American Society for Clinical Investigation and the Association of American Physicians. He published extensively in the medical literature.

During the Howard era, C.A. Peters was the third physician and assistant professor, until he retired in 1932. Numerous associate physicians supervised and taught on the medical wards. Junior assistant and assistant physicians attended the outpatient medical clinics.

In May 1936, Howard developed phlebitis, which was responding to treatment; however, he insisted on meeting a commitment for a lecture tour in California. He had started his lectures when there was an exacerbation of the phlebitis, and he died suddenly of a pulmonary embolus on 3 June 1936 in his sixtieth year. This was great shock to his family, patients, colleagues, and students at MGH. Howard was remembered for his teaching ability, his skill in medical practice, his investigative work, and for being the highest type of professional gentleman.

Succeeding Campbell Howard, Alva Gordon was appointed professor of medicine.[5] He was recognized as an outstanding physician and teacher. Born in 1876 on Prince Edward Island, Gordon enrolled at McGill in 1893 and graduated MD, CM in 1899 with the Holmes Gold Medal. He was an intern at MGH for one year, then worked as a paid assistant to a doctor in British Columbia for a year before returning to Montreal to open a medical practice. His McGill career started with an appointment as demonstrator in physiology and a junior appointment in medicine at MGH. Gordon advanced to become a physician at MGH, chief of one of the two medical services and assistant professor of medicine from 1924 to 1936. (The other physicians from 1936 to 1939 were C.C. Birchard, D. Grant Campbell, L.C. Montgomery, and J.B. Ross.)

In 1931 Gordon was a charter Fellow of the Royal College of Physicians and Surgeons of Canada (RCPSC), a member of Council from 1931 to 1939, and vice-president (medicine) from 1935 to 1937. When he was president of the Association of American Physicians, his presidential address was entitled "Montreal Medicine after Osler." He was granted an LLD (McGill and McMaster) and DCO (Acadia) during the course of his career. In 1939, at age sixty-two, as a part-time professor, Gordon retired from his university and MGH appointments and continued private and consulting medical practice for several years as a member of the MGH honorary consulting staff. He died in 1953 at age seventy-seven.

Lorne Cuthbert Montgomery Era, 1939–47

When A.H. Gordon retired in 1939, there were four physicians – C.C. Birchard, D.G. Campbell, L.C. Montgomery,[6] and J.B. Ross. The unanimous decision of the Medical Board was that Montgomery should be promoted from associate to professor of medicine to succeed Gordon. The Board of Management supported this recommendation, and the Joint Hospital Committee confirmed his appointment.

Lorne Montgomery was born in Richmond, Quebec, 5 August 1894. He attended Montreal High School and enrolled at McGill Medical School in 1913. He was overseas with the CAMC from 1915 to 1918, at first with No 3. Canadian General Hospital and then transferring to the 42nd Royal Highlanders. After returning to Montreal, he completed his medical studies at McGill, graduating MD, CM in 1920 with the Wood Gold Medal. After interning at MGH for two years, he was at Johns Hopkins Hospital from 1922 to 1923, was appointed junior assistant physician at MGH in 1923, where he advanced to assistant physician in 1924, associate physician in 1934, and physician in December 1936. In June 1931 he was granted FRCPC ad eundem gradum.

On 15 June 1940, Montgomery was granted indefinite leave of absence from MGH and McGill to serve with the RCAMC with the rank of lieutenant-colonel. He was officer in charge of medicine, consultant in medicine, and, after August 1942, director of medical services. He served in England, Italy, and Northwest Europe, returning to Canada in 1944 for health reasons. After demobilization and a period of convalescence, he resumed his duties at MGH and McGill.

Many other MGH physicians joined the armed services after 1939, and soon there was an acute shortage of staff. In 1940, there was a double cohort of medical graduates – the five-year course of 1935 and the four-year course of 1936. Many of them interned at MGH and promptly joined the military services instead of remaining at as senior resident staff. The same situation prevailed with the medical graduates of the classes of 1941 and 1942, and the two classes of 1943. Lester McCallum, a graduate of 1943B, recalls being a fourth-year medical student one week, and the next week being the intern on E.S. Mills's service on Ward E with no senior resident to guide him.

To make matters worse, J.B. Ross, one of three remaining physicians, developed *viridans endocarditis* in 1941. Born in 1900, Ross had been an outstanding medical student at McGill, graduating MD, CM in 1922. He joined the MGH staff in 1928 as a junior assistant physician. His promotion was rapid: assistant physician in 1930, associate physician in 1936, and assistant professor in 1937. He was secretary to the Medical Board from 1938 to 1942. In spite of treatment with penicillin, he died on 7 March 1942.

To fill the gap, J. Keith Gordon was recalled from overseas duty with the RCAMC and was promoted to physician and given a seat on the Medical Board. Edward S. Mills took over many of Montgomery's duties, including attending physician on Ward E with C.C. Birchard. As the senior physician, Birchard was chair of the MGH Department of Medicine. Mills was promoted to physician and associate professor of medicine and attended his first meeting of the Medical Board in September 1942. J.C. Meakins, dean of the medical faculty, professor of medicine, and chair of the McGill Department of Medicine, was on active military service. In 1943, Mills was acting chair of the McGill Department of Medicine.

During the war years, particularly from 1942 to 1945, some medical services were restricted and the scheduling of clinics at the central and western divisions of MGH were reduced due to shortage of staff. In 1945, some of the MGH staff began to return after demobilization from the armed services, and the usual medical services at MGH were continued.

After 1945, Montgomery resumed his activities at MGH and McGill. He was a member of the RCPSC Council from 1939 to 1947 and was president of Montreal Med-Chi in 1947.

In 1947, J.C. Meakins retired as dean, professor of medicine, chair of the McGill Department of Medicine, and director of the RVH University Medical Clinic. He held these posts on a full-time basis. Having been professor of medicine since 1939, Montgomery was offered the chair of the McGill Department of Medicine but on a part-time basis. He was unable to accept the offer and resigned as physician at MGH and from McGill. He was appointed to the MGH honorary consulting staff. This was unusual at his age of fifty-three. He continued his medical practice from his office on 1414 Drummond Street, admitting patients to the MGH until his health declined in the 1970s. During his last illness, he was a patient at Cedar Lodge, St Lambert, and died 4 March 1985 at age ninety-one.

Edward Sadler Mills Era, 1948–57

When Montgomery resigned in 1947, the remaining three physicians were C.C. Birchard, J. Keith Gordon, and E.S. Mills.[7] Birchard was the senior physician and chair of the MGH Department of Medicine.

In 1948, Mills was selected to be the professor of medicine at MGH. In keeping with the policy that the physician with the highest academic rank was automatically chair of the MGH Department of Medicine, Mills replaced Birchard. J. Keith Gordon was associate professor of medicine. In 1950, the Board of Management appointed Mills as the first MGH physician-in-chief, ending the tradition of two medical services, which started in 1882. The titles in the Department of Medicine were changed to: senior physician, associate physician, assistant physician, and junior assistant physician. C.C. Birchard and J. Keith Gordon were senior physicians.

Edward Sadler Mills was born on 1 October 1897, in Ormstown, Quebec, a town in the Chateauguay Valley south of Montreal, where the Sadlers were pioneer settlers. He enrolled at McGill in 1915, graduated BSc in 1919 and MD, CM in 1922. After internship at MGH, he was awarded a Cooper Fellowship and completed a thesis to qualify for MSc in 1926. The following year he was a resident at the Mallory Institute for Pathology at Boston City Hospital, where he was influenced by the work of Minot, Murphy, and Castle and developed special interest in diseases of the hematopoetic system. On returning to Montreal, he was appointed junior assistant physician at MGH and McGill demonstrator of medicine. He began his private medical practice by renting an office in Campbell Howard's building on Mackay Street.

In 1929 Mills married Marian Baile. They raised a son, John, who became a rheumatologist at Massachusetts General Hospital, and a daughter, Betty, who became a nurse at the MGH. Mills continued his interest in haematology and established a small laboratory at MGH. Later he obtained a grant from a pharmaceutical company and was able to hire a technician. He was promoted to assistant physician on the outdoor staff and, in 1939, to associate physician and lecturer in medicine on the indoor staff. In 1940, when Montgomery joined the armed services, Mills was promoted to physician, assistant and then associate professor, and, in 1943, was acting chair of the McGill Department of Medicine.

In 1943, Mills established and directed the subdepartment of haematology at MGH. S.R. Townsend joined the sub-department after the Second World War, and D.G. Cameron joined in 1949. In 1931, Mills was granted FRCPC ad eundem gradum. He was a member of the RCPSC Council from 1949 to 1957, vice-president medicine from 1953 to 1955, and chair of the Medical Division of the Credentials Committee. In addition he was honorary Treasurer of the CMA from 1950 to 1957 and CMA representative on a committee for nursing in 1951.

For many years, the MGH Board of Management had considered relocating the hospital from the Dorchester Boulevard site, and planning began in earnest after the Second World War. When C.C. Birchard was chair of the Medical Board from 1948 to 1950, land was purchased bordering Cedar and Pine avenues, and plans were developed for a new hospital building. The MGH Western Division was sold to Montreal Children's Hospital.

In the 1930s, Mills worked with Campbell Howard on various projects, and they co-authored numerous publications in the medical literature. When Howard died in 1936, Mills purchased the Mackay Street building. He continued his medical practice from there until 1953, when he moved his office to MGH and was the first geographical full-time physician-in-chief. He sold the Mackay Street building to the Canadian Red Cross.

Mills was chair of the MGH Medical Board from 1952 to 1956 and was very involved in the move to the Cedar/Pine Avenue site in May 1955. In

September 1957, Mills resigned from MGH, McGill, and the RCPSC Council and moved from his Grosvenor Avenue residence in Westmount to a waterfront property in Foxboro, Essex, Connecticut (near New London), where he pursued his interests in sailing and gardening. He died in 1970 at age seventy-three.

In 1952, N. Feeney was promoted to senior physician and continued as director of the EKG department, having replaced C.C. Birchard in 1949. C. Fullerton and H.S. Mitchell were promoted to senior physicians. In 1952, Mills established and directed the MGH University Medical Clinic (UMC), with D.G. Cameron and E.H. Bensley as assistant directors. In 1954, W. Bauld joined the UMC. While Mills was physician-in-chief, Townsend became the director of the subdepartment of haematology, and additional subdepartments were established: cardiorespiratory (D.J. MacIntosh), endocrine (A. Gold), and allergy (H.S. Mitchell).

Douglas George Cameron Era, 1957–80

When Cameron succeeded Mills as physician-in-chief,[8] professor of medicine, and director of the University Medical Clinic in September 1957, he intended to follow MGH's traditional objectives of patient care, teaching, and research, but he could not have anticipated the many changes that were to occur during the twenty-three years of his tenure. Cameron was born in Swift Current, Saskatchewan, on 17 March 1917. After graduating BSc with honours from the University of Saskatchewan in 1937, he joined the third-year class of McGill Medical School (five-year course), graduated MD, CM in May 1940, and was awarded a Rhodes Scholarship. He interned at MGH from 1940 to 1941, and then served with the RCAMC in England, Italy, and Northwest Europe until 1946, at which time he was discharged with the rank of lieutenant-colonel.

As a Rhodes Scholar, he studied and had postgraduate clinical training at Oxford University from 1946 to 1949. On returning to Montreal, he was awarded a National Research Council Fellowship, 1949–51, and was appointed assistant physician at MGH and assistant professor at McGill. In the next few years he advanced to associate physician and associate professor. When the MGH University Medical Clinic was established in 1952, Cameron was assistant director, with E.H. Bensley. He was awarded FRCPC in 1952 and was active in several medical organizations.

During the Cameron era, two government bills had an important effect on patient care – the Hospital and Diagnostic Services Act, 1959, and the Medicare Act, 1970. There were many developments in diagnostic and treatment facilities. As outlined in the following sections, the medical specialties developed and became divisions in the Department of Medicine. There were marked changes in the personnel of the department, with the appointment of geographical full-time physicians. This was accelerated when the MGH Nursing School closed in 1972, and Livingston Hall became available for specialty clinics and doctors' offices. Specialty units were established for coronary care (CCU), intensive care (ICU) ,and renal dialysis. Cameron directed two outreach programs: the McGill-CIDA-Kenya Medical Development Program, 1978–88; and the McGill Baffin Zone Project, 1965–75.

In the undergraduate teaching program, there was a transition from lectures to small group teaching with an emphasis on correlating basic sciences with clinical teaching. Other features were clinical clerkships in the fourth year, and elective periods in the third and fourth years. Cameron assigned responsibility for each component of the teaching program, and Lester McCallum, Stewart Polson, Gordon Copping, Michael Dixon, and John Ruedy played major roles.

Likewise there were major changes in the residency program for internal medicine: straight internships in medicine and graduated responsibility for residents throughout the four-year program. There was a transition in the control of the program from hospital to university to government (and the CPMQ). The residents developed effective national and provincial organizations, and this led to improved remuneration and working conditions.

The Department of Medicine was active in continuing medical education with fellowships and specialty courses, and there was a marked increase in research activities during the Cameron era. The UMC moved from the twelfth floor to larger facilities on the tenth floor, and, in 1973, the MGH Research Institute opened. There were many geographic full-time (GFT) appointments to the UMC, the doctors receiving financial support from numerous sources.

The most remarkable research development in the Cameron area was Freedman and Gold's description of carcinoembryonic antigen (CEA) – an achievement for which they received many honours. Freedman, Hollenberg, and McCallum were promoted to professors of medicine.

In 1980, Cameron felt that things were going well in the Department of Medicine, and he retired from his appointments one and a half years before

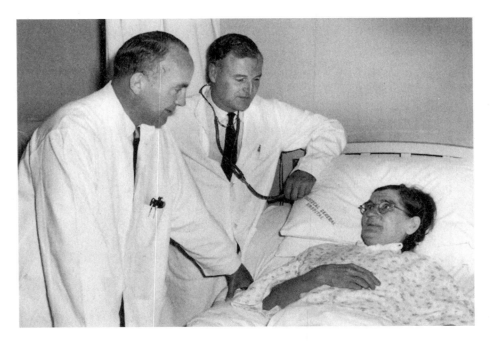

Fig. 3.1 H. Rocke Robertson, chief of surgery, and Douglas Cameron, chief of medicine, at the bedside. Photographer unknown.

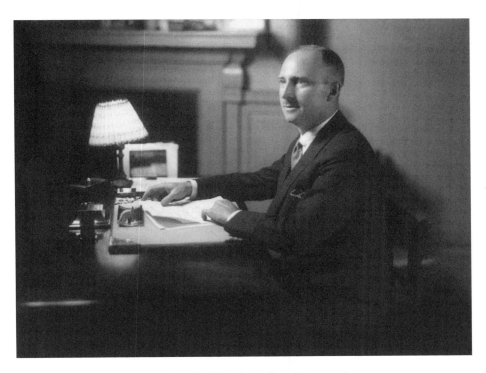

Fig. 3.2 Edward Mills, chair of medicine, 1948–57.

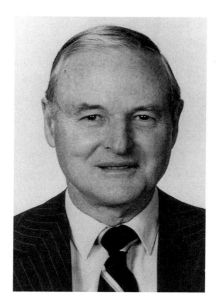

Fig. 3.3 Douglas Cameron, chair of medicine, 1957–80.

the usual retirement age. He continued his consulting and private medical practices from an office on the nineteenth floor of the hospital.

Phil Gold Era, 1980–95

Phil Gold was appointed to succeed Cameron as MGH physician-in-chief,[9] and was the first Douglas Cameron Professor of Medicine. Gold was born in Montreal on 17 September 1936. After high school he enrolled in McGill in 1952 and graduated BSc 1957 and MD, CM 1961. While in medical school, he enrolled in the Faculty of Graduate Studies and was awarded an MSc in 1961 and a PhD in 1963. He interned, underwent residency training in internal medicine at MGH, and was awarded an FRCPC in 1965. He was appointed to the MGH staff in 1965 at McGill, where he rose through the ranks to be senior physician and professor of medicine, physiology, and oncology.

He continued his research in immunology and, with Sam Freedman, isolated CEA, for which he received many honours. CEA is a blood test frequently used in the management of colon cancer.

During the Gold era, there were many changes in the clinical services at MGH – new divisions, centres, and units in the Department of Medicine. The new divisions were: internal medicine (Alex Miller and Laurence Green); clinical epidemiology (Walter Spitzer and Stephen Grover); geriatrics (McClaran and Sandra Richardson); palliative care (Ann A. Towers);

and infectious diseases and microbiology (Michael Libman). The new centres were: immune deficiency treatment; AIDS research (Chris Tsoukas); lupus erythematosis clinic (Ann Clark); and bone marrow transplant (Wytold Rybka). The new units were: medical oncology; tropical medicine clinic (McGill Ethiopia program, Dick MacLean); rheumatic disease (John Esdaile); and holter monitoring service (Michael Rosengarten).

The number of clinical teaching units (CTUs) was reduced. Some acute care wards became long-term care wards (16 E). Eleven E became a private medical care unit and was the first private unit without residents. The role of CTU directors was upgraded and they received financial support. CTUs were staffed by members of the general medicine division. Medical outpatient clinics were separated from the CTUs (Peter McLeod in charge). Gold made weekly rounds on the CTUs.

When Lester McCallum retired in 1982, Blair Whittemore was in charge of the undergraduate teaching program. Gold taught Introduction to Clinical Medicine (ICM basic and advanced). Following the 1992 Stoddart-Baier Report, the number of internal medicine residents at MGH was reduced from eighty to a total of sixty, with fifteen new appointments each year. MGH residents were withdrawn from QMVH, Reddy, and St Mary's. South American and Middle East residency programs were established. Teaching seminars and journal clubs were started for the residents, and they were encouraged to participate in research programs.

Research expanded during the Gold era, with Joe Shuster as director of the MGH Research Institute (MGHRI) and Harry Goldsmith as director of the Division of Experiment Medicine and the Bertha Levinschi Laboratories on the second floor of Livingston Hall. The MGHRI increased from eighteen thousand to 250,000 square metres. The number of basic and clinician scientists was tripled, and research funding was increased from $2.4 million in 1980 to $25 million in 1995. Under Albert Aguayo, neuroscience research was moved from the Montreal Neurological Institute to the MGH. Emil Skamene continued his research on host resistance, and Tom Hudson directed the genome centre. Outreach programs in the Baffin Arctic Zone (Nunavut, J.H. Burgess) and Africa (Brian Ward, Erwin Shurar, and J. Dick MacLean) continued. In 1995, with the formation of MUHC (not until 1997), Gold retired as MGH physician-in chief and became director of the McGill Oncology Centre. He continued as professor of medicine and oncology.

NOTES

1 J. Hanaway and R. Cruess, *McGill Medicine: The First Half Century, 1828–1885* (Montreal and Kingston: McGill-Queen's University Press, 1996), 171–2.

2 Frederick Gault Finley, MB, MD, CM (1861–1940).

3 Henri Amedee Lafleur, MD, CM, FRCPC, LLD (McGill and Queen's), (1862–1939).

4 Campbell Palmer Howard, MD, CM, FRCPC (1877–1936).

5 Alvah Hovey Gordon, BA, MD, CM, FRCPC, LLD (McGill and McMaster), DCO (Acadia), (1876–1953).

6 Lorne Cuthbert Montgomery, OBE, MC, VD, Legion of Merit, FRCP London, FRCPC, FRSM (Hon), (1894–1985).

7 Edward Sadler Mills, BSe, MD, CM, MSc, FRCPC, FACP (1897–1970).

8 Douglas George Cameron, OC, MC, BSe, BSe (Oxon), MD, CM, FRCPSC, MRCP (London), FRCP (London), MACP, FRACP, FRCP (Glasgow), (1917–89).

9 Phil Gold, CC, OQ, BSc, MSc, MD, CM, PhD, FRS (C), FRCPC, MACP, (1936–).

Department of Medicine, 1980–95

Phil Gold

Phil Gold succeeded Doug Cameron as physician-in-chief of the MGH and chair of
the Department of Medicine at McGill. He provides personal perspective on the years
leading up to the formation of the McGill University Health Centre.

Introduction

In the fall of 1980, very shortly after I had been asked to take the post of
physician-in-chief at the Montreal General Hospital, I received a call from
Harvey Barkun, the director general (CEO) of the hospital at that time. He
wanted to have a short talk, and I said that I would walk down the hall and
meet with him at his office. I had known Harvey for many years, we had become good friends, and he had been on the Search Committee that had
selected me for the position of physician-in-chief. After our usual exchange
of a few stories, in both directions, he said quite candidly, "I know what
you're like, and that you're going to go out and begin to hire people for every
kind of position. I just wanted to let you know that you should take it easy
because we have no space and no money." After a short discussion as to why
he hadn't mentioned this during the Search Committee process, I went back
to the business of the day. Some fifteen years later, after the Department of
Medicine had added well over two hundred people – as clinician-teachers,
clinician-scientists, and fundamental scientists – I stopped by Harvey's office to say, "*Now* we have no space and no money." It is the interval between
these two conversations that I try to summarize in the material that follows.

Nineteen-eighty was a milestone year for the Department of Medicine
at the MGH. After some twenty-two years of devoted service, Douglas G.
Cameron resigned the post of physician-in-chief at the hospital. It is worthy
of note that the original MGH had been the site at which McGill University

had begun in 1821, and so the hospital carried a great deal of historic moment. During Cameron's tenure, the Department of Medicine had evolved
from providing fine patient care and student teaching to being an outstanding academic medical department. The development of MGH's McGill
University Medical Clinic – initially under the directorship of Arnold S.V.
Burgen (now Sir Arnold), then Francis Chinard, and then Carl A. Goresky
– was a major step forward. The "Clinic" evolved into the Montreal General
Hospital Research Institute and provided the third leg of the academic tripod of patient care, teaching, and research. Thus, I was greatly honoured to
have been asked to take the post left vacant by Cameron, one of my former
teachers, and even more so to have been named the Douglas G. Cameron
Professor of Medicine.

Forward Planning of the Department of Medicine

After twenty-two years of a single stewardship, the Department of Medicine
required a bit of rethinking going forward. Between September and December of 1980, a parallel process of planning for the future of the Department of Medicine was undertaken. I asked Carl Goresky to chair a planning
committee for the department, with the other members being Joseph Shuster, Albert Aguayo, and Harry Goldsmith. I undertook a comparable task for
myself, and the final report of the department, and the roadmap we would
follow, was a blend of the recommendations that were forthcoming.

    This was the first such internal review that had been attempted by the
Department of Medicine for as long as anyone could remember. The mandates for both myself and the committee were to examine both the strengths
and weaknesses of the department and to project the needs in terms of
human resources, space requirements, and other necessities over both the
short-term (approximately two years) and the long-term (five to ten years)
in order to make our department one of the finest of its kind in the world.
Both the committee and I expended a great deal of time and energy reviewing the reports that had been requested from each division, interviewing
each of the divisional directors, and, finally, synthesizing the material into
unifying concepts that would serve as a blueprint for our department as we
entered the 1980s.

    The final report began with the words of Robert Petersdorf, who discussed
the evolution of departments of medicine as follows:

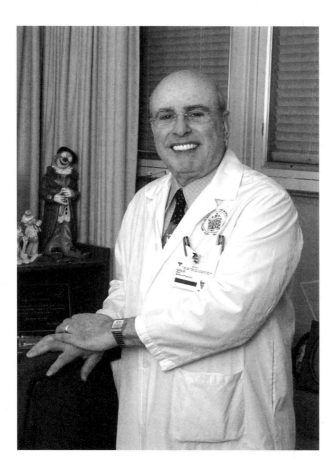

Fig. 3.4 Phil Gold, Chair of Medicine, 1980–95

Departments of Medicine are commonly described as the linchpins of medical schools. They are the largest departments in the medical schools and they are often the largest in the University. They have the primary responsibility for the education of medical students, they retain the largest house-staff, they train the greatest number of research and clinical fellows, and in most institutions they do the most research. Most have major service responsibilities. Perhaps because of their size they are also the most vulnerable to such external perturbations as changes in the level of external funding … and on certain levels of state appropriations. Moreover, because of their diverse functions, they are more vigorously buffeted by change than any other clinical departments.

In the fifteen years that followed, Peterdorf's words would prove prophetic as the department burgeoned in terms of staff members and the inextricable interactions of patient care, teaching, and research.

It is perhaps worth noting at this point, that, in 1980, the research activity of the hospital took place within a space of some sixty-six hundred square metres, with a budget of just under $2 million. I would learn sometime later that there was a good deal of anxiety among some of the staff of the department (and perhaps appropriately so) that, because of my background, my major thrust for the time of my tenure would be to *grow the research activity of the department*, perhaps to the detriment of the critical issues of patient care and teaching. After a time, I think it became quite clear that my philosophy was: if we could not appropriately care for patients, we had no right to teach; and if we could not teach well, we had no right to conduct research. Hence, research would only occur if the first two legs of the tripod were firm. That said, the major recommendations of the melded documents were fairly straightforward and are outlined below.

All new members of staff were to be of the highest academic calibre and were to have major commitments to patient care, and/or teaching, and/or research (one would hope for a combination of all three). It is interesting that, at the time that the report was written, there were some thirty-three principle investigators within the University Medical Clinic, twenty-seven of whom held MD degrees, or MD/PhD degrees, and only six of whom were PhD scientists. As MGH's research effort grew over time and kept pace with clinical care and teaching, this ratio would equalize and then begin to reverse. Hence, there was a major concern even at the time of the report that the clinician-scientist was, indeed, an endangered species, and that every effort had to be made to maintain programs that would involve clinicians in research.

The problem of personnel support was addressed in terms of income from both the university and the hospital, in addition to that generated by patient care. It was also felt that the more senior physicians in the department could contribute a substantial amount of money towards the base salaries of younger colleagues who were to be recruited. This concept would go through a number of iterations that would soften the blow vis-à-vis the more senior members of the staff.

There was a major concern regarding the amount of space available for recruiting new principle investigators into research, and it was projected that some twenty-four square metres of research space would be required.

Indeed, twice that much space would finally be built, but time was required to make it available and to have it properly equipped.

Excellence would have to be ascertained through peer review, be it in patient care, teaching, or research. It was strongly suggested that the concerns expressed in the report be taken to the MGH's Board of Directors. Indeed, this led to the development of the board's Strategic Planning Process. It was recommended that all divisions, and their directors, be reviewed every five years to determine if objectives had been met and, if not, what was to be done about this. Again, such reviews had not been carried out for a very long time and probably caused some degree of anxiety among some members of the staff. However, by 1984, all of the divisions had been reviewed, without major trauma.

It was obviously necessary to reallocate space within the confines of the hospital, particularly with regard to that already belonging to the Department of Medicine, in such a manner as to bring members of any one division into the closest possible proximity to one another. It was strongly recommended that the directors of the clinical teaching units of the medical wards be sited on those units in order to encourage more interactions with other professional groups – most particularly nurses and other consulting specialists – as well as patients, students, and residents. New forms were devised in order to improve the communication between doctors and nurses, and the hospital-based physician and his/her counterpart in the community. Still in the context of CTU activities, it was recommended that a rheumatic disease unit (RDU) consisting of four beds should be designated specifically for the treatment and evaluation of patients with a variety of rheumatic diseases. A similar recommendation was made for acute oncology beds. For various reasons noted below, these initiatives were instituted but then had to be abandoned.

It was anticipated that several new divisions/services would have to be established within the department and, indeed, planning for this began immediately. These units included:

1 *A Division of General Internal Medicine.* It was initially envisioned that this division would serve as an interface between the Department of Medicine and other departments of the hospital. As it turned out, however, that role would change over time, and this division would play an increasingly important part in the activities of the Department's CTUs.
2 *A Division of Geriatric Medicine.* This division was needed because of the aging of our population.

3 *A Division of Clinical Epidemiology.* This division was needed to conduct studies, or to assist in the establishment of studies, that focused on problems directly or immediately relevant to decision making on the part of clinicians in their medical practices. In addition, bio-epidemiologists would be critically important to many of the research groups in the hospital because of the ever-expanding databases that had to be analyzed in the work already under way and in that to come.

4 *A Palliative Care Service.* The establishment of this service was crucial to a population that was being underserved in every fashion, and for which adequate resources were, and are, unavailable in the community.

The report of the department concluded that this plan, if successful, would create within the MGH a tightly linked academic medical nucleus for patient care, teaching, and research rivalled by few other institutions. The concern was clearly expressed that if we did not meet the challenges facing our community by engaging in a frontal attack, then our institution would not progress our personnel base would not be renewed, and we would suffer a progressive loss of space. Indeed, if we continued along the path we were presently on, we would lose our place among the very best institutions. The objective, then, was to create an optimistic and forward-looking environment – one in which first-rate achievement on a continuous basis would, again, become commonplace.

Remarkably, this would occur.

As is the case with any recommendations, so it was with these: means, needs, and objectives changed over time. Many of the recommendations went on to grow and flourish, while others quietly atrophied, diminished, or changed direction when it was felt that they were no longer required as initially planned.

A number of the recommendations contained in the melded reports, and that required only intradepartmental approval, were implemented immediately. These included reallocation of space within the confines of the hospital to bring together members of any given division. Establishment of divisional objectives over the next five years were requested from each of the divisional directors and, indeed, the *five-year reviews* were actually completed by 1984. The reviews covered both the activities of the division and the divisional leadership. CTU directors were sited on their units, and six active and acute care CTUs were in place at the time (11 East, 16 East, 16 West, 10 East,

10 West, and 17 East). Stipends for the CTU directors were arranged. Again, with the changing needs within the system, the activities of the CTUs altered over time (see below).

An immediate effort was made to initiate the new divisions/services within the Department of Medicine. These included the following:

1 The Division of Clinical Epidemiology, which had begun as the Kellogg Centre under the direction of Walter O. Spitzer, was given full divisional status. Spitzer would subsequently be followed by Steven Grover, and the division flourished.

2 The Division of General Internal Medicine was established under the direction of Alexander Miller, and recruitment began from the superb chief medical residents that had come through (and would continue to come through) the department. The division's responsibilities virtually exploded as it took on responsibility for the functioning of the CTUs, for a good deal of both resident and student teaching, and for direct patient care on the wards. Members of this division, of course, continued to have their own clinics where new patients were seen. Moreover, such units as the Hypertension Clinic were spinoffs of the Division of General Internal Medicine. Miller's leadership was assumed by the then second divisional director, Laurence Green, who had, to my delight, been the first chief resident that had been appointed to the department at the time that I had taken on the post of physician-in-chief.

3 A medical oncology unit was established under the direction of Michael Thirlwell. An attempt was subsequently made to establish a department of oncology in the MGH and then in the hospitals of the McGill University system. A good deal of funding had come through the Fast Family Foundation, through the intersession of Carl Goresky and John Hinchey. This made possible a salary for the director of the unit and for the recruitment of young oncologists. Hence, Thirlwell was appointed as the first oncologist-in-chief at the MGH. Unfortunately, at that time, agreement could not be reached with the other hospitals of the system for the establishment of a department of oncology within the Faculty of Medicine. However, such a department was subsequently established at the university and at the hospital level. This awaited the development of the McGill University Hospital Centre (MUHC), but the Medical Oncology Unit, under Thirlwell's supervision, continued to function in a remark-

able fashion in those "early days," in concert with the Department of Radiation Oncology under the direction of Carolyn Freeman.

4 A need to consider medical ethics with regard to all the activities of the Department of Medicine became an obvious requirement. The route to this was made easier by the fact that Michael Kaye, director of the Division of Nephrology, had been ordained as a minister of the Baptist Church. Kaye worked with Joseph Lella, associate professor, medical sociology, Department of Humanities and Social Studies in Medicine at McGill University. The program began with two sessions during Medical Grand Rounds that were devoted to medical ethics. Subsequently, these rounds were initiated on a regular basis on 16 East, as a pilot program, for one hour a week. The concept was ultimately extended to all CTUs, and this became the forerunner of the Research Ethics Office at the MGH and, subsequently, the MUHC.

5 In 1981, the Department of Medicine opened the Extended Care Unit on 16 West under the direction of Lester McCallum. This unit would take on responsibility for the bulk of the long-stay patients who no longer required acute intervention from other CTUs of the Department of Medicine, allowing for better deployment of attending and resident staff in terms of patient care and education. This certainly provided a better level of care for the long-stay patients as well. Unfortunately, the problem of providing extended care would burgeon due to a persistent lack of chronic care facilities within the community, even though, over the years, these had been repeatedly promised by the Government of Quebec. This problem continues, and grows, to this day.

6 A university-based program in tropical medicine was established under the direction of the late J.D. MacLean and was based at the MGH. Members of the division would include physicians from a variety of disciplines from within the hospital, including infectious diseases, general internal medicine, and others interested in tropical diseases. In addition, close liaison was maintained with the Institute of Parasitology at MacDonald College. Under the same umbrella, a variety of activities were undertaken, including a McGill-Addis Ababa project, the provision of a service for the examination of immigrants from tropical countries, as well as the increased number of individuals traveling to the tropics and then returning to Montreal. It is certainly interesting that the service component of this unit had at its disposal the superb research capabilities that that been

built into the Centre for Host Resistance by Emil Skamene and his colleagues. They were examining the genetic control of host resistance at the research level, and this enormous undertaking will be further considered in a report from the Research Institute.

7 Services to the North have been provided by the MGH for a very long time. Suzanne Dubé has, for over twenty years, been providing an invaluable service in internal medicine to Val D'or and Rouyn Norandin. Her weekly visits to this area, which she has undertaken in a completely selfless manner, is valued by the residents for both her superb medicine and her warm care. Certainly the longest provision of care to northern Canada to be provided by any member of the MGH staff, and perhaps by any other centre in North America, has been provided by John Burgess. Burgess, a senior cardiologist at the hospital and professor of medicine at McGill University has provided a service in cardiology to Canada's Inuit community for over thirty years. This is a singular phenomenon, and it is often cited as an example for the younger physicians and students as they come through their training. Burgess has recently published his memoires, entitled *Doctor to the North: Thirty Years of Treating Heart Disease among the Inuit* (McGill-Queen's University Press, 2008). The book has been a virtual bestseller across the country, of interest not only to physicians but also to the lay public. Appropriately enough, an excerpt from Burgess's book may be found in the cardiology chapter of this book.

8 The Bone Marrow Transplantation Tissue Unit was established under the direction of Wiltold Rybka of the Division of Haematology. In doing so, Rybka ensured that the MGH was in a leadership position in the area of bone marrow transplantation in Montreal. When he took an important position in bone marrow transplantation in the United States, this activity shifted to the Royal Victoria Hospital.

9 Michael Rosengarten, both an engineer and a cardiologist, developed the superb Holter Monitoring Unit within the electrophysiological arm of the Division of Cardiology. Holter monitoring went on to utilize telecommunications (the evolution of electrophysiological activities is considered further in chapter 5).

10 The Geriatric Medicine Unit was established with the recruitment of a number of individuals trained specifically in this specialty. Indeed, under the directorship of Sandra Richarson, the 13 East unit became the Geriatric Medicine Program.

11 The need for beds for palliative care, mentioned above, became critical. This unit was established on 10 East under the directorship of Anna Towers and has now been expanded to the McGill Centre for Palliative Care.

12 The Immunodeficiency Treatment Centre was established within the Division of Clinical Immunology and Allergy by Chris Tsoukas. The centre initially dealt almost exclusively with HIV/AIDS patients but has since expanded its horizons to deal with primary immune deficiency problems as well. From the outset, both clinical and research arms were built into the functions of the centre.

13 There had been concern expressed about the calibre of grand medical rounds. For this reason, at least half of the rounds would subsequently be given by speakers invited from outside of the institution by the various specialties divisions, and these would include Nobel laureates.

The 3 Percent Solution

Quite obviously, the hiring of personnel and the expansion of MGH's Department of Medicine required support for infrastructure and salaries. I suppose it is always the perception of one taking on a leadership position that one's predecessor has stored away a significant amount of money to look after such contingencies. However, like Old Mother Hubbard, when I did go to the cupboard I found, as she had, that it was bare. Doug Cameron had maintained the Department of Medicine in good fashion with very little money in-hand. The budget from the university Faculty of Medicine covered those funds already committed to staff salaries, some secretarial support, and little else. There would, therefore, be no way to undertake recruitment and to fuel the aims that that had been established without seeking other sources of funding. The possibility that senior staff could provide "overage" for the support of younger members was, in many ways, a pipe dream. Hence, very early in my tenure, at a monthly departmental meeting, I brought the "3 percent solution" to the table. This involved the "taxation" of all clinical income, from all members of the department, by taking 3 percent off the top of all such earnings. This solution was met with overwhelming silence, but without apparent revolution. A finance committee elected by the membership of the department was put in place. All funds of the 3 percent tariff was handled by the committee and my use of these funds for departmental issues had to be approved by them at all times.

With this process in place, a light appeared at the end of the tunnel. Using the generosity of the staff as a medium, I was able to entice the MGH Foundation of the hospital to match a good part of these funds. Then, the Faculty of Medicine, under the extraordinary deanship of Richard Cruess, became critically important in the development of the department.

The process worked as follows: clinician-teachers, clinician-scientists, and basic investigators were brought on to the staff and funded by the income from the 3 percent solution, matched by funding from the MGH Foundation. Those recruited to tenure track at that time had three years of this kind of funding to successfully apply for independent support from a provincial, national or international organization, which would then provide the major source of their income. If they failed to do this within three years, they were aware that we would be unable to continue their support.

Under special circumstances an additional year of funding was provided, either to allow for one more attempt at external support or to provide some time for the individual in question to find another post. However, because of the care with which these young people were selected, well over 80 percent were able to find independent support as Medical Research Council (MRC) of Canada scholars and associates, Chercheurs Boursiers, Chercheurs Bourchier Cliniciens, and so on. They then went on for two or three more years, on tenure track, and then went forward for tenure at the associate professor level. At this point, then, and with the perennial support of Dean Richard Cruess, those at the associate professor level, with tenure, were moved onto the university payroll, and the funds that had been used for their support could then be recycled to younger colleagues coming on staff. Some fifteen new staff per year could be supported in this fashion, and many of the over two hundred to two hundred and fifty new staff personnel who joined us have remained at the MGH MUHC and have gone on to do exceptional, ground-breaking, and leadership work in research, teaching, and clinical care. Still others have been recruited to very important posts in other universities in Canada, the United States, and abroad.

I must underscore here the enormous generosity and support from different organizations both inside and outside of the hospital. Indeed, to this day, the named fellowships that are provided to the staff of the McGill University Health Centre carry the names of those philanthropic individuals, families, and organizations. Among these, during the fifteen years of my tenure, were the following:

- The Montreal General Hospital MGH Auxiliary
- The Fast Family Foundation
- The R.H. Webster Family Foundation
- The Levinichi Foundation
- The Edith and Richard Strauss Foundation
- The Markin Foundation
- The Rita and Morely Cohen Foundation

Moreover, I would be remiss not to mention particular individuals whose hard work in raising funds within the philanthropic community of the city must be recognized. These include: Rochelle Malus, who was critical in the establishment of the Inflammatory Bowel Disease Centre, and a chair in Gastroenterology. Morely Cohen, who spearheaded the Montreal General Hospital Campaign, in which he raised $3 million that would be used for a critical addition to the Research Institute on the top floor of Livingston Hall; and Sheila and Marvin Kussner, who, as always, were available to support fundraising within the McGill sphere.

"This Is No Job for One Person"

At the outset of taking on the post of physician-in-chief, it became quite obvious to me that, if there was to be any time available to actually think through the future of the Department of Medicine and to implement change, I would require a great deal of help from colleagues. The three main areas that would obviously need constant and careful care were the three inextricably linked legs of the medical academic tripod. Hence, I called upon three old friends and colleagues who took on enormous responsibilities within the department. These were:

1 Blair Whittemore, who took on the day-to-day running of the CTUs and the overall supervision of the patient care activities in the Department of Medicine. With Blair's movement to the Red Cross as the director and his subsequent return to the position of director of professional services at the MGH, his responsibilities passed on to Tim Meagher, who would later become a most critical player in the development of the McGill University Health Centre.
2 Peter McLeod, took on the responsibilities for the teaching program, both at the undergraduate and residency levels, and did an outstanding job in

this regard. Peter went on to a sabbatical in medical education at the University of Dundee, Scotland, to hone his educational skills, after which he returned to the MGH. He has subsequently gone on to the Department of Medical Education at McGill University, where he now spends the better part of his time doing outstanding work.

3 Joseph Shuster, who had already taken on the directorships of both the Division of Clinical Immunology and Allergy and the Division of Clinical Chemistry, agreed to take on the enormous responsibility for directing the Research Institute.

Had it not been for the priceless support of the individuals named, I think it is fair to say that the progress seen in the Department of Medicine during the period under consideration could never have occurred.

Research Activities in the Department of Medicine

Although the research accomplishments in the Department of Medicine are detailed in the material on the Research Institute (chapter 37), the following provides a brief overview.

In the beginning of the period under consideration (1980–81) the total research budget of the Department of Medicine, including grants in aid of research, grants for equipment, fellowships, scholarships, and associateships, totalled slightly over $2 million. At the end of the period under consideration (1994–95), the support had risen to well over $15 million per year. The space occupied by the research activities of the department in 1980–81 was largely that of the University Medical Clinic on the tenth floor of the hospital, which consisted of some nine thousand square metres, along with the Research Institute, which had been built just adjacent to the hospital. By 1995, space had increased in keeping with both the expansion of the research budget and the hiring of research staff, and the department occupied approximately forty-five thousand square metres. As already noted, a good deal of this space was obtained when new floors were built on top of Livingston Hall, providing an additional twelve thousand square metres of research space. Again, the funds raised by Morely Cohen, as well as the generosity of the Montreal General Hospital Foundation, enabled this to occur.

In addition, there was a major conversion, having to do with a variety of areas being transformed into laboratories because of alterations in activities in the hospital. These laboratories were built through the generosity of organizations already named, including the Bertha and Gustav Levinichi Foundation, the Edith and Richard Strauss Foundation, and the Rita and Morely Cohen Foundation. As one member of the department pointed out, "if there was an empty cupboard found, it became a laboratory."

Every division of the department made major contributions to research discoveries. As examples, the Division of Neurology under the directorship of Albert Aguayo, and with the able support of Garth Bray, Michael Rasminsky, and Samuel David, made ground-breaking discoveries in their work dealing with the regeneration of central nervous system tissue. This was, indeed, the beginning of the concept of neural cell plasticity and would earn great laurels for members of the group.

With movement of tumour immunology research to the McGill Cancer Centre, the Division of Clinical Immunology and Allergy refocused attention to the Centre for the Study of Host Resistance, under the direction of Emil Skamene. These studies were extended to the Department of Biochemistry at the McIntyre Sciences Building (Philippe Gros) and were a major stimulus to the ultimate construction of the McGill Genome Centre (Tom Hudson).

A program of National Networks of Centres of Excellence was established by the federal government, and in very short order, the department was successful in obtaining recognition and funding for four such centres:

1 Neurosciences: directed by Albert Aguayo
2 Respirology: involving Pierre Ernst, David Eidelman, Stewart Gottfried, and Arnold Zidulka
3 Genetics: involving Emil Skamene and David Rosenblatt
4 Bacterial Diseases: involving Daniel Mallaux

Still other members formed MRC and FRSQ research groups.

Those involved in the research activities of the Department of Medicine received numerous forms of recognition – locally, provincially, nationally, and internationally. Many members were the recipients of such prizes as the Killam Award, the Gairdner Foundation International Award, and appointments to l'Ordre national du Québec, and the Order of Canada, among others.

As already pointed out, there were numerous members appointed to the research staff who were initially funded by "in-house funds" and who then went on to get support from national and international organizations. Space that had become available was soon occupied and, of course, accounted for the increase in research funding. Many of these investigators would then form groups, and this led to an exponential increase in the funding of the department in their particular research area Nevertheless, one must take strength where it is found.

In terms of citations in the biomedical literature, our scientists continued to be among the most widely cited in the world. This, once again, attested, in an objective fashion, to the national and international regard in which the work of our scientists continues to be held.

The McGill University Health Centre

Beginning in 1992, the idea of the construction of a single centre that would house the Faculty of Medicine, all the hospitals of the McGill University system (the Montreal General Hospital, the Royal Victoria Hospital, the Montreal Children's Hospital, the Montreal Neurological Hospital and Institute, and the Montreal Chest Hospital Centre), and the research space that would be required to support the activities of both the Faculty of Medicine and the hospitals centres involved was put on the table. The effort was supported by Principal David Johnston, Dean Richard Cruess, and the boards of the various hospitals. Discussions were held regularly and frequently. This led finally, on 29 March 1994, to the *miracle of the annunciation*. By that time, the possibility the moving the Faculty of Medicine, the hospitals, and the various research institutes had been dropped as a possibility. The main focus of the Faculty of Medicine would remain at the McIntyre Medical Sciences Centre (although the dean's office would subsequently move to another building on the corner of Mountain Street and Penfield Street), while all of the hospitals would move to another site to comprise the McGill Mega-Hospital Centre (now the Glen Site). With this evolution, the MGH would remain open and active, as would the Montreal Neurological Institute and Hospital. It would then be the Royal Victoria Hospital, the Montreal Children's Hospital, and the Montreal Chest Hospital Centre that would be closed and move to the Glen site, along with the conjoint research institutes of the various hospitals. All MUHC faculty might well have activities at any or all of the MGH, the MNH/MNI, and the Glen site.

All that having been said, the "annunciation" on this occasion did not take place in a grotto in Nazareth but, rather, in a well appointed room in the Queen Elizabeth Hotel. Boyd Whittal, chair of the Montreal General

Hospital Board, and his counterparts from the other McGill University hospitals, signed the Resolution of Intent to go forward with the request for an Order-in-Council from the Government of Quebec to allow for the functional planning of the MUHC. However, it would not be until the spring of 2010, some eighteen years after the first meetings of the Steering Committee, that a hole would finally find its way into the ground at the new site for the MUHC.

Nevertheless, with the decision taken, it was necessary to begin to plan for the integration of the Department of Medicine across the hospitals of the university, for every division and for every service. Hence, we would all become part of the McGill University Health Centre. A task force from the MGH began to wrestle with the development of a template whereby each division could start to define its present status and future requirements for integration. The first of many Department of Medicine planning retreats took place in the autumn of 1994.

Governmental Interventions

The positive evolution in the areas of patient care, teaching, and research in the Department of Medicine transpired *despite* the governmental interventions described below. This inevitably led to the oxymoronic phrase: "How can things be so good if they are so bad?"

In the early 1980s, funding to the MGH, among the hospitals in the Montreal area, as well as to the Faculty of Medicine and McGill University as a whole, was curtailed, both relatively and absolutely. This led to a variety of changes, including nursing shortages and the subsequent closure of beds because of inadequate staffing. In addition to this problem, despite ongoing promises to the contrary, the persistent lack of chronic care facilities in the community outside of the hospital led to the increasing growth of extended care patients on the wards. In domino fashion, this led to further conversion of active, acute care, and clinical teaching beds (indeed, units) to extended care facilities; thus, fewer active beds would be available for patients gathering in the Emergency Room. The longer periods of waiting in the ER led to ever-increasing stress among both patients and staff.

Then, the government felt that, somehow, the manner in which residency training was being conducted had to be altered since the Island of Montreal had become too "flush," while the outlining areas were in need of different kinds of physicians. In order to achieve this aim, the full complement of resident and fellowship staff (which had peaked between the 1960s and the 1980s, when literally hundreds of medical internists and medical specialists were trained in the McGill system in all of the major university hospitals in Canada, the United States and abroad) was constrained – indeed, gutted.

In 1989, the first year without internships in Quebec, the departments of medicine *for all McGill hospitals* were allowed twenty-five first-year internal medicine residents. The number of subspecialty positions, at the time, was left untouched, but only the first shoe had dropped. Indeed, in that year, there had been two fellowships added to gastroenterology; one to medical oncology; two to nephrology; and two to respirology.

And then, in 1992, the second shoe dropped, with the invention of the ABC system, which, with little or no input from the medical profession, defined which subspecialties in medicine were to be the *priorities, relative priorities, or not really needed at all.* McGill was allowed a minimum number of slots for subspecialty fellows. By 2002, the smallest cohort would be admitted to the McGill Department of Medicine.

Those residents who wished to enter subspecialty training, where no slots were available, would remain as residents in internal medicine only and have no option of going on to subspecialty training. Seven (see above) slots were then allocated to residency training programs in different categories, which obviously allowed us to train far fewer specialists at the other end of the pipeline. The reason the government gave for this was that we required many more family physicians,; but, unfortunately, these were not forthcoming. Most graduates who could not enter the specialty programs in which they wished to train did not enter family medicine but, rather, left Montreal and went to other provinces in Canada or to the United States, where they could enter the program that they desired. This led to a marked shortage of both trained medical specialists and family physicians. Even those family physicians that have remained have filled their practices rapidly; frequently, they do not open offices but simply work as itinerant physicians in different emergency rooms and clinics around the city.

To continue with this draconic approach, then, the government further decided that it had to control the number of staff positions that were to be filled by specialists on the Island of Montreal and so introduced the phenomenon of *Effectifs Médicaux*. This was the beginning of government control over who would be allowed to work in hospitals on the Island of Montreal and, of course, at the MGH. Moreover, if these individuals would not agree to work in the "outlining areas" of the province, they would earn

only 70 percent of the usual tariff for their services. Again, this most unpopular approach led to further evacuation of specialists from the City
of Montreal and, indeed, from Quebec. Following the same line of logic,
the government introduced the phenomenon of PREMs (Plans régionaux
d'effectifs médicaux), which would determine the number of specialists
allowed to practise in any region of Quebec. Similarly, any doctor coming
onto the staff of the hospital would require governmental approval, or
PEMs (Plans des effectifs médicaux).

     With all of that having been said, however, we have, *remarkably*, contin-
ued to grow both in strength and in numbers. The mechanisms that allow
this growth to occur are tell a story of resilience and innovation on the part
of numerous members of the staff of the MGH's Department of Medicine
and of the entire MUHC. Indeed, it often seemed that our motto as a department should have been *Robor per Adversa* (strength through adversity).

4

Allergy and Clinical Immunology

Samuel O. Freedman

Sam Freedman initiated research as director of the Division of Allergy and Immunology before becoming dean of medicine at McGill.

The Division of Allergy and Clinical Immunology began as an allergy clinic shortly after the Second World War, when Howard (Cap) Mitchell returned to the Montreal General Hospital on Dorchester Boulevard after serving as a captain in the Canadian army overseas. Mitchell, a specialist in internal medicine, developed a major interest in allergic disorders through his friendship with Harry Bacal at a military hospital during the war years. Bacal was a paediatric allergist affiliated with the Montreal Children's Hospital. He was one of the few physicians in Montreal to have formal training in a specialty that, at the time, was not highly regarded.

Before the hospital was relocated in 1955 from Dorchester Boulevard to its present site on Cedar Avenue, the Allergy Clinic had the use of a small laboratory located in a converted washroom for the preparation of allergy extracts used in skin testing. Crowded outpatient clinics took place weekly and were staffed by Mitchell and Richard Laing. In 1957, Douglas G. Cameron was appointed physician-in-chief. One of his first priorities was to establish a divisional structure in the Department of Medicine. This decision was responsible for the creation of the Division of Allergy. Samuel Freedman joined the division in 1959, with the proviso that he had admitting privileges for allergy patients only. Previously, Mitchell had suggested to Freedman that he give serious thought to further training in allergy at the Institute of Allergy of Columbia University in New York because there was a pressing need for another allergist in the division. The director of the Institute of Allergy was

Robert A. Cooke, considered by his peers to be the leading allergist in North America. In addition, he had written the standard textbook on the subject. The method of instruction at the institute was in many ways unique to Cooke and his colleagues. Each afternoon he would sit at a large conference table adjacent to his office at Roosevelt Hospital and the residents and research fellows would come and go depending on their responsibilities elsewhere. The discussions around the table would be either clinical or research orientated, as decided by Cooke. He often brought one of his patients to the room to demonstrate his methods of diagnosis and treatment. The remainder of the session was devoted to current research projects in progress at the institute. Each participant was usually asked a question about one of the topics under discussion and was expected to give a five-minute response without prior notice. If Cooke was not satisfied with the answer, he let the speaker know in no uncertain terms. At the conclusion of each resident's training period, Cooke would present a framed and signed photograph taken of an oil painting of himself. However, this was only given to those residents who met with his approval. Because it was a painting, Cooke's eyes appeared to be looking at the viewer from any position in the room. Freedman hung the painting in every office that he occupied in order to feel that Cooke was still evaluating his diagnostic and therapeutic decisions.

In its new location, the MGH Allergy Division was provided with much better facilities, eventually occupying one-half of the seventh floor of the Cedar Avenue wing together with rheumatology. Under Cameron's leadership major changes were taking place in the Department of Medicine. At the time of his appointment, the MGH had few full-time physicians since its focus was on excellent patient care rather than on clinical or fundamental research. In order to achieve the latter objective, Cameron founded the University Medical Clinic shortly after his twenty-three-year term of office began. One of his first recruits to the university clinic and the Department of Medicine was Freedman, who replaced another young allergist who relocated because of an insufficient number of referrals. Fortunately, Freedman was able to achieve recognition in his chosen field of allergy shortly after his appointment in January 1959.

The opening ceremony for the St Lawrence Seaway took place in St Lambert on 24 June 1959 in the presence of Queen Elizabeth and President Dwight Eisenhower. The president of the St Lawrence Seaway Authority arrived in Montreal a week before he was scheduled to give a thirty-minute opening address on international television. The Queen and President Eisen-

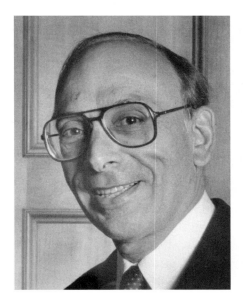 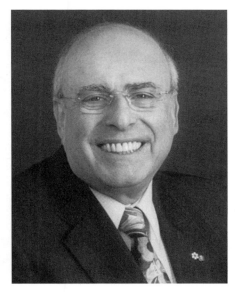

Fig. 4.1 Sam Freedman, chair, allergy and immunology, 1960–75
Fig. 4.2 Phil Gold

hower participated in a more ceremonial capacity. Lorne Montgomery, a senior member of the Department of Medicine at the MGH, held the honorary position of the Queen's Physician in Canada. Unfortunately, the seaway president, who had suffered from moderate asthma for many years, developed severe symptoms three days before the opening. On the advice of no less a personage than Her Majesty, he consulted Montgomery about having treatment that would enable him to speak to millions of listeners. Montgomery admitted him to hospital and asked Freedman to assume responsibility for his treatment, with the admonition that the patient had to be able to speak to a worldwide television audience within forty-eight hours. Freedman spent most of those forty-eight hours at the patient's bedside, and the result was positive. The speech was made, and Freedman's reputation as an allergy consultant was firmly established after six months in practice.

After obtaining a Medical Research Council grant to support his own research, Freedman began to recruit additional clinician-scientists for the renamed Division of Allergy and Clinical Immunology. In 1968, he was fortunate enough to be able to attract three outstanding young recruits in the same year: Phil Gold, Joseph Shuster, and David Hawkins. Gold and

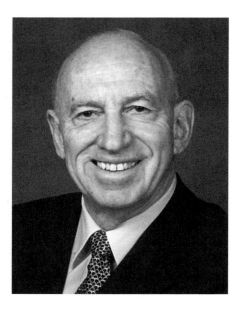

Fig. 4.3 Joe Shuster

Hawkins had been first in their medical school classes at McGill and Dalhousie universities, and Shuster had the second highest marks at the University of Alberta. Of interest is the fact that Joe Martin, who was a neurologist at the MGH for several years and, later, became dean of medicine at Harvard, was first in Shuster's medical school class. Predictably, Freedman had considerable difficulty with both the hospital and the university regarding the budgetary aspects of hiring of three new staff members for one small division in a single year. After much discussion, it was finally agreed that all three would be allowed to submit applications to the Medical Research Council for salary support. To everyone's surprise, except Freedman's, the awards were granted and the financial problems were solved. One of the first contributions of this group of four colleagues was the joint writing and editing of a textbook entitled *Clinical Immunology*.[1] The first edition appeared in 1971 and the second in 1976. It was a great success in the 1970s and was regarded as the best textbook on the subject, especially for physicians preparing for certification in clinical immunology. The publisher of the second edition deemed it a bestseller in its category, and it was translated into Spanish and Italian.

During the same period there was a large increase in the number of productive physician-scientists, which led to an inevitable competition for laboratory space (already in short supply) on the tenth floor of the hospital. A joint planning committee consisting of members of the medical staff and the

Board of Directors was established to find a solution to the space problem. The outcome of their deliberations was the establishment of the Montreal General Hospital Research Institute, with Freedman and the Honourable Mr Justice G. Miller Hyde playing key roles in its founding. The building for the Research Institute was completed in 1973, at a cost of approximately $2 million, at a location on Pine Avenue adjacent to Livingston Hall.[2] It was subsequently extended, with two additional floors built above Livingston Hall. Cameron was somewhat less than enthusiastic about this decision, but the prevailing opinion was that departments other than medicine were also engaged in excellent research projects. The relationship between the Research Institute and the University Medical Clinic remained unclear for several years afterwards.

Phil Gold graduated in medicine at McGill University in 1961. Freedman had been Gold's PhD supervisor in McGill's Department of Physiology during his residency in internal medicine. Although there was no formal MD-PHD program at the time, an ad hoc procedure was arranged with the university, making Gold one of the first at McGill to obtain the joint degree. Following the common practice at the time, Gold was arbitrarily assigned an investigator in the field of haematology at the University Medical Clinic as his PhD supervisor, but he preferred to have Freedman as his mentor. The problem was eventually solved by his trading supervisors with another resident. The collaboration between Freedman and Gold exceeded all expectations with their joint discovery of the carcinoembryonic antigen (CEA).[3] CEA is a glycoprotein with a molecular weight of approximately two hundred thousand detected by techniques such as immunoprecpitation in gel media from entodermally derived human cancers, and in the embryonic and foetal gut, pancreas, and liver in the first two trimesters of gestation. Since 1969, a number of sensitive and reproducible radioimmunoassays for CEA have been developed that are capable of detecting nanograms of CEA in the serum or plasma of patients with a variety of malignant tumours. Important areas for the clinical application of the CEA test are the postoperative prognosis and management of colon cancer with "second-look surgery" or chemotherapy. It is now generally agreed that elevated levels of CEA should not be used as a screening test for cancer.

The publication of their results in the *Journal of Experimental Medicine* in 1965 attracted worldwide attention, and the paper was listed as one the top five journal articles in the Medical Citation Index for the next several years. Gold subsequently became director of the Division of Allergy and Clinical

Immunology in 1977, when Freedman was appointed dean of the Faculty of Medicine. In 1980, Gold was chosen as physician-in-chief at the MGH by a selection committee chaired by Dean Freedman. Thus, the professional lives of these two physician-scientists, who had somewhat different personalities, intersected in many endeavours to the great benefit of medical science, the MGH, and McGill University.

After completing his training in internal medicine at the MGH, David Hawkins spent three years as a research fellow at the Scripps Research Institute in La Jolla, California, under the supervision of C.G. Cochrane, investigating immunological factors related to human disease. He joined the Division of Allergy and Clinical Immunology, which, at that time, included rheumatology. After the recruitment of additional staff members, including John Edsdaile, a separate Division of Rheumatology was created in 1971. Hawkins was appointed as the first director of rheumatology. The principal treatment and research interests of that division concerned the immunologic mechanisms involved in the pathogenesis of rheumatoid arthritis and related diseases.[4] Over the years, many important articles on this topic were published in widely read journals. Hawkins was born in St John's, Newfoundland, and received his MD degree from Memorial University. In 1987, he returned to his native province as dean of the Faculty Medicine at the Memorial University of Newfoundland, where he provided outstanding leadership in medical education and research.

Joseph (Joe) Shuster obtained a PhD in biochemistry from the University of California at San Francisco after completion of his medical studies. He then returned to the MGH with his young family following a hazardous automobile trip that took him through Vancouver and along the Trans-Canada Highway in midwinter. Unfortunately, the family was stranded in western Ontario during a record-breaking snowfall, and there was no obvious way of digging out the car. It was left in the snow to be retrieved at a later date, and the remainder of the journey was undertaken by a flight from Thunder Bay.

Following his return, Shuster became the founding director of the Clinical Immunology Laboratory that replaced the former Allergy Laboratory, and he has remained in that position throughout his professional career. There was a close working relationship between his laboratory and the Division of Medical Biochemistry. From 1986 onwards, he was director of both divisions. Shuster had several research interests in the immunological aspects of tumour antigens, blood disorders,[5] and viral disease. He published extensively and served as scientific director of the Montreal General Research Institute from 1981 to 1999. Despite time-consuming administrative duties, he continued to function as a much sought after consultant in allergy and immunology.

David Thomson received his medical degree cum laude at the University of Western Ontario, and this was followed by a postgraduate position as a resident in internal medicine and allergy at the MGH. He then undertook further training in cancer immunology with Professor Peter Alexander at the Chester Beatty Research Institute in London, England, and was granted a PhD in 1973. His interest in cancer immunology began as the result of attendance at weekly divisional seminars while he was a resident in allergy and immunology. On his return to Montreal, he became a physician-scientist who continued his cancer research projects with numerous grants and awards throughout his career.[6] Colleagues and patients alike regarded him as a highly competent allergist. In addition, he had many other clinical interests, including: chronic fatigue syndrome, environmental allergy syndrome, and sick building syndrome. He was considered an expert on these topics and frequently acted as a consultant to referring physicians or organizations who had an interest in illnesses with vague symptoms and causation. His many contributions to the division were much appreciated by all concerned.

Emil Skamene first attracted the attention of Freedman when the medical director of the MGH asked his opinion of an application received for a residency position in the Department of Medicine. On reviewing the documentation, Freedman quickly realized that, after obtaining his MD degree at Charles University in Prague, the applicant had been a PhD student of Professor Milan Hasek. Professor Hasek had been a strong candidate for a Nobel Prize in 1960 due to his discovery of immunological tolerance. The original objective of the CEA project was to determine the relevance of immunological tolerance to the development of cancer cells in humans. At the time of his application, Skamene was a postdoctoral fellow in Boston but was unable to return to Czechoslovakia because of the Soviet invasion of 1968. He completed his clinical training at the MGH in internal medicine and allergy and immunology in 1973. He then quickly established a world class laboratory in immunogenetics.[7] The McGill Centre for Host Resistance, which he founded with several outstanding colleagues, was an instant success, producing 205 papers in frequently cited journals published from 1976 to 1996. In addition to his clinical practice and extensive research activities, he more recently served as director of research for the McGill University

Health Centre. He was also very much in demand as an invited speaker at major scientific meetings throughout the world.

Abraham (Abe) Fuks's first contact with the Division of Allergy and Clinical Immunology was in the capacity of a summer student in the laboratory of Freedman and Gold, who were involved with a project related to human tumour antigens. He graduated from the Faculty of Medicine at McGill in 1970 and followed this with residency training in internal medicine and allergy and clinical immunology at the Royal Victoria Hospital and the MGH. Fuks then spent two years with Gold as a research fellow, followed by an additional three years in the laboratory of Jack Strominger at Harvard University working on a project involving the study of histocompatibility antigens. He returned to McGill and the MGH in 1978 as an assistant professor of medicine. In addition to his clinical appointment in the Division of Allergy and Clinical Immunology, Fuks served as acting director of the McGill Cancer Centre, located in the McIntyre Medical Building, from 1984 to 1987. His principal research interests were related to several aspects of the carcinoembryonic antigen and the ethics of clinical research.[8] Fuks was appointed dean of the Faculty of Medicine at McGill and served in this position from 1995 to 2006.

Deborah Danoff received her medical degree in 1973 from McGill University followed by residency training in internal medicine and allergy and clinical immunology at the RVH and MGH. She joined the division in 1978 and was a caring and compassionate physician who was much admired by both her patients and her colleagues. Her special clinical interest was in the autoimmune diseases such as lupus erythematosus and Wegener's granulomatosis.[9] In addition, she played a major role in the modernization of medical education. Danoff was appointed associate dean for Medical Education and Student Affairs at McGill from 1989 to 1997, with a special interest in the assessment of clinical competence and provision of humanistic heath care. In keeping with her educational objectives, she occupied important administrative positions relating to the education and assessment of practising physicians in both Washington and Ottawa from 1997 onwards. In recognition of her many accomplishments, she subsequently served as McLaughlin Professor of Medical Education at the University of Ottawa.

Before receiving his MD degree at the University of Athens in 1977, Christos (Chris) Tsoukas had pursued undergraduate and graduate studies in microbiology and immunology at McGill and the University of Hawaii. He completed his residency training in 1983 in both internal medicine and allergy and clinical immunology at the MGH, and was appointed to the attending staff the same year. Recognition of the onslaught of the AIDS epidemic was in its first stages in the early 1980. Tsoukas, who has achieved worldwide recognition as one of the pioneers in AIDS research, founded the Immune Deficiency Treatment Centre at the MGH. In 1983, the HIV virus had not yet been discovered, but there was widespread interest in blood product safety issues in relation to transfusion and related procedures. Tsoukas played a major role in sounding the alarm that led to the establishment of the Commission of Inquiry on the Blood System in Canada (Kreiver Report). More recently, his research activities have been concentrated on HIV/AIDS vaccine development and immune-based strategies for the prevention and treatment of a disease that has caused millions of deaths on a global basis. Tsoukas joined the Division of Allergy and Clinical Immunology in 1990 and succeeded Shuster as director in 2007.[10]

Ann Clarke graduated in 1984 from Memorial University of Newfoundland with an MD degree, followed by postgraduate studies in health research and policy at Stanford University, California. Her resident training in internal medicine and allergy and immunology at the MGH was completed in 1990. After joining the division, she pursued her research interests in rheumatic diseases such as lupus erythematosus and rheumatoid arthritis.[11] In addition, she collaborated with colleagues in epidemiology on the topic of health economics as it relates to autoimmune diseases. She also had a long-standing interest in peanut allergy. In a well designed study, she was able to demonstrate that, contrary to conventional wisdom, the prevalence of peanut allergy had not increased in incidence over a five-year period. One of her most widely quoted conference presentations is entitled "Nuts to Peanuts." Equally important was her broad range of clinical skills and her meticulous care and kindness to numerous patients with allergic and rheumatic conditions.

The Royal Victoria Hospital and the Montreal Children's Hospital had comparable allergy divisions led by Bram Rose and Harry Bacal. Relations between these three divisions were mutually friendly and cooperative largely due to the efforts of Rose, who was the senior member of the group. For example, monthly journal club meetings were held at Rose's home to exchange viewpoints on recent publications relating to allergy and immunology. There was also a frequent exchange of information about patients who consulted one or more members of the three divisions. Freedman and Rose were frequently asked for an opinion by the same patient. There was an unofficial agreement that duplication of tests and treatment plans between hospitals was a waste of time and money for all concerned. An arrangement was made for the rapid transfer of patient records between hospitals, and each allergist simply added his opinion to the same chart. The group led by Rose had an extensive research program largely devoted to the identification of the allergen in ragweed pollen. Alec Sehon, who was a physical chemist, was an important collaborator in this research project, which was extended over several years. At the Montreal Children's Hospital the emphasis was on superb clinical care for infants and children afflicted with life-threatening allergic disorders.

During the period under discussion there were many advances in the treatment of asthma and allergic rhinitis. For example, when Freedman joined the division, oral corticosteroids had yet to be discovered by the pharmaceutical industry, although adrenocortic trophic hormone (ACTH) could be administered intravenously. The problem in severe asthmatic crises was that ACTH took eight hours or more to exert a beneficial effect and was usually accompanied by intravenous aminophylline. However, at that time, methods for the laboratory measurement of blood levels of a potentially toxic bronchodilator were not available. That meant that the treating physician or resident was required to take the patient's blood pressure and pulse at thirty-minute intervals, often while sitting at the bedside for several hours, until there was clinical evidence of improvement in lung function. Desensitization to a wide variety of pollens, animal dander, and foods was widely used for the long-term treatment of asthma and rhinitis at considerable inconvenience and expense to the patient. Since the introduction of prednisone in the mid-1960s, desensitization to pollen, food, or animal dander has been gradually restricted to patients with asthma or rhinitis that are unresponsive to antihistamines or bronchodilators. There was also much discussion in allergy journals and meetings concerning the relative merits of intradermal testing and scratch testing for the diagnosis of asthma and hay fever. The so-called Eastern Group of allergists, led by Cooke, favoured intradermal testing on the basis of more reliable results, whereas the Western Group, led by Samuel Feinberg from Chicago, insisted that scratch testing was superior because there were fewer associated anaphylactic reactions.

The importance of the Western Group is highlighted by the recent endowment of the Feinberg School of Medicine at Northwestern University in Evanston, Illinois. In more recent years, both methods have been supplanted by a prick test developed by Jack Pepys of the Royal Brompton Hospital in

London, England. Another important contribution of the division was the introduction of sophisticated testing for autoimmune diseases in the Clinical Immunology Laboratory under the supervision of Shuster.

Over the years, the members of the Division of Clinical Immunology have been widely recognized for their many contributions to scientific knowledge and the administration of highly regarded research institutes. In addition, numerous prizes and honours have been awarded to its members. The Gairdner Foundation Annual International Award was received by Freedman and Gold in 1978 for their joint discovery of the carcinogenic antigen. The Prix Armand Frappier was awarded to Freedman and Skamene by the Quebec government for their roles in building and administering outstanding research institutes in the province. Freedman, Gold, and Tsoukas were inducted into the Order of Canada; and Freedman, Gold, and Skamene were awarded the Order of Quebec. In addition, Freedman, Fuks, and Hawkins became deans of medicine at McGill and Memorial universities. As a result of all of the accomplishments described in this Chapter, the division rapidly became known as one of the leading centres for the research and teaching of clinical immunology in North America.

NOTES

1 S.O. Freedman, P. Gold, D. Hawkins, and J. Shuster, *Clinical Immunology* (New York: Harper and Row, 1971).

2 Interview with Raymond Groulx, 2010.

3 P. Gold and S.O. Freedman, "Demonstration of Tumor-Specific Antigens in Human Colonic Carcinomata by Immunological Tolerance and Adsorption Techniques," *Journal of Experimental Medicine* 121 (1965): 439–62; P. Gold and S.O. Freedman, "Specific Carcinoembryonic Antigens of the Human Digestive System," *Journal of Experimental Medicine* 122 (1965): 467–81.

4 D. Hawkins. R.N. Pinckard, and R.S. Farr, "Acetylation of Human Serum Albumin by Acetylsalicylic Acid," *Science* 160 (1968): 780–5.

5 H.K.B. Silver, P. Gold, S. Feder, S.O. Freedman, J. Shuster, "Radioimmunoassay for Alpha-fetoprotein in the Diagnosis of Human Cancer," *Proceedings of the National Academy of Sciences* 70 (1973): 526–32.

6 D.M.P. Thomson, "The Isolation and Characterization of Tumor Specific Antigens of Rodent and Human Tumors," *Cancer Research* 36 (1976): 3518–25.

7 E. Skamene, P. Gros, A. Forget, et al. "Genetic Regulation of Resistance to Intracellular Pathogens," *Nature* 297 (1982): 506–10.

8 A. Fuks, C. Banjo, J. Shuster, et al. "Carcinoembyonic Antigen: Molecular Biology and Clinical Implications," *Biochemica et Biophysica Acta* 417 (1975): 123–52.

9 D. Danoff, L. Lincoln, D.M.P. Thompson, P. Gold, "Big Mac Attack," *New England Journal of Medicine* 298 (1978): 1095–6.

10 C. Tsoukas, F. Gervais, J., Shuster, et al. "Association of HTLV-III Antibodies and Cellular Immune Status of Hemophiliacs," *New England Journal of Medicine* 311 (1984): 1514–15.

11 A.E. Clarke, D.A. Bloch, D. Danoff, and J.M. Esdaile, "Deceasing Costs and Improving Outcomes in SLE: Using Regression Trees to Develop Health Policy," *Journal of Rheumatology* 21 (1994): 1218–24.

5

Cardiology: The Road to the First Subspecialty of Internal Medicine

John H. Burgess

Cardiology became the first division in the Department of Medicine in 1960. It arose from the Department of Electrocardiography and a subsequent cardiology specialty clinic.

The Osler Years, 1874–84: Cardiovascular Disease Holds Centre Stage in Pathology and Internal Medicine

Sir William Osler is remembered as the greatest clinician and teacher of his era – the man who brought pathology and bedside teaching to the practice of medicine. Osler started medical school at the University of Toronto in 1868. He transferred to McGill in 1870, where there were better facilities for hospital work. Following graduate training in London and Europe he returned to McGill and the Montreal General Hospital as "Lecturer upon the Institutes of Medicine." He was active as both a clinician and a pathologist at the MGH before being officially appointed as the first pathologist in 1876. For ten years he performed all the autopsies.[1]

Osler was a general internist living in an era when there were no subspecialties of internal medicine. However, one-third of all his publications concerned diseases of the heart and circulation. His first clinical presentation was to the McGill Society of Montreal, 24 November 1877, on "the influence of position for hearing heart murmurs." He had a special interest in rheumatic valvular disease, pericarditis, infective endocarditis, and arterial aneurysm. In 1885 he was the youngest Fellow of the Royal College of Physicians of London to give the world-famous Gulstonian Lectures. He based these on MGH autopsy studies of infective endocarditis, which contained the first comprehensive account of the disease in the English language.

Osler's classic textbook, *The Principles and Practice of Medicine*, published in 1892, contains one hundred (out of 1,092) pages devoted to cardiovascular disease. These were based on his clinical and autopsy studies at the MGH. The weighting towards cardiology demonstrates its predominance in internal medicine. And, indeed, Osler established the importance of cardiology in internal medicine at the MGH.

Maude Abbott at McGill, 1898–1936: Cardiac Specimens from the MGH Form the McGill Medical Museum

Maude Abbott is recognized as the world pioneer of congenital heart disease. Her classic *Atlas of Congenital Heart Disease* (American Heart Association, 1936) is based on early MGH autopsy specimens. She obtained her MD from Bishop's University in 1894 – the McGill Medical School did not admit women at that time. However, all of the teaching was in Montreal and the clinical work was at the MGH. Following graduate studies in England and Europe, Abbott returned to McGill in 1898 to take up the position of assistant curator of the McGill Medical Museum under Professor J.G. Adami, the chair of pathology. The specimens collected by William Osler during his ten years at the MGH formed the basis for the museum, and it was Abbott's job to organize and catalogue them. She was encouraged in this task by Osler after meeting him in Philadelphia. Osler, like many of his male chauvinist colleagues of the time, felt that there was no place for women in clinical practice: "That a larger proportion of women than men are unfit to practice, will I think, be acknowledged; on the other hand, a relatively larger proportion of the former are adapted to scientific work, and it is a most encouraging feature to see so many women taking up laboratory life – what they lack in initiative and independence is counterbalanced by a more delicate technique, a greater patience with minutiae, and a greater mastery of detail."[2] He had an enormous influence on Maude Abbott's life, directing her into cardiac pathology. In Abbott's case, Osler's view of women in medicine resulted in her becoming an international authority in the field of congenital heart disease.

Abbott never held an official appointment at the MGH, but her pathologic contributions furthered the development of cardiology at the hospital.[3] In 1905, Osler asked her to write the section on congenital heart disease for his textbook *Osler's Modern Medicine*. Both during her life and since her death Abbott has remained one of Canada's most internationally renowned cardiologists. Her former pupil, Harold N. Segall, would play an important role in the formation of a cardiac clinic at the MGH – the first subspecialty clinic within the Department of Medicine.

Electrocardography: A Major Impetus to the Development of Cardiology as a Subspecialty

The first electrocardiographic (ECG) instrument in Canada came to the MGH in 1914 courtesy of Thomas Forest Cotton. Cotton was born in Cowansville, Quebec, graduated from McGill Medical School, and, on Sir William Osler's advice, trained with the great Thomas Lewis in London, England, where he was introduced to the early ECG recorders. He returned to the MGH in 1913, but his hopes of obtaining an instrument were poor. However, Osler wrote a supporting letter to the MGH Board of Governors. The board offered eleven hundred dollars, and Osler contributed twenty-five dollars himself. The chief of medicine, H. Lafleur, gave fifty dollars and one of Cotton's colleagues produced one hundred dollars. Funds were now sufficient to purchase a primitive Cambridge instrument. Thomas Cotton was the first Canadian to obtain training in electrocardiography, and he set up the service at the MGH. He probably recorded an ECG only a few days or weeks before tracings at the Royal Victoria Hospital in Montreal and the Toronto General Hospital.[4]

C.R. Bourne and C.C. Birchard shortly joined Cotton. Birchard ("Birch" to his friends) was an intern (first year out of medical school) at the time of the instrument's arrival. He found the technique a natural outlet for his mechanical ingenuity and recognized that an early problem with ECGs was due to electrical interference from the nearby laundry. Birch soon corrected this by having the laundry turn off its machinery during recordings. He took charge of the apparatus after Cotton's return to England and, by 1915, was using it as a valuable clinical and research tool, particularly for studying heart changes at the time of death. Birch became director of the Department of Electro-Cardiography in 1920. According to MGH Board of Management minutes, it is noted: "That Dr Birchard be, and he is hereby appointed as director of the Electro-Cardiographic Department with Dr Bourne as assistant, it being understood that he will have the use of beds for the observation of heart cases." "That in the notice for the Annual

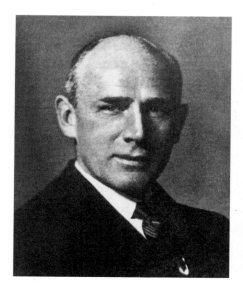 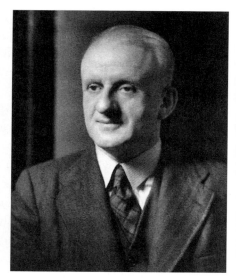

Fig. 5.1 Thomas Forest Cotton, performed the first ECG in Canada at MGH, 1914
Fig. 5.2 C.C. Birchard, first MGH director of electrocardiography, 1920

Meeting of the Governors to be held on February 17th, 1920 notice will be given of the change in the By-Laws." "That the Director of the Electro-Cardiographic Department shall have a seat on the Medical Board."[5]

Birchard showed in one patient that the heart continued to have electrical function after it stopped beating.[6] This phenomenon is now known as electromechanical dissociation, or pulseless electrical activity. Although not published, this may be its first description as a cause of sudden death. The phenomenon became recognized worldwide with the application of bedside ECG monitoring during the early 1960s.[7]

The first ECGs were recorded with the patients' hands and feet in buckets of salted water and took about an hour to produce (as opposed to fewer than five minutes today). Other physicians outside this select group of three were concerned that the new technique would have a negative financial impact on their practices. They needn't have worried. The fee schedule for ECGs in 1932 was as follows:

- Public patients $3.00
- Semi-private patients $6.00 (½ to the doctor and ½ to the hospital)
- Private patients $10.00 (½ to the doctor and ½ to the hospital).[8]

In 2004 the fee set by the Quebec Health Insurance Board was $1.13 for all patients – such is the price of progress. During the first year the ECG laboratory took in eighteen dollars.

The beginning of an ECG recording service set the scene for the foundation of a cardiac clinic by Birchard, Bourne, and Segall and, ultimately, a cardiology subspecialty service. C.C. Birchard was medical director of the Sun Life Assurance Company of Canada and established the tradition that he and other Sun Life cardiologists would have staff positions at the MGH. He was a brilliant clinician and well known as the typical absent-minded professor. On one occasion he took his son Tommy with him to the Sun Life Building on a Sunday morning and forgot to bring him home at lunch. Fortunately, his wife Lucille was used to this behaviour and quickly rescued the six-year-old boy from the vacant downtown building. In 1931, the company donated a new Cambridge instrument to the hospital, and ECGs became routine. Birch's other important contribution to the MGH was as chair of the Medical Board, when he championed the hospital's move from old Montreal to its present Cedar Avenue location.

The Cardiac Clinic: An Important Move towards the Creation of a Division of Cardiology

Harold N. Segall was instrumental in establishing the cardiac clinic – the first subspecialty clinic within the Department of Medicine. He was appointed an assistant to Maude Abbott immediately after his graduation from McGill in 1920. He did further training in pathology at McGill and then clinical training at Harvard in Boston. After two more years in London, England, he returned to Montreal. He was interested in establishing a cardiac clinic at the MGH, but the physician-in-chief, Campbell Howard, and other internists were resistant to a fragmentation of their specialty. Segall had learned persistence from Abbott and prepared a brief emphasizing the future of electrocardiography and other research as needing an identifiable group of cardiac patients. This was presented to the Medical Board and both the clinic and Segall's appointment were approved. C.C. Birchard was named chief of the Cardiac Clinic, with Bourne and Segall as assistants: "The Secretary read to the Meeting a letter from the Medical Board in connection with the establishment of a Cardiac Clinic under the Directorship of C.C. Birchard, and also a letter recommending the appointment of H.N. Segall as Junior Assistant in Medicine to be attached to the proposed Clinic, both of which were

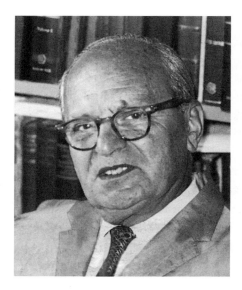

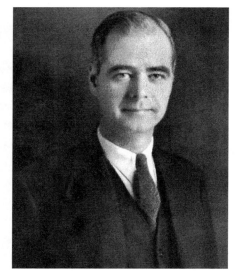

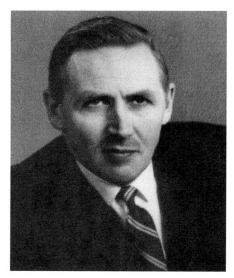

Clockwise from top left
Fig. 5.3 Harold N. Segall, instrumental in starting Cardiac Clinic at the MGH
Fig. 5.4 Neil Feeney, first director, Division of Cardiology, 1960–63
Fig. 5.5 E.A. Stewart Reid, director, MGH Division of Cardiology, 1963–73

approved by the meeting."[9] Their work in the clinic was unpaid and did not impinge on the practices of internists without subspecialty cardiac training.[10] In 1951, Neil Feeney succeeded Birchard as director of the Department of Electro-Cardiography.[11]

Although there were no medical subspecialty training programs, the number of physicians taking a special interest in, and confining their practice to, cardiology increased over the next thirty years. Following the tradition set by C.C. Birchard, almost half of them were associated with the Sun Life Assurance Company. At the MGH they identified themselves with the Department of Electrocardiography and the Cardiac Clinic. By 1960, medical subspecialty training programs were developing in the United States and Canada. The time was coming for the creation of a clinical division.

Cardiac Catheterization: Further Identifying Cardiology as a Subspecialty of Internal Medicine

Cardiac catheterization began in New York City under Andre Cournand and Dickinson Richards in the early 1940s.[12] They received the Nobel Prize along with W. Forssman. As cardiac surgery became possible for congenital and valvular heart disease it became an essential technique in all medical schools.

E.A. Stewart Reid introduced this technique to the MGH. He received his MD from McGill in 1942 during the middle of the Second World War. Stewart Reid had enlisted after his internship and served in Italy and Europe. He trained in internal medicine at the MGH during 1946 and then spent a year in cardiology at the Massachusetts General Hospital. He then went to the Hammersmith Hospital in London, England, where he acquired the technique of cardiac catheterization, still in its infancy. He then returned to the MGH to set up cardiac catheterization as part of a cardiorespiratory laboratory.[13] The first patients were studied in a Department of Radiology fluoroscopy room after the last barium enema of the day was cleaned up.

Cardiac catheterization was a prelude to cardiac surgery at the MGH. Stewart Reid, in his tenacious style, played a role in getting the surgeon-in-chief to reluctantly agree to a closed mitral commissurotomy operation a few years after the first one in Canada was performed by Edouard D. Gagnon at Notre Dame Hospital in 1950.

The Division of Cardiology

A Large Subspecialty within the Department of Medicine

By 1959, the creation of subspecialties within the Department of Medicine became inevitable. The physician-in-chief, Douglas G. Cameron, recognized that medical laboratory services – electrocardiography and metabolism – had the title of separate departments. To keep them under the umbrella of his Department of Medicine he devised the creation of subdepartments.[14] Cardiology was the first.

Following upon a recommendation of the Medical Board concerning the establishment of a Sub-department of Cardiology, it was, upon MO-TION, duly SECONDED,
    RESOLVED that:

a) the present Department of Electrocardiography and the Cardiorespiratory Sub-department of the Department of Medicine be both established as of June 30, 1959,
and that:

b) A Sub-department of Cardiology of the Department of Medicine be established as of July 1, 1959; this new sub-department to include the electrocardiography and cardiorespiratory laboratories and assume responsibility for the Cardiac Clinic in the Outpatient Department and the Public Indoor Consulting Service in Cardiology.
and that:

c) the following be appointed to the Staff of the Sub-department of Cardiology-

Neil Feeney	Director
E.A.S. Reid	
I.G. Milne	Associates
D.J. MacIntosh	
D.H. Woodhouse	
T.R. Hale	Assistants
R.F.P. Cronin	

Neil Feeney was general internist with a special interest in cardiology. He had joined the Department of Electrocardiography in the 1930s and became director in 1949. He became the first director of the new subdepartment in 1959. It encompassed the ECG service, the cardiac clinic, catheterization and cardiorespiratory laboratories, and a newly established consultation service. Medical residents could spend one of their five years of internal medicine training in cardiology.

    In 1961, all subdepartments in the Department of Medicine became divisions: "The Board was advised that with the Medical Board's approval, all Sub-departments within the Department of Medicine will be re-designated as Divisions of the Department of Medicine."[15] Douglas Cameron had now consolidated his power over the largest department in the MGH.

E.A. Stewart Reid was director of the Division of Cardiology from 1963 to 1973. He was famous at Department of Medicine meetings for sitting at the far end of the table and squaring off with the physician-in-chief. It was from this position that he usually got his way in furthering developments within his division.

Subspecialty Beds in Cardiology

There was considerable opposition from internists and other subspecialists to the creation of subspecialty beds in the Department of Medicine. However, by 1964, the beginning of coronary care units (CCU) for the treatment of patients during the first critical days of an acute myocardial infarction could not be avoided in any hospital. Stewart Reid's first projects were the building of a CCU and the expansion of space on the fifth floor to accommodate the increased volume of cardiac activities – EEGs, cardiac catheterization, and respiratory labs and office space for the first full-time hospital cardiologists as well as the part-timers who were spending about one-half their time on inpatient duties.

Code 99

The realization that many cardiac deaths were due to transient electrical phenomena, not necessarily related to the amount of irreversibly damaged heart muscle, led to the creation of a roving cardiac arrest team in 1964. Stewart Reid arranged for John H. Burgess – a senior medical resident who had returned from two years of cardiac research training in Birmingham, England – to put this team in place. The first "code 99" for a cardiac arrest was called at night on a patient in a single room. In those days the cardiac defibrillators required four hundred volts of alternating current. Burgess assembled his team-nurses, two other medical residents, and an anaesthetist – around the patient, who was being given closed chest massage. When he pressed the red button on the defibrillator instead of a shock being delivered through the patient's chest to restart his heart all the lights went out on the floor. The fuses were unable to carry the necessary current, and the life-saving attempt degenerated into a shambles. Fortunately, none of the code 99 team received a shock. Future code 99s were more successful. The first good result made the front pages of the *Montreal Gazette*.[16] What we used to call death was now a cardiac arrest, which could be reversed if reached in time. The principle of the early treatment of sudden death due to a cardiac arrest translated into the benefits of continuous monitoring of all patients with heart attacks and the creation of the Coronary Care Unit. C.C. Birchard would have been proud to see his early work on electrical cardiac deaths translated into successful resuscitation.

The Coronary Care Unit

The Coronary Care Unit opened in 1966. Six beds were created by knocking down the wall between two four-bedded rooms and installing bedside monitors and a central monitoring system operated by the nurses. All patients with acute cardiac problems – heart attacks and life-threatening arrhythmias – were under the care of an attending staff cardiologist, a cardiac resident, and medical residents on rotation. The nurses were given authority to initiate resuscitative measures and electrical defibrillation for cardiac arrest. The MGH Coronary Care Unit, like other newly established units across the country, resulted in the in-hospital mortality for acute heart attacks dropping from 30 to 10 percent. This resulted from immediate treatment of life-threatening arrhythmias before irreversible heart and brain damage could occur. We had come a long way from the days when heart attack patients were treated in an oxygen tent in unmonitored single rooms. Patients with hearts too young to die were no longer found dead during routine nursing rounds.

The Modern Academic Division of Cardiology

Subspecialties within internal medicine had been certified through examination by the Quebec College of Medicine since the early 1950s. By the mid-1960s, they were also recognized by the Royal College of Physicians and Surgeons of Canada. This paved the way for two-year specialty training positions within the Division of Cardiology. Formal postgraduate teaching by members of the division for future cardiologists was now added to that of internal medicine residents and undergraduates. The additional teaching as well as clinical and laboratory demands increased the need for full-time university and hospital based cardiologists.

John H. Burgess became director of the Division of Cardiology in 1973 and remained in this position for twenty-one years. This was a time of further expansion. Burgess actively recruited for the attending staff, increasing the university full-time positions to three, hospital full-time positions to six, and part-timers to eight. The position of associate director of the division (M. Godin) was created as well as directors of the Coronary Care Unit and Cardiac Catheterization Laboratory.

Three step-down beds were added to the Coronary Care Unit, bringing the acute cardiac care capacity to nine. Ten cardiac subspecialty beds were created on 11 East in 1990. These were the first elective subspecialty beds within the Department of Medicine, much to the envy of other divisions. Most MGH cardiac patients were now under the direct care of cardiologists.

The number of cardiology residency training position increased to seven. Second- and third-year medical residents rotated through the division, and four final-year medical students were regularly assigned for one-month elective periods. The cardiology residency-training program became integrated with the Royal Victoria Hospital, the Montreal Children's Hospital, and the Jewish General Hospital to form a McGill program. The cardiology outreach program also expanded with dual staff appointments at St Mary's Hospital, the Reddy Memorial Hospital, the Queen Mary Veterans Hospital, the Brome-Missisquoi-Perkins Hospital, the Verdun General Hospital, and the Lakeshore General Hospital. ECG interpretation services were supplied to the Baffin Arctic region and northern Quebec.

During his tenure as director of the Division of Cardiology, Burgess began making monthly cardiac consulting visits to Ormstown and Lachute and, for many years, was the cardiac consultant to the Baffin Region (later Nunavut) and northern Quebec (later Nunavik). He visited these regions and their settlements for two weeks each year and, in between visits, fielded telephone consults several times a week. All Inuit patients requiring hospitalization for cardiac care in the Eastern Arctic came to the MGH. Burgess was awarded the Order of Canada in 1987 for this clinical activity. It also led to the publication of his autobiography, *Doctor to the North: Thirty Years Treating Heart Disease among the Inuit* (McGill-Queen's University Press, 2008).

Burgess also served as chief examiner in cardiology for the Royal College of Physicians and Surgeons of Canada, chaired the Committee on Examinations, and was president of the Royal College from 1990 to 1992. He received international recognition with fellowships from the Royal College of Physicians of Edinburgh, the Royal College of Physicians of Australia, the College of Medicine of South Africa, and the Royal College of Physicians of London as well as a mastership from the American College of Physicians.

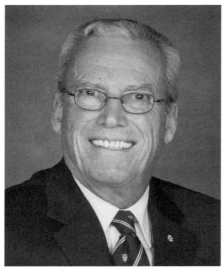

Fig. 5.6 John H. Burgess, director of
Division of Cardiology, 1973–94

Below
Fig. 5.7 Monaural stethoscope – a modern
version of Laennec's first tube stethoscope
of 1819

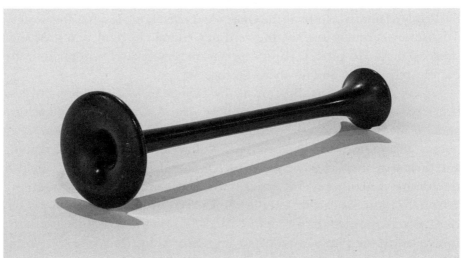

Research within the Division of Cardiology
Until 1960, cardiology research at the MGH was mostly clinical, relating to
patient reports. R.F. Patrick Cronin was the first university full-time cardiologist to join the division. He carried out basic animal research on the coronary circulation as well as clinical investigation. He was a leading researcher,
clinician, and teacher of his day. He later became dean of the McGill Faculty
of Medicine. Cronin encouraged John H. Burgess to pursue a career in aca-

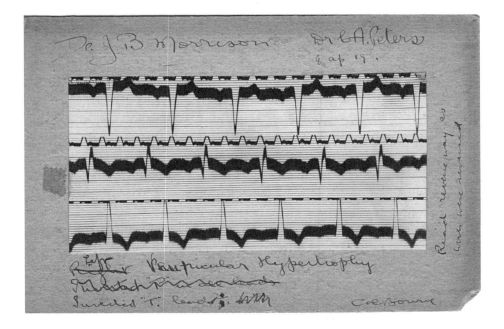

Fig. 5.8 Early ECG with right and left arm leads reversed.

demic medicine. Burgess – the second university full-time cardiologist – on his return from the University of California, San Francisco, in 1966 began both basic and clinical investigations involving the pulmonary circulation system. Burgess also initiated a series of clinical investigations of patients in the coronary care unit and in cooperation with the Department of Surgery in the surgical intensive care unit. In cooperation with Cronin and Carl Goresky of the Medical University Clinic, he applied the multiple indicator dilution technique to the study of fluid exchange in the pulmonary circulation system. Colin P. Rose worked with Goresky studying transcapillary exchange. Jean-Lucien Rouleau, on becoming director of the CCU, began a series of clinical studies on patients with heart failure. He later gained international recognition at the University of Sherbrooke, University of Montreal, and University of Toronto continuing this early interest. H.F. Mizgala and J.W. Warnica participated in important multicentre drug trials before moving to senior cardiology positions in western Canada. T. Huynh continued division participation in a series of multinational trials. By the early 1990s, five to six original research publications per year were being produced by members of the MGH Division of Cardiology.

The MGH Becomes Part of the McGill University
Health Centre (MUHC)

By 1990, the decision was made to combine the administration of the MGH, the Royal Victoria Hospital, the Montreal Children's Hospital, the Montreal Chest Hospital, the Montreal Neurological Hospital, the Montreal Maternity Hospital, and the Allen Memorial Institute into a single McGill University Health Centre. The original plan was for the activities of all these institutions to be combined under one roof at a McGill super-hospital. The new site was planned on the Canadian Pacific Railway's Glen Yards. As plans unfolded, it appeared that the MGH would remain open as a separate site of the MUHC.

In 1994, John Burgess stepped down as director of the MGH Division of Cardiology, and Michael D. Rosengarten replaced him for one year as acting director. In 1995, John L. McCans became the first MUHC director of cardiology. He left for a position at Queen's University three year later. Richard Haichin became acting director for one year, and, in 1999 Jacques Genest became MUHC director of cardiology. Genest brought a large cardiac genetic research enterprise with him, which was located at the RVH site.

Cardiology at the MGH has come almost full circle. Beginning as a laboratory ECG service and subsequent cardiac clinic it expanded into a full division and, with the formation of the MUHC, retreated to a smaller but essential service.

NOTES

1 H.N. Segall, *Pioneers of Cardiology in Canada, 1820–1970* (Willowdale, ON: Hounslow Press, 1988), 31–4.

2 W.O. Osler, "In memoriam of Mary Petnam Jacobi," *New York Medical Records* 66 (December 1907): 3–8.

3 D. Waugh, *Maudie of McGill* (Toronto: Hannah Institute and Dundurn Press, 1992), 53–66.

4 Segall, *Pioneers of Cardiology*, 76–7.

5 Minutes, MGH Board of Management, 21 January 1920, MGH Archives.

6 H.E. MacDermot, *A History of the Montreal General Hospital* (Montreal: Montreal General Hospital, 1950), 97.

7 H.A. Fozzard, "Electromechanical Dissociation and Its Possible Role in Sudden Cardiac Death," *Journal of the American College of Cardiology* suppl. B (1985): 31.

8   Minutes, MGH Board of Management, 11 August 1926, MGH Archives.

9   Segall, *Pioneers of Cardiology*, 124–5.

10 Minutes, MGH Board of Management, 22 November 1932, MGH Arcives.

11 Ibid., 21 February 1951.

12 A. Cournand and H.A. Ranges, "Catheterization of the Right Auricle in Man." *Proceedings for the Society of Experimental Biology* 46 (1941): 462.

13 Segall, *Pioneers of Cardiology*, 285–6; Minutes, MGH Board of Management, 21 January 1953, MGH Archives.

14 Ibid., 17 June 1959.

15 Ibid., 19 November 1961.

16 *Montreal Gazette*, 10 June 1964.

6

Dermatology

R. Roy Forsey, William Gerstein, and John H. Burgess

Roy Forsey succeeded Fred Burgess as head of the Department of Dermatology. Bill Gerstein succeeded Forsey. The Skin Clinic, which was started in 1879 by Thomas Roddick, was soon taken over by Francis Shepherd, who made dermatology a subspecialty at the MGH and established it as specialty in Canada. He was a surgeon/anatomist at McGill and did this as a sideline. Dermatology became a Department in 1924, and, in 1928, J.F. Burgess was appointed the first fully trained dermatologist and later became a founding member of the Canadian Dermatological Association. A resident program was started in 1946, Roy Forsey was appointed in 1950, and the department expanded after the move to Cedar Avenue in 1955. William Gerstein was the first full-time dermatologist-in-chief, 1981.

In 1879, the medical faculty at McGill University established what is known as the "University Dispensary" on St Urbain Street. Thomas Roddick, a surgeon, later Sir Thomas Roddick, was put in charge of the skin clinic. Within a few months Francis J. Shepherd returned from Europe, where he had spent some time at the Stanford Street Skin Hospital under Jonathan Hutchison. Shepherd soon took over the clinic. In 1883, he was appointed to the indoor staff of the Montreal General Hospital, and he transferred the clinic to that institution. Shepherd also gained fame as an anatomist and as a surgeon, but he continued to run the skin clinic until he retired in 1921.

It has been said that dermatology was a hobby for Shepherd; nevertheless, of his 122 papers at least nineteen of them concern skin diseases. He was sufficiently recognized as a dermatologist that he was elected to membership in the American Dermatological Association, and he served both as vice-president and president of that organization and was subsequently elected to honorary membership. He served as vice-president of the International Congress of Dermatology in 1907 and was made an honorary president as one of the forerunners of the Canadian Dermatological Association (the Canadian Branch of the British Dermatological Association). Shepherd was the father of dermatology at McGill and at the MGH. He established dermatology as an important part of the hospital and, when he retired, dermatology had attained the status of an independent department within the MGH. It is interesting to note that the first two dermatologists were both surgeons and, indeed, it was thought at the time that dermatology was more or less a surgical specialty. In fact, when the Royal Victoria Hospital opened, dermatology was so much considered a surgical specialty that it was finally taken over by the physicians. Several clinicians worked in Shepherd's clinic, and J.D. McGovern subsequently became chief of dermatology at St Mary's Hospital. A.O. Freedman, W.R. Bourne, and C.A. Peters all worked in the skin clinic. Peters was appointed visiting professor of dermatology at the University of Vermont and went down on regular occasions to teach the medical students there.

In 1921, when dermatology became a department, Gordon G. Campbell was made the first dermatologist-in-chief. Campbell came to Montreal from the Maritimes and was a botanist of some repute. His collections of specimens from the Maritime provinces still reside at McGill. He was particularly interested in bacteriology and the pathology of the skin. He was a sound clinician and an excellent photographer. In 1921, he published the first Canadian textbook on dermatology: *Common Diseases of the Skin*. He was one of the founders of the inter-urban dermatological association and was its first president. This was the beginning of what became the Canadian Dermatological Association.

In 1924, John Frederick Burgess joined the department and succeeded Campbell, becoming the second dermatologist-in-chief in 1927. Burgess graduated in medicine at the University of Toronto in 1913 and had aspirations in surgery. While serving as a medical officer in France during the First World War he was severely wounded and, as a result, lost his left arm at the shoulder. This ended his surgical career. Following a long period of rehabilitation he spent the years from 1920 to 1923 in postgraduate training in dermatology in London and Vienna. He returned to Canada and was appointed to the attending staff at the MGH in 1924. He was the first fully trained dermatologist and began some basic research. He was particularly interested in fungus diseases, and he also became an excellent photographer. His work at the hospital was of course voluntary, and he supported himself with a private practice, which, at that time, was a slow process. He even considered giving up dermatology and taking an administrative post with the Department of Veterans Affairs in Ottawa. When Campbell heard of this, he took Burgess to his office, showed him a copy of *Common Diseases of the Skin*, and encouraged him to stay. Campbell then urged his colleagues to send patients to Burgess instead of to him. From then on, Burgess's practice began to grow. This act, I believe, shows the high regard in which Campbell held Burgess. When Campbell retired, Burgess succeeded him.

Burgess was also a founder of the Canadian Dermatological Association and of the Montreal Dermatological Society. He, too, was elected to the American Dermatological Association, and he served as its vice-president in 1939. In 1946, with the return of the veterans from the First World War, Burgess was one of those to see the need for a residency training program, and R. Roy Forsey and C.W.E. Danby were appointed for residency training.

No history of dermatology at the MGH would be complete without at least mentioning the contribution of Barney David Usher. Barney was a Montrealer and a graduate of McGill. He did postgraduate training in Cleveland and in Chicago under the great William L. Pussy. It was in Pussy's office that he met Francis Sinear, and together they published a paper on what has become the Sinear-Usher syndrome. Usher returned to Montreal and joined the MGH's Department of Dermatology in 1926, where he taught generations of students for the next fifty years. He also conducted basic research, and he stimulated others to do so as well as to publish. He was a great bedside teacher and was revered by all the dermatologists who carne to the MGH for postgraduate training.

In the late 1930s, Donald Strange Mitchell, a graduate of the University of Chicago, joined the staff at the MGH. During the Second World War, Mitchell was chief dermatologist in the Royal Canadian Navy and stimulated an interest in dermatology in a number of young medical officers who served on the east coast. He was an inspiring teacher. By late 1943, he had become very interested in wool as a cause of skin eruptions, and this led him down the path of what is now known as environmental medicine. This dedication led him away from orthodox dermatology and cost him dearly. His appointment was terminated at the department in the late 1950s, but he continued to explore his new interest until his death.

Robert Roy Forsey, a veteran of the Royal Canadian Navy, first became interest in dermatology when he was exposed to the teachings of Don Mitchell in 1942. After six months with Mitchell he was sent to St John's, Newfoundland, to take care of the patients with skin diseases and those with venereal diseases. While in Newfoundland he developed administrative skills and became assistant principal medical officer at the RCN hospital in St. John's. He was also sent to Montreal in 1945 for further training in dermatology. On demobilization he became resident at the MGH in January 1946, and he completed his training at the University of Michigan in 1947. He was appointed to the staff of the MGH in 1947. While in Michigan, Forsey was appointed to the staff and he became an associate of Burgess in his private practice in January 1948. In December 1950, Burgess retired and Forsey was appointed the third dermatologist-in-chief at the MGH.

While dermatology was and still is an independent department at the hospital, it is a subdepartment of medicine at McGill. At that time, half of the medical students at McGill took their medicine at the MGH and half at the RVH in their third year and alternated in their fourth year. Forsey, working with the physician-in-chief, revised the teaching at the MGH. Didactic teaching was drastically reduced, and bedside and clinical teaching was increased. At one time, if a student took his/her medicine at the MGH he/she would receive at least seventy-two hours in dermatology. With the emergence of other specialties, this time was gradually eroded. The elective program was developed for both undergraduates and non-dermatological postgraduates.

The residency training program was expanded. At one point there were seven residents in dermatology. There had always been a close liaison with the Department of Pathology at the hospital and dermapathology was a key feature.

A rotation was established with the Montreal Children's Hospital and the Queen Mary Veterans Hospital, where Forsey was in charge of the indoor service. When the Queen Mary Veterans Hospital ceased to be, the rotation was transferred to the Jewish General Hospital. During Forsey's tenure over sixty-five dermatologists received at least one year of their training at the hospital. It was a policy at that time that the residents should receive a broad experience, and they were encouraged to spend at least one year away, usually in and American program. It was felt that this was a good experience for the residents and that it helped to develop strong ties with our American colleagues.

In 1967, Forsey encouraged the Ottawa group to begin to train dermatologists. The Ottawa program began as an offshoot of the MGH, first with one resident for one year. These residents completed their training at the MGH. The Ottawa program gradually grew and reached independent status in ten years. The Ottawa group not only trained a number of residents but also established Ottawa as an important dermatological centre.

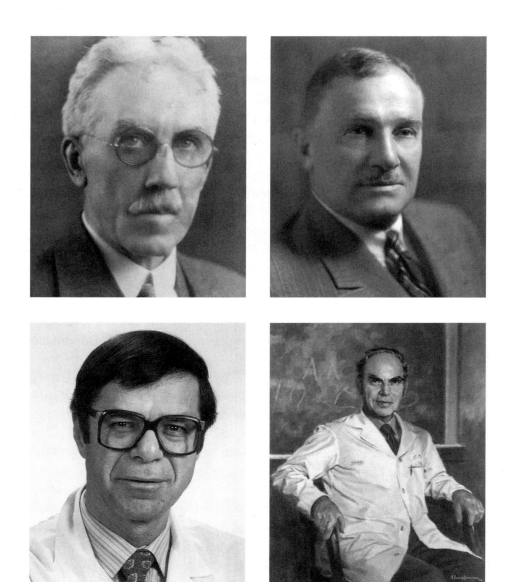

Clockwise from top left
Fig. 6.1 G. Gordon Campbell, 1921–27
Fig. 6.2 John Frederick Burgess, the second dermatologist-in-chief, 1927–50
Fig. 6.3 R. Roy Forsey, dermatologist-in-chief, 1950–81
Fig 6.4 William Gerstein, dematologist-in-chief, 1982–97

At that time the postgraduate program was hospital-based; nevertheless, there was a closed association with the Royal Victoria Hospital. Many activities, such as the journal clubs, rounds, and so on, were combined, and, on occasion, residents rotated between the two programs. In the late 1980s the hospital-based programs were discontinued in favour of the central McGill program.

The increased activity in the department demanded an increase in staff. Anna Flint was appointed in 1959. Flint became an excellent clinician and an able teacher. She developed a large private practice but always found time for her service and her teaching commitments. She remained on the staff until she retired in 1981. Flint now resides in Israel.

Thomas L. Sullivan spent three months in the department on rotation during his senior internship in medicine. Following this he decided to become a dermatologist and took his training at Stanford University in California and returned to join the staff in 1959. Tom was a good clinician and a good teacher, but he had an abiding interest in music and this sometimes interfered with his teaching assignments. Nevertheless, he made a worthwhile contribution. In 1973, he resigned from the staff to move to California.

William Gerstein also rotated through the service while a senior in medicine. He completed his training in Philadelphia and London, England, and joined the staff in 1963. At that time he took over the research laboratory and did some basic research. He continued at the hospital and succeeded Forsey as the fourth dermatologist-in-chief in 1981.

Dorothy June Irwin, a graduate of the program, joined the department in 1967 and taught in the clinic until 1981. During this time she established her practice on the West Island. Otto Schlapner, also a graduate of our program, completed his training in Philadelphia and joined the staff in 1972. Otto was a keen teacher and made a significant contribution. In 1977 he resigned from the staff to move to Vancouver, British Columbia. Katheline Moses, a graduate of Ottawa and the program, joined the staff in 1973 and continued until 1983, when she moved back to Ottawa. David Gratton, another graduate of the program, was appointed to the staff in 1975, followed by Audette Fornier-Blake in 1978 and Elizabeth O'Brien in 1980. Forsey reached the mandatory age of retirement in 1980, and William Gerstein was appointed the fourth dermatologist-in-chief in January 1982. Forsey played a guiding role in the Department of Dermatology for over thirty years and was instrumental in leading the department to its present location in Livingston Hall.

Following the move to new quarters on the eighth floor of Livingston Hall, William Gerstein became the first full-time dermatologist-in-chief. The department now occupies most of the North Wing of the eighth floor. The clinical facilities include seven fully equipped examining rooms, a residents room, a clinic secretary and nurses' area, and a large treatment room with an overhead ultraviolet therapy unit that can be raised and lowered above the patient. These facilities are in constant use. The department has an active immunodeficiency clinic and has developed educational computer programs that are used throughout North America. The graduates of the training program are to be found coast-to-coast, from St John's, Newfoundland, to Victoria, British Columbia, and south of the border.

7

Endocrinology, Metabolism, Toxicology, and Clinical Chemistry

Guy Joron, Donald Douglas, and John H. Burgess

Guy Joron and Donald Douglas were staff members at the inception of the Division of Endocrinology and Metabolism. John Burgess used their notes to write this chapter.

Started by house officer Israel Mordecai Rabinowitch in 1919, the Department of Metabolism was created in 1921, with its main focus on diabetes. Alan Fowler (1929) and Edward Benseley (1932) also came to work on diabetes, which continued to be the main interest of the group for years. This interest expanded into toxicology, thyroid disease, and general endocrinology. Joron, Bauld, Douglas, Hollenberg, Tonks and Gardiner, and Pierson-Murphy are people who made major contributions to what was the Department of Metabolism, then the Department of Metabolism and Toxicology, and eventually the Department of Endocrinology and Metabolism, with toxicology and clinical chemistry laboratories.

The founder and first director of the Department of Metabolism was Israel Mordecai Rabinowitch (1891–1983), known as Rab. The department's development reflected Rab's foresight and numerous talents, which he demonstrated throughout his career. After his MD, CM degree from McGill University in 1917, he went to the Montreal General Hospital as an intern and resident. His laboratory career started as a house officer in 1919, when he started conducting biochemical tests in a corner of the residents' clinical laboratory. He could test blood sugar (BS), urea nitrogen (BUN), non-protein nitrogen (NPN), and creatinine, and he tied these to a variety of diseases. His colleagues were so impressed with the application of these tests that he was appointed a pathological chemist in the Department of Pathology in 1920 and was given a small laboratory. The usefulness of these tests also led to the establishment of a diabetic clinic – the forerunner of the Department of Metabolism.

The MGH Department of Metabolism was created in 1921, with Rab as the director and head of the Diabetic Clinic. Fortuitously, Banting and Best isolated insulin the same year, and Rab obtained it from Fred Banting for use at the MGH. He and Banting were among the first to use insulin on patients in Canada, and Rab published his results in 1923.

One of Rab's major contributions to the treatment of diabetes was a diet program. Patients were previously prescribed diets very low in carbohydrate (CHO), very high in fat, and low in protein. These diets had to be weighed for individual meals. Rab claimed that food values were approximations and that scales could be replaced by linear descriptions illustrated by wooden models and drawings resulting in the development of food exchanges. This concept greatly simplified the lives of patients and increased their compliance. With insulin treatment the general pattern was to increase the CHO and caloric value of the diet while still maintaining a high fat content. He also noted that the plasma cholesterol was elevated in most diabetics, which he attributed to poor control and the high fat diet. This led him to conclude that the protein content should be increased. He later proposed a moderate CHO, low fat, and high protein diet. He was one of the first to note the relation of cholesterol and arteriosclerosis.

Edward R. Bensley graduated from the University of Toronto Medical School with a gold medal in 1930 and came to the MGH for his internship and residency training. Within two years he was offered a position as assistant–physician in the Department of Metabolism. His responsibilities were in the laboratory and Diabetic Clinic. In 1929, Alan Fowler (MD, CM 1927) had joined the department as assistant and began work in diabetes, as did everyone who worked under Rab.

The demand for chemical analyses of blood and urine increased in the 1930s with the development of new tests, machines, and the general progress of scientific medicine. Rab also became interested in the toxicology of heavy metals and poisons, which his laboratory was asked to investigate.

Research in the treatment of diabetes and its complications continued. A significant contribution involved a simple and effective way to treat diabetic coma – a method that could be used in any hospital laboratory facilities. This was a major contribution for a country like Canada, with a large rural population and many small local hospitals.

Canada entered the Second World War in 1939, and Rab was sent to Great Britain by the Canadian army to study chemical warfare in a mobile unit that he had developed. Bensley also went overseas with the No. 14 Canadian General Hospital. He later became advisor in nutrition to the Canadian army overseas, retiring as a major and as a Member of the British Empire. Fowler was left at the MGH to run the department and to supervise the laboratory and diabetic clinic.

Rab returned to civilian life in 1943 and wrote a series of pamphlets on how to deal with chemical weapons. He continued as director of the department that saw an increasing number of poison cases brought to the ER, dramatically changing this aspect of the department's work. In 1945, the Department of Metabolism's name was changed to the Department of Metabolism and Toxicology.

Rab retired as director of the Department of Metabolism and Toxicology in 1947 and took a job as director of the McGill Institute for Special Research and Cell Metabolism. He retired from this position for health reasons but continued a limited practice until 1955. He died at age ninety-two on 2 November 1983, having published over 150 articles. according to the editor of the Canadian Society of Clinical Chemists News, this established him as the father of clinical chemistry in Canada.

Ed Bensley succeeded Rab as director of the Department of Metabolism and Toxicology in 1947 and devoted himself to the clinical laboratory and his interests in nutrition and toxicology. Fowler continued as director of the Diabetic Service. In the same year, the Department of Medicine created a subdepartment of endocrinology, with R. Palmer Howard (the grandson of Osler's teacher and mentor Robert Palmer Howard, 1823–89) as its director. Since the Department of Medicine had no laboratory facilities of its own, Howard was given an appointment as assistant in the Department of Metabolism and Toxicology to develop and supervise the assays required for endocrine function. He resigned in 1951 to accept a position at the School of Medicine of the University of Oklahoma. Allen Gold (MD, CM, McGill 1942) replaced him as endocrinologist. Gold had a particular interest in thyroid disease and introduced the use of radioactive iodine to the MGH.

Guy Joron (MD, CM, McGill 1941) was appointed an assistant in the Department of Medicine and Toxicology in 1951. His duties were to assist Alan Fowler in the care of diabetic patients, participate in the care of patients with nutritional problems, and, most important, in the care and evaluation of poison cases. This aspect of the department's activities became so important that Bensley and Joron wrote a small manual on poisoning entitled *Handbook on the Treatment of Acute Poisoning* (London: E&S Livingstone Ltd., 1953). This little classic was the first of its kind in Canada and was meant to complement the course being taught to medical students. It was a small gem, used by residents, staff, and students, and went to a third edition in 1963. In addition to cases of intentional poisoning with drugs or chemicals, doctors had now to be concerned with unexpected toxic side-effects of new legitimate drugs. Poisoning in the home and/or workplace were common. An increasing concern was intentional overdose of barbiturates and other sedatives.

William S. Bauld (MD, CM, McGill 1949; PhD, Edinburgh 1953) was appointed as assistant in the department with a main interest in estrogen metabolism and endocrinology in general. When the MGH moved to Cedar Avenue one of his major responsibility's was planning, equipping, and implementing the new laboratories. Automation in clinical chemistry was at hand, and Bauld introduced the Technicon Autoanalyzer in 1957, the first one in Canada. Under the supervision of Mr John Knowles, who had been trained by Technicon Inc. of Terrytown, New York, the machine was designed to do many blood tests (e.g., routine blood sugar and BUN tests were conducted daily). This was a far cry from the time when Fowler persuaded Rab to use a Fisher Electrophotometer in the lab (which, at that time, was a big advance).

Donald Douglas, PhD, joined the department in 1957 to develop a toxicology laboratory, principally to identify the substances responsible for the numerous poisonings that came to the MGH ER and other hospitals in the McGill medical system. He had been working in the Biochemistry Department at McGill when Rab recruited him in 1946 to join his new project, the Institutes for Special Research and Cell Metabolism. Pending the opening of the institute, he went to Chalk River to learn how to use radioisotopes in lab work. When the institute's work was transferred to McGill, he resigned in December 1955. He worked for Merck and Company, retaining an informal connection with McGill. In the summer of 1957, Bauld invited him back to work in the MGH Department of Metabolism and Toxicology. His task was to develop the toxicology laboratory to serve the MGH and other hospitals. Unfortunately, his efforts to obtain a Provincial Public Health Grant for this project were unsuccessful. However, he set up the lab with equipment purchased by special funds (Fowler had raised about fifty thousand dollars from his grateful patients). The work of the lab soon required help from another chemist, and Irene Dobuschak was recruited.

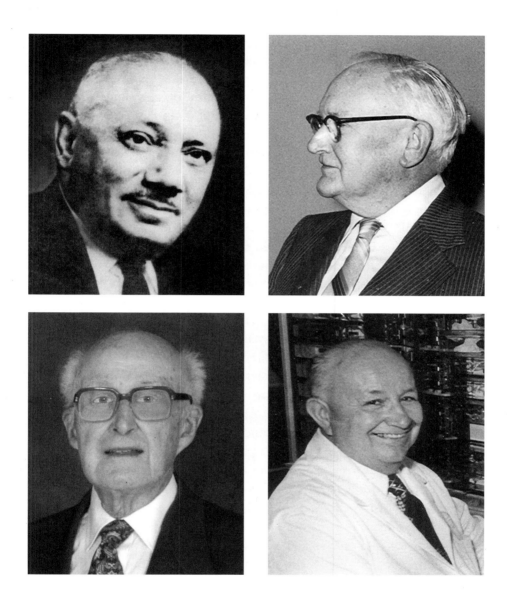

Clockwise from top left

Fig. 7.1 Israel Mordecai Rabinowitch, first director, Department of Metabolism, 1924–47

Fig. 7.2 Edward Benseley, Gold Medalist from Toronto, second director, Department of Metabolism, 1947–60

Fig. 7.3 David Tonks, director of clinical chemistry, 1961–87. He established the first laboratory self-testing program in Canada to calibrate the laboratory apparatus.

Fig. 7.4 Guy Joron, assistant director of endocrinology and metabolism, 1951–75, was primarily interested in poisoning – chemical and drug – seen in the ER.

The department suffered a severe blow on 20 July 1958, when Bauld and his wife and family were killed in a highway accident in New Brunswick. Since he joined the department in 1954 he had reorganized and extended the biochemical and endocrinological services. At the time of his death, Bauld was associate director of the Department of Metabolism and Toxicology, assistant director of the University Clinic, and assistant professor of medicine at McGill. Donald Douglas took over the direction of the biochemical laboratories.

In October 1957, Ronald Hobkirk, PhD, joined the department as a temporary special research assistant. He had obtained his PhD in 1955 in biochemistry at Edinburgh University with a primary interest in steroid chemistry. He had met Bauld, who was lecturing at Edinburgh, and in 1957 came to work at McGill with R.H. Heard, who died suddenly and left Hobkirk stranded. Bill Bauld came to the rescue and offered him space in the MGH laboratory. In 1958, Hobkirk was given a staff appointment in the department. He became director of the endocrine laboratory and assumed responsibility for Bauld's graduate students. In April 1959, he was appointed a biochemist, extended the endocrine services, and even attracted new graduate students. In 1970, Hobkirk accepted a position at the University of Western Ontario.

In October 1960, two major changes occurred in the Department of Metabolism and Toxicology. A subdepartment of diabetes and endocrinology was established in the Department of Medicine under A.F. Fowler, with responsibility for the diabetic clinic and endocrine laboratory. Of equal importance, Bensley resigned to accept a position as associate dean under Lloyd Stevenson. He had been an excellent chief, fair-minded, even-tempered, decisive, and always willing to help. Among his new duties he became interested in the history of medicine at McGill and the MGH and published many interesting articles.

In 1963, Dean Stevenson resigned to accept a position as medical historian at Yale University, and Ed Bensley became acting dean for two years until the appointment of Ronald Christie. He stayed on as vice-dean to help smooth the medical school's transfer to the new McIntyre Medical Sciences Building, and then he retired for health reasons. But this was not the end of Ed Bensley's career at McGill. He moved, as curator, to a small office in the Osler Library, where he devoted himself full time to the history of medicine. He wrote an excellent book of short biographical sketches, *McGill Medical Luminaries*, which was published as the first volume in the Osler Library Studies in the History of Medicine series. He advised, corresponded with many, conducted research on various projects, and, on his final retirement, was made honorary curator of the Osler Library and emeritus professor of the history of medicine. He died in 1959 after an outstanding career at McGill.

Bensley's retirement from the MGH Department of Metabolism and Toxicology led to its demise in 1961. Its functions were assumed by the Department of Medicine, and, as part of a general reorganization, two divisions were created: the Clinical Chemistry Division under David Tonks and the Metabolic Diseases Division under Fowler. A search committee was formed to find a successor to Bensley. The leading choice was Slater from the Hospital for Sick Children in Toronto. Slater wanted Tonks to come as his assistant. This was agreeable to the MGH, but Slater dragged his feet because he was also being sought by the University of Vermont. Fortunately, the job was then offered to Tonks who wanted to come to Montreal. He was made director of the Division of Clinical Chemistry, created in 1961 in the Department of Medicine. This would supersede the Department of Metabolism and Toxicology.

Throughout his career, David Tonks took a keen interest in quality control. He was one of the early members of the American Association of Clinical Chemistry, founded in 1951, and a founding member of the Canadian Society of Clinical Chemists, founded in 1956. He established a testing program for 170 laboratories in Canada and would send specimens to each laboratory to check for accuracy and precision. His 1963 publication in the *Journal of Clinical Chemistry* describes this program as program as a first in Canada. He was involved in several proficiency testing programs in the United States and internationally. He was assisted by Paul Koch.

In 1961, Michael Kaye, a nephrologist, took over the renal section of the lab. The volume of tests continued to increase with further automation and, by 1985, had reached 1,670 daily. The annual report of the clinical chemistry laboratory in 1969 revealed that 613,905 tests were performed. In 1971, 1 million were conducted, and the number rose to over 3 million in 1985.

Donald Douglas retired after thirty-five years of service in the toxicology laboratory, and David Tonks retired in 1987. Joseph Shuster qualified as a clinical chemist in 1974 and later took over the division.

Fowler retired in 1968 and was succeeded by Charles Hollenberg as director of the Division of Endocrinology and Metabolism. Hollenberg, a former Markel Scholar, gained an international reputation as an endocrinologist and became a full professor at McGill University. He left to become

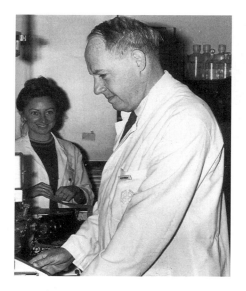

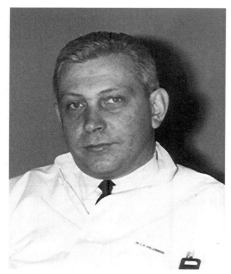

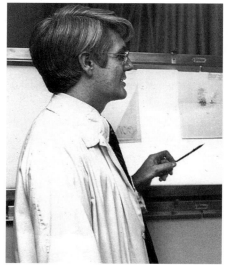

Clockwise from top left
Fig. 7.5 Donald Douglas, director of the
Toxicology Laboratory, 1957–92
Fig. 7.6 Charles Hollenberg, director
of Department of Endocrinology and
Metabolism, 1968–69. Famous endo-
crinologist before he got to the MGH
Fig. 7.7 Robert Gardiner, director of
Department of Endocrinology and
Metabolism, 1969–97

chair of medicine at the University of Toronto in 1969. He was succeeded by
Robert J. Gardiner, a Canadian authority on diabetes, who served as director
until it became the McGill University Health Centre Division in 1997.

During the 1980s and 1990s, research in the Division of Endocrinology
and Metabolism was mostly carried out by Beverly Murphy. Her early research
was mainly concerned with the development of new assays for hormones.

When she started, no hormones could be measured directly until she developed a new method for the estimate of plasma cortisol. A year later she applied a similar method to the measurement of thyroxine, the main hormone secreted by the thyroid gland. Murphy was the first to demonstrate that premature babies with respiratory distress syndrome were deficient in cortisol, and its supplement became a promising treatment for prevention of this disease. Psychiatrists applied her cortisol assay method to depressed patients who were found to have an excess of this hormone. Initial clinical trials in the use of antiglucocorticoid drugs in the treatment of major depression proved promising. Murphy became a widely cited researcher for her pioneering assays of cortisol and thyroxine.

8

Gastroenterology

Douglas G. Kinnear

Doug Kinnear was the first director of the Division of Gastroenterology.
He was a nationally famous teacher and clinician.

Gastroenterology started as a clinic in 1960 and as a consult service with weekly meetings in conference room number 1022, which drew students, residents, and staff. A fellowship program started in the early 1960s. In 1968, a GI division was started with increased staff, all GFT. In this chapter, I discuss procedures such as endoscopy, upper and lower; Crosby Capsule research; gluten free diet, and Flagyl treatment for antibiotic-induced enterocolitis. I founded the Division of Gastroenterology and retired from it in 1988.

In Canada, the establishment of separate divisions in the various disciplines of internal medicine took place largely after 1960. Prior to this, academic centres had an umbrella department of medicine in which attending staff worked in all areas. Many of those physicians had a special interest in one body system, which served as the precursor for the coming development of the subspecialties.[1]

At the MGH, G.W. Halpenny was the first postwar member of the attending staff to take a significant interest in diseases of the digestive tract. He was also physician-in-chief at the Queen Mary Veterans Hospital and very active in medical politics, rising to the presidency of the Canadian Medical Association.

These other commitments prevented him from taking a more active role in GI diseases, but he was still the person one turned to for consultations. When he returned from service with the 14th Canadian Field Hospital after

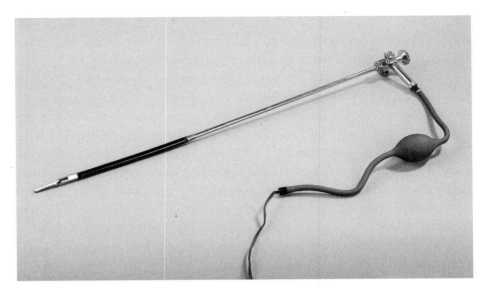

Fig. 8.1 The Eder-Cameron gastroscope used by J.C.G. Young for years until the
GI Service was established in the early 1960s.

the Second World War, he brought back one of the earliest gastroscopes, a
Wolf-Schindler.

Gastroscopy in that era was the equivalent of sword swallowing: the image
was transmitted up from a distal lens/light bulb through a series of lenses,
the main shaft would bend only thirty degrees in one plane, only a side view
was available, biopsies could not be done, and usually the view was confined
to glimpses of the anterior wall of the stomach. Needless to say, the information yield was not great. As a junior intern in 1952, I recall being the head
holder for Young while conducting gastroscopies in the operating room of
the old hospital on Dorchester Street east. I continued this role through residency training in internal medicine and developed an interest in the evolving field of gastroenterology.

I was the last chief resident in medicine, 1956–57, under then chief E.S.
Mills, who was not a strong advocate of subspecialty training. I was left on
my own to pursue my interest in GI. There were no Canadian training programs in GI at that time, and so, with the support of the new incoming chief,
D.G. Cameron, I spent two years in Boston in the Harvard training program
in gastroenterology. Cameron was an advocate, if not the leading innovator,

of the concept of geographic full time, whereby young internists with a bent for academic medicine were given offices in the hospital. He also promoted the concept of clinical teaching units in university hospitals.

Returning to the MGH in 1960, I established a service in GI. The first step was an outpatient clinic held once per week in the medical outdoor consultation service. A parallel indoor consultation service was soon over-subscribed, and a weekly clinical teaching conference, held in room 1022, became one of the best attended and popular teaching sessions in the hospital. Real live patients were wheeled into the conference room, and a multidisciplinary free-for-all would ensue, much to the delight of the residents and medical students. Active participants, apart from the GI attendings, included Alan Thompson, Larry Hampson, and John Hinchey from GI surgery; John Lough from pathology; and Fleming McConnel and (later) France Bourdon from radiology.

I was soon joined by other McGill MD graduates who had done their core training in internal medicine in Montreal followed by further training in diseases of the GI tract in the United States and overseas. D.L. Thomson joined the service in 1963, a highly trained and competent clinician and researcher who had trained in the United Kingdom and at the Karolinska Institute in Sweden. In 1968, he became director of the GI Division when I moved to the McIntyre Building as associate dean of faculty. Thomson's career came to a premature ending in 1970 when illness forced his resignation. He died several years later, and I returned to lead the division.

H.A. Warner, who had trained in GI at the Mayo Clinic, had returned to the staff of the MGH in 1963 and elected to pursue private practice. In 1970, he was persuaded to move from his outside office to a geographic full-time position in the hospital and played a vital role as a clinician and teacher.

Eldon Shaffer, a graduate of Queen's University, came to the MGH for core training in internal medicine and then trained in GI in the MGH program, which he followed up with three years further research in hepatology in Boston, Massachusetts. He then returned to the MGH and joined the attending staff of the GI Division. He was successfully lured away in 1977 to head up the GI Division of the newly formed University of Calgary, where he has had an illustrious career, including serving as chief of medicine and, subsequently, dean of the faculty.

Mansour Jabbari, graduating from the University of Teheran in 1960, and all too aware of the political and social unrest in his country, moved to the United States, where he trained in Buffalo and Jersey City in medicine and

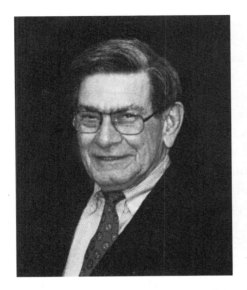
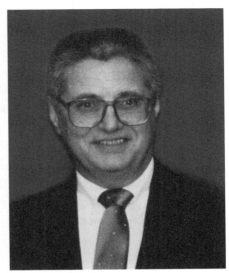

Fig. 8.2 Douglas Kinnear, founder and first director of the Division of Gastroenterology
at the MGH, 1960–88

Fig. 8.3 Carl Goresky, third director of the Division of Gastroenterology, 1988–97.

D.L. Thompson, the second director, 1968–70, was forced to retire after two years
because of chronic illness.

GI. He then moved to Kingston, Ontario, as a fellow in GI and subsequently accepted a position as staff gastroenterologist at the Queen Mary Veterans Hospital in Montreal. He was jointly appointed to the GI Division at the MGH and moved to this site following government closure of the QMVH. He retired in 2000.

Carl Goresky, a graduate of McGill in 1955, joined the staff of the MGH in 1961 and pursued a brilliant career as a career investigator for the Medical Research Council of Canada. Apart from his primary research interests he remained active in the clinical field, his main focus being liver disease. In 1988, he succeeded me as director of the GI Division and encouraged an expansion of research activity in GI disease.

Donald Daly, a native of British Columbia and a graduate of Queen's, came to the MGH in 1966 and did his core training in internal medicine. He then trained in GI in Kingston and returned to the MGH to work in Carl Goresky's lab for one year. He was then recruited to the attending staff of the GI Division at the MGH in 1972 and rapidly achieved a reputation as a no-nonsense first-rate clinician, a superb endoscopist, and an excellent teacher.

After twenty-five years of service he relocated to his native province, settling in Victoria, British Columbia.

Paul Cleland and Raeleen Cherry joined the staff of the GI Division in the 1980s, Cleland as a well trained hepatologist and Cherry as an all-round first-rate consulting clinician. Gary Wild, a superb researcher and excellent clinician, joined the division in 1988 and established his laboratory in the University Clinic on the tenth floor. Valued contributions to the basic understanding of intestinal malabsorption ensued, with the corollary of advancing expertise in the area of inflammatory bowel disease.

The above core of geographic full-time gastroenterologists constituted the GI Division at the MGH from 1960 onward. In addition, Norman Goldberg, who was on the staff of the Jewish General Hospital, was on the part-time staff of the MGH, participating in the endoscopy lab and the GI outpatient clinic.

In its early years, the 1960s, the GI Division endured a somewhat nomadic existence. Endoscopy was a prime example. Gastroenterology at the "old" General, on Dorchester Street east, was conducted in the operating room. This tradition continued with the move in 1955 to the present site, and I recall having to formally book gastroscopies in the daily OR poster, scrub and gown, and later check the patient's status in the recovery room. After several years of this, with no particular administrative blessing we took the bull by the horns and started performing all our gastroscopies in the treatment room on the 10 East Medical Ward.[2]

This worked beautifully, and complications were virtually unknown. Subspecialty beds in the Department of Medicine were not in vogue, the subspecialty attendings acting as internal medicine "rounders" on the medical teaching units. The GI Division attendings were all assigned to 10 East, and this became the hub of our activities. We had no GI nurse at the time, but the assistant head nurse on 10 East, a young woman from Barbados named Olga Clarke, was always willing to help us out during endoscopies. We all got along famously, and finally, when budgets allowed, Clarke joined the GI Division as our first full-time nurse. This was a union made in heaven as Clarke spent the next twenty years working with us, finally retiring in 1993. She was the real heart and soul of the group, and, to this day, one of the first comments from our past staff or residents remains: "How is Olga? Say hello to her for me."

From the 10 East treatment room, endoscopy moved to 6 West, which was then a ward used for concerted medical testing. Then, in the early 1970s, we were finally able to set up a multi-room endoscopy lab on 11 West. Our offices, however, were in Livingston Hall, the old nurses' residence, and this required a lot of to-and-fro travel. After several years on 11 West, a patient floor became available with the closing of the obstetrical unit on 7 West on the Cedar Avenue side of the building. GI moved in and was joined by the Tropical Disease Service and the Division of Respiratory Diseases, and, for the first time, our offices, the GI Clinic, and the endoscopy rooms were adjacent to one another, complemented by a conference room and nurses' office.

The GI endoscopy lab, under the supervision of Daly, became an extremely active area. New techniques became commonplace (e.g., gastroscopy of upper and lower GI bleeds and injection of bleeding sites). Portacaval shunt surgery was rendered obsolete by endoscopic sclerosing injection of esophageal varices. Closed needle biopsy of the liver was initiated in the early 1960s.

Advances in endoscopy were made possible by the introduction of fiberoptic technology in the early 190s, and sentinel articles elaborated on such new entities as Schatzki rings; the watermelon stomach[3] – a key description of the endoscopic appearance of the duodenal mucosa in gluten sensitive enteropathy; and the inlet patch in the upper esophagus. I recall attending "sprue" conferences in the early 1960s and meeting with William Crosby, who had designed the Crosby capsule for peroral biopsy of the upper small bowel. A spare capsule changed hands, and, over the next year, some one hundred patients with adult celiac disease underwent the procedure, the diagnosis was confirmed, and the prescribed gluten-free diet led to resolution of this disabling malabsorption syndrome.[4] Likewise, Jabbari was the first to introduce endoscopic retrograde cholangiopancreatography into the country and became a pioneer in the diagnosis and management of diseases of the biliary tree and pancreas. Cherry was one of the first persons to describe the use of Flagyl (Metronidazole) in the treatment of antibiotic associated diarrhea, or pseudomembranous enterocolitis, and this continues to be the basic treatment for this condition.[5]

The residency training program in gastroenterology was established in the 1960s and was one of the earliest in the country. Quebec certification and Royal College Fellowship accreditation were obtained, and in excess of one hundred trainees subsequently went through the MGH program. The program was merged with that of the Royal Victoria Hospital, our sister McGill hospital, in 1980, and this allowed greater exposure for our trainees. A special bond was established in Quebec City as Laval Faculty of Medicine had elected to forgo establishing a GI training program, and a succession of trainees subsequently came to the MGH and then returned to Quebec City, where they currently constitute a substantial part of the GI cadre.

Of note, is the formation of the Canadian Association of Gastroenterology in June of 1962. I was one of twelve founding members and served as president from 1969 to 1970.

From its formation in the early 1960s, the activities of the GI division focused on service and teaching. I stepped down as director in 1988 and was succeeded by Goresky, whose interests were mainly in the research area. Illness forced Goresky to step down and, in 1997, Alan Barkun was appointed head of the division. Barkun was a McGill graduate and had done his undergraduate and subsequent training in internal medicine and gastroenterology at the MGH. He then obtained his master's in epidemiology, which he followed with additional training in interventional endoscopy in Europe and the United States. The division continued to flourish under his guidance, and new recruits included Baffis, Deschenes, Fallone, Bitton, Parent, and Mayrand.

The staff of the GI Division at the MGH were, and remain, a cohesive group. It was a place where practice and teaching were enjoyed and disagreements were rare. At the end of the twentieth century, the division is strong and the friendly family-like atmosphere of the old General still manifests itself.

NOTES

1 H.E. MacDermot, *The Montreal General Hospital: The Years of Change, 1945–80* (Montreal: Montreal General Hospital, 1970), 27.

2 I.T. Beck. "Canadian Gastroenterology, Yesterday, Today and Tomorrow." *Clinical and Investigative Medicine* 5 (1982): 93–107.

3 M. Jabbari, R. Cherry, J.O. Lough, et al. "Gastric Antral Vascular Ectasia: The Watermelon Stomach," *Gastroenterology* 87 (1984): 1165–70.

4 M. Jabbari, G. Wild, G. Goresky, et al. "Scalloped Valvulae Conniventes: An Endoscopic Marker of Celiac Sprue," *Gastroenterology* 95 (1988): 1518–22.

5 R. Cherry, D. Portnoy, M. Jabbari, et al. "Metronidazole: An Alternate Therapy for Antibiotic Associated Colitis," *Gastroenterology* 87 (1982): 849–51.

9

Geriatrics

Sandra Richardson and Jacqueline McClaran

Sandra Richardson was a staff physician at the beginning of the Division of Geriatrics and its second director. Jacqueline McClaran was the first director of the division.

Introduction

Geriatric medicine is a relatively new subspecialty. The idea of a subspecialty for elderly persons began in the United Kingdom in 1936 when Margery Warren systematically reviewed the cases of several hundred inmates of the workhouse ward of the West Middlesex County Hospital. On the basis of her findings, she advocated the creation of a medical specialty in geriatric medicine as well as the establishment of specialized geriatric units in the general hospitals.

In Canada, the earliest academic interest in aging occurred here at McGill in 1944, when D.E. Cameron, professor of psychiatry, established a gerontological laboratory to study the changes in memory that occur with aging. The first clinical geriatric services were established in Winnipeg in 1963. It wasn't until the early 1980s that the McGill teaching hospitals began to support the development of geriatric services.

Training in the care of the elderly can be obtained in one of two ways. The most common involves three years of training in internal medicine followed by two years of subspecialty training in geriatric medicine. After certification, those recruited by academic hospitals such as the Montreal General Hospital also take further subspecialty training. The first Canadian Royal College subspecialty exams in geriatric medicine were held in 1986. Quebec subspecialists were certified the same year. The second way of obtaining training in the care of the elderly involves spending six to twelve months of Supplementary Training in Care of the Elderly after qualifying in family medicine.

Geriatric Medicine at the MGH

In 1981, Phil Gold, chief of medicine, established an allocation of beds on 16 West as an extended care service (i.e., patients awaiting placement in a nursing home) with a mandate to initiate geriatric services. L. McCallum was the initial service chief. John Rostant, in turn, became service chief in 1983. Ann Smith was the head nurse.

In 1983, Jacqueline McClaran was recruited by Gold to develop a program of "gerontology" at the General – that is, a comprehensive geriatric service with an inpatient unit, outpatient services, research, as well as consults to outlying regions concerning health care delivery to the frail elderly.

In 1986, the Division of Geriatric Medicine within the Department of Medicine was formally established, with McClaran as director. Over the next few years, the organization of the inpatient unit was reorganized and a team consult service was put in place in the ER. At that time, Richard Monks was appointed director of geriatric psychiatry and became an integral part of the service. Three geriatricians – Julian Falutz, Elliot Kravitz, and Michael Bonnycastle – were recruited.

The Community Consult Team

One of McClaran's outstanding achievements was the manner in which she created the Community Consult Team in 1983–84. At that time, the Home Care Services provided by local community service centres were restricted to nurses with a small number of social workers who had little expertise in the assessment and care of the frail elderly. McClaran was able to obtain government funding to create an outpatient consult team with a nurse, physiotherapist, occupational therapist, and social worker. Several family physicians provided the medical input. When a consult was requested by a physician, nurse, or social worker from the local community, two team members would assess the patient in his or her home. The purpose of a general geriatric assessment is to evaluate not only the physical and mental health of the patients referred but also to assess their social situation and their relative safety in that setting as well as their ability to make decisions to protect their best interests. For this reason, a home evaluation is invaluable. The homes visited varied from the poorest, dirtiest apartments to huge Westmount mansions or even to someone living at the Ritz Carlton. Not surprisingly, this has resulted in very colourful and challenging situations. For example, on one home visit to a high-rise on Peel Street, when the physician and the occupational therapist got off the elevator there was smoke billowing out of the patient's door. She had very bad rheumatoid arthritis deformities in her hands and had set her mattress on fire while lighting a cigarette. She was trying to put it out with a little pot of water. They called firefighters, who came and threw the mattress out the window into the snow. It seems that's the only thing to do with a burning mattress. When the firefighters left, the physician and OT then spent quite some time on the phone trying to find a place for the woman to stay until she could get a new bed. They finally found La Porte du Ciel in Old Montreal, but she refused to go and insisted she was fine where she was. They finally left her there after having taken her cigarettes and matches away and threatened the depanneur across the street with the police if it sold her any more cigarettes. They heard afterwards that she had spent the night riding the elevator and bumming cigarettes from neighbours.

Such situations, in which the professional must tread a fine line between a patient's safety and his or her legal right to autonomy, arise not infrequently. It can sometimes be heart-wrenching to witness a patient's vulnerability but not have enough evidence to legally take away her/his rights for her/his own protection. Even being in a nursing home does not always protect a patient from him or herself. Ferrier was once asked to see a very demented woman in a small private nursing home in NDG. One of the employees had called the patient's cousins in Ontario, told them that he was travelling to where they lived, and asked if they would like him to bring the patient for a visit. They thought that this was a very thoughtful, generous offer and agreed. After the visit, on the way back to Montreal, he stopped off in Cornwall, where he married the patient. His cousin conveniently happened to be there to serve as a witness. Ferrier was asked to evaluate her mental competence to consent to the marriage after it had occurred. When asked who this man was, the patient replied, "I don't know." The "husband" said: "Don't you remember? I'm your husband and you love me." So she replied: "He's my husband and I love him." There was no evidence of abuse or neglect, and the cousins in Ontario did nothing to intervene. In the end, the "husband" left her in a public nursing home and took off with her savings.

The Inpatient Unit on 16 West

Although 16 West may have initially served as an extended care unit, it quickly evolved into a geriatric rehabilitation unit. At that time, outside rehab hospitals had strict admission criteria and would not admit the frail elderly. This unit was organized to answer this need. The ward was divided into a rehab service, which had the majority of beds plus four beds reserved for admissions for geriatric assessment upon referral by the Community Consult Team, as well as four beds reserved for those patients referred by the geriatric team in the ER.

Inpatient Consults

A geriatric consult service provided by the staff geriatricians has been available since 1983. For a period of time, there was also a geriatric team in the ER, consisting of a geriatrician, nurse, physiotherapist, and an OT. In 1998–90 there were 902 consults. Due to budget constraints, the team was later disbanded. Since that time the ER had been staffed by a geriatric nurse consultant with consults from geriatricians as needed.

Consultation to Regional Services

At a time when regional health care services didn't have access to geriatric expertise, McClaran also served as a consultant in analyzing the resource needs of the elderly in Temiskcaming, Ormstown-Huntington, and Mont Laurier.

The Service Evolves

In 1992, McClaran became discharge planning officer for the Montreal General Hospital, and Sandra Richardson became service chief of geriatric medicine. George Kuchel was also recruited to the service at this time.

In 1995, the administration of the MGH, the Royal Victoria Hospital, the Montreal Chest Hospital, the Montreal Neurological Hospital, the Montreal Children's Hospital, and the Allen Memorial Hospital combined into the McGill University Health Centre. Although the leadership of the geriatric service changed over the subsequent years, the geriatric service at the MGH has continued to evolve in response to the changing needs of the patients, hospital, and community.

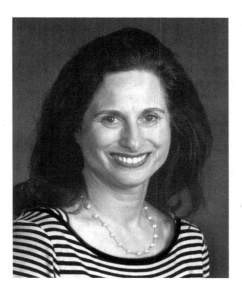

Fig. 9.1 Jacqueline McClaran, first director of the Division of Geriatric Medicine, 1986–92

Outpatient Services

By 1992, when Richardson became service chief, the needs of the community health care workers for geriatric consultation had changed. The community CLSC services had expanded to include physio- and occupational therapists who were able to provide their own home assessments and treatments. The expertise of the community workers in caring for the frail elderly had also increased, in part as a consequence of the monthly McGill Geriatric Rounds as well as the collaborative teaching over cases referred to the Community Consult Team. The physiotherapy and occupational therapists were therefore transferred to the inpatient unit, where they were greatly needed.

While the outpatient "general geriatric assessments" have continued to be requested, subspecialty clinics have also been developed in response to need. As a result, the Community Consult Team continues to expand under the management of Guylaine Bachand, who became the nurse on the team in 1990.

Urinary Incontinence

The first geriatric subspecialty clinic was started by George Kuchel in 1993. The demand was great and the size of the clinic increased exponentially until Kuchel accepted a position at the University of Connecticut in 2000. The service has been continued on a part-time basis by Cara Tannenbaum.

Memory Clinic

Gary Inglis started the Memory Clinic in 1998. Patients with cognitive problems, or those who are concerned that they may be developing a problem,
are referred for assessment. Lisa Koski, a neuropsychologist, joined the service in 2004. This has provided the opportunity to more precisely document
the areas of strength and weakness in the patient's cognitive ability and has
also assisted in diagnosis. Providing counselling to patients and families as
well as linkages to community resources are also a part of the service.

In 2008, with funding support from the Alzheimer's Society, Guylaine
Bachand led a family support group for care-givers of patients with cognitive impairment.

Pain in the Elderly

In 2003, David Lussier returned from three years of training in New York to
set up the Geriatric Pain Clinic. He works in collaboration with the pain
service already in place at the General. The demand for this service has
grown exponentially since its initiation.

Competency

Catherine Ferrier, who has been on the Community Consult Team since
1984, provides a consultation service to help patients with cognitive impairment deal with issues of "competency" from a legal and ethical perspective.

The Inpatient Service

In 1993, the Geriatric Unit moved from 16 West to 13 East. The mandate of
the inpatient unit is to provide a holistic approach not only to the medical
needs of the patient but also to their psychosocial and rehabilitation needs.
A creative approach is often necessary. To give just one example, when a confused elderly man who had habitually eaten lunch every day at the Ritz refused to eat in hospital, his family wisely arranged for his customary waiter
to bring his favourite food and personally serve him for several days until he
started to eat again. Caregivers often become part of the treating team in arriving at innovative solutions to help patients. Unfortunately, in rare case,
they can also be part of the problem, which presents an added burden when
attempting to assure the patient's well-being. Legal protection from so-called
caregivers has to be arranged if a serious problem is identified. In such in-
stances, collaboration with community social corkers is invaluable.

The Patient Population
Over the almost three decades since the Geriatric Unit was started in 1981, the patient population admitted to it has become much older as well as more medically unstable and functionally disabled. The service has evolved in response to these changing needs. In many respects, the unit now looks more like an acute medical ward. Happily, at the same time, many of the aspects of the geriatric approach have been adopted in medicine, orthopaedics, and surgery.

Rehabilitation on the Geriatric Unit
The Inpatient Geriatric Unit on 13 East was the first unit at the General to institute the concept of early mobilization and functional assessment both at the bedside and on the unit. We were fortunate in obtaining a donation from John Cole, which gave us the opportunity of creating a small gym on the unit. Previously, a porter had to transfer patients by wheelchair from the sixteenth floor to the second-floor gym for their therapy, after which they had to wait for a porter to take them back to the unit. The severity of illness and disability of the patients increased over the years until, by 1993, most were too frail to make this arduous trip. With the institution of a small gym on the unit, short sessions of rehab appropriate to the stamina of the patient could be instituted either in the gym or at the bedside. The early mobilization and assessment of self-care needs also resulted in more timely discharge. Although the Geriatric Ward was the first to have a gym, the benefits were obvious and the practice soon became standard on other wards.

Demonstrating That the Most Disabled Can Also Benefit
Beginning in 1993, all patients admitted to the Geriatric Unit were assessed for their cognitive and functional ability through the use of the four short standardized measures of the McGill Geriatric Profile at admission and discharge. At the time, most geriatric services, both in practice and in the literature, were targeting geriatric rehabilitation services for those with mild to moderate disability in the belief that severely disabled patients would be unable to benefit. The Geriatric Unit on 13 East admitted patients of all levels of disability. After three years the data were analyzed by Karen Beazley, the physiotherapist. They showed that even those with the most severe disability benefited from a geriatric rehab approach. Most improved their level of independence, which resulted in improved self-esteem and a significant

decrease on caregiver burden. Forty percent of those who were in the lowest functional category at the time of admission were eventually discharged into the community.

Equally important, the data showed that patients with significant cognitive impairment could also benefit from a specialized geriatric approach. These informal studies played an important role in changing the approach towards the most vulnerable group of elderly patients both at McGill and elsewhere in Canada.

Pharmacy
In 2004, Louise Papillon, a pharmacist with specialty training in medications for the elderly, joined the team on the Geriatric Unit. She has played an essential role in the education of physicians, nurses, students, patients, and their families as well as in the prevention of medication errors.

Donors and Volunteers

By 1993, in spite of the excellent nursing and rehab team, patients and their families were still often reluctant to be transferred to "Geriatrics." This was partly due to the fact that the term "geriatric" signified old age, and many declared that they did not want to be with "old people." The run-down appearance of the Geriatric Unit was also a major hurdle.

The Helen McCall Hutchison Fund, set up by her family in memory of one of the founding members of the Women's Auxiliary, provided the opportunity to renovate the nursing station, conference/family meeting room, and the patient dining room. The inspiration for the project came from Helen Hutchson's daughter, Janet Hutchison.

To finish off the renovation, another Women's Auxiliary member and former MGH nurse, Jean Bradwell, spoke to Fred Burbage, chair and CEO of CP Rail, about our need. He, in turn, explained our problem to Tania Richie, head of CP Rail Volunteers. After seeing the state of the unit for herself, she organized forty-three volunteer painters, including the executives, to spend five weekends repainting the entire ward. When finished, the unit was the most attractive in the hospital at the time and a great buffer against the negative connotations of the word "geriatric." Gradually, patients and families were asking to be transferred to "Geriatrics." It was also a wonderful boost to staff morale.

The Geriatric Unit continues to benefit from its donors. Since 1995, the Levinschi Foundation has been an invaluable resource for innovative projects that would otherwise not have been be possible. Pilot projects, such as having a senior nurse as coordinator of care of the elderly (including transfer of care to the transitional care unit), were initially funded by the Levinschi Foundation and later, after the value of the position had been demonstrated, picked up by the hospital. We have also been able to initiate nutrition and mobility projects, a pilot project to demonstrate the value of a pharmacist on the unit, and support for a database. The outpatient Incontinence Clinic and Pain Clinic have also been supported. A small sum is available each year for those patients who cannot afford such items as foot care or special shoes. This support has made an invaluable contribution to the well-being of the elderly patients at the MGH.

Since 1987, each year the Helen McCall Hutchison Foundation provides research funding for projects related to aging or the care of the elderly. This funding goes to two young investigators who are at the beginning of their careers. Many scientific careers have been made possible because researchers were provided the opportunity to obtain the initial data that enabled them to apply for further funding from large national agencies.

In 1994, the first Janet Hutchison Lectureship was held in Livingston Hall. Every year an internationally renowned leader in geriatric medicine is invited to speak and to participate in seminars related to his or her specialty.

Our Community Partners

A regular geriatric consult service is provided to the Montreal Extended Care Hospital as well as to the Catherine Booth Hospital and the Julius Richardson Rehabilitation Hospital. We have also participated in the planning of the services to the elderly at Centres de santé et de services sociaux Cavendish.

"An Elderly Friendly Hospital"

While 9.2 percent of the population is over the age of sixty-five, this age group accounts for 28 percent of hospital admissions and 63 percent of bed-days. These numbers are expected to increase dramatically in the coming years. Those over the age of eighty-five are the fastest-growing segment of the population.

The reason for the greater number of admissions and longer hospital stays of the elderly is related to the increasing prevalence of chronic disease and disability that occurs with age. In spite of a small but significant decrease in functional disability in the elderly over the past few decades, the facts concerning our declining years remain sobering. There is little general awareness that only 15 to 20 percent of us will remain relatively well and fit until we die suddenly or after a short illness. Most of us will be unable to avoid a significant period of disability in our last years of life. Perhaps of even greater concern is the fact that the prevalence of dementia in Canada has been shown to rises exponentially with age, reaching 29 percent in men and 37 percent in women over the age of eighty-five. This means that a significant proportion of elderly patients are already disabled – either physically, cognitively, or both – at the time of admission. It has also been well documented that elderly patients admitted to hospital are at high risk of becoming acutely confused (delirious) or more functionally disabled during their stay. In some cases, they are no longer capable of returning to their homes and, as a result, remain in hospital for a prolonged period.

While the care of the elderly at the MGH has improved significantly over the past twenty-five years, much remains to be done. *The new MUHC must be an "elderly friendly hospital" – medically, culturally, and architecturally.* The goal is to provide a safe and effective milieu for those admitted who are already disabled, to prevent new confusion or disability from occurring while in hospital, and to promote a timely discharge to an appropriate setting – optimally, a return home. Treatment must be tailored to the needs of each individual patient rather than rely on a textbook approach focused solely on diagnosis and treatment. Recent advances in the field of geriatric medicine provide an opportunity to address these challenges.

In 1985, 16 East was converted into a long-term care ward for patients awaiting transfer to a nursing home. This service is situated within the Division of Internal Medicine, with Alex Miller as service chief and Cathy Robinson as head nurse.

10

Haematology

John H. Burgess

No haematologist was able to write this chapter. John Burgess authored it with the help of Cindy Lee, a long-time senior secretary in the Division of Haematology. Laurence Hutchison, the second director of the division, read and approved the manuscript.

Haematology became a division of the Department of Medicine at the Montreal General Hospital in 1957. It originated with the University Medical Clinic. Prior to this, Edward Mills had established a very small laboratory in 1925 at the old Central Division on Dorchester Street, with the encouragement of Campbell P. Howard who, after a notable career at the University of Iowa, returned to his alma mater to become professor of medicine at McGill University and director of the Department of Medicine at the MGH. Mills was Howard's first resident and the first physician to have an interest in haematology. In his laboratory, blood counts and differential counts of the white cells were made by hand. Hematocrits were determined and red cell indices calculated. The blood bank was part of the Pathology Department at the Central Division.

When the move to the new MGH Mountain site occurred in 1955, both the blood bank and haematology labs were located on the fifth floor, Pine Avenue wing of the building directly over the boiler room. Mills had now become physician-in-chief at the MGH. Stuart R. Townsend, Mills's last resident, then became the first chief of the newly created Division of Haematology. In a note behind a photograph of Mills in the Haematology Conference Room, Townsend writes as follows: "After serving as a resident interne [sic] at The Montreal General Hospital, he [Campbell Howard] went to John's [sic] Hopkins Hospital where he served under William Osler. He then studied in Munich, Berlin, Paris and London. A man of vigorous physique and giant intellectual

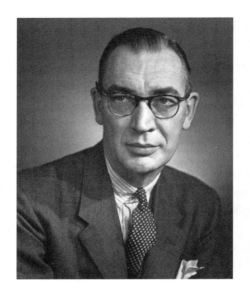

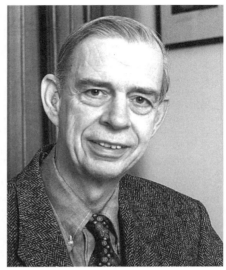

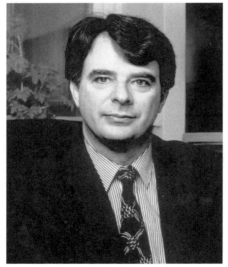

Clockwise from top left
Fig. 10.1 Stewart Townsend, first director
of the Division of Haematology, 1955–72
Fig. 10.2 J. Lawrence Hutchison, second
director of Division of Haematology,
1972–92
Fig. 10.3 Jacques Leclerc, director of
Division of Haematology, 1992–97

distinction he was especially known to me, his last resident, for his human
qualities as a wise friend and counsellor. His support in founding a laboratory in Hematology almost 50 years ago, in the presence of not a little opposition, is gratefully acknowledged by the present Division of Hematology of
the Department of Medicine."[1]

In addition to bringing the laboratory and blood bank into the modern
era, Townsend greatly expanded the clinical services. The haematology con-

sulting service became very active, and an anticoagulant clinic was established. The latter was particularly important as warfarin treatment became
available for patients with thrombotic disorders, artificial heart valves, and
cardiac irregularities. Townsend retired as director of the division in 1972
and J. Lawrence Hutchison succeeded him.[2]

Hutchison recalls the early days in the new laboratories:

> The lab was hotter than hell with no air conditioning – it did not im-
> prove the quality of the work or the disposition of the working staff.
> Differential staining of blood smears was introduced and counts re-
> ported, when requested. Red cell indices were calculated by hand, when
> requested. Since the red cell counts were unreliable, the hemoglobin
> little better, and the hematocrit read carelessly, the indices were far
> from reliable. I might add that the technical staff were straight out of
> high school, with no training and little motivation to improve their
> skills. Most of the lab discussions were about social dates etc. The blood
> bank was fortunate to have a chief tech from England who was trained
> and competent. At least one or two other blood bank techs had some
> training. Thank God for that or we would have lost patients.[3]

There was a rumour, not confirmed by Hutchison, that some technicians,
in addition to spending their spare time discussing social activities, also set
up an apparatus to distil alcohol for personal consumption. Fortunately, the
beginning of the Quebec Colleges d'Enseignment Generale et Practiques
system, requiring two years of further education after high school, resulted
in improved formal training in all areas of medical technology.

An important occurrence during the Hutchison era was the development
of bone marrow transplantation. Witold Rybka was director of this program
from 1990 to 1991.[4] The first marrow transplant in Quebec was performed
on the seventeenth floor of the MGH. Unfortunately, a decision was made
to move organ transplants to the Royal Victoria Hospital, and Rybka left for
the University of Pittsburgh in 1991.

Hutchison was director of haematology for twenty years and oversaw
many advances in clinical services, laboratory techniques, and research. During his tenure, Geoffrey Blake (associate director of haematology), Denis
Cournoyer (a Quebec Chercheur–Boursier trained in molecular genetics),
Susan Solymoss, and Linda Lacroix were recruited to the division. Another
senior member, Blair Whittemore, took over the blood bank and later became

the director of professional services at the MGH. Hutchison stepped down in 1992 and was replaced by Jacques Leclerc from McMaster University, where he had made major contributions to the field of thrombosis. Leclerc resigned in 1997, and the leadership passed to a McGill director when the McGill University Medical Centre was established.

NOTES

1 Note on Edward Mills by S.R. Townsend on back of picture in Haematology Conference Room, seventh floor, MGH.
2 Personal Communication, Cindy Lee, secretary of Division of Haematology.
3 Personal Communication, Lawrence J. Hutchison.
4 Minutes, Division of Haematology, 31 January 1990, seventh floor, MGH.
5 Ibid., 2 September 1992.

11

Infectious Disease

Michael Libman

Michael Libman was a director of the Division of Infectious Diseases and was instrumental in its early development.

The Division of Infectious Diseases is one of the youngest divisions created at the MGH. Indeed, as a specialty, it was only recognized by the Royal College of Physicians and Surgeons in 1980. Until that point, infections were simply part of general medicine, and, indeed, in the pre-antibiotic era much of internal medicine involved the diagnosis and management of infections. The various more severe or complex infections were handled mostly by specialists in the organ systems involved as well as by generalists. In some cases, by convention, certain specialties became responsible for infections outside of their "organ system." For example, sexually transmitted infections became the domain of urologists in the United Kingdom and dermatologists in many other countries. The emergence of progressive antimicrobial resistance and the introduction of multiple new antibiotic classes in the late 1960s and early 1970s led to increasing complexity in the management of infections. In addition, around the same time, there was an increasing prevalence of iatrogenic immunosuppression, largely driven by aggressive new anti-neoplastic therapies as well as treatments for various auto-immune conditions. This, in turn, led to the emergence of many new and/or poorly described pathogens, and increasingly unusual presentations related to previously known agents. These phenomena highlighted the commonalities among many types of pathogens, regardless of the organ system or systems involved, and led to the notion of a specialty in diagnosis and treatment of infections in general.

The Concept of a Specialty in Infectious Diseases

In most of the country, the job of diagnosing and treating complex infectious problems fell at first to the medical microbiologist. In many areas, microbiologists were not MDs, and their clinical experience was limited. In Quebec, however, a more European model was followed, whereby most microbiologists were MDs and had clinical as well as laboratory training, and microbiologists became prominent consultants for infection-related problems in all the major hospitals in the province. At the MGH, the first microbiologist to take an active role consulting on the medical wards was Geoff Richards, who arrived from the United Kingdom in the late 1960s. He was later joined by David Portnoy, who had trained in Belgium, returned to work at the MGH as a microbiologist in 1974, and established an active outpatient consultation service as well as seeing inpatients. In this, he followed in the footsteps of his brother, who established a similar practice at the Jewish General Hospital.

At the Royal Victoria, Hugh Robson, who had trained in infectious diseases in the United States, began working to have the specialty recognized in Canada and at McGill. However, at the MGH, consultations in infectious diseases took a different tack. Through the 1970s the medical specialty of clinical pharmacology developed a strong presence in the hospital. The idea was that the increasing complexity of pharmacotherapy, especially in the field of antibiotics, required specialists who understood pharmacokinetics, pharmacodynamics, and the mechanisms of action of the multitude of newly available agents. Thus, generalists and other specialists commonly sent people who needed consults for complex infections either to microbiologists or to the Division of Clinical Pharmacology. At the same time, the MGH began developing expertise in tropical medicine and the related microbiological specialty of clinical parasitology. The McGill Centre for Tropical Medicine was established in 1980 and was given divisional status within the Department of Medicine. Infections thought to be "imported" by immigrants and travellers were dealt with by this rapidly growing and highly reputed unit.

The Specialty of Infectious Disease at McGill and the MGH

The specialty of infectious diseases was established in the United States in the early 1970s. After the Royal College of Physicians and Surgeons formally established the specialty of infectious diseases in 1980, the first Montrealers who had trained in the United States (including Hugh Robson from the Royal

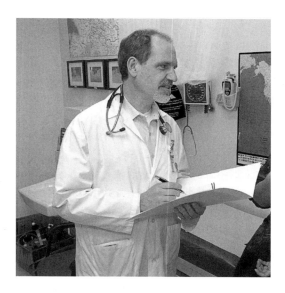

Fig. 11.1 Michael Libman, director of the Division of Infectious Diseases and Department of Microbiology, 1996–2005

Victoria and Jack Mendelson from the Jewish General) returned to their respective hospitals in Canada. At the MGH, this service continued to be controlled by the Department of Microbiology and the Division of Clinical Immunology until the arrival of Francois Lebel in 1984. Lebel had trained in microbiology in Quebec as well as in infectious diseases in Boston. The Division of Infectious Diseases at the MGH was formed by Phil Gold around Portnoy and Lebel, with part-time help from new Canadian trainee Kathleen Knowles. Richards participated in the provision of service but did not formally join the division. The Division of Infections Diseases swiftly began adding personnel as the clinical pharmacology service began to lose members and influence in this domain. Brian Ward, who was also trained in infectious diseases in the United States, returned to complete his training in medical microbiology but worked primarily in the Tropical Disease Centre with Dick MacLean as well as the parasitology lab, which was functioning independently of the general microbiology lab.

MGH Division of Infectious Diseases

From this point onwards, the Division of Infectious Diseases steadily grew, always by recruiting physicians who were also trained in medical microbiology. Lebel became head of the division and recruited Mark Miller in 1988, the first combined infectious disease/medical microbiologist at the MGH to have trained in both specialties at McGill. There was a lull when Richards left to practise in Saskatchewan, Lebel chose to continue his career in industry, and Miller left to bolster the new division at the Jewish General.

Michael Libman joined part-time in 1992, coming from St Mary's Hospital, then became full time in 1994. He was named interim head of the division as well as the Department of Microbiology in 1996 on the departure of Lebel. During almost nine years as interim head, Libman expanded the division by formally bringing in Brian Ward as well as Vivian Loo from the Royal Victoria and Pierre Lebel from Ste Justine Hospital. He also began formal negotiations for merging the clinical microbiology services at the Royal Victoria (which had been based in the McGill University Department of Microbiology across University Street) and the Montreal Children's Hospital as well as the divisions of infectious diseases in the two adult hospitals. He also organized the incorporation of the Division of Tropical Diseases into the Division of Infectious Diseases, and the parasitology lab into the Department of Microbiology, although the latter two remained functionally independent under Dick MacLean.

MUHC Division of (All) Infectious Diseases

As of 2013, the now combined MUHC Division of Infectious Diseases is made up of sixteen physicians, with nationally and internationally recognized specialists in all branches of the specialty, including tropical medicine, mycobacterial infections, fungal infections, vaccination, epidemiology, infection control, and the immunology of infectious diseases. The division, including medical scientists cross-appointed from several specialties, is one of the most productive in terms of research of any in the Department of Medicine, also providing leadership in education and administrative roles at the university both regionally and internationally.

12

Medical Genetics

David Rosenblatt

David Rosenblatt was the first director of the Division of Medical Genetics. He brought it to international prominence.

Medical genetics as a clinical discipline has its roots in basic science departments. At McGill, Clarke Fraser pioneered the area of clinical genetics at the Montreal Children's Hospital, starting in the 1950s. For a long time there had been an attempt to initiate activities in "adult genetics" at the McGill teaching hospitals. Leaders in human genetics and medicine initiated a search for someone to head such an activity about five years before the division was established. Leonard Pinsky, the head of the Centre for Human Genetics at McGill – with the support of Peter Macklem, physician-in-chief at the Royal Victoria Hospital; Roger Hand, director of the McGill Cancer Centre; and Dean Sam Freedman – attempted to recruit George Sack for this position in 1981. In 1984, the Toronto General Hospital approached David Rosenblatt, who at the time was a medical geneticist at the Montreal Children's Hospital, to establish a genetic service. The seeds for the development of a division of medical genetics in the Department of Medicine at the MGH were sown in a May 1985 letter from Rosenblatt to Phil Gold, physician-in-chief at the MGH. In this letter Rosenblatt states: "the very presence of a geneticist in the department will encourage both the staff and the trainees to think in terms of heterogeneity and the uniqueness of each patient's genetic/environmental interaction."[1]

During the fall of 1985, discussions among Phil Gold, Peter Macklem, Dean Richard Cruess, Harvey Barkun, Mr Steven Herbert, and Joseph Shuster resulted in the following proposal: "to open, at the earliest possible time, Genetic Counselling Services at the M.G.H. and the R.V.H. in areas

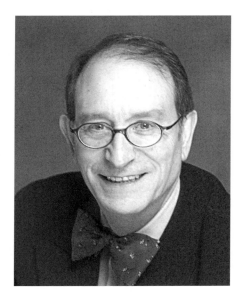

Fig. 12.1 David Rosenblatt, first director of
Medical Genetics, MGH, 1985 to the present

of clinical strength and interest … that would allow for interfaces with clinical investigation and basic biomedical studies."[2] This resulted in a proposal
from Dean Cruess: "Drs. Macklem and Gold will, with great enthusiasm,
create at both the levels of the Department of Medicine and within both
Hospital departments, a formal Division of Adult Genetics equivalent to
existing divisions."[3]

The initial space for the new division was a locker in the physicians'
locker room at the MGH. With time, the clinical service migrated from the
fourth floor of Livingston Hall to the ninth floor of the main hospital to
the eighth floor of Livingston Hall before finally settling on the tenth floor
of Livingston Hall. With the announcement of the creation of the Adult
Medical Genetics Service at the MGH, the first Division of Medical Genetics in a department of medicine in Canada was established. David Rosenblatt was appointed as its founding director, a position he holds to this day
(August 2015).

The first year saw the hiring of Shari Miller (MS, Sarah Lawrence) as the
first genetic counsellor in the adult service, Estelle Lamothe (MS, Utah) as
the clinical laboratory manager and biologist, and Maria Materniak as the
shared secretary. Access to clinical space for one day per week was arranged
with the generous support of Shuster in the Division of Allergy and Immunology. This clinic arrangement has persisted to this day.

As the determination of the location of laboratory space had not been finalized, the clinical laboratory was initially located in the Stewart Biology Building of McGill University. Techniques were set up for the study of families with adult polycystic kidney disease and haemophilia. The original intent was to put Rosenblatt's research laboratory in the Royal Victoria Hospital and the clinical laboratory in the MGH. A substantial amount of the funding for the research laboratory was to come from funds requested by Charles Scriver as part of the Medical Research Council of Canada Group in Medical Genetics, of which Rosenblatt was a principal investigator.

Due to the evacuation of National Research Council space, W.D. Dauphinee, the physician-in-chief at the RVH, proposed that "a total of approximately 2,000 sq. ft. which would include the original promised space for research but also the displacement of the service lab from the Montreal General ... be assigned to Medical Genetics."[4] This established the structure that was to remain in force until the formal creation of the McGill University Health Centre and the eventual move of the laboratory to the MGH site. The space was identified in the Hersey Building of the RVH on H5, adjacent to the Ludwig Institute in Cancer Genetics. As noted, funds for new construction and the outfitting of the laboratory came from a number of sources, including the MGH, the RVH, the Medical Research Council of Canada, and the Faculty of Medicine. No space for the clinical services, except for the laboratory, was provided at the RVH. At the MGH, four small offices were eventually provided on Livingston 10.

A major event in the life of the division was the donation of $1 million to McGill University to establish the Hess and Diane Finestone Laboratory in memory of Jacob and Jenny Finestone. This endowment's purpose is to promote activities in the area of medical genetics at McGill and, in particular, to support the laboratory activities of David Rosenblatt. Mr Finestone made this donation in honour of his fiftieth birthday, and a plaque commemorating this donation, which was made in 1988, still hangs in the laboratory on Livingston 3 at the MGH. A website for the Finestone Laboratory was established. and all the division's annual reports may be found at www.mcgill.ca/finestone.

One of the division's first initiatives was to become the Quebec centre for predictive testing for Huntington disease. A national structure had been created in Canada, its base being at the University of British Columbia. The national collaborative study on the predictive testing for Huntington disease was activated in Quebec in 1989 with the hiring of Suzanne Dufrasne, MPs, as clinical coordinator. A portion of her salary initially came from the National Study, but she was subsequently funded, first, by a transition grant from les Fonds de la Recherche en Sante du Quebec and, later, by the Finestone Endowment. The Montreal component of this national study consisted of Eva Andermann, MD, PhD; Vema Bound, PSW; Suzanne Dufrasne, MPs; Estelle Lamothe, MS; Shari Miller, MS; Paul Pepin, MD; David Rosenblatt, MD; Madeline Roy, MD; and Ghislaine Savard, MD. This team combined health professionals from both the McGill and University of Montreal systems. At that time, genetic counselling for adult polycystic kidney disease was introduced as a clinical service, and the laboratory provided predictive testing for this disease in facilities in which linkage studies were possible.

The year 1989 marked the recruitment of Guy Rouleau to the Division of Neurology of the MGH with a cross-appointment in medical genetics, providing expertise in gene mapping in conjunction with facilities for the establishment of permanent lymphoblast cell lines for the indefinite storage of genetic material from large kindreds. Rouleau went on to become one of the most prominent neurogeneticists in Canada, identifying a large number of genes involved in inherited neurological disease.

The most significant accomplishment of 1991 occurred in the area of recruitment. Steven Narod became the first physician recruited to the division to conduct research and service in the area of cancer genetics. This was a turning point for the Division, establishing it as a leader in both Quebec and Canada in the area of hereditary cancer. Narod had received his medical degree at the University of British Columbia. After training in community medicine, he completed a fellowship in genetics at the Hospital for Sick Children in Toronto, followed by two years at the International Agency for Research on Cancer in Lyons, France. Patricia Tonin, PhD, joined Narod as a fellow in 1993 and began working on the search for the breast/ovarian cancer gene.[5]

During this period, the molecular diagnostic laboratory continued to offer testing for the molecular diagnosis of myotonic dystrophy and adult polycystic kidney disease by linkage analysis as well as for apolipoprotein E disorders and MEN2. A thriving neurogenetics clinic with Rouleau and Shari Miller operated at the MGH. Thanks to the work of Paul Goodyear, a nephrologist based at the Montreal Children's Hospital, a genetics/bone clinic maintained regular activity at the MGH. The major function of this clinic was the management of patients who had been followed since childhood in the Quebec Network for Genetic Medicine. Theresa Rheade, a nurse with extensive experience with these patients, was instrumental in maintaining the viability of this clinic. With her departure, the clinic was integrated into the MGH's regular renal clinic in 1992.

One of the most exciting things to happen during this period at McGill was that concrete steps were beginning to be taken to convert the Centre for Human Genetics into the Department of Medical Genetics. This was finalized in 1993. The department is considered both a basic science and a clinical department in the Faculty of Medicine.

Because of the rapid growth in counselling activities, approval was given for a second genetic counsellor, and Ophira Ginsburgh, MSc, was hired in 1991. She served for several years with great distinction before leaving to return to medical school and eventually training as a medical oncologist.

Nineteen ninety-one and 1992 marked the years in which Dana Lasko, PhD, and David Watkins, PhD, were hired as assistant professors in the division. Lasko had an interest in DNA replication and, at that time, Watkins was involved with linkage analysis and worked closely with Rouleau. After several years, Lasko left McGill, but Watkins has continued to play a major role in the Vitamin BJ2 diagnostic laboratory and, with Rosenblatt, in the investigations of inborn errors of folate and cobalamin metabolism. In addition, Laura Humphries became the first full-time clinical secretary in the Division of Medical Genetics at the MGH site, joining Yasmin Karim, the administrative secretary based at the RVH site.

Ken Morgan, PhD, moved his laboratory to the MGH in 1992. He and Mary Fujiwara, MS, moved into offices on Livingston 10, adjacent to those of Narod. This provided a critical mass of investigators at the MGH in the area of linkage analysis, population genetics, and genetic epidemiology. This concentration of excellence in such a highly sought-after area of research was a major accomplishment of the Division of Medical Genetics.

Brian Gilfix was appointed to the faculty in medical biochemistry in 1993 and was cross-appointed in medical genetics. Over the years, Gilfix introduced testing for a number of genetic conditions and played a major role in developing molecular diagnosis in the two divisions. Eleanor Elstein was recruited by cardiology and also given a cross appointment in human genetics. Paul Matthews was recruited to the Montreal Neurological Hospital; his interest was in mitochondrial disease. He maintained an affiliation with the division before being recruited back to the United Kingdom.

The year 1994–95 was one of great accomplishment in the area of research. Steven Narod and his postdoctoral fellow at that time, Patricia Tonin, were co-authors of a paper in published in *Science* describing the successful isolation of a gene BRCA1 (responsible for hereditary breast and ovarian cancer C 4). This gene had been the object of an international hunt since 1990, when its existence was first suggested on the basis of the study of families with early onset cancer. The discovery of BRCA 1 received a great deal of attention in the press and was highlighted in *McGill News* in a story entitled "Race of Life."[6]

Because of the close interaction between the clinical and research activities of the Division of Medical Genetics, methodology for the detection of additional affected members in families in which the first mutation had been found was successfully transferred to the clinical laboratory. Procedures were established whereby genetic counselling and the results of molecular testing for hereditary cancer susceptibility could be provided to families at risk. The year 1994–95 was a year of transition for the clinical service. Shari Miller, MS, the first and, for a long time, only, genetic counsellor of the division took a leave of absence and moved to Florida. Ophira Ginsburg, MSc, also took a leave of absence to attend medical school at Queen's University. Three new graduates of the McGill program in genetic counselling were hired: Corinne Serruya, MSc; Gordon Glendon, MSc; and Chia Chia Sun, MSc. In the clinical laboratory, Estelle Lamothe, MSc, took a leave of absence because of illness. Her replacement, Maria Galvez, has occupied this position since that time. This year also saw the introduction of PCR-based testing for Huntington disease, removing the requirement for linkage analysis. The defect in Huntington disease had been shown to be associated with an expansion of a triplet repeat of the nucleotides CAG. Because virtually all Huntington disease patients have the expansion, testing became possible for confirmation of diagnosis as well as for predictive testing.

The year 1995–96 saw a great scientific accomplishment as both Narod and Tonin played an important role in the successful isolation of a second gene for hereditary breast and ovarian cancer (BRCA2).[7] Unfortunately, despite their major contributions to the science, neither investigator was included on the patents filed for these major discoveries. They also found that two mutations in the BRCA1 gene are commonly found in hereditary breast/ovarian cancer families in which there is an Ashkenazi Jewish background. This observation has been validated over the years, and it became the basis for ethnic-specific mutation testing. In the fall of 1995, Narod left McGill to become chair of breast cancer research at Women's College Hospital at the

University of Toronto. He had been instrumental in making the Division of Medical Genetics a world-class centre in the area of hereditary cancer. Of great importance, Narod was responsible for the postdoctoral training of both Patricia Tonin and William Foulkes, both of whom have gone on to be major figures in cancer genetics in Quebec and Canada.

Genetic counsellors have proven to be both in great demand and highly mobile. Both Gordon Glendon and Chia Chia Sun moved to Toronto, and Lidia Kasprzak, MSc, a new graduate of the McGill program, was hired as a genetic counsellor. Shortly after, Jennifer Ozaki, MS, a graduate of the University of Michigan replaced Corrine Serruya.

This history ends in 1996, and it is in that year that Thomas Hudson returned to McGill from Michigan and was cross-appointed in the Division of Medical Genetics at the MGH. Thomas went on to become the best known Canadian scientist in the area of genomics. This ushered in a golden era for genomics at McGill, which culminated with the opening of the McGill University-Genome Quebec Innovation Centre.

In 1996, Gail Graham became the first McGill trainee to complete the Royal College training program in medical genetics and to receive her fellowship in this field. Although medical genetics had been recognized as a primary specialty by the Royal College of Physicians and Surgeons of Canada in 1986, it was not until 1997 that it was so recognized in Quebec. Graham had begun her training in medical genetics in Ontario and transferred to the McGill program in her second year of residency. Until 1997, this was the only way to gain entrance into the program. Today, McGill has one of the largest residency programs in medical genetics in Canada. Vitamin B12 Laboratory David Rosenblatt's work has focused on inborn errors of vitamin B12 (cobalamin) and folate metabolism. His laboratory is an international referral centre for these diseases and one of only two in the world specialized in diagnosing patients with these diseases. It receives one to two cell lines weekly from around the world and has succeeded in describing new steps in the cobalamin pathway and five new diseases. Over the years, the genes for a number of these have been identified. Most are diseases of infants and children, but, surprisingly, several of these diseases have had adult onset. Because the laboratory collects clinical information on all referred samples, it has been able to correlate laboratory and clinical findings. Over the years, Rosenblatt, alone or with collaborators, has written the definitive chapters for these diseases in major texts in the areas of metabolism, haematology, neurology, prenatal diagnosis, and biochemical genetics. This laboratory is known throughout the world for excellence in the area of inherited metabolic disease.

Model for the MUHC

From the beginning, the Division of Medical Genetics was a cooperative activity between the departments of medicine at the MGH and the RVH. Both hospitals contributed to the construction of the facilities, and Rosenblatt was appointed as division head at both hospitals. In this sense, medical genetics can be seen as a model for other divisions as it provided the first example of a fully integrated unit – the precursor for the McGill University Health Centre.

NOTES

1 David Rosenblatt to Phil Gold, letter, 17 May 1985, MGH.
2 Phil Gold to David Rosenblatt, letter, 4 October 1985, MGH.
3 Dean Richard Cruess to David Rosenblatt, letter, 18 October 1985, MGH.
4 W. Dauphinee to David Rosenblatt, letter, 16 January 1987, MGH.
5 T. Miki, J. Swensen, D. Shattuckeidens, P.A. Futreal, K. Harshman, S. Tavtigian, Q.Y. Liu, C. Cochran, L.M. Bennett, W. Ding, R. Bell, J. Rosenthal, C. Hussey, T. Tran, M. McClure, C. Frye, T. Hattier, R. Phelps, A. Haugenstrano, H. Katcher, K. Yakumo, Z. Gholami, D. Shaffer, S. Stone, S. Bayer, C. Wray, R. Bogden, P. Dayananth, J. Ward, P. Tonin S. Narod, P.K. Bristow, F.H. Norris, L. Helvering, P. Morrison, P. Rosteck, M. Lai, J.C. Barrett, C. Lewis, S. Neuhausen, L. Cannonalbright, D. Goldgar, R. Wisemaj, A. Kamb, and M.H. Skolnick, "A Strong Candidate for the Breast and Ovarian-Cancer Susceptibility Gene." *Science* 266, 5182 (1994): 66–71.
6 Louise Gagnon, "Race for Life." *McGill News* 75, 2 (1995): 20–1.
7 R. Wooster, G. Bignell, J. Lancaster, S. Swift, S. Seal, J. Mangion, N. Collins, S. Gregory, C. Gumbs, G. Micklem, R. Barfoot, R. Hamoudi, S. Patel, C. Rice, P. Biggs, Y. Hashim, A. Smith, F. Connor, A. Arason, J., Gudmundsson, D. Ficenec, D. Kelsell, D. Ford, P. Tonin, D.T, Bishop, N.K. Spurr, B.A.J. Ponder, R. Eeles, J. Peto, P. Devilee, C. Comelisse, H. Lynch, S. Narod, G. Lenoir, V. Egilsson, R.B. Barkadottir, D.F. Easton, D.R. Bentley, P.A. Futreal, A. Ashworth, and M.R. Stratton, "Identification of the Breast-Cancer Susceptibility gene BRCA2," *Nature* 378, 6559 (1995): 789–92.

13

Nephrology

Michael Kaye and Michael Laplante

Michael Kaye was the first director of the Division of Nephrology. He started one of the first chronic dialysis programs in Canada. Michael Laplante was a urologist who played a major role in the renal dialysis and transplant programs.

Introduction

Nephrology as a subspecialty started at the Montreal General Hospital in 1957. Backed by the innovative chief of medicine, D.G. Cameron, the service started a dialysis program for chronic renal disease and, in a special unit, patients were soon being treated day and night. The many problems with chronic dialysis were confronted: the AV shunt problems, the strain on the blood bank, the use of anticoagulants for the artificial kidney, the development of a home dialysis program, the kidney transplant program, and research on the effects of chronic renal disease and dialysis on bone metabolism are discussed. This very successful clinical and research program attracted outstanding house staff and fellows, a number of whom had leading careers in nephrology.

Background

Perhaps to some, the history of medical kidney disease (nephrology) at the MGH would date from the time that dialysis was started there. However, this is not the case. L.J. Adams, who had done postgraduate training in Boston, had an interest in hypertension and renal diseases. Interest in this area was minimal because the number of patients was small and treatment was limited.

M. Kaye had become interested in the kidney during the two years (1952 to 1954) he spent training at the Royal Victoria Hospital. He spent the next

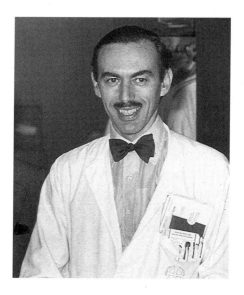

Fig. 13.1 Michael Kaye, first director, Division of Nephrology, 1957–98

two years at the Queen Mary Veterans Hospital in a small renal unit on a medical ward studying calcium metabolism in chronic renal failure. This led to a paper in the *New England Journal of Medicine*. Kaye was then introduced to D.G. Cameron, who had recently replaced E.S. Mills as physician-in chief at the MGH. Kaye joined the MGH staff in 1957 and formed a renal labora-tory in the clinical chemistry area. He also initiated a renal consulting serv-ice and outpatient clinic with Adams.

Early Years
An essential role was played by senior house staff Faye Inman (later to be-come the wife of John Dirks, the future chief of nephrology at the RVH). Others included G.A. Posen, P. Cordy, and A. Shimazu, all of whom went on to have distinguished careers in nephrology in other Canadian medical centres. There was plenty of activity, with an active research program, con-sultations, and the clinic, but very significant changes were imminent.

Haemodialysis
Successful human dialysis was initiated by William Kolff in Holland during the Second World War. The rotating drum kidney, a cumbersome giant al-most the size of a hospital bed, was made possible by a semi-permeable membrane (like a sausage casing) and heparin (a Canadian discovery) to

prevent the blood from clotting outside the body. Kolff settled in the United States after the war, where he developed a Twin-Coil Dialyser, the first practical small-sized unit suitable for acute dialysis. In 1961, the MGH Women's Auxiliary donated two thousand dollars for our first artificial kidney. In 1962, 147 dialyses were carried out, averaging three per week. Some of these procedures were for acute renal failure and some for poisonings.

Sometime in 1962, Charles Hollenberg (later to move to a distinguished career at the University of Toronto) told Kaye that Scribner at the University of Seattle had been treating patients with end-stage renal failure by repetitive haemodialysis using a small volume dialyser and permanent shunts for vascular access. Lindsay Ogilvy (a general surgeon) and Kaye went to Seattle for several days and were impressed by the possibility of chronic dialysis. The vascular shunts in the forearm could stay open for months, and the dialyser used required no blood priming or pump.

On returning to Montreal it was decided to embark on a program for permanent, long-term dialysis. Posen and Kaye modified a system so that two patients could be dialysed simultaneously from a single bath. They then built a two hundred-litre tank capable of six simultaneous dialyses. The next step was to build a permanent dialysis unit. This consisted of six beds and a large preparation area. Arlene Thompson became the head nurse and remained in that position for the next thirty years. The unit functioned six days per week, twenty-four hours per day. Patients who worked during the day came in after work, had dinner, were dialysed overnight, had breakfast the next morning, and returned to work. The whole project moved ahead because of the ongoing support of Douglas Cameron and the approval of executives in nursing and administration.

A major problem was the Teflon access in the forearm, which was prone to clotting and infection. We were indebted to Jerry Innes, a vascular surgery resident, who provided care for these catheters at any time of the day or night. Eventually they were replaced by more flexible silicon catheters, but all artificial catheters became obsolete with the introduction of surgically created forearm arterio-venous fistulae. These became the gold standard for long-term access in the subsequent decades, only being supplanted by synthetic vascular grafts or indwelling central venous catheters. The creation of fistulas and synthetic grafts was assumed by the Department of Urology, with Douglas Ackman and Michael Laplante the usual surgeons. Later, as we moved into long-term peritoneal dialysis, they also assumed responsibility for inserting those catheters that would remain in the abdomen for months or years. Later, Roger Tabah from the Department of Surgery was pivotal in providing central venous access, and over one hundred such catheters were inserted by him.

As more patients were taken on it became apparent that we would run out of space. Even if space were available there were patients who were travelling hundreds of kilometres each week to come in for dialysis. This led to the decision to embark on home dialysis, which was initially entirely haemodialysis. In 1966, the first patient went home, and, in a short time, we were looking after patients all over Quebec and east to New Brunswick, eastern Ontario, Vermont, and northern New York State. The home program required special skills and time commitment.

Initially, Arlene Thomson and Joan Briggs did the training and follow-up; subsequently, Glenda Oscar started in 1969 and retired after thirty years. Oscar shared the work with Betty McClosky, who remained for twenty-six years. Over one hundred patients went home over this period. In 1967, we abandoned standard routine transfusions, which reduced the risk of transfusion hepatitis and iron overload. This policy, unique in Canada at the time, was continued until recombinant erythropoietin became available in the 1990s. During this period we were also treating children. One fourteen-year-old female was 40 percent below her ideal weight and blind from hypertensive retinopathy. Six months after starting dialysis, she could see again and had regained her normal weight. She went on home dialysis and was eventually transplanted.

Peritoneal Dialysis

Intermittent peritoneal dialysis has been present and used for some time. However, because of its low efficiency, it was not the method of choice for acute dialysis at the MGH, and repeated insertion of intra-peritoneal cannulas made it undesirable for long-term use. Nevertheless, we used it by choice for initial treatment of patients in chronic renal failure.

The modern era of long-term peritoneal dialysis began in 1978. Between 1979 and 1999, 265 patients were trained and sent home. Patients requiring long-term dialysis could now make an informed choice as to which modality they preferred because each one was compatible with good survival and permitted eventual transplantation if required.

Research

From the beginning we were fortunate in being able to combine clinical work with an active research program that led to over 140 publications. We were able to examine in the laboratory setting any clinical problems encountered, with the active assistance of several laboratory workers. Ms B. Butler, Ms J. Henderson were there for almost thirty years, the latter leaving eventually to take a doctorate in experimental medicine and become a distinguished academic in her own right. Ms Malynowski, in addition to helping with other research projects, was pivotal in the study of the histology of uncalcified bone to elucidate bone metabolism in renal disease. At the outset, ours was the sole facility in Canada to use this technique and the only one of a handful in the world.

In the early decades, we were probably the most active group in Canada engaged in clinical research in nephrology. Initially, the emphasis was on the development of various techniques and the study of phosphorus, magnesium, and calcium and other dietary constituents in renal disease. We were also studying the role of Vitamin D and parathyroid hormone in the characterization of bone disease in these patients. Later, with the recognition of the magnitude of aluminum poisoning and with the use of bone biopsies, we were able to provide a diagnostic service to many other institutions.

Personnel

The vital role that our medical residents played in the early years has been mentioned. Subsequently, we were fortunate in having the opportunity to work with a number of research fellows, most of whom went on to important careers in nephrology, some at the MGH but mostly elsewhere. Among these were A. Shimizu, T. Ng, G.A. Posen, D. McDade, G. Cohen, S. Sagu, S. Borra, R. Mangel, P. Cordy, R.F. Gagnon, T. Wiegman, P. Lemaitre, L. Dufresne, P. Sommerville, J. Lien, P. Bourgouni, D. Churchill, and others. Mangel, Dufresne and Gagnon all returned to the MGH full-time staff after further training elsewhere.

Transplantation

The first renal transplantation at the MGH was performed in October 1971. This initiated an ambitious program developed almost single-handedly by Roman Mangel, with the enthusiastic support of Michael Kaye. Support from the RVH was considerably less enthusiastic as the pioneering work in renal transplantation in Canada had been done there. Nevertheless, it seemed reasonable that this form of treatment for end-stage renal disease should be available to complement the MGH dialysis program. Transplanted patients enjoy a better quality of life than do those on chronic dialysis.

On returning to Montreal after transplant training in Boston, Stanford, and London, England, Mangel was determined to establish a transplant program at the MGH. He was personally responsible for the selection of potential recipients and the organization for obtaining donor kidneys. He monitored the entire medical care of these complex patients. This had its frustrations. He once presented himself to Air Canada Freight to obtain a donor kidney shipped from the United States only to be given a bureaucratic run-around by a customs agent who did not have a "donor kidney" on his list of "admissible imports."

In the first year, ten cadaver donor transplants were carried out, all on patients from the MGH dialysis unit. The results were excellent, and there followed twenty-five years of transplants of both cadaver and live donor kidneys for a total of 372. Forty of these were from living related donors and three from non-related living donors.

The Greek Connection

Before the establishment of a well structured program of national and international organ sharing a kidney would become available with no suitable candidate in Quebec. Mangel had been approached regarding the transplantation of Greek patients with end-stage renal disease. For a few years Greek patients travelled to Montreal for assessment and could be placed on a "long-distance" wait list. When a kidney became available, and there was no Quebec or Canadian candidate, they would come to the MGH for transplant. Seventeen Greek patients were successfully transplanted. On one occasion a Quebec resident was located travelling in Europe and brought back to Montreal to receive a cadaver kidney from Bermuda.

The initial surgical team included a urologist, either Douglas Ackman or Michael Laplante, and one of several vascular surgeons, including H.G. Scott, David Mulder, and Peter Blundell. After the first year the urologists became comfortable performing the vascular component of the transplant procedure. Once the MGH program was well established the RVH was keen to integrate. This was firmly resisted by Mangel.

In early 1988, Lawrence Rosenberg, a McGill graduate and trained transplant surgeon, returned to the MGH. Having a highly trained kidney/pancreas transplant surgeon on board greatly enhanced the MGH program. He began performing the majority of these procedures.

In 1997, an administrative decision was taken to merge the two McGill transplant programs and move the MGH patients to the RVH. Mangel remained very active in the merged program, but the MGH surgeons were not integrated into the "combined" program. With the formation of the McGill University Health Centre and the integration of many services within the adult sites, the combination of the transplant program was inevitable, albeit slightly premature in the eyes of the MGH team.

14

Neurology and Neuroscience Research

Garth M. Bray and Donald W. Baxter

Donald Baxter was the second director of the Division of Neurology. He established
a world class academic program. Garth Bray followed him when he moved to become
chief at the Montreal Neurological Institute.

Introduction

Interest in diseases of the nervous system at the Montreal General Hospital
began informally in the 1870s, with Osler's clinico-pathological correlations,
and in the 1980s, with a clinic. Neurology was officially recognized in 1903 as
a department in the MGH. For the next fifty years, clinical service was the
main emphasis and research was confined to clinico-pathological observations. In the 1950s, new leadership in the Department of Medicine and the
Department of Surgery at the MGH provided increasing support for research. In the 1960s, this shift towards research included a quest for clinician-scientists in neurology. During the second half of the twentieth century,
MGH neurology evolved into an academic specialty that embraced neuroscience research and emphasized clinical and basic science teaching as well
as patient care.

Neurology at the MGH can be traced on the latter half of the nineteenth
century, when a few physicians developed special interests in patients with
neurological disorders. William Osler, physician and pathologist at the MGH
from 1874 to 1884, wrote detailed clinical and pathological observations on
many neurological conditions.[1] In 1888, James Stewart, another physician interested in neurological disorders,[2] decided to hold clinics on two afternoons
each week to see "cases of diseases of the nervous system." This is the first
record of a specific clinic at the MGH for such patients.

Department of Neurology

In 1903, the MGH became the first hospital in Quebec to recognize neurology as a specialty.[3] The minutes of the Medical Board record that the by-laws were altered to permit the appointment of "a specialist in Neurology" and the establishment of "a special clinic for Diseases of the Nervous System." David A. Shirres (fig. 14.1),[4] a native of Aberdeen, was named the first "Neurologist to the Hospital." Shirres was an imaginative clinician who reported many clinico-pathological studies in the *Montreal Medical Journal*.[5] He continued as MGH neurologist until 1921, when he was succeeded by Fred Holland Mackay (fig. 14.2).[6] Mackay, who was a highly regarded clinician and teacher, held that position until his death in 1947. MGH neurologists also provided consultations at the Western Division of the MGH (merger 1924) when neurologist George Robbins retired in 1930.[7]

Many of the patients seen by the neurologists during the first four decades of the twentieth century had disorders that would now be classified as psychiatric. Norman Viner and C.A. Porteous,[8] an assistant neurologist who was also superintendent of the Verdun Hospital for the Insane, had major interests in mental illness. Other neurologists with such interests were F.H. MacKay (hysteria and malingering), A.A. MacKay (alcoholism), and G. Paterson-Smyth.

Growth of the Department of Neurology

After the Second World War, Preston Robb (fig. 14.4), who had served in the Canadian navy, was appointed in 1945. Towards the end of the 1940s, C. Miller Fisher,[9] who was a medical officer in the navy and who had been a prisoner-of-war for four years, was appointed in neurology (1948) and pathology (1949). Working at the MGH and the Queen Mary Veterans Hospital, Fisher did meticulous clinico-pathological studies on carotid artery and cerebro-vascular disease. He left Montreal for an appointment at the Massachusetts General Hospital in 1954 when it was apparent that his work on stroke was misunderstood by the chief of medicine and was felt to be a bad choice for research.

Another postwar appointee was neurosurgeon Harold Elliott (1946) (see chapter 21), who was the first neurosurgeon to perform most of his procedures at the MGH rather than at the Montreal Neurological Institute.[10] In 1948, at the urging of Elliott, the name of the department was changed to the Department of Neurology and Neurosurgery.[11] Dr Francis McNaughton

Table 14.1
Department of Neurology, 1903–48

Neurologists	Associates Neurosurgeons	Assistants Neurosurgeons	Junior Assistants	
			Neurosurgeons	Neurosurgeons
David A. Shirres 1903–21		B.W.D. Gillies 1903–07		
		Aubrey Mussen 1903–10		
		William Winfrey 1903–10		
		Norman Viner 1909–25	G. Robinson 1918	
		A. Armour Robertson 1909–25[2]	H.V. Robinson 1919–22	
Fred H. MacKay 1921–47		C.A. Porteous[3] 1922–25	A. Armour MacKay 1922	
		A. Armour MacKay 1922–25		
George E. Robins[1] 1926–30	Norman Viner 1926–52	Aegret A. MacKay 1926–45		
	Wilder Penfield[4] 1928–34		William V. Cone[4] 1928–34	Arthur E. Elvidge 1930
			Arthur E. Elvidge 1931–33	

G. Paterson-Smyth
1931
Francis L. McNaughton
1935

C.A. Porteous
1931–47
G. Paterson-Smyth
1932–40

Arthur E. Elvidge
1933–47

Francis L. McNaughton
1936–45

Travis E. Dancey
1945

Francis L. McNaughton
1945–48
Aegret A. MacKay
1945–48

Travis E. Dancey[5]
1946–47
Allan A. Bailey
1946
J. Preston Robb
1946–47

Harold Elliott[6]
1946–48

Allan A. Bailey
1946–47
J. Preston Robb
1948–51

Francis L. McNaughton
1948

NOTES

1 Robins was the neurologist to the Western Division of the MGH until he retired.
2 Robertson, a McGill graduate of 1894, died in 1925 (Medical Board Minutes, vol. 49, p. 154. 7 April 1925).
3 C.S. Porteou in the Medical Board minutes but C.A. Porteous in the Board of Management minutes.
4 After 1934, Penfield and Cone were reappointed annually as "Consulting Neurosurgeons."
5 In 1947, Dancey's appointment was transferred from Neurology to Psychiatry
6 "Clinical assistant" is an appointment category that was introduced in 1935 (Board of Management Minutes, vol. 3, p. 549, 25 September 1935).

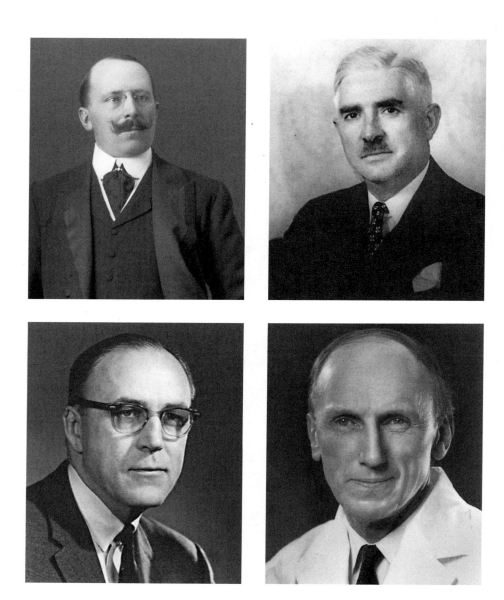

Clockwise from top left
Fig. 14.1 David Shirres, first neurologist at the MGH, 1903–21
Fig. 14.2 Fred McKay, first fully trained neurologist at Queen Square, 1921–47
Fig. 14.3 Francis McNaughton, first chief of neurology/neurosurgery, 1948–51
Fig. 14.4 Preston Robb, second chief of neurology/neurosurgery, 1951–54

(fig. 14.3),[12] who had been a member of the Department of Neurology since 1935, was appointed director of the renamed department with Elliott as associate director. Other members of the renamed department are listed in table 14.2.

In 1951, McNaughton resigned the MGH. Preston Robb succeeded McNaughton as chair of the joint department, but this decision was reversed with objections from Elliott, who was appointed director of the department, with Robb as neurologist to the hospital.[13]

A New Hospital

As early as 1945, there were many discussions concerning the inadequacies of the MGH building on Dorchester Street (now René Lévesque Boulevard). Two weeks after the end of the war in Europe, F.H. Mackay, chair of the Medical Board, wrote the Board of Management stating: "A new hospital on a new site is the one solution that assured the future life and efficiency of the Montreal General Hospital." There were also discussions with the dean of the McGill Faculty of Medicine and with the leadership of the Royal Victoria Hospital concerning possible mergers with other institutions. In March 1948, the Board of Management decided to build a new hospital on a site that was separate from the RVH, thereby deferring attempts to amalgamate McGill's teaching hospitals for the next fifty years. Within two months of this decision, the MGH started negotiations that led to the purchase the estate of Judge Alexander Cross on Cedar Avenue. The 1940s ended with a sense of excitement generated by the prospect of a new building for the MGH.

1950s – Neurology in Turmoil

Although the planning and eventual move to the Cedar Avenue site were invigorating activities for the hospital as a whole, neurology at the MGH made little progress during the 1950s. There were numerous staff departures. Norman Viner retired in 1952 after forty-three years; Preston Robb left in 1954 to become an assistant director at the MNI/MNH; and C. Miller Fisher accepted a position at the Massachusetts General Hospital in 1954. Bernard F Graham, appointed in 1952, moved to the MNH as registrar in 1954, and Joseph G. Stratford went to the University of Saskatchewan in 1956 after only one year as a junior neurosurgeon. By the end of decade, the only neurologists on staff at the MGH were W.F.T. "Bill" Tatlow,[14] appointed by the Medical Board in 1952 in charge of the EEG laboratory, and David Howell, who had been a neurologist and neuropathologist since 1954.[15]

Table 14.2
Department of Neurology and Neurosurgery, 1948–61

Neurologists	Neurosurgeons	Associates Neurosurgeons	Assistants	Junior/Clinical Assistants Neurosurgeons	Neurosurgeons
Francis L. McNaughton[1] 1948–51	Harold Elliott[2] 1948–61	Norman Viner 1948–52 J. Preston Robb 1948–51		C. Miller Fisher 1949–50	Keasley Welch[3] 1950
J. Preston Robb 1948–51		C. Miller Fisher 1952–55	C. Miller Fisher 1951–52 H.A. Bowes[5] 1952 W.F.T. Tatlow 1952–55 Bernard F. Graham 1953–55	Otto Magnus[4] 1950 Bernard F. Graham 1952 W.F.T. Tatlow 1952 David Howell 1954	

W.F.T. Tatlow
1955–61

David Howell
1955–61

J.G. Stratford
1955
Hugh Samson
1956–62

J.G. Stratford[6]
1955–56

Ruth McDougall
1957–59
Allan Morton
1958–61

NOTES

1 Director of the department
2 Associate director, 1948–51; director, 1951–61
3 *Locum tenens* for Elliott
4 In charge of the Sub-Department of Electroencephalography.
5 "Voluntary assistant."
6 Stratford left for Saskatoon in April 1956.

When the MGH moved to Cedar Avenue on 29 May 1955, the Department of Neurology and Neurosurgery was assigned thirty-five beds on its own ward (15 East). Because these beds were not fully utilized, and in spite of Elliott's objections, neurology and neurosurgery patients were moved to separate wards in 1959; neurology was assigned ten beds on a medical ward (initially 11-West, then 11-East) while neurosurgery was given ten beds on the ward of the Traumatic and Reparative Service (a.k.a. the Trauma Service) created by the newly appointed surgeon-in-chief, H. Rocke Robertson.

On 21 November 1960, Elliott wrote the Medical Board requesting the Department of Neurology and Neurosurgery return to a single ward. A special committee chaired by D.G. Cameron was created to decide on the fate of the combined department. After many discussions, letters, and outside consultations it was decided to disband the department and to create a division of neurology in medicine and a division of neurosurgery in surgery. By June 1961, the Medical Board and the Board of Management had ratified the recommendations of this committee to disband the Department of Neurology and Neurosurgery and to create divisions of neurology and neurosurgery in the departments of medicine and surgery, respectively.

Early Neuroscience Research at the MGH

The clinico-pathological studies on nervous system disease conducted by Osler between 1874 and 1884 constitutes the earliest neuro-research at the MGH. Such studies remained the main research activities of the neurologists at the MGH for the first half of the twentieth century and peaked with the extraordinary observations and conclusions of neuropathologist C. Miller Fisher on stroke phenomena between 1950 and 1954.

During the 1950s the MGH began to recognize that research should be a hospital priority. Resistance to a research commitment persisted among senior physicians, who felt that the MGH was a clinical centre and wanted to remain independent of any McGill-controlled research clinic. This attitude changed dramatically in the late 1950s with the appointments of Doug Cameron, chief of medicine, and Rocke Robertson, chief of surgery.[17]

1960s: Neurology Transformed

The influences of such strong and visionary leaders as Doug Cameron and Rocke Robertson were apparent in the divisions of neurology and of neurosurgery by the early years of the 1960s. In 1962, Robertson persuaded

Joseph G. Stratford to return from the University of Saskatchewan as director of the Division of Neurosurgery and the first full-time neurosurgeon at the MGH. Elliott had continued as director of neurosurgery until he retired in 1962. Stratford managed the neurosurgical service alone until Robert M. Ford was recruited as the second full-time neurosurgeon in 1965. Cameron also promoted changes in the Division of Neurology. When the division was created in 1961, William F.T. Tatlow (fig. 14.5) was acting director.[18] Peter K. Thomas was recruited in January 1962, but he returned to London later the same year, and, in 1963, David Howell also left for England. Obviously frustrated by the situation in neurology, Cameron created a committee early in 1963 to examine the direction of the division.[19] As a consequence, Donald W. Baxter (fig. 14.6) was recruited as the full-time director of neurology as of September 1963.[20] Baxter's vision of a division staffed with "physician-scientists" was exactly what Cameron wanted to solve the problem with neurology,[21] and he strongly supported Baxter. By the end of the 1960s, Baxter had recruited four new physician-scientists to the Division of Neurology (table 14.3).

Matthew W. Spence joined the Division of Neurology in 1965. Matt, an MD from Alberta, interned at the MGH and obtained a PhD in neurochemistry with Leon Wolfe at the MNI. He established a laboratory in the MGH University Medical Clinic in 1965, where he worked for four years before he left in 1969 to become director of the Atlantic Research Centre for Mental Retardation at Dalhousie University and capped his scientific career as president and CEO of the Alberta Heritage Foundation for Medical Research from 1990 to 2004.

Albert J. Aguayo (fig. 14.7) was persuaded to come to the MGH in 1964 for the final year of his residency through contacts with Jerzy (George) Olszewski, the neuroanatomist-neuropathologist who was a colleague of Baxter and Stratford in Saskatoon. Albert graduated in medicine from the University of Cordoba in Argentina in 1959 and immigrated to Canada the following year. After an internship at the Port Arthur General Hospital (Ontario), he was accepted into the neurology program at the University of Toronto, where his residency was supervised by J.C. Richardson (neurology) and Jerzy Olszewski (neuropathology).

With the support of a McLaughlin Fellowship, Aguayo did further clinical and research training with Professor John Walton (later Lord Walton of Dechant) and his colleagues at the University of Newcastle-upon-Tyne. He returned to Montreal in September 1967 as an assistant professor of

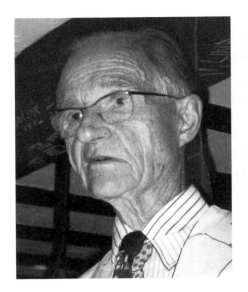

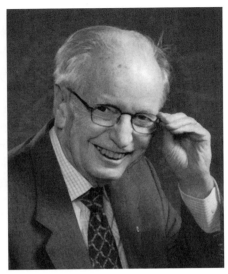

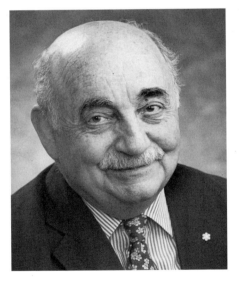

Clockwise from top left

Fig. 14.5 William Tissington Tatlow, acting director, Division of Neurology, 1961–63

Fig. 14.6 Donald Baxter, first GFT director, Division of Neurology, 1963–79

Fig. 14.7 Albert Aguayo, director, Division of Neurology, 1979–90

neurology and neurosurgery and as director of the section on diseases of nerve and muscle at the MGH.

Morrison H. Finlayson, an MD graduate from Alberta, was recruited to the MGH as a neurologist and neuropathologist in 1966. "Fin" had completed training in clinical neurology at the National Hospital, Queen Square, London, and in neuropathology at the MNI. Fin's premature death in 1982 was a great loss to the Division of Neurology, to the McGill Program, and to the MGH.

The final recruit of the 1960s was Garth M. Bray, a medical graduate from Manitoba who had trained in neurology and neuropathology with the famed Maurice Victor and Betty Banker at the Cleveland Metropolitan General Hospital. Garth's research was initially focused on muscle pathology, but, after 1971, he collaborated with Albert Aguayo on morphological studies of axon-Schwarm cell interactions and axonal regrowth.

Patient Services and Facilities

In September 1966, a new neurology-neurosurgery clinical teaching unit opened with thirty beds (including an eight-bed intensive-care area) for neurology and neurosurgery patients, space for EEG and EMG laboratories, and two small offices. This was the first ward in the MGH in which there was no distinction between "public" and "private" or "semi-private" beds.

The MGH had acquired its first electro-encephalograph (EEG) machine in the 1950s,[22] and Tatlow took charge of the EEG laboratory after 1961. P.K. Thomas performed EMGs and nerve conduction studies in 1962, which were not offered again until 1967 by Aguayo.

In 1967, the hospital created a neuroradiology suite in the Department of Radiology and purchased new equipment for cerebral angiography, pneumoencephalography, and myelography. In the pre-CT scan days, radioisotope brain scans and echoencephalography were used frequently as brain-imaging tools. Leonard Rosenthal cooperated with the neurologists and neurosurgeons on the applications of nuclear medicine to clinical problems. Echoencephalograms were initially performed by Robert M. Ford, neurosurgeon, in his small office. When Fred Winsberg joined radiology in 1972, that department assumed responsibility for echoencephalography.

1970s: Expansion Based on Recruitment of Physician-Scientists

During the 1960s, the Medical Research Council of Canada introduced policies and personal support programs to foster the recruitment and retention of "physician-scientists." The Division of Neurology elected to recruit additional colleagues who would be candidates for such awards by developing a practice model that would permit physician-scientists to devote the required 80 percent of their time to research activities. Members of the group also

Table 14.3
Division of Neurology, 1961–2010

Directors	Clinical Neurologists (GFT)	Neuroscientists[1]
W.F.T. Tatlow,[2] 1961–63	David Howell, 1961–63	
	P.K. Thomas, 1962	
	Fred Andermann, 1962–69	
Donald W. Baxter, 1963–78	W.F.T. Tatlow. 1963–2005	Matthew Spence, 1965–69
	Morrison Finlayson,[3] 1966–82	
	Albert J. Aguayo,[4] 1967–present	
	Garth M. Bray,[4] 1968–2007	
	Joseph B. Martin, 1970–1978	
	Donald G. Lawrence, 1972–2000	Paul Brazeau, 1972–77
	Michael Rasminsky,[4] 1973–present	
	Leo P. Renaud,[4] 1973–90	
Albert J. Aguayo,[4,5] 1979–89	John D. Stewart, 1978–89	Bruce Livett, 1977–82
	Calvin Melmed, 1979–83	Alan C. Peterson, 1979–86
	Yves Lapierre, 1981–98	Ian Duncan, 1980–82
	Robert Côté, 1983–present	Samuel David, 1983–present
	Myra Sourkes, 1984–98	Salvatore Carbonetto,[7] 1984–present
	Martin Veilleux, 1989–2003	Pierre Drapeau,[6] 1985–2005
	Guy Rouleau,[4] 1989–2005	Charles Bourque, 1987–present
		Jean-Pierre Julien, 1989–2003

Garth M. Bray, 1990–2004

Colin Chalk, 2004–present
Jeff Jirsch, 2006–09
Stuart Lubarsky, 2010–present
Eric Ehrensberger, 2010–present

Colin Chalk, 1991–present
Lucy Vieira, 1999–present
Richard Riopelle,[6] 2000–12
Anne-Louise Lafontaine, 2000–present
Ron Postuma, 2004–present

Rob Dunn, 1989–2007
Lisa McKerracher, 1992–97
Michael Ferns, 1995–2003
Yong Rao. 1998–present
Don van Meyel, 2003–present
Keith Murai, 2004–present
David Stellwagen, 2007–present
Brian Chen, 2009–present
Jesper Sjöström, 2011–present

NOTES

1 Neuroscientists were appointed to the Centre for Research in Neuroscience after 1986.
2 Acting director.
3 Died in 1982.
4 Jointly appointed at the Centre for Research in Neuroscience starting in 1986.
5 Director, Centre for Research in Neuroscience, 1986–2001
6 Director, Centre for Research in Neuroscience, 2001–05
7 Director, Centre for Research in Neuroscience, 2005–present
8 Chair, Department of Neurology and Neurosurgery, McGill University, 2000–10

agreed to pool their academic and clinical earnings – a practice-plan that was ahead of its time.

With the 1970 introduction of Quebec's version of the Canada Health Act (Canada's Medicare Act of 1966), the infamous "Bill 65," which took over the management of all hospitals and their finances, and the Health Services and Social Services Act (HSSS), 1971, staff associations and financial management of each Department was now necessary.

Joseph B. Martin was the first physician-scientist recruited to the MGH in the 1970s. A graduate of the University of Alberta, he completed neurology training at Western Reserve University Hospital in Cleveland and obtained a PhD in neuroanatomy with Seymour Reichlin at the University of Rochester. With an MRC scholarship, Joe and his family arrived in Montreal in September 1970 – in time to experience the political crisis (October Crisis) precipitated by the FLQ murder-kidnappings and the doctors' strike over Quebec Bill 65's, fee restrictions of specialty care and no added billing clause (see chapter 48 regarding government health legislation). In spite of these events, Joe soon established a laboratory and became a valued participant in the division's patient care and teaching efforts. Joe Martin remained with MGH neurology until 1976, when he became neurologist-in-chief at the Montreal Neurological Hospital. He was appointed chair of the McGill Department of Neurology and Neurosurgery the following year but unexpectedly went to Boston to become chief of the neurology service at the Massachusetts General Hospital (the "other" MGH) and a professor of neurology at Harvard University. He was subsequently recruited to the University of California, San Francisco, as dean of medicine and later as chancellor. In 1997, Joe returned to Harvard as dean of the School of Medicine, a position he held until his retirement in 2007.[23]

Donald G. Lawrence was recruited in 1972. An MD, CM from McGill, Don completed his neurology training at Western Reserve University Hospital in Cleveland and spent three productive years as a research fellow with Hans Kuypers in the Department of Anatomy at Western Reserve, describing the organization of the descending motor pathways in the brainstem and spinal cord. After a year's postdoctoral fellowship at Oxford University, and another with Kuypers in Rotterdam, he returned to Montreal, jointly appointed to the MGH Division of Neurology and the neuroanatomy laboratory at the MNI. In 1973, he became director of the "CNS Course" – the main undergraduate neuroscience course in the Faculty of Medicine. Because of his efforts it was one of the most highly rated courses in the undergraduate medical curriculum. Don also served as associate dean for admissions from 1984 to 1993. He retired in 2000.

Two more physician-scientists joined the Division of Neurology in 1973: both were awarded MRC scholarships. Michael Rasminsky, a Harvard University medical graduate, did a neurology residency at the Albert Einstein College of Medicine. While a PhD student with Thomas A. Sears at the National Hospital, Queen Square, Mike developed a technique to record conduction patterns in single nerve fibers in laboratory animals. He was soon applying this technique to experimental models of demyelination and became a close collaborator with Albert Aguayo and Garth Bray in studies of models of dysmyelination and neural regeneration.

Leo Renaud graduated in medicine from the University of Ottawa. Following internship and residency, Leo studied neuroanatomy at the MNI with Jacques Courville, completed a PhD in neurophysiology at McGill with Kasamir (Kris) Krynevic, and trained in clinical neurophysiology with Pierre Gloor (electro-encephalography) and Albert Aguayo (electromyography). In his research laboratory, he developed sophisticated techniques to study hypothalamic function *in vivo* and *in vitro*. Renaud's laboratory soon attracted cohorts of graduate students who have gone on to distinguished careers. In 1990, Leo Renaud returned to the University of Ottawa as head of the Neuroscience Group at the Loeb Research Institute.

Neuroscience Research in the 1970s

As the research accomplishments of the MGH group became increasingly recognized, funding from local to international agencies permitted the recruitment of new investigators and the acquisition of specialized research equipment. Three PhD scientists were recruited during the 1970s: Paul Brazeau completed his postdoctoral training in neuro-endocrinology at the Salk Institute and worked closely with Joe Martin and Leo Renaud from 1972 to 1977, when he moved the University of Montreal; Bruce Livett, a neurochemist from Monash University in Australia, arrived in 1977 and investigated the neurobiology of adrenergic neurons with a novel in vitro approach using bovine adrenal glands before returning to Australia as a professor of biochemistry at the University of Melbourne; and Alan Peterson, with a PhD in genetics from the University of British Columbia, came to the MGH in 1979 and moved to a cancer research laboratory at the RVH in 1986.

With the completion of the MGH Research Institute in 1973, neurology was given the first two floors for research space, making it the leading hospital-based neuro-research facility in Canada.

Clinical Recruitment

Towards the end of the 1970s, the Division of Neurology recruited additional colleagues whose activities were mainly clinical and teaching. John D. Stewart, a graduate of the University of the West Indies, joined the division in 1978 after completing the final year of his neurology training at the MNH. He took over the EMG lab and worked at the MGH until 1989, when he went to the MNH. Calvin Melmed, a medical graduate from the University of Manitoba and of the McGill Neurology training program, was recruited from the JGH in July 1979. In September 1979 he was named director of the MGH Neurology Clinical Teaching Unit. He returned to the JGH as chief of neurology in 1983.

The practice model of the Division of Neurology, initiated on 1 March 1970, was based on two clinical teams: a *ward team* responsible for up to fifteen patients admitted to the CTU (7-East Pine) and a *consultation team* that responded to requests concerning patients in the Emergency Department or on the wards of the hospital. The clinician-scientists of the division mainly saw office patients during their rotation on the consultation service, but they also held a weekly office time or clinic to see follow-up patients.

Regarding the resident training program, in 1974, Henry J.M. Barnett from the University of Western Ontario visited the division as part of the accreditation process of the Royal College. In response to Barnett's recommendation that the program needed more didactic sessions, a series of one-hour teaching sessions were organized for two mornings each week.

In 1978, the MGH acquired its first CT scanner, which was a great advance in head scanning for many conditions; and, sadly, the Queen Mary Veterans Hospital, which a number of the neurology staff had attended for years seeing chronic neurological problems, closed.

1980s – New Leadership – Growth of Neuroscience Research and Neurology Subspecialties

In 1979, Baxter left the MGH as neurologist-in-chief at the MNI/MNH and subsequently chairman of McGill neurology and neurosurgery. In June 1979, Albert Aguayo was appointed director of the Division of Neurology, marking the end of one remarkable era and the beginning of an equally exciting new one. In 1980, Phil Gold succeeded Doug Cameron as physician-in-chief and continued the Department of Medicine's strong support of neurology. The neurologists recruited to the Division of Neurology during this decade contributed to the continued growth of subspecialty neurology by bringing expertise in multiple sclerosis (Yves Lapierre), cerebrovascular disease (Robert Coté), clinical neurophysiology (Myra Sourkes, Martin Veilleux, and Allan Ryder-Cook) and neurogenetics (Guy Rouleau).

Neuroscience Research in the 1980s

In 1978, Albert Aguayo created a neuroscience unit within the Division of Neurology to further the successful research already accomplished. In the 1980s, he developed techniques to make CNS fibers myelinate in peripheral nerve environment and, with tracing techniques, demonstrated that, under the right circumstances, CNS neurons in the injured cord model could grow axons.[25] The group also cleverly showed that axons in nerve grafts could be guided to CNS targets to form synapses.

These important discoveries in 1986 led McGill to form the Centre for Neuroscience Research (CRN), headed by Aguayo. This led to greater funding for research as well as to funding for the Neural Regeneration and Functional Recovery Network as part of the federal government's Network of Centres of Excellence Program. This, of course, led to more space for the MGH centre's research elsewhere in the hospital complex.[26] In 1984, plans were initiated for the hospital to purchase an MRI scanner. The MRI did not materialize for seven years, but a second CT scanner was acquired in 1985.

1990s: Living with the Uncertainties of Impending Change
With the plans to form the McGill University Health Centre after 1992 (it was officially established in 1997), there were concerns about the future of the MGH Division of Neurology and the Neuroscience program. The 1990s also brought repeated budget cuts with consequent reductions of hospital services, bed closures, and government-enforced attempts at the "rationalization" of services. The minutes of the Division of Neurology record concerns about delays in admitting elective patients, the waiting lists for office and clinic appointments, reductions in the number of residents, and the impact of Article 12, which strictly regulated the number of "on-calls" allowed for residents.

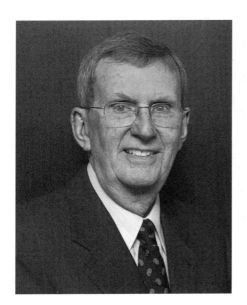
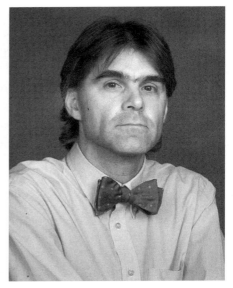

Fig. 14.8 Garth Bray, director, Division of Neurology, MGH/MUHC, 1990–2004
Fig. 14.9 Colin Chalk, director, Division of Neurology, MGH/MUHC, 2004–

Garth Bray (fig. 14.8) followed Albert Aguayo as director of the Division of Neurology in 1990 (Albert continued as the director of the expanding Centre for Research in Neuroscience). Colin Chalk (fig. 14.9), an MD, CM graduate of McGill, was recruited in 1991. Colin trained in neurology at the Mayo Clinic and Oxford University and then did a fellowship in peripheral nerve diseases with Peter Dyck. In 2004, he became director of the Division of Neurology.

By 1990, non-invasive techniques (CT scanning, MR imaging, and diagnostic ultrasound) had replaced myelography, pneumoencephalography, and angiography as the main tools to investigate patients with brain and spinal cord disorders. Prior to 1990, most patients with strokes were admitted to the medical CTU; only the more complicated or unusual stroke patients were admitted to the Neurology service. After 1992, care for stroke patients was coordinated by a multidisciplinary team and unit that was initially part of a general medical ward and was eventually incorporated into the neurology CTU. By the end of the decade, the Cerebrovascular Clinic, under the direction of Robert Cote, was functioning four half-days each week.

The Future of Neurology at the MGH

In a strictly legal sense, MGH neurology ended when the McGill University Health Centre was created in 1997. But because the MUHC took seventeen years to complete, MGH neurology and research survived with changes in personnel at the MGH and the MUHC, and it will remain on Cedar Avenue for the foreseeable future.

NOTES

Minute books and correspondence from the committees and departments of the MGH are found in the McGill University Archives (MUA).

1 Osler's autopsy reports from his years at the MGH (1874 to 1884) included descriptions of intracranial aneurysms, cerebral haemorrhage, meningitis, multiple sclerosis, brain abscesses, and various types of brain tumours.

2 James Stewart, who joined the staff of the MGH in 1883 after postgraduate studies in Vienna, had a major interest in neurology and psychiatry. In 1887, he became the first physician-in-chief at the RVH and, in 1888, started the first clinic for nervous diseases at McGill and was appointed professor of medicine at McGill.

3 P. Robb, *The Development of Neurology at McGill*, Montreal: privately published, (1989), 9.

4 David Alexander Shirres, a graduate of Aberdeen University, came to Canada in 1893 as surgeon to the governor general, the Earl of Aberdeen. After postgraduate studies in Europe, Shirres settled in Montreal, where, by 1902, he was a "Clinical Assistant in Neurology" at the RVH and a "Demonstrator of Neuropathology at McGill University." In 1903, Shirres became the first neurologist at the MGH. By 1905, he was also professor of neurology at the University of Vermont in Burlington, where he travelled regularly to lecture.

5 After eighteen years, Shirres resigned his position at the MGH. H.E. MacDermot, in his*History of the Montreal General Hospital* (Montreal: Montreal General Hospital, 1950), 96–7, describes Shirres as "a man of great energy [who] did not keep abreast of developments." He died in Montreal on 28 December 1945 at the age of eighty-two.

6 Fred Holland MacKay was born on Prince Edward Island in 1884, graduated MD, CM from McGill, and interned at the RVH .While serving in the Canadian army during the First World War, he developed an interest in malingering, "shell-shock," and traumatic nerve lesions. After the war, he studied

neurology at the National Hospital, Queen Square, London. On his return to Montreal in 1921, MacKay succeeded David Shirres as head of the Department of Neurology at the MGH, a position he held until his death in 1947.

7 Robb, *Neurology*, 10–14, 37, 79–89, 101–2.

8 Norman Viner was born in Romania, came to Montreal, and graduated in medicine from McGill in 1902. His son-in-law, the late Allan Gold, reported that Viner developed a keen interest in neurology from David Shirres while working in the Outdoor Neurology Clinic at the MGH. In 1924, Viner went to Vienna to study with Sigmund Freud and other psychoanalysts. When he returned to Montreal in 1925, he practiced neuropsychiatry. He was also a consultant at the Verdun Protestant Hospital and was the first neurologist on staff when the Jewish General Hospital opened in 1934. He died in 1970.

9 Charles Miller Fisher graduated from the University of Toronto in 1938. He joined the Royal Canadian Navy in 1940 while a resident in medicine at the RVR Later that year, the boat to which he was assigned was torpedoed and he spent four years in a German prisoner-of-war camp.

10 During a postwar refresher course, Wilder Penfield encouraged Fisher to study neurology. He spent two years (from 1946 to 1948) as a fellow in neurology at the MNI, and another in neuropathology (1949–50) with Raymond Adams at the Boston City Hospital, where he identified the link between haemorrhagic infarcts and atrial fibrillation. In 1950, he returned to the MGH and for the next four and a half years continued to investigate strokes in the neuropathology laboratory and clinic. During this period, he described transient ischemic attacks, carotid artery disease, "watershed" infarcts, and hypertensive cerebrovascular disease and laid the foundation for his career as a specialist in cerebrovascular disease. He also described the variant of Guillain-Barre known as the Miller Fisher syndrome.

11 Despite Fisher's pioneering work at the MGH, the chief of medicine, not understanding the importance of what had been done, suggested to him that stroke had little promise for future research. Ray Adams at Harvard thought differently and invited Fisher to join him at the Massachusetts General Hospital in 1954, where he became his generation's leader in understanding stroke and its presentations.

12 In 1928, Wilder Penfield and William Cone were appointed to the "subdepartment" (subdepartments were renamed divisions in 1961) of neurosurgery at McGill. Because the arrangement (insisted upon by MGH surgeons) that they operate at the MGH had proven unsatisfactory, the MGH agreed to support a trainee in neurosurgery, Arthur R. Elvidge, with the understanding that he

would return to the MGH in charge of neurosurgery. After completing his training with Penfield and Cone, and in London and Lisbon, Elvidge took up his appointment as an associate in neurosurgery in 1933. However, he transferred most non-trauma patients to the MNI, where the treatment was superior to what the MGH could offer.

13 In 1948, the MGH created the Department of Neurology and Neurosurgery with the neurologist as director and the neurosurgeon as associate director.

14 Francis Lothian McNaughton, a Montrealer, graduated MD, CM from McGill in 1931. After postgraduate studies in Boston and London, McNaughton became a research fellow at the MNI and was appointed to the MGH in 1934. In 1948, he succeeded MacKay, who resigned from the MGH to become neurologist-in-chief at the MNH, a position he held until 1969. Known as St Francis M., few will forget his remarkable personality.

15 James Preston Robb was born on 14 April 1914. After his McGill MD, CM, Robb interned at the MGH and trained in neurology at the MNI as well as at hospitals in the United States. In 1941, he joined the Royal Canadian Navy and held the rank of surgeon lieutenant commander when he was demobilized in 1945. He was first appointed to the MGH in 1945. After McNaughton resigned in 1951, Robb was given the position of neurologist to the hospital. In 1954, Robb left the MGH to become director of Hospitalization at the MNI and, eventually, chief of neurology.

16 William "Bill" F. Tissington Tatlow graduated from St Bartholomew's (Bart's) Hospital Medical School in 1939. A few days after joining the Royal Army Medical Corps in May 1940, he was the medical officer on a paddle steamer that made three harrowing journeys across the English Channel in the troop rescue from Dunkirk. After the war, Bill trained at the National Hospital, Queen Square, and at the Royal Infirmary in Bristol. During this period, he co-authored a textbook, *A Synopsis of Neurology*. In 1951, he joined the staff of the MGH and Queen Mary Veterans Hospital, became head of the MGH neurology service in June 1954, and served as acting director of the Division of Neurology from 1961 to 1963. When he was eighty-seven years old, he published *A Doctor's Life*, which describes the events of his remarkable life.

17 David Howell was an assistant neurologist and neuropatholgist at the MGH from 1954 to 1961, when he returned to England.

18 Report of a Special Committee. On 20 February 1961, the Special Committee recommended that the Department of Neurology and Neurosurgery be disbanded and replaced by divisions of neurosurgery and of neurology in the departments of surgery and of medicine, respectively.

19 D.W. Baxter and J.G. Stratford, "Neurology and Neurosurgery at the Montreal General Hospital, 1960–1980," *Canadian Journal of Neurological Sciences* 27 (2000): 79–83.

20 Full-time physicians and surgeons (GFT, geographical full-time) had "ceilings" on their total clinical income, carried out their entire practices in the hospital, and were paid salaries by the hospital or the university for their work in teaching, research, and administration. The hospital usually provided office space and secretarial support. Two categories of full-time appointments were subsequently developed at the McGill teaching hospitals: GFT-H (hospital) and GFT-U (university).

21 Early in 1963, Cameron named a committee to study the reorganization of the Division of Neurology which needed new leadership. The result was to invite Donald Baxter, from Saskatchewan to be the new Director of the Division of Neurology.

22 Donald W Baxter graduated MD, CM from Queen's University (Queen's ceased awarding the MD, CM for the MD only in 1960). He spent a year as a research fellow in neuroanatomy with Jerzy Olszewski at the MNI, when they produced their folio-sized histology atlas, *Cytorchitecture of the Human Brainstem,* in which they showed nuclear groups in the reticular formation of the pons and midbrain. He had further training in medicine at the KGH (1953–54), in neuropathology (Joseph Foley, 1954–55), and neurology (Derek Denny-Brown, 1955–57) at the Boston City Hospital.

  a. In 1957, he joined the Department of Neurology and Neurosurgery at the University of Saskatchewan and, after a few years, went to Temple University in Philadelphia. In 1963, he was recruited to the MGH as director of the Division of Neurology and as an associate professor in the Department of Neurology and Neurosurgery as well as the Department of Medicine at McGill.

  b. Over the next fifteen years, he built a division of clinical scientists that reinstated Neurology at McGill. In 1979, he moved to the MNI/MNH as neurologist-in-chief and chair of the McGill Department of Neurology and Neurosurgery and became director of the MNI in 1984. As the leading neurologist at McGill, he was president of the Canadian Neurological Society from 1969 to 1970, chair of the policy-making Royal College Committee on Neurology from 1970 to 1975, was made an Officer of the Order of Canada in 1996, and was given a Lifetime Achievement Award from the MNI in 2005. He died on 24 July 2012.

23 D.W. Baxter, "The J.C. Richardson Lecture: "Prospects for Canadian Medical Neurology," *Canadian Journal of Neurological Sciences* 2 (1975): 101–7.

24 On a request from McNaughton, in 1950, the hospital agreed to establish an EEG laboratory and to put Otto Magnus in charge of the laboratory.

25 J.B. Martin, *Alfalfa to Ivy: Memoir of a Harvard Medical School Dean*, Edmonton: University of Alberta Press, 2011.

26 S. David and A. Aguayo, "Axonal Elongation into Peripheral Nervous System 'Bridges' after Central Nervous System Injury in Adult Rats," *Science* 214 (1981): 931–3.

27 P. Richardson, U. McGinness, and A. Aguayo, "Axons from CNS Neurones Regenerate into PNS Grafts," *Nature* 284 (1980): 264–5.

15

Medical Oncology

Michael Thirlwell

Michael Thirlwell was the first director of the Division of Medical Oncology and chair of the original tumour board of the MGH.

Introduction

Medical oncology is a relatively young subsubspecialty of medicine. It has its origins in the use of medications or chemical agents for the treatment of cancer. This idea has been around since the days of the ancient Greeks,[1] and there are recorded attempts dating back to the first century AD.[2] However, the scientific basis for the use of the chemical treatment (chemotherapy) of cancer did not develop until the twentieth century. Dogmagk's 1935 discovery of sulpha drugs for antibacterial chemotherapy stimulated research in cancer chemotherapy.[3] Further impetus for research in the field derived from observations that exposure to mustard gas led to hypoplasia and aplasia of lymphoid organs and bone marrow. Those observations were made in soldiers exposed to sulphur mustard in the First World War and in sailors exposed to mustard gas when Allied ships in the Port of Bari carrying poisonous war gas were destroyed during a bombardment.[4]

Goodman and Gilman et al. conducted the first clinical trial of nitrogen mustard in patients with malignant lymphomas.[5] The dramatic regressions of the lymphomas seen in this study generated tremendous excitement in this new field of medicine. The results, published in 1946,[6] could be said to mark the beginning of modern chemotherapy. Soon thereafter, Farber et al.,[7] building on studies of the effect of folic acid antagonists on leukemia cells, conducted a clinical trial of aminopterin in children with lymphoplastic leukemia and were able to achieve temporary remissions of the disease. Five years later, the less toxic folate antagonist, methotrexate, was introduced, and it produced the first example of a drug-induced cure of a metastatic solid tumour, viz. gestational chorio-carcinoma.[8]

Nitrogen mustard was the prototype for the development of other alkylating agents, while the anti-folate antagonists led the way to the development of other antimetabolites, including the pyrimidine analogue, 5-Fluorouracil, which showed clinical effect in breast and colon cancer. During the 1950s and 1960s, several other classes of anticancer drugs were developed and introduced into clinical practice, and a whole new expertise in the management of cancer patients with chemotherapy was required. Thus, there arose the need for a discipline consisting of physicians trained in internal medicine with subspecialty expertise in neoplastic diseases and its treatment by drugs. These specialists would complement the already established roles of specialists in surgery and radiation treatment in the management of patients with cancer. The use of chemotherapy is congruent with the fact that surgery and radiation therapy are local or regional forms of therapy but do not control metastatic disease, which systemic therapy (i.e., chemotherapy) is directed towards.

Development of Chemotherapy at the Montreal General Hospital, 1950s to 1975

Lawrence Hutchison, director of the Division of Haematology of the MGH from 1972 to 1997 provided some personal recollections.[8] Between 1952 and 1955 in the old MGH (where he worked), Douglas Cameron, who himself had an interest in haematology, used crude adrenocorticol extracts to treat leukemia. This met with little success. Following the move to the new MGH, the major development was the joining of the Acute Leukemia Group B (ALGB) by Stuart Townsend, who had become the head of haematology in 1956. The ALGB was comprised of a group of physicians from different institutions in North America who had joined forces to conduct scientific clinical trials on the treatment of leukemia. In subsequent years it changed its name to the Cancer and Leukemia Group B (CALGB) as it expanded its activities to include studies of the treatment of non-hematologic malignancies. Participation in this group's activities effectively brought the MGH into the mainstream of the treatment of leukemia and other hematological malignancies, including lymphomas. With respect to the latter, Hutchison distinctly recalls telling medical students in 1970 that Hodgkin's disease was a uniformly fatal disease, only to read in a publication shortly there-after that Vera Peters at the Princess Margaret Hospital had achieved lasting remissions equivalent to cure with the use of radiation therapy. Although the treatment used was radiation therapy, it was later shown by DeVita et al that combination chemotherapy could also cure Hodgkin's disease.[9] In 1972, on the retirement of Stuart Townsend, Hutchison became principal investigator of CALGB trials for the MGH. Also around that time, Bernard Cooper replaced S. Lowenstein as head of haematology at the Royal Victoria Hospital. Hutchison subsequently became the principal investigator of the CALGB trials for McGill University, representing the MGH and the RVH.

In the late 1950s, as other chemotherapeutic agents became available, such as thiotepa (an alkylating agent) and 5-Fluorouracil (an antimetabolite), sur-geons became interested in chemotherapy for the treatment of cancer, either as an adjunct to surgery[10] or in metastatic disease.[11] Among the surgeons at the MGH, John Palmer participated in studies involving the perioperative treatment of patients with intravenous thiotepa in the hope of reducing the number of circulating tumour cells and the formation of micrometastases.[12] This paved the way for subsequent adjuvant chemotherapy studies in early breast cancer as part of the National Surgical Adjuvant Breast Project Group (later expanded to National Surgical Adjuvant Breast and Bowel Project). Further expertise in the area of chemotherapy was provided by the recruit-ment from Harvard University of Ian W.D. Henderson, a surgeon with knowledge of chemotherapy for cancer patients. Henderson applied his sur-gical expertise to the treatment of various solid tumours including breast, colon, and sarcomas. On a personal note, one of his patients included a teen-ager with limb sarcoma treated with surgery and chemotherapy who remains alive to this day. This patient, a farmer's daughter from Glengarry County, Ontario, adjoining the Quebec border, is a cousin of my wife. Henderson subsequently moved to Ottawa to head the Drug Directorate of the Health Protection Branch of Canada.

In 1969, John K. MacFarlane, an MGH surgeon, returned from MD An-derson Hospital and Tumor Institute following training in surgical oncol-ogy and brought further expertise back to the MGH, including knowledge of the technique of regional chemotherapy.[13] In this technique, there is site-directed perfusion of specific regions of the body directly affected by the can-cer. In particular, this method was applicable for the treatment of primary liver cancer, or metastases from colorectal cancer, and for the perfusion of limbs bearing malignant melanoma as the primary site.

Leading up to 1975, those particularly involved in chemotherapy were K. MacFarlane, L. Hutchison, N. Blair Whittemore, Barbara Lipowski (a part-time hematologist), Peter Mansell (a part-time surgeon chemotherapist from RVH), and Peter Blahey (a gynaecologist). Blahey specialized in the treatment of gynaecologic cancers. Among the new drugs being introduced were dactinomycin D and cyclophospamide. These drugs were beneficial for gynaecologic cancers such as ovarian cancer and gestational chorocarcinoma and were used by Peter Blahey. Of note, Blahey was also trained in radiotherapy and, in particular, the technique of brachytherapy for the treatment of uterine cancer.

In passing, a comment should be made about the use of endocrine therapy for the treatment of malignancies arising in organs normally under the influence of sex steroid hormones – namely, breast, endometrium, and prostate. The development of endocrine therapy began following Beatson's 1896 observation of the successful treatment of metastatic breast cancer by oophorectomy.[14] Other hormonal ablative procedures were later introduced. Beatson was later awarded the Nobel Prize for his work. As the field evolved, additive therapies using androgens, estrogens, and progestins were also developed, culminating in the introduction of the first anti-estrogen (ICI-I46474, tamoxifen) in the early 1970s. Used as a catholic definition, the term "chemotherapy" includes not only cytotoxic drugs but also hormonal agents and other chemicals. In fact, the current term used for the use of any type of oral or parenteral medications for the treatment of cancer is "systemic treatment."

Concurrent with advances in chemotherapy, the field of radiation therapy, which had been introduced in the 1930s, also progressed. Cobalt 60 units providing super voltage were introduced in the early 1950s and replaced orthovoltage machines for most types of cancer treatment. In turn, cobalt 60 units were later supplanted by even higher energy machines, the linear accelerators.

It was evident that, increasingly, the treatment of cancer required a multidisciplinary team approach. In the area of radiotherapy at the MGH, Marvin Lougheed was a driving force and an important member of the team. Working with him was Julio Guerra, a fully trained radiation therapist (the term "radiation oncologist" was introduced in the late 1970s). Early specialists in radiation therapy arose from the ranks of radiology specialists. At the MGH those involved in radiation therapy included Ross Hill and Leonard Rosenthall. With the retirement of Lougheed and concurrent with plans for modernization of the Radiotherapy Department, J. Webster was recruited in the early 1970s from Rosewell Park Memorial Institute in the United States to head the Department of Radiation Therapy. Completing the cadre of surgeons closely involved in the treatment of cancer were Roberto Estrada, Lawrence Hampson, E. John Hinchey, Andrew Hreno, Lindsay Ogilvy, and Alan Thompson.

Through the influence of John Palmer, and following the guidelines of the American College of Surgeons Committee on Cancer (ACSCC), then the only certifying body for hospital based cancer programs, the Tumour Board and Multidisciplinary Tumour Policy Committee was set up in the late 1950s to add to the third element for certification, the Tumour Registry, which was already in place. Another specialty playing an important role in the Tumour Board and Tumour Registry was pathology. The Department of Pathology was headed by W. Matthews and subsequently by W. Duguid in the mid-1970s. Conforming to the guidelines of the ACSCC was essential with regard to accreditation of the training program in surgery. Estrada and Hutchison were active in overseeing the collection of data for the Tumour Registry, which operated out of the Medical Records Department under the direction of Edith Cole and her staff. Cole was also responsible for organizing the weekly Tumour Board and the monthly Tumour Policy Committee meetings held in a conference room on the second floor of the hospital. Of note, for all cases presented at the tumour boards, patients under review were presented, questioned, and examined. Unfortunately, for logistical reasons, this is a practice that no longer occurs.

To complete the picture of what was in place up to 1975, the different treating specialists held separate ambulatory clinics. For chemotherapy, the outpatient clinic (Oncology/Chemotherapy Centre) occupied one wing of the seventh floor of Livingston Hall, which had been the former nurse's residence. MacFarlane, and to some extent Hutchison, saw patients with cancer who were receiving chemotherapy there. The drugs were administered by one chemotherapy nurse, Monica MacDonald, later assisted by Janet Ong, and there was one clerical assistant/secretary, Anne Dougherty. Thus the various pieces were in place to further advance the cancer program from 1975 onward.

Laying the Foundation for a Division of Medical Oncology, 1975–84

It is against the preceding background that there was, in the early 1970s, an increasing realization of the need to recruit a properly trained chemotherapist (medical oncologist) for the MGH. To this end, it was fortuitous that, through the writings of Kennedy[15] and others[16] a fourth-year internal medicine resident, Michael Thirlwell, had become interested in the developing new specialty of medical oncology in the United States.

In 1989, Kennedy, Regents' Professor of Medicine and Masonic Professor of Oncology at the University of Minnesota Medical School, was honoured by the Royal College of Physicians and Surgeons of Canada by being selected to deliver the annual Parke-Davis Lecture. This lecture was entitled "Medical Oncology: The Past, Present and Future.[17] With the encouragement of Douglas Cameron, physician-in-chief of the MGH, Thirlwell went to train in medical oncology in the United States at the MD Anderson Hospital and Tumor Institute in Houston, Texas, in the Department of Development Therapeutics as a fellow under the directorship of the renowned Emil Freireich. At that time (1973), it was, and remains, one of the leading institutions in the world conducting clinical trials on cancer treatment and, in particular, on new anti-cancer drugs in Phase 1 and Phase 2 studies.

Having completed his training at the MD Anderson, Thirlwell was appointed as assistant physician at the MGH in the Division of Haematology, Section of Medical Oncology, commencing July 1975. This was a geographical full-time hospital position with an appointment as assistant professor in the Department of Medicine at McGill University. Cronin was dean of the Faculty of Medicine at the time. Of note, Thirlwell was cross-appointed to the department of surgery at the MGH and McGill University with the support of Alan Thompson, surgeon-in-chief. This latter appointment was a very far-sighted one as it enabled the closer collaboration of the rapidly solid tumour chemotherapy activities in medical oncology with the activities of the surgeons involved in cancer care. Thirlwell was the first fully trained medical oncologist recruited to McGill University. The primary tasks that lay ahead for Thirlwell following his arrival were to oversee the development of the new specialty of medical oncology at the MGH so as to provide care to patients; to provide teaching to medical students, residents, and others; and to foster research and scholarly activity in the field.

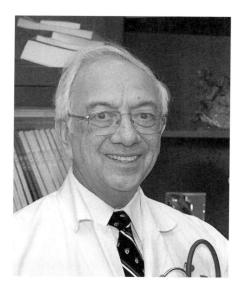

Fig. 15.1 Michael Thirlwell, director, Section of Medical Oncology, Division of Haematology, 1975–84. A separate division of medical oncology was created at the MGH in 1984, with Thirlwell as director until 2005. The MUHC was formed in 1997, and medical oncology became an MGH/MUHC division.

Developing medical oncology care for patients required having an outpatient (ambulatory) facility, with adequate space and staffing and an inpatient ward service. The outpatient clinic had become inadequate for the number of patients being seen. Additional nursing help was needed too. Fortunately, as part of the expansion of the Radiation Therapy Department, space became available on the fifth floor adjacent to this department and to the Radiology Department. This, in fact, made for great convenience for patients scheduled for visits to radiotherapy and radiology. It also made for easy interaction between the physicians delivering chemotherapy and their radiotherapy colleagues. The medical oncology chemotherapy clinic moved in 1977 to an expanded facility on the fifth floor Cedar west wing. This provided the opportunity, and indeed it was a necessity, to recruit additional nurses and clerical staff to supplement the two chemotherapy nurses and single secretary. Among the additional nurses recruited was Lois (Holly) Hollingsworth, who had worked in the ambulatory chemotherapy clinic at the RVH. Her role evolved into that of head nurse in the new Oncology Centre. She played a vital role in the continued development of the delivery of chemotherapy and the supportive care of patients, including attention to the psychological and social aspects of the care of cancer patients and their families. Another secretary, Antonella (Toni) Carriero, joined the team and has provided dedicated service over the years. An additional physician, Guy Boileau, was also recruited. He had completed his medical oncology training at the Harvard Medical Centre (Peter Bent Brigham Hospital) and had

been working at the Notre Dame Hospital in Montreal. Both medical oncologists worked in collaboration with their haematology colleagues with
regard to the on-call and ward coverage assignments. In the latter regard it
became evident that, for optimal nursing and medical care to be provided
to patients with hematologic malignancies or solid tumours admitted to hospital for treatment, complications, or essential investigations, it would be
best to cluster them together on a single ward. Thus a combined general
medical-haematology/medical oncology clinical teaching unit was created:
the 16 East Ward.

Nevertheless, as chemotherapy treatment became even more complex,
and with the introduction of very high-dose chemotherapy and bone marrow transplantation regimens, it became essential to have a specially designed
ward devoted entirely to patients with malignancies. It required staffing by
trained expert nurses and exclusive supervision by a team of hematologists
and medical oncologists. Around this time (1979), Witold Rybka had just returned from Seattle, where he had trained under E.D. Thomas and his colleagues at the Washington University Medical Centre, the leading institution
for bone marrow transplantation in North America. This method of treatment required the construction of separate laminar flow rooms to provide
a "sterile" air environment to reduce the risk of infection in these patients.
This requirement helped to hasten the creation, on 17 East, of a haematology-medical oncology unit consisting of twenty beds and two laminar flow
rooms. In the early days of the MGH, before Medicare was introduced, the
17 East ward was assigned to "private" paying patients and all the rooms were
single. This made 17 East well suited for the admission of patients ill with
febrile neutropenia and requiring protective isolation. Besides leading the
bone marrow transplantation program, Rybka also assisted in the treatment
of medical oncology patients.

As a spin-off from the need to provide bone marrow transplantation
patients with blood product support, intravenous fluids, antibiotics, and,
in many cases, parenteral nutrition, the development of central venous
catheters was introduced. These were inserted through a skin tunnel on the
chest wall into the subclavian vein and right atrium. The catheter permitted a long-term reliable venous access for these patients. It stimulated research in the whole area of venous access systems, culminating in the
development in the early 1980s of subcutaneous implanted ports, which are
now widely used in patients with any type of malignancy requiring prolonged intravenous infusion of chemotherapy and repeated blood sample

analyses. The insertion of these external catheters or implanted ports required the expertise of surgeons and reflects again the multidisciplinary approach to the care of cancer patients. This was also exemplified by the interdisciplinary collaboration provided by the highly skilled nurses on the Haematology-Medical Oncology Unit headed by Joyce Constatin. It should also be noted that the nursing groups in the United States and Canada in the 1980s formed the Oncology Nursing Society, followed by the Canadian Association of Nurses in Oncology, respectively, to foster the development of oncology nursing. Certification examinations for this nursing specialty are held annually.

As the medical oncology service grew, it exerted its presence through teaching and consultations, provided internally (in the MGH) and externally to hematologists and other physicians from many centres (e.g., Rouyn-Noranda, Gaspesie, Ormstown, St Mary's Hospital, Montreal Chest Hospital, Queen Elizabeth Hospital, Reddy Memorial Hospital, Santa Cabrini Hospital, Lakeshore General Hospital, and Lachine General Hospital). Through medical oncologists rounding on the wards, teaching medical students and residents, and making presentations at specialty and Medical Grand Rounds, internal medicine residents became interested in medical oncology. Some chose to do electives in medical oncology and expressed their wish to become medical oncologists. This provided the impetus to develop a training program at the MGH. Our first trainee in 1978 was A. Maksymiuk, a graduate of the University of Saskatoon who had done his internal medicine training at the MGH. He went on for further training at the MD Anderson. Maksymiuk was subsequently recruited back to his alma mater in Saskatoon, where he became the head of the Division of Medical Oncology. It should be noted that trainees have come from Quebec and other provinces as well as from the United States and other countries, including Panama, Mexico, Israel, China, Kuwait, Saudi Arabia, and the United Arab Emirates. In 1978, there was still no recognized specialty of medical oncology in Canada. Nevertheless, there were stirrings across Canada due to the creation of a medical oncology specialty, with certification by the Royal College of Physicians and Surgeons of Canada.

Among the early proponents of medical oncology were Daniel Bergsagel of Toronto and Neil MacDonald of Edmonton. MacDonald had moved from McGill to Edmonton to head the W.W. Cross Cancer Institute in the early 1970s. In 1982, the Council of the Royal College of Physicians and Surgeons of Canada established the Nucleus Committee for Medical Oncology, and

Michael Thirlwell was one of the members. This committee defined the new specialty of medical oncology and the training required to be eligible for certification in this specialty. It set the guidelines required for training programs that had to be taken in order to be accredited for training. The Board of Examiners in Medical Oncology was established, and Thirlwell sat on it as a member between 1990 and 1993 and was its chair between 1994 and 1996. The University of Toronto was the first medical faculty in Canada to have its training program (based at the Princess Margaret Hospital) recognized by the Royal College (in 1984). McGill University, with its training program based at the MGH, was the second Canadian centre, and the first in Quebec, to be accredited by the Royal College (1985) and, by extension, the American Board of Internal Medicine. Thirlwell was the first director of the McGill University training program in medical oncology.

The first Royal College written examination for the specialty of medical oncology took place in 1985. Candidates had to be certified in internal medicine before they could be eligible for the examination. For a grace period, recognized experience and expertise in the field (without formal training in the specialty) was accepted to allow "grandfathers" to sit for the examinations.[18]

In Quebec, disappointingly, although a medical oncology specialty eventually came into being, this did not happen until 1993. There had been a prolonged debate, over several years, regarding whether (medical) oncology should remain linked to haematology (as most hematologists involved in the care of hematologic malignancies had expanded their interests to solid tumours) or whether it should continue its development and separate into a specialty of its own (as had already occurred across North America). Medical oncology was also a separate specialty in Europe. Although most of the hematologists on the francophone side were in favour of a single specialty of haematology-oncology in Quebec, a strong proponent for a separate medical oncology specialty was Joseph Ayoub of Notre Dame Hospital. It is alleged that it required the intervention of Premier Bourassa, himself suffering from malignant melanoma and being treated by a non-haematology medical oncologist (Jacques Jolivet, who had trained at the National Cancer Institute in the United States) to intervene to halt the debate and to ensure ministerial approval for this new specialty. McGill was represented on the Corporation Professionnelle des Médecins de Quebec Nucleus Committee for Medical Oncology (1991–93) by Thirlwell. The first certifying examination of the new specialty was held in 1995.

Nevertheless, at the present time only the McGill teaching hospitals have separate divisions of medical oncology, while all the other university hospitals in Quebec still have combined divisions of haematology-oncology and combined haematology-oncology training programs. Debate aside as to the merits of having a separate or a combined specialty with regard to patient care, teaching, research, and the advancement of knowledge, there is no arguing the fact that there is more financial advantage to being certified as a hematologist-oncologist in Quebec.

With the recognition of medical oncology as a specialty across Canada, the additional recruitment of medical oncologists, and the increasing role of medical oncology in the care of patients with non-hematologic malignancies at the MGH, it was natural for medical oncology to evolve and separate off as a division in its own right. Thus the Medical Oncology Unit, which had been recognized in 1981, officially became the Division of Medical Oncology in 1984, with Thirlwell as its director. This was the first Division of Medical Oncology formed in any Quebec hospital.

Growth and Consolidation of Medical Oncology, 1984–97

In succession, the other members appointed to the unit/division were Gerald Batist, Jane Skelton, Gerald Boos, Pierre Major, Andre Veillette, Francisco Dexeus, Marc Trudeau, Ingrid Hings, Christine Legler, Wahbi Hammouda, Brian Leyland-Jones, Pierre Desjardins, Nini Wu, Jean Viallet, Raghu Rajan, Louise Craig, Vera Hirsh, Peter Gruner, Linda Ofiara (respirologist), Paul Ahlgren, Neil MacDonald, Christopher Trettor, Adrian Langleben, Steven Ades, Marie-Claude Gouttebel, Pierrre Boutin (gastro-enterologist), Thierry Alcindor (2004), and Jean-Pierre Ayoub. Two members appointed, not as medical oncologists but as clinical associates, to assist in the daily care of the cancer patients in the outpatient centre were Barbara Roback and Julie Cournoyer. The Medical Oncology Division was the first to introduce this model to the MGH, its purpose being to reduce the burden of patient care for the specialist members of a division, freeing them to devote more time to academic activities, including clinical research. Recruitment and retention of staff has been a challenge over the years due to various external factors, but, nevertheless, a critical core of medical oncologists has remained in place since the formation of the division. Part of the solution to the problem has been the cross-appointment of specialists from other disciplines who are specifically trained in chemotherapy (e.g., Linda Ofiara for lung cancer and Pierre Burtin for gastrointestinal cancers).

With regard to research, although "wet lab" research has been conducted by various members of the division (M. Thirlwell, G. Batist, P. Major, A. Veillette, and L. Vialet), the major emphasis has been on clinical research. Beginning with participation in the clinical trials of the CALGB and the NSABP, there has always been strong involvement in clinical research. This expanded to participation in other cooperative group trials (National Cancer Institute of Canada and Radiation Oncology Treatment Group) and industry-sponsored trials of new agents. There have also been internally originated MGH clinical trials.

Worth mentioning with regard to published research from the MGH is the use of hepatic arterial infusion chemotherapy for cancer of the liver[19] and the initial North American studies on a slow-release formulation of morphine.[20] The former established the MGH as a referral centre for this form of regional chemotherapy, while the latter helped to provide the basis for the approval of the drug in Canada and preceded the development of a succession of other slow-release opioids for the treatment of cancer pain.

A major development in 1978 was the creation of the McGill Cancer Centre in the Faculty of Medicine. One of its roles was to coordinate cancer clinical research activities across the McGill teaching hospitals. Its first director was Phil Gold. The clinical research activities of the division then grew and involved more frequent collaboration with other medical oncologists across the McGill teaching and affiliated hospitals.

The McGill Cancer Centre later became the Department of Oncology. The creation of the Department of Oncology at the university level in 1982 engendered much debate across the McGill hospitals (in which the Division of Medical Oncology participated) as to whether a similar organizational structure should exist within the hospitals. A hospital oncology department would bring together a number of specialists in cancer care – namely, surgeons, gynaecologists, radiation oncologists, medical oncologists, palliative care, and others. A departmental structure also had implications in terms of recruitment and appointment of staff, income, resident coverage, hospital beds, infrastructure support and space (for clinical work and laboratory research), among other issues.

The final outcome was that the structures at both the MGH and the RVH remained as they were – namely, oncology services with simply a coordination function headed by a director (John MacFarlane at the MGH and Dr Henry Shibata at the RVH). MacFarlane left for Vancouver's St Paul's Hospital in 1984 and was replaced by Thirlwell. At the Sir Mortimer-Davis Jewish General Hospital a department was formed, headed by Richard Margolese. At St Mary's Hospital a department was ultimately formed under the leadership of Jaraslov Prchal. This debate surfaced again at the MGH in the early 1990s and culminated in a decision to form a department of oncology in 1993. Jean Viallet was selected to be the director of the new department. This engendered a fair bit of controversy within the MGH milieu. The divisions of medical oncology and the Department of Radiation Oncology were grouped together in this new department. Members of the Division of Medical Oncology were cross-appointed to the Department of Medicine. Jean Viallet departed in 1995 to take up a position in industry and Thirlwell was asked and agreed to be acting director.

Beginning in 1992 there were serious discussions concerning the merger of the MGH and the RVH with the Montreal Neurological Institute, the Montreal Chest Hospital, and the Montreal Children's Hospital.[21] This merger became official in 1999, and the new entity was later named the McGill University Health Centre. As the RVH was still operating as an oncology service, discussions began as to how to reconcile this with the departmental structure at the MGH. This culminated in a decision to abolish the Department of Oncology at the MGH in 2000 and to form a joint oncology committee for the MGH and the RVH co-chaired by Thirlwell and Shibata. A 2002 task force, chaired by Mostafa Elhalali, to examine the best organizational structure for the MUHC, recommended that an oncology program be established. Carolyn Freeman, head of radiation oncology, was appointed as the acting-director of this program, and a search committee was formed to recruit a director. In summer 2003, Joseph Ragaz, a prominent senior medical oncologist from the British Columbia Cancer Agency, was selected.

Across the various divisions of the MGH and the RVH, clinical integration committees were formed, including one for medical oncology and palliative care. Palliative care was well established in the RVH under Balfour Mount, a palliative care physician (formerly a urologist) with an outstanding local, national, and international reputation. However, this aspect of care for cancer patients was not formally organized at the MGH. Attempts had been made, notably by Michael Kaye (senior nephrologist), to establish a palliative care team in the early 1980s, but this had stalled over issues of bed assignment, lack of human resources, and other matters. Nevertheless, as palliative care is such an important component of the trajectory of care in cancer patients from diagnosis to death, the cry for a service at the MGH similar to that at the RVH rose again. A committee to examine the state of palliative care at the MGH, chaired by Joseph Stratford (1996), recommended the formation of a palliative care service with assigned beds and physician staffing under the leadership of Balfour Mount. Together with a number of physicians, the push for palliative care services at the MGH came from several sources, including nurses, social workers, patients and families, auxiliary and board members, and community representatives. Earlier in 1990, members of these groups were also instrumental in the creation of a support program for cancer patients and their families. The core committee involved in the formation of the program consisted of Lois Hollingsworth (nurse), Barbara Himsel (social worker), Joan LaMontagne (director, community relations), Carol Shea (MGH volunteer and auxiliary member), and Michael Thirlwell (medical oncologist). With financial support from the Elaine Peters' Fund, the first director, Dawn Halmay, RN, was recruited. This program, called the Volunteers for Oncology Program (or, affectionately, the VOP Squad), grew and expanded over the years. Following in the footsteps of the MUHC merger movement, in 2002 the program joined forces with the highly successful Can Support Program of the RVH, founded by Gwen Nacos, and supported by the Cedars Cancer Institute.

Integration across the RVH and the MGH was also occurring in pharmacy services. Leading this process was Madame Patricia Lefebvre, who became the first chief pharmacist for the MGH and the RVH.

Medical Oncology into the Twenty-First Century, 1997–2005

By the mid-1990s, it became increasingly evident that the facilities on the fifth floor Oncology Centre were inadequate to cope with the increasing number of cancer patients requiring chemotherapy. This was a reflection of the increasing success of chemotherapy in different advanced cancers and in the adjuvant treatment of early cancers, initially breast cancer, later colorectal cancer, and, more recently, lung cancer. These three malignancies, plus prostate cancer, make up the four most common cancers in North America. Also, the newer standards for drug preparation and safe handling of the drugs necessitated the introduction of specific ventilation hoods and proximity to the treatment care. Furthermore, to function as an appropriate teaching and training facility, to accommodate the increased number of personnel working in the centre, and to allow a more comfortable and less crowded environment for treating patients, more space was urgently needed. With increasing participation in clinical research trials, space was also needed for the data managers (now called clinical research associates) to facilitate their work with the medical oncologists in identifying patients for trials and to follow them during their course of treatment.

With regard to clinical research, it is important to note that the level of review of the scientific and ethical aspects of clinical trials was becoming increasingly stringent, and a strong institutional review board, which met regularly, was a necessity. A site for these weekly meetings was required, and the J.L. Hutchison Library/Conference Room in the Oncology Centre was chosen as the appropriate venue.

Some of the impetus for improving the crowded treatment environment derived from patients themselves, who had experienced unpleasant chemotherapy side effects (e.g., a patient vomiting violently while sitting right next to another patient receiving chemotherapy). Support also came from various members of the community. A strong supporter from the lay community was Vicki Hodgson, a member of the Webster family and an MGH auxiliary and board member. Through the efforts of the MGH Foundation and its productive president, Ron Collett, a commitment was made for a sizeable donation ($1 million) from the Webster family for the construction of a new oncology centre named after G. Howard Webster.[22] In this regard, another major contributor to the needs of the Medical Oncology Division was the Peters family. Charles Peters had established the Elaine Peters Fund in memory of his wife, Elaine Peters, who had been a patient cared for by Thirlwell.

Finally, with regard to the economic use of personnel and facilities, it was logical that the separate haematology outpatient treatment facilities – for the chemotherapy of hematologic malignancies, phlebotomies, blood transfusions, and other procedures – should be merged into a new oncology/haematology ambulatory centre.

The new comprehensive G. Howard Webster Ambulatory Centre was duly opened in July 1997 with the most up-to-date design and facilities for patient care, teaching, and clinical research. This centre has facilitated our functioning in the modern era of systemic anticancer therapy, which now involves many complex regimens of chemotherapy as well as the use of biologic agents and molecularly targeted drugs. Concomitant with, and, indeed, essential, to this has been close collaboration with pharmacists and oncology nurses as they further develop their expertise in the use of anticancer drugs. The improved environment for administering chemotherapy to patients (less crowding and more privacy) and additional beds and comfortable chairs ("lazy boys") for patients receiving prolonged chemotherapy or other treatments has been greatly welcomed by patients and staff alike. Much appreciated too has been the improved waiting area and a separate family "quiet" room for patients or families requiring moments of privacy or general relaxation away from the waiting area. The new centre also provides a trainees' room for residents and medical students and a library/conference room named after L. Hutchison.

Accompanying the advances in chemotherapy has been an increase in the number of patients treated, particularly those with the most common cancers. As noted earlier, the results from clinical trials have established the benefit of adjuvant treatment in early breast, colo-rectal, and lung cancer. Furthermore, in contrast to earlier days, patients with metastatic lung, colo-rectal, and prostate cancer can benefit from chemotherapy. These, among other factors, including the aging population, have all contributed to the increase in the number of patients treated in the ambulatory centre. The number of outpatient visits in the year 2005 totalled twenty-two thousand. Of note, at any time, patients with cancer-related problems make up 35 percent or more of the census of patients admitted to the MGH wards.

With the new centre, clinical research activities have increased, including participation in trials of new anticancer drugs. As noted earlier, the requirements for approval criteria for studies by institutional review boards, or research ethics boards as they are now called, have become more stringent, precise, and comprehensive. Of particular concern are the ethical issues relating to potential benefits versus risks and the obtaining of proper informed consent from research participants. The weekly board meetings are chaired by Denis Cournoyer and Michael Thirlwell and are organized very efficiently by Esher Boyle, the administrative coordinator.

Among the major challenges as we entered the twenty-first century was, and still is, the struggle to provide new and effective but highly expensive drugs for our patients. The recruitment and retention of medical oncologists, aggravated by the shortage of medical oncologists across the country and our heavy workload, has been challenging as well. This personnel problem became particularly poignant at the RVH when all three of its medical oncologists departed in succession over several months in late 2001 and early

2002. This necessitated, among other actions, the intervention of the MGH Division of Medical Oncology, which provided services while frenetic efforts were made to recruit replacement medical oncologists. This period precipitated the unification of the divisions of medical oncology at the MGH and the RVH, and Michael Thirlwell served as acting-director. Concurrent with this development, and in keeping with the recommendations of the Elhalali Task Force to create an oncology program, a search committee was formed to seek a director for the oncology program As mentioned earlier, in the summer of 2003, Joseph Ragaz, from the British Columbia Cancer Agency, was chosen. Over the next several months, three medical oncologists – Catalin Mihalcioiu (from Winnipeg), Martin Chasen (from South Africa), and Thierry Alcindor (from Sherbrooke) – were recruited as well as a clinical associate, E. Garoufalis.

The Medical Oncology Division has continued to play an important role in the activities of the Department of Oncology at McGill University, chaired by Gerald Batist, who replaced Brian Leyland-Jones, the first chair of the department. Leyland-Jones had been recruited from the National Cancer Institute (in the United States) in 1990. The division has contributed to the clinical research program, the conduct of the medical oncology training program, the teaching of medical students and residents, and the deliberations of the Management Committee of the Oncology Department.

In October 2005, Thirlwell stepped down as director of medical oncology. Jeremy Sturgeon, a prominent senior medical oncologist from Princess Margaret Hospital, Toronto, was recruited to succeed him. As we enter the next phase of development of medical oncology as a unified MUHC division we can look back with satisfaction and pride on all that has been accomplished in the past thirty years thanks to the input of numerous people, some of whom are mentioned in the previous pages. To these must be added the succession of senior administrators (Harvey Barkun, Gerard Douville, Blair Whittemore, and Francoise Chagnon) and physician-in-chiefs (Phil Gold and Tim Meagher) who encouraged and supported the development of medical oncology at the MGH. It has been an exciting three decades, coinciding with the establishment of the role of chemotherapy and of medical oncology as a specialty. There have been major advances in the systemic treatment of patients with cancer. Over the years, the members of the Medical Oncology Division have made their mark locally, nationally, and internationally. They have continued to conduct teaching, clinical research, and other academic activities, while providing service to patients and undertaking administrative duties expected of the members of a specialty division. The Medical Oncology Division is firmly grounded, and we can look forward to its continued success as plans proceed for its move to the new Glen Yards site of the MUHC.

ACKNOWLEDGMENTS
I gratefully acknowledge the encouragement of John Burgess, Gweneth Audrey, and the secretarial assistance of Esther Boyle in the production of this manuscript.

APPENDIX
MGH Medical Oncology Trainees 1978–2005
1 Dr Andrew Maksymiuk
2 Dr Darcy Spicer
3 Dr Jane Skelton
4 Dr Francisco Dexeus
5 Dr Helen Keable
6 Dr Christine Legler
7 Dr Carlos Gonzales
8 Dr Hilla Baytner-Zamir
9 Dr Rita Trujillo
10 Dr Robert Sunenblick
11 Dr Nelson Adamson
12 Dr Ti QiWang
13 Dr JeffChiarro
14 Dr Wahbi Hammouda
15 Dr April Shamy
16 Dr Sonya Brisson
17 Dr Jean Viallet
18 Dr Safika Al Awade
19 Dr Linda Ofiara
20 Dr John Goffin
21 Dr Shaheena Dawood
22 Dr Munir Al Rafee
23 Dr M. Seebag

NOTES

1 M. Dolliner, E.H. Rosenbaum, and G. Cable, *Everyone's Guide to Cancer Therapy*, 3rd ed. (Sommerville House, 1997).

2 J.H. Burchenal, "The Historical Development of Cancer Chemotherapy," *Seminars in Oncology* 4 (1997): 135–46.

3 M. Peckham, H.M. Pinedo, and U. Veronesi, *Oxford Textbook of Oncology* (Oxford: Oxford Medical Publications, 1995).

4 M. Abeloff et al., *Clinical Oncology*, 3rd ed. (Amsterdam: Elsevier Churchill Livingston, 2005).

5 A. Gilman and F.S. Philips, "The Biological Actions and Therapeutic Applications for B- Chlorethyl Amino Acid Sulfates," *Science* 103 (1946): 409–41.

6 L.S. Goodman et al. "Nitrogen Mustard Therapy: Use of Methyl-Bis (Beta-Chlorethyl) Amino Hydrochloride and Tris (Beta-Chlorethyl) Amino Hydrochloride for Hodgkin's Disease, Lymphosarcoma, Leukemia and Certain Allied and Miscellaneous Disorders," *Journal of the American Medical Association* 132 (1946): 126–32.

7 S. Farber et al., "Temporary Remissions in Acute Leukemia in Children Produced by the Folic Acid Antagonist, 4-Aminopteroyl-Glutamic Acid," *New England Journal of Medicine* 238 (1948): 787–93.

8 J.L. Hutchison, interview by the author, 11 February 2008.

9 V.T. DeVita, A.A. Serpick, and P.P. Carbone, "Combination Chemotherapy in the Treatment of Advanced Hodgkin's Disease," *Annals of Internal Medicine* 73 (1970): 891.

10 D.S. Martin and R.A. Fugman, "A Role of Chemotherapy as an Adjunct to Surgery." *Cancer Research* 17 (1957): 1098–101.

11 U. Veronesi, "Breast Cancer," in *Oxford Textbook of Oncology*, ed. M. Peckham, H.M. Pinedo, U. Veronesi, 1243–89 (Oxford: Oxford University Press, 1995).

12 Ludwig Breast Cancer Study Group, "Prolonged Disease-Free Survival after One Course of Perioperative Adjuvant Chemotherapy for Node-Negative Breast Cancer," *New England Journal of Medicine* 320 (1989): 491.

13 J.K. MacFarlane, recollections, July 2008, personal communication.

14 G.T. Beatson, "On the Treatment of Inoperable Cases of Carcinoma of the Mammae: Suggestions for a New Treatment with Illustrative Cases," *Lancet* 2 (1896): 104–7.

15 B.J. Kennedy, "Training in Medical Oncology," *Archives of Internal Medicine* 121 (1963): 189–91.

16 S.C. Taylor III, "Cancer and the Internist" (editorial), *Annals of Internal Medicine* 65 (1966): 189; W.P.L. Myers, J.H. Krakoff, and B.D. Clarkson, "The Train-

ing of Internists in Cancer," *Medical Clinics of North America* 55 (1971): 647–52; 18 B.J. Kennedy, P. Calabresi, E. Frei III, J. Holland, A.H. Owens, M.H. Sleisenger, and J.H. Beck, *Annals of Internal Medicine* 78 (1973): 127–30; Editorial, "Medical Oncology," *Lancet* 2 (1971): 419.

17 B.J. Kennedy, "Medical Oncology: The Past, Present and Future," *Annals Royal College of Physicians and Surgeons of Canada* 23 (1990): 39–44.

18 Personal communication, Office of Royal College of Physicians and Surgeons of Canada, February 2008.

19 M. Thirlwell, M. Hollingsworth, M. Herba, G. Boileau, G. Boos, and J. MacFarlane, "Ambulatory Hepatic Arterial Infusion Chemotherapy for Cancer of the Liver," *American Journal of Surgery* 151 (1986): 58.

20 M. Thirlwell, P. Sloan, G. Boos, et al., "Pharmacokinetics and Clinical Efficacy of Oral Morphine Solution and Controlled Release Morphine Tablets in Cancer Patients," *Cancer* 63 (1989): 2275–83.

21 Minutes of the Executive Committee and Quarterly Meetings of the Council of Physicians, Dentists and Pharmacists, Montreal General Hospital, MGH Archives.

22 Mr R. Collett. Recollections, June 2008, personal communication.

16

Respirology

Neil Colman and John H. Burgess

Neil Colman was the second director of the Division of Respiratory Diseases. John Burgess combined his manuscript with notes from his predecessor, Donald MacIntosh.

"Progress" said the director of the Division of Endocrinology. "Progress" echoed the director of the Division of Allergy and Immunology. "Progress" chanted the director of the Division of Gastroenterology, and so on around the rich mahogany table of the boardroom at the Montreal General Hospital. It was 1975. Division directors were assembled for the monthly meeting of the Department of Medicine. At the head of the table was D.G. Cameron, the chair, a man who ruled the department with an iron fist cloaked in a mailed glove. As was the custom, each chief reported by that single word the developments of the past month for his or her respective division. This was inevitably followed by Cameron's lengthy and uninterrupted review of the department's activities.

Donald MacIntosh stood to speak; a hush fell over the room. It was not clear to many why MacIntosh was taking the floor. It soon would be. "The Division of Respiratory Medicine," he announced, "wishes to propose the appointments of two new members to the Department of Medicine." And the respiratory division was born. Until that moment, respiratory medicine was an adjunct to the Division of Cardiology, under its director, John Burgess. With the recent recognition of respiratory medicine as a distinct specialty for the purposes of accreditation by the Royal College of Physicians and Surgeons of Canada, Cameron had decided to inaugurate the Division of Respiratory Medicine at the MGH in 1975.

The service actually had its origins in 1953. On 13 November 1953, L.A. Caswell, who was the chief of the Cardio-Respiratory Department, wrote to

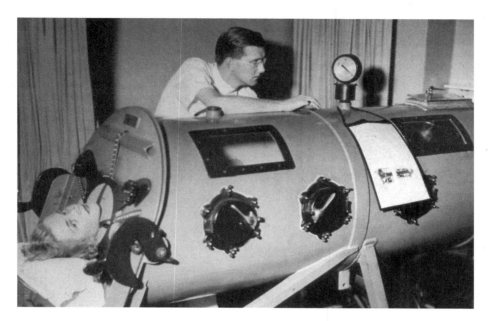

Fig. 16.1 The Iron Lung, or Negative Pressure Ventilator, invented in 1927 at Harvard, was first used at the Peter Bent Brigham Hospital in 1929. Used mainly for polio victims, it was in use in the United States and Canada from 1927 to 1959, when the positive pressure respirators replaced them and polio was only a minimal threat. Last used at the MGH in 1960.

Edward Mills, the physician-in-chief of the MGH, then located on Dorchester Boulevard East, suggesting that a chest clinic would offer a useful service in the Department of Medicine and the hospital as whole … such a clinic would serve as a diagnostic and consultant clinic; as such, the cases would be returned to the referring clinic as quickly as possible. On the same day, he proposed that Donald J. MacIntosh be appointed as an assistant in the Cardio-Respiratory Department. A research cardio-respiratory laboratory had been established in the previous two years at the MGH, but, by 1953, the techniques developed there were being translated to patient care. The measurement of maximum breathing capacity was available at a cost of ten dollars (five dollars for public patients); the vital capacity could be measured for six dollars (three dollars for public patients). In 1956, a single pulmonary paper was produced for publication. Lung volume was measured seventy-three times during the course of the year in the laboratory. By contrast, current publications are innumerable, three thousand full lung function studies are conducted at the MGH during the year, as are more than five thousand spirometric studies. The fee schedule, however, has gone down, even in absolute dollars.

Prior to 1975, MacIntosh had been the de facto head of service and now assumed formal responsibility for the development of the division's activities. The other members of the service included Magdy Younes, David Bruce, Stan Eidinger, and Richard Kennedy. Eidinger and Kennedy were part-time clinicians in the department and had major responsibilities elsewhere. MacIntosh, an astute clinician, was also the chief of medicine at the Royal Edward Chest Hospital, which later became the Montreal Chest Hospital Centre only to assume its most recent designation, the Montreal Chest Institute. David Bruce was GFT-H at the MGH. The burden of research was borne by Magdy Younes, a physiologist, who had already announced his decision to move to Winnipeg at the end of the academic year. Clearly, there was work to be done.

The appointments announced by MacIntosh were those of Neil Colman and Arnold Zidulka. Colman had trained in the respiratory program at the Royal Victoria Hospital and in Nancy, France. He was in the process of completing a year as chief resident at the Royal Edward Chest Hospital. Arnold Zidulka was on the staff of the RVH. His major appointment was at the Queen Mary Veterans Hospital and he was joining the MGH as a researcher and clinician. Both joined the staff in July 1976. Colman was appointed medical director of inhalation therapy. Zidulka became director of the lung function laboratory.

Two developments in those early days are of historical interest. The first was the initiation of a fiberoptic bronchoscopy service at the MGH. Until then, bronchoscopy was performed only with rigid bronchoscopes and only by cardiothoracic surgeons in the surgical suites. The thoracic surgeons at the hospital welcomed their new colleagues and agreed to develop this service with them. This was in the early days of fiberoptic instrumentation. Patients were examined in a treatment room on the thoracic surgery floor, 15 East. They sat in a modified dental chair. Recovery occurred in the corridor. Consequently, little sedation was used and, fortunately, little was required. It wasn't clear that the service was ever formally approved or developed by the administration. David Mulder, who was the surgeon responsible for the service at the time, was a firm believer in developing facts on the ground. It was a daring strategy, and he succeeded here, as at other times and in other situations, in dragging a ponderous administration reluctantly into the world of late twentieth-century medical innovation.

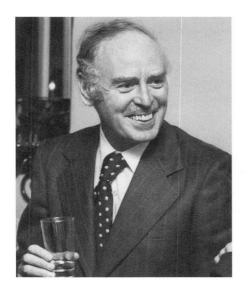
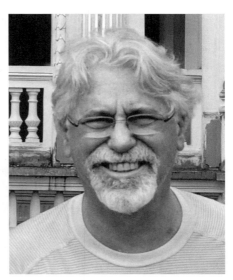

Fig. 16.2 Donald MacIntosh, director, Division of Respiratory Medicine, 1975 to 1978, when he went to Dalhousie. He was de facto head of the respiratory service for years.
Fig. 16.3 Neil Colman, director, Division of Respirology, 1978–97

In 1976, inhalation therapy was a small hospital service. Its major activity consisted of the administration of aerosol therapy to patients with the aid of a Bird ventilator – intermittent positive pressure breathing (IPPB). By then, it was apparent that bronchodilator therapy could be given with equal efficacy and lower cost by the use of hand-held devices or by aerosol mask administration. A new role for inhalation therapy was needed and new services were required. The field of intensive care was being developed. Surgical, neurosurgical, and medical intensive care units (MICUs, SICUs, and NICUs, respectively) had been opened. The MICU was on 11 East and under the direction of the Division of Clinical Pharmacology. The SICU was on the eighth floor adjacent to the operating theatres and recovery room, while the NICU was on the fourteenth floor. Mechanical ventilation was being increasingly used as a life-saving intervention in the critically ill. Under medical direction, the inhalation therapists developed expertise in the monitoring and management of these patients in the critical care areas. This became one of their major responsibilities in the hospital and has remained so to this day.

In 1976, the Parti Québécois won its first provincial election, and the separation of Quebec from Canada seemed imminent. Forty members of the Department of Medicine at McGill left Montreal in the following year. The optimists remained and were soon joined by Eli Matouk, who became a part-time member of the division.

In about 1978, MacIntosh left Montreal and took a position in Halifax at Dalhousie University. New leadership was required. Cameron demonstrated stunning foresight in his appointment of J.A.P. Pare as chief of the Respiratory Division. Pare became chief of the division at the RVH and the Montreal Chest Hospital Centre at the same time. This was the first integrated division of medicine at McGill University and foreshadowed the development of the MUHC and the division's current structure. The division's role at the time was to provide a clinical service at what would eventually be known as the MGH site. There was an active consultation service and a very small ambulatory care service, shared with the MOD on the second floor of the Pine Avenue wing. Joseph Braidy joined the division as a part-time clinician. Kennedy, Bruce and Eidinger had left Montreal. Zidulka was the sole researcher in the division; he had a small laboratory in the Research Institute and also worked in the Meakins-Christie Laboratories. Pare wrote the second edition of what was the standard text in the field of pulmonary medicine, *Fraser and Pare's Diagnosis of Diseases of the Chest*.

In 1982, Pare retired. Phil Gold had replaced the now-retired D.G. Cameron as chief of medicine at the MGH. In 1982, Neil Colman was appointed director of the division at the MGH. Although the division remained an integrated one, especially in the areas of training of fellows and of research, its leadership was now divided. Gold instructed Colman that his mandate was to develop the clinical, teaching, and research activities of the division. In the absence of computers and palm pilots, Colman carried a single sheet of paper in the left-hand pocket of his suit jacket. It served as a reminder of "things to do" and as a personal agenda. The first items on the list in 1982 consisted of: (1) recruit new members, (2) get new space, (3) get money for new space, (4) build clinical activity, and (5) department meeting, 8:00 AM on Thursday.

The 1980s were a period of important growth for the Division of Respirology. Pierre Ernst, who had a background in respiratory epidemiology and became an international authority in his area, joined the division. He also made a major contribution to the development of the lung transplant program (see below). Andre Gervais was a part-time clinician for a few years in the early 1980s, as was Mario Rizzi, who soon left to work full time at Santa Cabrini Hospital. David Lockhat did part-time duty in the division; his major area of activity was in intensive care, where he was among the first of the "respiratory intensivists" at McGill. Braidy left to join the staff at St Luc hospital while Jim Gruber joined the staff at the MGH. Zidulka continued as director of the laboratories and became medical director of inhalation therapy. He developed a sleep disorders laboratory, carved out of the EEG facility in the department of neurology. At a later time, this laboratory was integrated with the laboratory at the RVH to form the sleep laboratories of the MUHC, currently housed in the RVH's Woman's Pavilion. The department was growing, but its space was confined to a small cul-de-sac on the fifth floor. "Offices" consisted of wire baskets on the desk of the division's sole secretary. To say that the space was inadequate was no exaggeration. When the division eventually moved from that area, the latter was offered to the laundry service for repair of patient curtains and so on. They refused to take the space until renovations were completed as it was simply too shabby.

It was the National Hockey League that provided the solution to the space problem, at least for a time. Clarence Campbell, who was a patient of Colman and the recently retired president of the league, facilitated Colman's introduction to Bill Wirtz, who was a friend of his (Campbell's) and president of the NHL Board of Governors. Mr Wirtz was sympathetic to Colman's suggestion that the league honour Mr Campbell by funding the development of new equipment and space in the hospital for the respiratory division. Each of the twenty-one teams donated US$10,000, which was used in the construction and equipping of the current office and laboratories on the seventh floor of the Cedar wing.

The unit opened in 1985 shortly after Campbell's death. It was anticipated that ambulatory care activity would include two thousand patient visits, but, within several years, there were eight thousand patient visits and the facilities became (and remain) severely cramped.

In the late 1980s, David Eidelman joined the Division of Respirology and became director of the laboratories. He was a clinician-scientist who conducted major work on the pathogenesis of asthma at the Meakins-Christie Laboratories. At about the same time, Stewart Gottfried was recruited as a research scientist. He worked out of a small lab in the research institute and at the Meakins-Christie. His interest was in lung mechanics, in developing novel methods of mechanical ventilation, and in the utility of non-invasive mechanical ventilation in patient management. By the end of the 1980s, division members were contributing about thirty articles annually to the medical literature. With the reduction of hospital beds, there had been a major shift in care and diagnostic services to ambulatory care, and the service had developed to provide it. Training of fellows shifted to the ambulatory care areas, long before it became fashionable to do so.

In 1988, the first Canadian lung transplantation was performed at the Toronto General Hospital. In 1989, a lung transplantation program was instituted at the MGH under the direction of Hani Shennib, a newly recruited thoracic surgeon who had trained in Toronto. Pierre Ernst became the co-director of the program on the medical side. With Shennib, an infrastructure was carved from virtually non-existent resources. As the success of the program grew, the administration reluctantly allocated more resources to the support of this high-profile activity, but it is fair to say that it was never properly funded. The entire division lent its support, and, eventually, a transplant service rotation became a particular clinical responsibility for division members. In 1995, Paul Corris was recruited from Newcastle-upon-Tyne to co-direct the transplant program. He was a prominent researcher and clinician in the transplant world and his joining the staff constituted a real strengthening of our resources in this area. Nevertheless, in the face of underfunding and personality conflict, the program was soon transferred to Notre Dame Hospital, where it has remained (it should be noted that Corris was never part of the problem, only part of the solution).In the mid-1990s, Ash Gursahaney was recruited to the division. An outstanding teacher and clinician, he later became director of the now integrated intensive care unit and oversaw the development and construction of its current state-of-the-art facilities on the ninth floor of the hospital.

In 1993, the first asthma unit at McGill and one of the first in the province was developed by Colman and Ernst at the MGH. It became a model of the multidisciplinary care of patients and involved collaboration with the allergists, lung function technicians, and pharmacy and inhalation therapists. An active clinical trials program developed in parallel with the increasing clinical load and expertise in this area. In 1995, Colman resigned as division director. He was now writing the fourth edition of *Fraser and Pare's Diagnosis of Diseases of the Chest,* which was published in 1999.

In the MUHC accreditation, the Division of Respirology was singled out as providing the best quality of patient care at the MUHC. Its research activities are broad and constitute a place of excellence at the university. It is difficult to believe that this is what Caswell had envisioned on that cold November day fifty-two years ago.

17

Rheumatology

David Hawkins and John Esdaile

David Hawkins was the second director of the Division of Rheumatology. He was succeeded by John Esdaile. The editors combined their contributions.

Early Treatment of Rheumatic Diseases at the MGH

In the 1950s and 1960s, rheumatology at the Montreal General Hospital was primarily a clinical service, staffed by John Martin and Eva Arent-Racine. Martin and Arent-Racine carried on a large consulting practice in rheumatology and provided teaching to medical students and house staff in the context of care of patients with rheumatic diseases. David Hawkins established the first Division of Rheumatology at the MGH, which became a funded clinical /research division and has thrived with many changes in staff.

In 1970, Martin was approached by the New Medical School at Memorial University of Newfoundland to come and establish the first rheumatic diseases unit or arthritis centre at that institution. There were, at the time, rheumatic disease units (RDUs) at every medical school in Canada, and the one at Memorial was proposed to be established at one of its teaching hospitals, St Claire's Mercy Hospital. Martin left the MGH and became professor of medicine at Memorial University, established the new rheumatic diseases unit, and proceeded to recruit a team of academic rheumatologists, one of whom included John Lochead, whose father was a consultant internist at the MGH. John Lochead himself had done his residency at the MGM and was chief resident under the then chair of the department, Douglas Cameron. Lochead went on to do postgraduate training in rheumatology with Morris Ziff in Dallas, Texas, and was then recruited by Martin to Memorial.

In 1971, Cameron approached David Hawkins of the Division of Clinical Immunology and Allergy to see if he might be interested in establishing an academic division of rheumatology at the hospital. Hawkins had been a resident in internal medicine at the MGH from 1962 to 1964, and he returned from a postdoctoral fellowship at Scripts Research Institute in California in 1968 to join the then fledgling division of clinical immunology and allergy. That divison's development was critical to subsequent developments in rheumatology. In 1968, Sam Friedman was head of the Division of Clinical Immunology and Allergy, and he recruited three former MGH residents to put together an academic clinical immunology group. These people were David Hawkins, Phil Gold, and Joe Shuster. Hawkins's fellowship in allergy, immunology and rheumatology at Scripts Research Institute had kindled an interest in connective tissue diseases and inflammation.

A Division of Rheumatology at the MGH

Because of his interest in this area, Cameron felt that he might be willing to expand into the clinical realm by establishing the Division of Rheumatology. This, in fact, took place in 1971. One of the first moves Hawkins made was to approach the Canadian Arthritis Society in Toronto to explore the possibility of obtaining its support, particularly for recruitment of additional faculty and for research in the area of rheumatic diseases. Arent-Racine remained at the MGH as an active clinical rheumatologist until her retirement. Over the next few years, Hawkins was able to successfully recruit three young academically trained rheumatologists, all of whom came with salary support from external agencies and external research funding. These individuals were John Esdaile, Hyman Tannenbaum, and Charles Bruneaut. Hawkins already had a functioning lab in the MGH/McGill University Research Institute, and Esdale, Bruneaut, and Tannenbaum quickly established their research presence, largely in the clinical realm. By the mid 1970s, the division was able to attract trainees in rheumatology through the McGill program. It carried on a positive relationship with its sister division at the Royal Victoria Hospital and continued to have very strong linkages to the Division of Clinical Immunology at the MGH. It is fair to say that, without the support of the group in clinical immunology, the Division of Rheumatology would not have been established, let alone prospered. That support was not only tangible but also highly collegial in the full spectrum of academic activities and not an inconsiderable number of social ones as well. The presence of two vibrant divisions

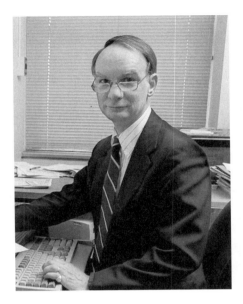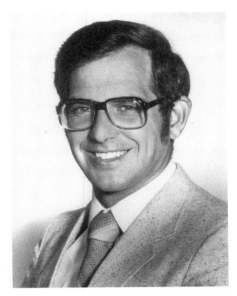

Fig. 17.1 John Esdaile, director, Division of Rheumatology, 1980–96
Fig. 17.2 Hyman Tannenbaum, director, Division of Rheumatology, 1996–97

with close linkages – namely, rheumatology and clinical immunology – provided an attractive milieu for trainees, research fellows, and future faculty.
These developments are described in chapter.

Changing Staff in the Division of Rheumatology

By 1978, the division had matured and was stable and well funded. Hawkins
took a sabbatical leave at the National Jewish Hospital and Research Center
in Denver, Colorado, to continue his research on mechanisms of inflammation. During that year he had the opportunity to work with J. Roger Hollis-
ter, at the time the only paediatric rheumatologist in the Rocky Mountain
catchment area, and, over the course of 1978–79, he began to participate increasingly in activities in paediatric rheumatology by carrying out consults
at the University of Colorado Medical Center and clinical trials at the NJH.
When Hawkins returned to McGill in the summer of 1979, the individual at
the Montreal Children's Hospital who had been running the juvenile arthritis clinic went on medical leave, and he (Hawkins) was asked if he would run
the arthritis clinic on an interim basis. With his recent Denver experience in
paediatric rheumatology he accepted this challenge and opportunity, and he

and John Esdaile carried the clinic on a monthly basis through 1979 to the summer of 1980, at which time Hawkins left McGill and the MGH to accept a position of professor and chair of medicine at Memorial University of Newfoundland.

Interestingly enough, when Hawkins went to Memorial in 1980 he became part of the rheumatic diseases unit that Martin had founded in 1971 and, in fact, became a colleague of Martin's and they eventually practised rheumatology together at the new health sciences centre in St John's. In 1987, Hawkins became the third dean of medicine at Memorial's Faculty of Medicine and, in 1995, took on the executive directorship of the association of faculties of medicine in Canada (located in Ottawa). Since then his clinical practice has been confined to paediatric rheumatology sited at the Children's Hospital of Eastern Ontario. John Esdaile remained at the MGH as the leader of the rheumatology group until 1996, when he was recruited to the University of British Columbia as professor of medicine, head of the Division of Rheumatology, and director of the Mary Pack Arthritis Centre in Vancouver. Esdaile went on to establish an international reputation for outstanding clinical research in rheumatic diseases and eventually formed the Arthritis Research Centre of Canada, establishing it as the premiere arthritis research unit in western Canada. In 2007, he became the chief executive officer and scientific director of the Canadian Arthritis Network, one of the federally funded Networks of Centres of Excellence. Charles Bruneau left the MGH in the late 1980s (?) and took a position with the Ministry of Health in France. He eventually became one of the top-ranking medical bureaucrats in France and was largely responsible for the accreditation of health institutions in that country.

Hyman Tannenbaum left his full-time university position at McGill to establish a multi-purpose arthritis centre in downtown Montreal. This, to my knowledge, was the first free-standing such centre that employed not only rheumatologists but also allied health professionals, providing "one stop shopping" to arthritis sufferers in the City of Montreal and the Province of Quebec. One of Tannenbaum's daughters graduated from McGill University in medicine and is a family practitioner in Ottawa.

When Hawkins left the MGH for Memorial University, the headship of the division passed to Hyman Tannenbaum. Tannenbaum had trained with Peter Schur at the Brigham and Women's Hospital, Harvard Medical School, and brought back to the MGH a research interest in immunologic responsiveness in rheumatoid arthritis. Interestingly, his wife, Marion, would also carry on a long-time career as a research associate at the MGH Research Institute. Tannenbaum set up many aspects of the clinical rheumatology program. In 1986, he gave up his position as academic head to develop a multi-disciplinary private practice rheumatology clinic, which continues to provide outstanding rheumatologic care to this day.

John Esdaile took over as head of the division. He had recently returned from Yale University Medical School, where he had participated in the Robert Wood Johnson Clinical Scholars Program under the supervision of Alvan Feinstein, completed a master's of public health at the Laboratory of Epidemiology and Public Health at Yale, and left having been appointed visiting associate professor of medicine.

Esdaile joined the recently created Division of Clinical Epidemiology at the MGH. He was involved in the considerable growth and success of the division in leading very applied research. In 1991, Esdaile was appointed division head for both the MGH and RVH programs. Both divisions had always functioned together well, but having a single director allowed for a stronger training program.

With Esdaile's departure to head the rheumatology program at the University of British Columbia in 1996, the division's headship was taken on by Mary-Ann Fitzcharles, a clinician and researcher from the RVH. In turn, she would be replaced by Henri Menard, an eminent basic scientist from the University of Sherbrooke whose work on the anti-Sa antigen is widely known.

In its first two decades, the Division of Rheumatology trained a number of eminent scientists who would go on to great success nationally and internationally. These included: Jean-Pierre Pelletier, who pioneered in the basic science of osteoarthritis at the University of Montreal; Robert Terkeltaub, an international authority on crystal-induced arthritis, who became a professor of medicine at the University of California at San Diego; Karin Straaton, a clinical scientist at the University of Alabama at Birmingham; Chenchen Wang, a Metro A. Ogryzlo Fellow funded by the Canadian Rheumatology Association who became a leader in research on alternative health care at Tuft's University, Boston; Jacques Pouchot, another Metro A. Ogryzlo Fellow, returned to Paris and became a leading clinician scientist in Europe; Liana Fraenkel went on to additional training at Boston University and is an associate professor and clinical researcher at the Yale University School of Medicine: Sydney Brandwein trained at Boston University before returning to the MGH, where he developed a successful. basic science laboratory in autoimmune research but would eventually immigrate to the United

States as a leader in clinical investigation at Abbott Laboratories; Simon Helfgott became an internationally recognized clinical teacher at Harvard Medical School; Paul Fortin returned to the MGH following research training with Matthew Liang at Harvard and started a national program in lupus research before becoming a professor of medicine at the University of Toronto.

Jeffrey Shiroky went on to additional training at the National Institute of Health, Bethesda, Maryland, and returned to the MGH to set up a research program focusing on inflammatory muscle disease and rheumatoid arthritis. He performed pioneering work on the safe use of methotrexate before joining the Mayo Clinic in Boca Raton, Florida. Shiroky's premature death from cancer was a great loss to the arthritis community.

Julie Paquin trained as an adult rheumatologist at the MGH and went on to additional training in New York with the noted paediatric rheumatologist Jane Schauer. Paquin returned to McGill and established the Division of Paediatric Rheumatology at the Montreal Children's Hospital. The division has grown to be one of the most successful groups in North America.

The division attracted two eminent PhD scientists, Joyce Rauch and Marianna Newkirk. Rauch trained with Robert Schwarz in New York, where she identified the antiphospholipid antibodies and recognized the phospholipid epitopes in anti-double-stranded DNA. She performed landmark research on antiphospholipid antibodies, which would lead to the eventual recognition of a distinct clinical syndrome: the antiphospholipid antibody syndrome.

A host of clinicians were trained and almost all have continued as academics actively involved as teachers, and many are widely published. These include James Angle, Michel Bergat, Vivian Bykerk, Denis Choquette, Martin Cohen, Alan Duby, Karen Duffy, Marc Favreau, Catherine Flanagan, Mark Hazeltine, Nancy Hudson, Jiri Krasny, Sophie Ligier, Veena Nayak, Michael Starr, Craig Watts, Lucino Yu, and Michel Zummer. The MGH Division of Rheumatology is proud of its contributions to other divisions across Canada.

18

Tropical Medicine

J. Dick MacLean

J. Dick MacLean was the first Director of the Division of Tropical Diseases. He became internationally known for his clinical work, teaching, and research prior to his untimely death.

Introduction

Tropical medicine has been defined as a subspecialty of medicine dealing with diseases acquired in the tropics and imported into Europe and North America. Its basic sciences include microbiology (especially parasitology) and clinical epidemiology. Its clinical challenges are the care of and the understanding of the diseases of travellers, expatriates, immigrants, refugees, missionaries, and volunteers.

Tropical medicine is not a recognized subspecialty in Canada, although masters degrees and certification in clinical tropical medicine can be acquired in Europe and the United States. Clinical training is almost always acquired in tropical, developing countries, where the volume of clinical exposure is large. As a result most tropical medicine clinicians have developed an appreciation for the preventive side of tropical medicine and an understanding of community and international health and the challenges of inequity in reference to health. Unlike subspecialties that reflect pathologies associated with a particular organ system, tropical medicine is like the subspecialty of infectious disease, both in its multi-organ orientation and in its microbiological and epidemiological underpinnings.

In the industrialized world the specialty of tropical medicine has been driven, as in other specialties, by demand. Colonialism and imperialism, both real and economic, were associated with the movement of large numbers of individuals from the industrializing "West" to the tropics. The diseases that they suffered drove the development of the specialty in Europe and the United States at the end of the nineteenth century and led to the creation of institutes, schools, and centres dedicated to the development and the teaching of the science of tropical medicine. Canada lacks this colonial history but, over the past forty years, has seen a gradually increasing demand for service from its burgeoning population of immigrants who have arrived (and are arriving) from tropical countries. Montreal was an appropriate site for the development of a tropical disease specialty because of its size, its large salt-water port, its large number of international engineering firms, and the long tradition of Quebec missionaries in underdeveloped countries.

The MGH has developed the subspecialty of tropical medicine for several reasons, including Canada's changing demographics: 80 percent of all immigrants to Canada now come from developing or tropical countries. Also important has been the long history of the MGH in serving immigrant populations, beginning in 1823. Eighty-eight percent of the MGH's first four years of admissions were immigrants, of whom 66 percent were Irish economic refugees. They arrived in a city lacking sewers or clean water and brought with them (and suffered in Montreal from) the diseases that are now considered tropical and that are associated with developing countries. The times were important. Canada's increased developmental assistance to tropical countries in the 1960s under Prime Minister Lester B. Pearson made possible MGH's involvement in this process, led by the then physician-in-chief Douglas Cameron. Finally, there are the characters that have become entangled, serendipitously or otherwise, in the process of developing a tropical disease profile at the MGH.

Changing Demographics

Canada's history is the history of its immigrants and its Aboriginal hosts. France, and then Great Britain and Europe, supplied immigrants that, at times, came in overwhelming waves. However, prior to 1960, less than 10 percent of immigrants and refugees arriving in Canada came from what could be defined as a tropical or a developing country. Canada was not open to immigration from countries other than the United States or Europe. When an unprecedented wave arrived in the first fifteen years of the twentieth century, less than 3 percent were from developing or tropical countries (fig. 18.1). However, after the Second World War, Canada began an unprecedented and prolonged period of immigrant intake. Unlike all previous waves of immigrants to Canada, these immigrants were increasingly from tropical countries and, since 1990, more than 75 percent have been from tropical or developing countries (fig. 18.2). During the same period, Canadians were travelling in continually increasing numbers to tropical countries. Most important, the immigrants to Canada who had arrived in the previous fifty years are travelling back to their tropical countries of origin with their families, thus once again exposing themselves to the infectious diseases of the tropics. These "tourists" are now defined as a risk category of their own – the VFR (visiting friends and relatives).

MGH and Montreal History

The development of Canada and the MGH has always been influenced in a major way by Canada's and Montreal's immigrants. The very first patient admitted to the hospital in 1822 was an Irish immigrant with viral hepatitis. During the first four years of the MGH's existence, when the population of Montreal was approximately thirty thousand, of the recorded 3,665 admissions, 82 percent were immigrants, 66 percent were Irish immigrants, and 70 percent of all admissions had infectious diseases (table 18.1). The infectious diseases (tuberculosis, typhus, typhoid, cholera, malaria, leprosy, dysenteries, etc.) were not, at that time, considered "tropical," yet they were, in fact, the diseases we see in tropical countries today (table 18.2). Waves of immigrants, in particular Irish immigrants, continued to arrive for the next thirty years. The MGH was their hospital. In the early years of the twentieth century, a massive wave of European immigration from countries other than Ireland arrived in Canada, many attracted to new railway-accessible land in western Canada.

In the nineteenth century, Montreal was an "underdeveloped" city. It lacked a sewage system and safe potable water. Infant mortality (death of infants in the first year of life) was at approximately 33 percent, which is what is seen in the least developed countries of Africa today.[1]

In Canada and other industrialized countries, prior to the twentieth century, morbidity and mortality were predominantly of infectious origin, while, since the First World War, non-infectious chronic diseases have predominated. The introduction of the public health measures of sanitation, clean water, and pasteurization in the last quarter of the nineteenth century and the first quarter of the twentieth century were influential in reducing the huge impact of infectious diseases – the diseases of underdevelopment –

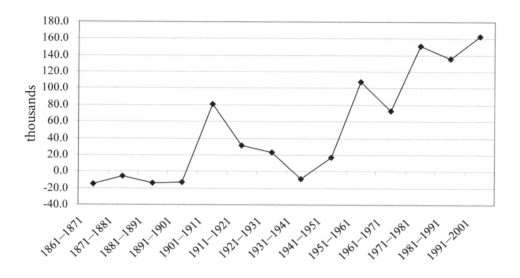

Fig. 18.1 Annual immigration less emigration

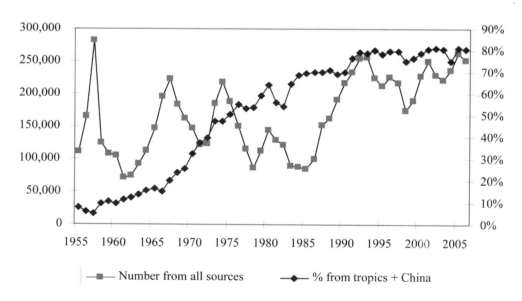

——■—— Number from all sources   ——◆—— % from tropics + China

Fig. 18.2 Immigration and emigration from Canada since statistics became available

on the health of Montrealers. This change from predominantly infectious diseases to chronic diseases was being seen throughout the industrialized world in the early twentieth century and has been called the "epidemiological transition."[2]

William Osler, in the fourteen years that he spent at McGill University's MGH as a student and then a professor, continued his naturalist interests in parasites, which, in fact, began even before he started his first two years of medical training in Toronto. His published manuscripts on trichinosis,[3] echinococcal disease,[4] malaria, and typhoid were ground-breaking at the time. He played a pivotal role in defining the need for the science of parasitology at McGill.[5] This resulted in the creation of the Institute of Parasitology (on the Macdonald Campus) led by founding director Thomas W.M. Cameron, PhD, a parasitologist trained at the universities of Edinburgh and Glasgow.[6] Finally, it has been William Osler's model of the clinical laboratory that has guided the development of today's interactive lab-clinic facility at the Tropical Diseases Centre.

After the First World War, European immigrants to Canada were no longer bringing with them the malaria, typhus, typhoid, and cholera that had been the cause of summer epidemics in Canada before the epidemiologic transition. There were medical officers from the First World War who returned with "tropical" and battlefield infectious disease experience and were the experts of their time at the MGH. Between the First World War and the Second World War immigration from the tropics remained low, and, while there were disabled veterans from the tropics, the lack of a patient load from the tropics led to a decrease in interest in, and knowledge of, tropical medicine. The Second World War again saw an increase in imported infectious diseases and in medical expertise returning from the tropics, and this once again fuelled the interest in "tropical diseases." It was this expertise that became the early core and stimulus for the present era of tropical medicine development at the MGH.

International Development

Several forces led to the early development of tropical medicine at the MGH during the 1960s and 1970s. It was the era of the beginning of the Canadian International Development Agency (CIDA) under Prime Minister Mike Pearson, when Canada was examining its international aid responsibilities. Hospitals and medical faculties saw significant funds made available from

Table 18.1
Country of birth of admissions to MGH, 1822–25

MGH admissions
1822–25 (3,665)

	%
Hibernus	66
Canadensis	12
Anglus	8
Scotus	8
Americanus	2
Germanicus	1
Welsh	1
Swiss	0.1

Table 18.2
Frequency of diagnoses in two MGH eras (infectious diseases in bold)

MGH 1822–25	%	MGH 1989	%
februm continuum	17	Acute coronary disease	11
synochus	16	cerebrovascular	5
ulcera	6	congestive heart failure	4
rheumatism	6	gastroesophageal	3
typhus	5	lymphoma/leukemia	3
pneumonia	3	lung cancer	3
diarrhea	3	**pneumonia**	3
malaria	3	peripheral vascular disease	2
dyspepsia	3	gastrointestinal haemorrhage	2
dysenteriae	3	obstructive lung disease	2

CIDA for international development projects. Rates of immigration had reached their highest levels since the boom of 1890 to 1910, but the origins of these immigrants were tropical rather than European. Socialized medicine meant that new immigrants were welcomed into an increasingly multi-ethnic medical system. Perhaps influenced by these forces, a number of McGill faculty began to look abroad. In the late 1970s, these were Doug Cameron, MGH physician-in-chief; Pat Cronin Dean of the Faculty of Medicine; Alan Ross, paediatrician-in-chief; and William Storrar, executive director of the MGH.[7] Funded by Canada's Department of External Affairs, the MGH and the Montreal Children's Hospital partnered with the University of Glasgow and the University of Nairobi to develop a medical school in Kenya. The University of Glasgow took on the responsibility for surgery and obstetrics, while the MGH and the MCH took on medicine and paediatrics. The project, from 1968 to 1978, placed thirty-nine McGill faculty and senior medical and paediatric residents in Nairobi for periods of a year or more. The success of this project had an impact on many MGH staff and may have been the most important stimulus to the development of a tropical disease centre at the MGH.

Beginning in the 1980s, funds were secured from CIDA by Douglas Cameron and the Faculty of Medicine's dean, Patrick Cronin, to begin a project in Addis Ababa, Ethiopia, with the University of Addis Ababa and the Black Lion Hospital. The link with Addis Ababa was through Edemarian Tsega, an Ethiopian trained at McGill and the MGH in medicine, internal medicine, and gastroenterology. He had returned to Ethiopia and, as physician-in-chief at the University of Addis Ababa's Black Lion Hospital had requested McGill's help. The project assisted in the development of an academic Department of Medicine; ten McGill faculty were sent to that hospital for a year each over an eight-year period, and ten Ethiopian residents from the growing internal medicine program at the Black Lion Hospital were brought to the MGH for a year of subspecialty training. Dick MacLean managed the project and secured the two funding renewals from CIDA that allowed it to reach completion. This project, in its final year, sent the MGH community health specialist Yves Bergevin to the Black Lion Hospital. He, with the support of Walter Spitzer, chair of McGill's Department of Epidemiology and Biostatistics, secured funding from both CIDA and the International Development Research Centre (IDRC) to develop the master's in community health program in the Department of Community Health at the University of Addis Ababa. This project continued from 1987 to 1998 and saw the engagement of a series of McGill faculty at the Black Lion Hospital for periods of one to four years each. The program trained seventy-five Ethiopians in a two-year field-research master's program in community health; 125 short-term (six-month) certificants in community health; and brought to Canada, the United States, and Britain twelve Ethiopians for master's and PhD degree training in a range of public health specialties.

In the 1990s, CIDA revised its approaches to foreign aid and reduced its commitment to the lowest level in thirty years. Medical education and health were of lower priority, and, as a result, McGill's Faculty of Medicine's enthusiasm for these large international projects declined. Consequently, the Centre for Tropical Diseases refocused its attention to both local and international research projects, led by Theresa Gyorkos and Brian Ward.

The Characters

After the Second World War, tropical medicine benefited as a consequence of military physicians returning from a variety of tropical fronts and continuing to enlarge on the experience they gained in caring for soldiers in theatres of war. In 1946, Phil Edwards, who had won five bronze medals over three Olympics (the last being the 1936 Berlin Olympics), and who had served with the Royal Canadian Army in Europe, became the resident tropical medicine expert at McGill, working at both the Queen Mary Veterans Hospital and the Royal Victoria Hospital. Returning from Europe after the Second World War, Hugh Starkey was made responsible for the laboratory resources that would screen the Canadian soldiers returning from Japanese prison camps.[8] No specialized diagnostic laboratory procedures other than the routine examination of feces, stool, and blood specimens, were available in those early years; however, over the next twenty years, the parasitology laboratory at the QMVH on Queen Mary Road developed a high level of excellence under Cliff Law, a medical laboratory technologist who had returned from the war and worked under Starkey. In 1970, Stanley Seah, an internist with a medical degree from the University of Manitoba and a PhD in parasitology from the London School of Hygiene and Tropical Medicine, was recruited by MGH physician-in-chief Douglas Cameron to fill retiring Phil Edwards's shoes in the MGH service of the QMVH. He continued the work of Phil Edwards, who retired in 1971. In 1978, with the closing of the

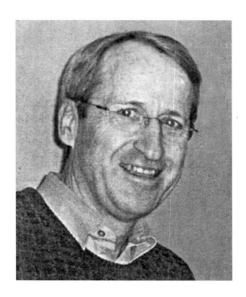

Fig. 18.3 Richard MacLean, first director of the MGH Centre for Tropical Diseases, 1980–2008

QMVH, Doug Cameron moved Stanley, with Cliff Law, to the MGH to start a tropical medicine centre in a tiny office and laboratory on the second floor.

In 1980, when Stanley Seah took up a position in Saudi Arabia, the then physician-in-chief Phil Gold appointed Dick MacLean as his replacement. MacLean, a medical graduate from Queen's University, had obtained his internal medicine at the MGH and a one-year diploma in clinical medicine of the tropics from the London School of Hygiene and Tropical Medicine. He had worked in Malaysia and Indonesia for two years with CARE-Medico, in Japan for a year with the University of Hawaii, and had been in Kenya for a year with the McGill team that, with Glasgow University, helped to build the University of Nairobi Medical Faculty.

The development of tropical medicine at the MGH met challenges of space, funding, and personnel, but crucial to this development was the creation of an integrated clinical laboratory that allowed the on-site diagnosis of tropical infections such as malaria, filariasis, and intestinal protozoa and helminths. Support for laboratory development came from the Institute of Parasitology in Saint Anne de Bellevue, possibly Canada's most important parasitology research centre. Its director, Neil Croll, PhD, MD, was an important supporter of the Tropical Disease Centre when it was starting up and, in fact, briefly joined it as a clinician before his premature death in 1982 at the age of thirty-nine.

The dean of the Faculty of Medicine, Dick Cruess, appreciated the need for a high-profile name and, in 1982, with the support of Phil Gold, accepted the name "McGill Centre for Tropical Diseases," a pretentious-sounding name for a one-physician clinic with a one-technologist laboratory. However, the name was seen as both a form of advertising and a stimulus to expansion and improvement.[9]

In 1985, the development of the seventh floor west wing of the hospital as an outpatient facility opened up the possibility of an expanded location for the TDC. Alcan Company of Canada contributed $250,000 to cover the costs of building an integrated clinical and laboratory facility situated between the gastrointestinal and respiratory medicine outpatient services on this floor, and the TDC had a new home. The space consisted of three clinical offices, a nurse's office, secretarial spaces, two laboratory spaces, one "wet" specimen preparation room, and one microscopy room. This remained the site of the TDC for twenty-five years until 2007 when a move to the tenth floor Livingstone Hall almost doubled the available space.

The staffing of the centre grew and evolved most significantly from 1985 to 2000. There was a need for clinical faculty and researchers, both bench and epidemiologic. McGill faculty who had worked in the tropics made up the initial wave. These were either internists or infectious disease specialists. David Dawson, back from the Congo, and Richard Lalonde and Laurence Green, who both worked in Ethiopia in the McGill-University of Addis Ababa Internal Medical linkage project, were early faculty, while Joyce Pickering, who spent three years in Ethiopia with the McGill-Ethiopia Community Health Master's Program and Brian Ward who had spent almost three years in Thailand, arrived in the early 1990s. The most recent staff additions have been Mike Libman and Chris Greenaway, who spent a year in the Gambia. Characteristics of each faculty have been their exposure to work in the tropics and their part-time involvement in the centre. The clinical load of the centre is approximately one GFT equivalent or ten half-day clinics. While Dick MacLean managed five half-days of outpatient work per week, each of the other five staff managed one half-day per week. All staff required financial support from a clinical or research base outside the centre. In fact, however, their "outside" activities were of significant benefit to the TDC because of the evolving seniority of their McGill academic positions. Both Brian Ward and Mike Libman became, at different times, directors of the MUHC Division of Infectious Diseases, Joyce Pickering became associate dean of medical education and student affairs, and Laurence Green was director of the Division of Internal Medicine. The influence that these academic/ administrative positions had on preserving space and funds for tropical medicine, especially during the period of budget contractions from 1990 to 2005, was significant, although difficult to define.

The initial research development in the Centre for Tropical Diseases was in epidemiology. With a master's degree in parasitology and four years of epidemiology research experience at the Institute of Parasitology, Theresa Gyorkos completed her PhD in epidemiology on the impact of parasitic infections among Southeast Asian refugees arriving in Montreal in the late 1980s. After a postdoctorate in 1988 at Université de Montréal with Pierre Viens, and as a new assistant professor in epidemiology at McGill, she was given a cross-appointment in the Centre for Tropical Diseases. This led to collaborative research with Dick MacLean in malaria and in indigenous Canadian parasitoses (e.g., Arctic trichinosis and North American liver fluke). In the 1990s, she worked on malaria in Brazil and Ethiopia, helminths in Guinée, and Chagas' disease in Paraguay. Her year with the Schistoso-miasis and Intestinal Parasite Unit at WHO, focusing on intestinal parasite prevention and control in Africa, and her recent research on hookworm during pregnancy in Peru, gave her an enviable reputation that reflected well on the TDC.

The long-term plan for strengthening both epidemiologic and bench re-search occurred when, in 1991, Brian Ward joined the TDC. A McGill med-ical graduate and Rhodes Scholar, with three years' experience working in the tropics (Thailand, Peru) and seven years of postgraduate and research training at Johns Hopkins, he changed the centre's profile from clinical re-search to bench research. His research activities in immunovirology and immunoparasitology attracted funding from several national and interna-tional sources, and his drive was a very positive addition to the TDC. With his new space in the MGH Research Institute expanding with master's and doctorate students, new opportunities arose. The Institute of Parasitology at MacDonald College (later named MacDonald Campus) had managed what was called the Parasitology Reference Service for the Laboratory Cen-tre for Disease Control (of Health Canada) in Ottawa. In a period of re-structuring, the Institute of Parasitology divested itself of this federally funded reference responsibility, and the TDC won the contract, taking it over under Brian Ward's management. In 1996, Bouchra Serhir, DVM, PhD, was recruited from Université de Montréal and led the National Centre for Parasitology (NCP) through two federal accreditations during a period when the government was closing other centres. In 2000, Serhir joined the Laboratoire de santé publique de Québec (LSPQ) and was replaced by Momar Ndao, a DVM, PhD originally from Senegal who completed his doctoral work on African trypanosomiasis at the Tropical Medicine Institute in Antwerp, Belgium. Together, Ward and Ndao expanded the NCP's range of serologies, PCRs, and parasite cultures, eventually putting the centre on an equal footing with the Centres for Disease Control (CDC) in Atlanta. In 2007, he was offered a McGill faculty position in recognition of his work and potential.

As the clinical and research development of the TDC progressed, the core clinical parasitology laboratory evolved and developed a reputation, first locally and then worldwide. The initial arrival of Cliff Law and his laboratory skills and equipment was somewhat unusual. Doug Cameron and the executive director of the MGH at that time, Harvey Barkun, set up the lab to operate independently of the Department of Microbiology with the aim of situating both the clinical and the laboratory operations within the Department of Medicine. The plan was to avoid the split between the Department of Medicine and the Department of Microbiology that made the development of the infectious diseases specialty at McGill so difficult. This policy, of fully integrating the laboratory and the clinic, both administratively and physically, had important benefits. First, the problems and challenges in the laboratory were constantly vetted by the clinical staff, and this promoted clinical laboratory research. Second, the close link between the clinician user and the laboratory was an ongoing quality assurance program that led to a better laboratory and, in the end, produced the best parasitology laboratory in Quebec. This was recognized after 2000, when the laboratory took over the responsibility for parasitology specimens from all the MUHC hospitals. Finally, the juxtaposition and integration of clinic and laboratory made an ideal teaching environment for residents, allowing their access to the daily flow of parasitology specimens and the teaching of working laboratory technologists. This clinic-laboratory linkage, the only one in the MUHC, was evaluated by residents (ID/micro, internal medicine, paediatrics and family medicine) as an ideal learning environment and attracted residents from the Université de Montréal, the Université de Sherbrooke, and, indeed, across Canada. In the 2000s all twenty-six available four-week elective slots for residents were filled before the academic year began.

The clinic-laboratory linkage led to another teaching innovation. Cliff Law, upon his retirement in 1991, was replaced as chief technologist by Evelyne Kokoskin. Because of the growing reputation of the laboratory under her management, in 1994 she was able to negotiate LSPQ support for a malaria quality assurance (QA) program for Quebec. The LSPQ funded a half-time technologist at the TDC to review all Quebec hospitals' malaria smears and to run courses for the province's malaria smear-reading technologists. The funding provided by this QA program freed up technologist teaching time for our residents and, with growing funds obtained from the sale of parasitology specimens for QA, QC (quality control), and teaching materials in the United States, it was possible for Kokoskin to devote the majority of her time to teaching. Her lab teaching reputation grew and led to invitations to teach laboratory parasitology courses in Australia, England, the United States, Peru, and India. Her teaching has also led to a TDC commitment to teach the laboratory component at the annual Gorgas Tropical Medicine Course in Lima, Peru. This course has become the pre-eminent tropical disease course in the world. Ward has also served as a core member of the Gorgas Course visiting faculty since its inception in 1996. In 2006, Mike Libman and Evelyne Kokoskin were invited to serve as visiting faculty to help in the development of a similar international health course in Lahore, India. During the past twenty-five years, the clinical parasitology laboratory survived and thrived while others shrank or closed across Canada. This has been in no small part due to strong technologists with very high standards. These standards have been attained through decades of experience gained from service and teaching in the clinical parasitology laboratory. Technologists Cliff Law, Evelyne Kokoskin, and Lynne Cedilotte have been at the centre of this excellence that helped to protect the centre from the past two years of shrinking MUHC budgets.

Besides the tropical focus of research, teaching, and the clinical activities of the centre there has been a simultaneous link to the Arctic. The challenges of health delivery to northern communities and tropical communities are similar. The diseases, in particular the parasitic diseases, have attracted the attention of the centre's clinical parasitology and reference laboratories. The discovery and definition of a new clinical disease (secondary trichinosis) and the North American liver fluke disease by MacLean, Ward, and Gyorkos have been as a consequence of this northern interest and attraction.

Not only has the Centre for Tropical Diseases developed its clinical and laboratory teaching and research but it has also developed and expanded its national and international responsibilities. A biannual tropical medicine CME course, the only one in Canada, has been offered for the past twenty years. With attendees from around North America, tropical and travel medicine advisory councils to both provincial and federal governments have, since their inception in the early 1990s, been chaired by Brian Ward or have had members from the centre (MacLean, Green, Greenaway). The centre's malaria QA program has expanded to include half of Canada's provinces. Dick MacLean has chaired the Clinical Group of the American Society for Tropical Medicine and Hygiene. Brian Ward and Momar Ndao sit on the National Blue Ribbon Panel on Blood Safety. Theresa Gyorkos has managed WHO research and development projects abroad. Dick MacLean managed the ten-year McGill-University of Addis Ababa internal medical linkage project in the 1980s, the eleven-year Community Health Master's Program in the Department of Community Health at the University of Addis Ababa in the 1990s, and a four-year primary health care training program with the University of the West Indies in the 1990s. Brian Ward presently co-manages a thirteen-year HIV research project in Zimbabwe. More than thirty-five manuscripts have come from this work to date, with Brian authoring more than half, and it is widely recognized as a highly influential project in HIV circles. All of these international projects have been funded by CIDA or the IDRC.

Pre-Travel

In the 1980s, guided by the perception that a tropical disease centre should be involved in preventive as well as curative medicine, a nurse was hired, initially two days per week and then three days per week, to give travel advice, malaria prophylaxis, and vaccines. The intent was that the pre-travel clinic would advertise the tropical diseases clinic and also inform the clinicians in the Tropical Diseases Centre on the larger issues of tropical disease prevention and control. Nurse Elaine Cyr worked for eighteen years, and the pre-travel clinic was always full. Provincial governments later declared that such pre-travel health care was not a government insured medical act or service, and travellers were required to pay for not only their vaccines but also for the medical advice that was billed as part of these visits.

Summary

Tropical medicine at the MGH became a tangible entity in the 1970s at a time, and possibly as a result, of a changing political climate in Canada. Prime Minister Lester Pearson reaffirmed and increased Canada's commitment to increasing foreign aid to developing and, in most cases, tropical countries. The involvement of the MGH in international projects created an environment that was receptive to the development of a tropical medicine specialty at the hospital. Over the past twenty-seven years of the Tropical Diseases Centre's existence, the demographic profile of Canada has changed.[10] Over the first 140 years of the MGH's existence, 95 percent of all immigrants to Canada were from Europe. In the past ten years, 80 percent of all immigrants have been from the tropics or China. Canadian physicians are increasingly required to have a knowledge of the diseases of their patients' homelands. The centre was built on the Oslerian model of a close association between clinical practice and clinical laboratory to the benefit of research, patient care, and resident teaching. The centre has a strong international profile in research and teaching and is one of the two largest tropical medicine clinics in North America. It also currently runs the federally funded National Reference Centre for Parasitology, which provides diagnostic services across Canada, and the provincially funded Quality Assurance Program for malaria in Quebec.

NOTES

1 P.A. Thornton, S. Olson, Q.T. Thach, "Dimensions sociales de la mortalité infantile à Montréal au milieu du dix-neuvieme siècle," *Annales de Demographie Historique* (1988): 299–325.

2 R. Omran Abdel, "The Epidemiologic Transition: A Theory of Epidemiology of Population Change," *Milbank Memorial Fund Quarterly* 49 (1971): 509–38.

3 W. Osler, "Trichina Spiralis," *Canadian Journal of Medical Science* 1 (1876): 135–6, 175–6.

4 W. Osler, "On Echinococcus Disease in North America," *American Journal of the Medical Sciences* 84 (1882): 475–280.

5 W. Osler, "Christmas and the Microscope," *Hardewicke's Science-Gossip* 1 February 1869, 44; H.M. Malkin, "The Influence of William Osler on the Development of Clinical Laboratory Medicine in North America," *Annals of Clinical and Laboratory Medicine* 7 (1977): 281–97.

6 T.W.G. Cameron, "The McGill University Institute of Parasitology," *McGill News*, March 1933.

7 E.-M.L. Rathgeber, "The Movement of Paradigms of Medical Knowledge and Research between Canada and Kenya: An Investigation into the Sociology of Knowledge Transfers" (PhD diss., State University of New York, 1982).

8 D.H. Starkey, "Problems of Tropical and Exotic Diseases Affecting Canadian Medicine: A Perspective," *Canadian Journal of Public Health* 64 (1973): 103–6.

9 Ibid., and "50 Years of Interest in Tropical Diseases in Canada," *Tropical-Canada* 2 (1983): 7.

10 Population and growth components, 1851–2001, Canada Census, extracted 20 July 2007; and Population and growth components (1851–2001 censuses), adapted from Statistics Canada CANSIM database http://cansim2.statcan.ca, table 051-00061, 2, extracted 11 July 2007.

SECTION 3

Department of Surgery and Its Divisions

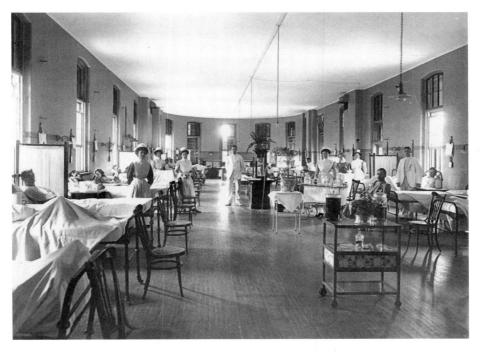

S.3 Open thirty-bed Surgical Ward L in Old MGH, 1910

19

General Surgery

Rea Brown and Joseph Hanaway

Rea Brown was a senior surgeon at the MGH and a leader in trauma surgery.
His manuscript was edited by Joe Hanaway.

Introduction

In 1882, general surgery became a subspecialty at the MGH when Thomas
Roddick declared that he would only practise surgery. Anaesthesia and
antiseptic surgery had already been introduced to set the stage for general
surgeons to explore the abdomen, pelvis, and chest without fatal infection.
It took a good decade for the surgeons to learn proper anatomy and new
procedures. Most of the early abdominal operations in the 1890s were ap-
pendectomies. X-ray came in 1896. I take readers through decades and the
lives and contributions of many surgeons, particularly F.B. Gurd, F.N. Gurd,
and H. Rocke Robertson who arrived in 1958 and led the department into the
modern era of surgery. I discuss the problems created by Bill 65 in 1970 and
by Bill 101 (the language bill) in 1977 as well as the appearance and research
of young, well trained new staff in the 1980s and 1990s.

Early Surgeons, Anaethesia, and Antiseptic Surgery

Surgery, in the early years, was seriously limited by the ever-present threat
of infection when treating burns, casting fractures, draining abscesses, doing
amputations, and/or removing superficial tumours.[1] Working under circumstances that are hard to imagine today, William Caldwell (1782–1833),
William Robertson (1784–1844), John Stephenson (1794–1842), and Andrew

Fernando Holmes (1798–1860) offered the highest level of care that was available at the time. Henry Loedel was in the group but became ill and died of typhus in 1825.[2]

There was no mention of an operating room (OR) in the two early converted homes of 1818 and 1819 (see chapter 2), but there was one in the Dorchester Street hospital under the cupola.

The first practical surgical teaching involved the appointment of "dressers" who were senior students and whose job was to follow the attending and assist in any minor procedures. Their duties are described in the 1823 Rules and Regulations of the MGH.

In 1823, the staff founded a small medical school, the Montreal Medical Institution (MMI), which was associated with the MGH, and the first official professor of surgery was John Stephenson. The MMI lasted until June 1829 when the staff agreed to be the founding faculty of McGill University. Stephenson kept his position until he died in 1842. He was replaced by the very capable George Campbell (1810–82), who retired in 1875. All the staff performed surgery, but Stephenson and Campbell were the appointed professors of the subject offered to students.

Exactly when anaesthesia was introduced to the MGH is not certain. In 1847,[3] Holmes published an account of the successful use of chloroform in a procedure outside the MGH. It is assumed that it was used in the hospital soon after. Ether anaesthesia, first reported by Crawford Long in Georgia in 1849,[4] was used at the MGH soon after chloroform. Senior students and other staff were the anaesthetists for decades until there was enough interest to make it a specialty in the late 1880s. According to Shepherd, H.B. Carmichael was the first trained anaesthetist, and he was appointed in 1885. Ether, from a bottle, was dropped onto a gauze mask, which was placed over the patient's nose and mouth until there was no response to pain. Induction was usually violent for a few minutes, and the patient had to be held down.

The old OR, under the cupola, had a wooden floor crusted with dried blood and other dried materials that had rarely been scrubbed clean. The wooden OR table was also crusted and had been wiped off but rarely scrubbed. Instruments and hands were washed after surgery, and the idea of sterilizing anything to be used by the surgeons had not yet occurred to anyone. The surgeons wore old frock coats left at the hospital, and they were usually stiff from the dried blood. Street clothes were worn by curious people walking into the OR to see what was happening. The students in the gallery came in wearing street coats, and in all weather, to witness the few operations that were performed. There was light from the cupola windows, otherwise oil lamps were the source of light. It is little wonder that the infection rate was so high until Joseph Lister came out with his monumental 1867 publication describing the results of his antiseptic OR procedures.[5]

The 1870s brought two major advances in surgery. One came from an unknown student from Toronto who transferred to McGill in 1870 because of its strong anatomy tradition and the MGM's relatively open-door policy with regard to students. William Osler graduated in 1872 and, like many Canadians, went to Europe to "walk the wards" – but in a different way. He became interested in pathology as a way to understand disease, studied with Rudolph Virchow (1821–1902) in Berlin, and heard Carl Rokitansky (1804–1878) in Vienna. On returning to the MGH in 1874 he started to perform autopsies and was soon appointed pathologist to the hospital (1877), where he performed 780 autopsies in ten years. He also studied surgical specimens, which gradually helped the correlation of clinical diagnosis and pathological processes. Before this, surgeons had had no way to verify their pre-op diagnoses.

Antiseptic Surgery

The second surgical advance in the 1870s was Roddick's introduction of antiseptic surgical technique. He made two trips to study with Joseph Lister, first in Edinburgh (1872) and then in London (1877). This discovery, promoted by Roddick, was the single most important development in surgery not just in his lifetime but probably in the history of surgery.

In the case of Roddick's amputations alone, the mortality from infection in 1877–79 decreased from 80 percent to less than 4 percent. He was not the first to use antiseptic technique in Canada, but, but with his articles, he was one of its most effective promoters.[6]

The procedure was simple. A gallon tank of water was heated with an alcohol flame, and steam through a narrow rubber tube was sprayed into the OR. A pint bottle of phenol (carbolic acid) solution was attached to the system so that it was sucked up into the steam tube and sprayed into the room as a mixture. Everything and everyone were drenched and dripping with phenol. It worked, despite having to operate in a fog, and the results far outweighed the inconvenience. Reactions to the phenol occurred on the skin and in the kidneys and lungs. The spray was abandoned by the late 1880s for a better aseptic technique (for both instruments and OR assistants), along with dry dressings and bandages. Hands and instruments were washed in alcohol and a chloride solution. Surgical gloves were introduced to protect the skin on the arms from allergic reaction to phenol, and they extended up to the upper arm. It was a resident in Obs/Gyn at Johns Hopkins, Hunter Robb, who mentioned using gloves for antiseptic reasons.[7] We do not know when the surgical mask was introduced, but it was in the last quarter of the 1800s.

Early MGH Surgeons

George Fenwick (1825–1894), who followed George Campbell as professor of surgery from 1875 to 1890, was an eccentric but capable surgeon who co-founded the *Canada Medical Journal* (1864–72) and continued it under another title, the *Canada Medical and Surgical Journal* (1872–79). He was also vice-president of the Canadian Medical Association from 1881 to 1882.[8] He embraced antisepsis and published many case reports. His greatest contribution, however, was to convince young Tom Roddick, who was on his way to medical school in Edinburgh in 1864, to enter McGill instead. Roddick was number one in his class for four years, was valedictorian, and won the Holmes Gold Medal in 1868.[9]

Francis Shepherd (1851–1929), a contemporary of Roddick and Fenwick, was never professor of surgery because he had the professorship in anatomy. For this reason he had to be content to be a lecturer in surgery. Despite this anomaly he became world famous for his series of thyroid surgeries and a number of first operations at the MGH. He was also a great teacher and embraced antisepsis. Shepherd made many contributions, but one of the most important was to support the need for professional nursing at the MGH. In 1890, after a run of head nurses, he convinced a neighbour, Elizabeth Gertrude (Nora) Livingston (1848–1927), to accept the position as head nurse in 1890.[10] Nora Livingston established nursing standards at the MGH and in Canada, demanding that nurses have a greater role in the care of patients and better pay. To top it off, she started a nursing school in December 1890 and graduated six women in April 1891.[11] The first operating nurse (Alicia Dunne) was appointed in 1887, and she dominated the OR, being quite independent of Livingston, who had the good sense to leave her alone.

Many years before Nora Livingston, in 1832, the nursing attendants were increased to six day and two night nurses. This number varied depending on the hospital finances and could be as low as two nurses with wards closed

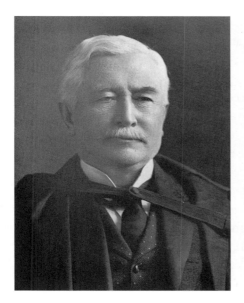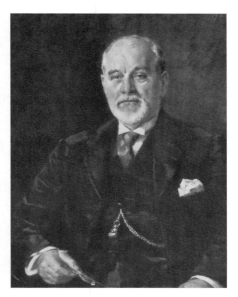

Fig. 19.1 Thomas George Roddick, chief of MGH surgery, 1890–93 (went to the RVH)
Fig. 19.2 Francis John Shepherd, chief of surgery, 1893–1913

to reduce expenses. But with each new wing (Reid, 1848, Fever, 1868; and More-land, 1875) more nurses were hired to care for the almost two hundred patients.

Roddick had incredible energy and physical stamina, which led to his being chosen to form a medical team to follow Major General Frederick Dobson Middleton and five thousand troops to the Canadian northwest in 1885 to quell the Métis rebellion led by Louis Riel. He attributed the minimal loss of life to being in the great outdoors rather than in the roach-ridden MGH. James Bell (1852–1911), another Holmes medalist (1887) from McGill, accompanied Roddick to western Canada in 1885 and published articles on new treatments for gunshot wounds of the chest and male genitalia. My colleagues, specialists in urology at the MGH, have read these reports and agree they set standards for the treatment for these injuries.[12]

Roddick declared surgery his only practice in 1882 and became the first general surgical subspecialist at the MGH. He was professor of surgery (1890–1907), dean of medicine (1901–08), president of the British Medical Association (1896–98), honorary president of the Canadian Medical Association for life (1912), and was knighted by King George in 1914. His decision to practise surgery occurred five years after he introduced antiseptic operating techniques, which had extraordinary results and were adopted by most surgeons. These techniques made surgery a viable practice. By the mid-1880s, the OR had been renovated, with a new table, a tiled floor, sterilized instruments, and better hand-washing procedures. By 1892, with the Greenfield and Campbell Pavilion, the new OR was tiled and rendered easier to keep clean. Doctors washed their hands in alcohol and wore clean linen gowns – but no gloves until a few years later (see note 6).

Surgical Firsts at the MGH

The first operation at the MGH that the patient survived was an amputation for a fractured femur on 14 May 1823.[13] The first successful tonsillectomy was performed on 29 November 1838.[14] Antisepsis led to major advances in surgery at the MGH, but it took years before the surgeons learned their anatomy and new techniques and procedures to a degree that enabled them to freely operate in the abdomen and pelvis. A number of firsts in surgery in the 1880s were: in 1877, Frank Buller became the first aurist and ophthalmologist; in 1882, George Major (1851–1923) became the first larybgologist; and, in 1884, Wm. Gardner (1842–1926) became the first gynaecologist. The first hernia operation (hemiorophy) was performed in 1884, the first kidney surgery for an abscess in 1882 (performed by Roddick),[15] and the first nephrectomy in which the patient survived in 1884 (performed by Shepherd).[16] The first supra-pubic operation on the prostate was performed by Shepherd in 1885,[17] the first nephrolithotomy (an enormous staghom) was performed by Shepherd 1887,[18] and the first brain abscess was aspirated in 1886. There is no mention in the operative records of surgery relating to the stomach until 1892, and the first operation on a perforated gastric ulcer was in 1893. The first bowel operation was in 1887, the second in 1891. The first pre-diagnosed appendicitis and appendectomy was performed by Bell in 1889.[19] Most abdominal operations in the 1890s were for appendicitis because it had become easy to diagnose (McBurney's point, described in 1889, is a point measured half way between the umbilicus and the anterior superior iliac spine, in most cases over the appendix. Point tenderness and rebound tenderness at McBurney's point was diagnostic of appendicitis).[20] On an elective level the abdomen was not entered even in the 1890s without major consultations and opinions because, despite antiseptic procedures, infections still occurred. Keep in mind that gloves, masks, sterile gowns, and hats were not in general use until after the 1900s, which probably accounted for the infections.

The 1890s were boon years for the general surgeons at the MGH. Shepherd, Bell, Roddick, and Fenwick had the advantages of anaesthesia, antiseptic techniques, new developments in surgery pertaining to the body, electric lights in 1892, the new separate Greenfield and Campbell surgical pavilion and OR, and, most important, the gradual standardization of OR antiseptic procedures.

Early House Surgeons

It is not certain when the training of house surgeons or house officers began, but it was started when senior staff chose top McGill graduates to work in the hospital as cheap labour, training them in medical practice so they could eventually go out on their own. House surgeons are mentioned in the MGH Rules and Regulations of 1823. Essentially, they were apprentices in the hospital, following the staff around and watching them examine and treat patients and taking notes in the admission ledgers. There was no structured system or graded responsibilities. The candidates stayed long enough to think they could make it on their own and be trusted by the staff to take calls when the latter were on vacation. Roddick, as an example of a house surgeon in 1868, was an assistant to George Ross (1848–92) until 1872, then was full house surgeon for two years until he could support himself. The duties of the house staff (who were not paid but lived and dined in the hospital) were to admit new patients and to write their histories in large folio-sized ledgers that were kept in the apothecary office. Weekly follow-up notes were usually dictated by the attendings until discharge. The books also contained temperature charts (the clinical thermometer was introduced in 1870 by Allbutt).[21] By 1880, the house staff had been increased by four because of the development of subspecialties and the expanding clinic, bringing the total to eight.

The house staff rotated among the attendings and into the clinic. By 1883, when the hospital had an ambulance service, the house staff would answer a bell, racing to the lobby to see who would be the one sent out, on a first-come, first-go basis. By the early 1900s there was better organization and even an official handbook for house officers with all the rules and regulations as well as duty rosters for the ambulance and night staff. There were 108 calls in 1884, 350 in 1893, and 2000 in 1924. Joseph Wray, who had run the ambulance service since 1883, provided motor vehicles by 1912.[22] As of this writing,

I have been unable to determine when an ER department and entrance were established. By 1875, the outpatient clinic had expanded to the basements of the Reid and Moreland wings, with many rooms for the different specialties and an entrance on the side street. The arrangements to see either surgical or medical patients were informal in the 1860s and 1870s and were decided between the clinic attendings. After 1884, and the beginning of surgical sub-specialization, there were rooms and staff designated for each.

The Royal Victoria Hospital

By 1887, Montreal's increasing population led to plans for another hospital for the city and McGill. To honour Queen Victoria's Jubilee year, Sir Donald Smith and his cousin George Stephen made generous donations to construct the Royal Victoria Hospital, which opened in 1893 (modelled after the Royal Infirmary in Edinburgh). After seventy years, the MGH was no longer the only teaching hospital for the McGill Medical School: there was now real competition. Roddick was appointed chief of surgery at the RVH in 1893 for one year. James Bell, who left the MGH with Roddick, was his successor in 1894. Frank Shepherd and George Armstrong (1855–1933) remained at the MGH to balance the departments.

By this time, Armstrong, like Shepherd, had a wide reputation for his work in thoracic surgery, for the surgical treatment of bleeding ulcers, the for the use of endotracheal anaesthesia, the early use of the Bovey cautery system, and the first use of radium (which he bought himself after learning its uses at the Radium Institute in Paris in 1909) in Canada.[23] He was elected president of the Canadian Medical Association in 1910.

James Bell died in 1911 (of unoperated appendicitis).[24] Armstrong was appointed his successor and was dean of medicine from 1922 to 1923. He retired in 1923 and was remembered for his well organized and well presented surgical clinics and his surgical expertise. The MGH, despite all its problems with age and funding, was keeping up with the new Campbell and Greenshields surgical pavilion built south of the main hospital in 1892. Major renovations were undertaken in the other wings in 1894 as well as in a pathology building built east of the Richardson Wing.

Shepherd and Armstrong were followed by J. Alex Hutchison (1873–1923) and John Elder (1861–1921). Four other surgeons, Edward M. Eberts (1873–1945), Alfred T. Bazin (1872–1958), Fred Tees (1880–1946), and W.L Barlow (l872–1952) were to be the next generation of general surgeons at the MGH.

X-Ray at the MGH

The first use of x-ray at McGill was in February 1896, when Robert Kirk-patrick (1863–97), a surgeon, had physics professor John Cox (1851–1923), who had developed an x-ray apparatus in the Physics Building at McGill, take an x-ray of a patient's leg, which had received a gunshot wound. This was fewer than seventy days after Roentgen's December 1895 article describing the x-ray. The operation took forty-five minutes with a hand-cranked generator that made a feeble picture in which a dark object (the bullet) could be made out. The plate was under-exposed and probably needed sixty minutes. The authors rushed into print in March 1896 with their pictures in tow; however, but in their haste, they failed to mention which leg was involved. For some time this was believed to be the first case of x-ray use in the world, but it was not. It was, however, the first in Canada. The MGH purchased its own apparatus after the turn of the century, and, in 1908, Walter Wilkins (1878–1962) was the first trained radiologist to be appointed.[25]

Fraser Baillie Gurd, 1883–1948

A young graduate in 1906, Fraser Baillie Gurd (1883–1948), known as Fraser B., won a graduation prize and began a career that was to have a great effect on surgery at the MGH.[26]

His father, a general practitioner, did not influence Fraser B., who wanted to be a surgeon from the onset of his career. Unfortunately, the First World War started in 1914, so Fraser enlisted but was rejected by the Canadians because of his lack of experience and a fellowship from the Royal College. Undeterred, he was accepted by the British War Office, which wanted doctors. He joined the Royal Army Medical Corp. in 1915 and left for England in May. Once there he volunteered for a front-line clearing station located in Air-sur-Lys, France. It is here that Fraser B. had the experience of a lifetime treating major wounds, tetanus, infected wounds (covered in mud), shock, ghastly fractures, dismembered soldiers, and the list goes on. Gurd soon made a name for himself by changing the surgical dressing technique from the Carrel-Dakin irrigation technique (Alexis Carrel, 1873–1944, won a Nobel Prize in 1912 for contributions to vascular surgery and renal transplant) to the more effective Bismuth Iodoform Pariffin Paste (BIPP) technique. Used in two world wars, it was replaced by antibiotics in the Second World War.[27] He returned to the MGH in 1919 and began an academic career at

McGill and the MGH that led to his being surgeon-in-chief and receiving a professorship of surgery at McGill (1947–48). He introduced the McGill Diploma Course in Surgery involving all the McGill teaching hospitals and an MS in experimental surgery from McGill.

Gurd saw that resident training in surgery lacked progressive responsibility. The residents were still just watching the masters perform and were expected to learn from that. He lobbied for a program of increasing surgical responsibility for the residents in the upper years. This was met with opposition until it was accepted that surgeons had to operate, not just observe, in order to learn the trade.

Fraser B. became a regent of the American College of Surgeons in 1938 and delivered the Scudder Fracture Oration in 1938, presenting his success with walking casts for lower leg fractures, which he had pioneered.[28] He also had a great interest in thoracic surgery, which was taught by his mentor Ted Eberts. Traumatic empyema abscesses and Tbc of the lung were surgical problems on which he published to the point of being elected the third president of the American Association of Thoracic Surgeons in 1941. His 1941 paper entitled "The Treatment of Gunshot Wounds [of the chest]" is recommended.[29] He also talked the Central Surgical Association of the United States into including Montreal in its geographic territory, which was a geographical stretch but an example of the esteem in which Gurd was held.

Other Surgeons

John Elder, MD, CM, who had been in charge of surgery in the No. 3 McGill Hospital Unit in the First World War returned to the MGH in 1919 as chief of the "L" service. Elder was ill from the war and died in 1921. He was replaced by Alfred Bazin, MD, CM, who was a professor at McGill in 1923 and a figure around the MGH for years. In 1923 he and Tees, Scrimger, McKim, and Thompson published *A Students Guide to Operative Surgery*, which was well received and is now a collector's item. A worthy effort, it offers the principles of surgery according to a group of experienced general surgeons and was the first such publication at McGill.

Fred Tees ran the fracture clinic started by Fraser B. Gurd and was particularly interested in the care of athletic injuries in young people at McGill (1919–41). He was a founding member of the Canadian Amateur Athletic Association.

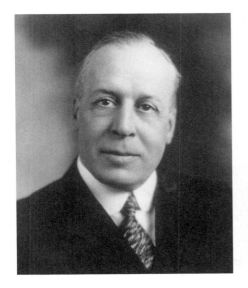

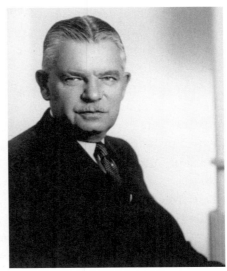

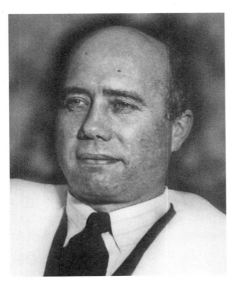

Clockwise from top left

Fig. 19.3 Alfred T. Bazin, chair of surgery, 1923–39

Fig. 19.4 Fraser B. Gurd, chair of surgery, 1947–48

Fig. 19.5 Ralph R. Fitzgerald, chair of surgery, 1948–53

Three McGill medical graduates from the 1930s, trained by Fraser B., are worth mentioning. Charles R. Drew (1904–50), had been an All-American football player at Amherst, an Olympic-level sprinter, and had an excellent academic record. Unfortunately, being black, he could not get into a US medical school in the 1930s, so he applied to McGill and, in 1930, was accepted.[30] He was second in the class. He had surgical training with Fraser B. at the

MGH in the 1930s. After surgical residency he went to the Rockefeller Institute in New York and worked on preservation of blood for transfusion. During the Second World War, in 1940–41, he was director of the American Red Cross Transfusion Service.[31]

After New York, Drew was appointed chair of the Department of Surgery and chief of surgery at the Howard University School of Medicine and Teaching Hospital in Washington, DC. His distinguished career was capped by being the first black (1943) to be an examiner for the American Board of Surgery.

The second 1930s graduate to have an outstanding surgical career was Fraser Newman Gurd (1914–95), who graduated in 1939. He trained in the MGH program and earned his fellowship in the late 1940s. Other notable graduates and MGH surgeons before the Second World War were Simeon James "S.J." Martin (1904–87), Campbell Gardner (1908–63), and Harold Rocke Robertson (1912–98).

Another 1930s graduate to have a distinguished career was Campbell Gardner, who served in the Second World War from 1940 to 1944 and saw more surgical trauma in four years than he did in the rest of his life. He became a lieutenant colonel and, after the war, became chief of surgery at the Queen Mary Veterans Hospital (1946), where he became famous for his work and teaching on shock. Others who enlisted at the beginning of the Second World War were Fraser N. Gurd (1914–95), Harry J. Scott, Donald Ruddick (1916–97), John D. Palmer (1917–2006), Campbell Dickinson (1916–87), Arnold Jones, and Alan G. Thompson, all of whom went overseas after taking their internships.

Larry Garth Hampson enlisted in the navy, and Fraser B. Gurd and Laurie McKim were senior surgeons who had consulting positions with the government. On returning to Montreal, the group who had not finished their training entered residency and the McGill Diploma Course headed by Gavin Miller at the RVH. With the help of Fraser B. Gurd, whose reputation was by now well established, each was also able to get a good position for a year in either pathology or research in the United States.

The two teaching units were "L" and "M" service. Herbert M. Elder (1898–1951) was chief of M service and died in 1951. F.B. Gurd and Ted Eberts were chiefs of L service. In 1948 F.B. Gurd died and Ralph Richard Fitzgerald (1897–1957) was appointed surgeon-in- chief (1948–52). His main contribution to the MGH was to require all new staff appointments in general surgery to have passed fellowship exams in Canada or the United Kingdom. This was an important decision for it assured the MGH would have qualified surgeons for the future. S.J. Martin replaced H.M. Elder on the M service in 1952, and F.N. Gurd went to the L service.

General Surgery in the 1950s

Phillip Rowe, MD, CM, was appointed surgeon-in-chief at the MGH (1952–58) and chair of surgery at McGill (Gavin Miller [1893–1964] from the RVH retired in 1952). This kind gentle man had a large private practice and was overwhelmed by his appointment. Unfortunately for him, a new MGH was to be built and it opened in 1955. This meant that he had to deal with a group of well trained junior surgeons who were vocal and wanted something to say about the course of the Department of Surgery at the MGH. Fraser N. Gurd, John D. Palmer, Harry Scott, Larry Hampson, Alan Tompson, Cam Dickinson, Don Ruddick, Eric MacNaughton, and Robert Estrada were going to be heard.

Rowe was unable to delegate any of his most trivial duties to his bright junior staff and, being in full-time private practice, did not devote enough time to the MGH program. His juniors had been through the Second World War and had had training in some of the leading university programs on the continent. Dissent gradually arose at the MGH and the RVH, where Surgeon-in-Chief Donald Webster, along with Phillip Rowe, were not providing the leadership to take the departments into the modem era. Principal Cyril James of McGill was made aware of the problem and requested a review committee consisting of three prominent academic surgeons. Professors R. Milnes Walker of the University of Bristol, Frederick G. Kergin of the University of Toronto, and Francis Moore of Harvard were invited to Montreal to evaluate the two programs. The committee report regretted the problem of poor departmental leadership (due to the distractions of private practice) and it recommended not renewing the contracts of P.G. Rowe at the MGH and of D.R. Webster (1902–87) at the RVH. Rowe, anticipating the report, resigned in 1958, while Webster carried on until replaced. S.J. Martin became the interim surgeon-in-chief at the MGH until Rocke Robertson arrived in 1958.[32]

House officers in surgery in the 1950s still had to have a "rotating internship" with medicine, surgery, paediatrics, and electives followed by a three- to four-year surgical residency. In 1960, if a resident was single, he or she lived in the hospital, was provided with meals, and was paid fifty dollars per

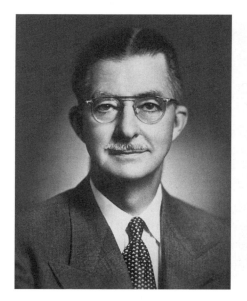
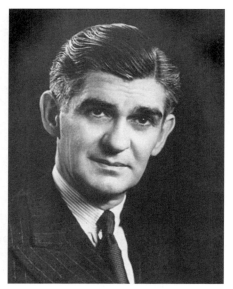

Fig. 19.6 Phillip Rowe, surgeon-in-chief, 1953–58
Fig. 19.7 S. James Martin, surgeon-in-chief, 1958

month. A married resident had a larger allowance of about $120 per month. Everyone wore white uniforms and was on duty every second or third night and weekend, depending on the service. The senior residents had better call schedules, and there were no limits on work hours, which were usually eighty to ninety hours per week. The house staff were assigned to different surgeons on rotation and were assistants until the third year. Then, gradually, they were allowed to operate on their own with close supervision from the attending staff.

Harold Rocke Robertson

Harold Rocke Robertson (1936), a McGill graduate and trainee of Fraser B. Gurd and a general surgeon by training, had a prewar fellowship from Edinburgh and a certification from the Royal College of Canada (1945). He completed his Second World War army service as a lieutenant colonel and accepted the chair of the Department of Surgery at the Vancouver Military Hospital in 1944. He became chief of surgery at the Shaugnessy Veterans Hospital and, finally, at Vancouver General Hospital in 1950. The medical school at the University of British Columbia (UBC) was being created in

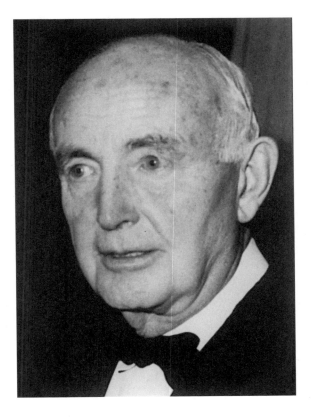

Fig. 19.8 Harold Rocke Robertson, full-time surgeon-in-chief, 1958–62. Rocke became the leading academic general surgeon in Canada and was appointed principal of McGill in 1962. He managed the university through its most tumultuous time.

1950, and Robertson was one of the first professors to be appointed to the UBC medical faculty. He was a driving force in the development of the new medical school and was acting dean of medicine in the late 1950s. His research interests focused on collecting data on wound infections, and this resulted in a better system for collecting and analyzing the variables and role of endothelial damage in veins in trauma situations.

After Rowe resigned, McGill looked for a leading surgeon who could revitalize general surgery at the MGH and head the McGill department. Robertson was the leading candidate and had the experience and skills to take on the task of bringing surgery at McGill and the MGH up to modern academic standards. By 1958, he was probably the most renowned academic surgeon in Canada, and there was a serious question of how to get him to leave UBC. This was mostly in the minds of the McGill people, though, because when Robertson understood he was the candidate for the MGH job he knew it was the opportunity of a lifetime.[33]

With his arrival in 1958 began a host of activities. He wasted no time getting his programs started and had a large surgical research laboratory, of which he was director, built on the ninth floor. The first paper from the laboratory was accepted by the American College Surgical Forum in 1963. It was by Mersereau and Ruddick and concerned venous endothelial damage in thrombosis. In 1959, the first geographical full-time salary (in addition to his own) was given to Fraser N. Gurd, who was vice-director of the laboratory and responsible for resident and medical school teaching. He abolished the McGill diploma course in surgery, centring the training (which he considered to be a hospital, not a university, responsibility) at the MGH and the RVH. He also had the ER redesigned with x-ray facilities – a first in Canada.[34] A surgical critical care unit was planned in 1960, based on a Johns Hopkins model, and F.N. Woolhouse, a plastic surgeon, was the trauma coordinator. In a short time, the morale in the MGH Department of Surgery was high as Robertson had an uncanny ability to get people enthusiastic about his reform program, which everyone knew was heading the department in the right direction.

Unfortunately for MGH surgery, just as the program was thriving in 1962, F.C. James, the principal of McGill, stepped down after twenty-two years, and Robertson was high on the list as a successor. He accepted the job and had to face one of the most tumultuous eras of student activism and unrest in McGill's history. To his credit, he remained in office for eight very stressful years, until many of the problems were settled.[35]

Fraser Newmen Gurd

Fraser Gurd assumed the vacated position of surgeon-in-chief at the MGH and chairman of the McGill department in 1962. Alan Thompson took Gurd's full-time position and became chief of L service on 9-East. M service passed from S.J. Martin to John Palmer, so all the personnel were in place to continue Robertson's program. It is of note that a windfall occurred at this time when Percy Randle Waters endowed the university surgical and medical research clinics on the ninth and tenth floors.[36]

This enabled a research team – Gustavo Bounous, Hope McArdle, L.G. Hampson, R. Chiu, and a group of talented surgical residents – to work on problems related to shock, resuscitation, and nutrition. Their observations pertaining to shock of phosphate mucosal metabolism in the gut, mucosal mucin production, alveolar surfactin action, and the grading of intestinal ischemic damage helped in understanding the consequences of "the low flow state." This resulted in an article: "The Prophylactic Use of an Elemental Diet in Experimental Hemmorrhagic Shock and Intestinal Ischemia." This ultimately led Mead-Johnson Pharmaceutical Company to produce and market a compound called "Flexical" for this purpose. It provided ancillary nutritional support for malnourished patients with surgical problems. McArdle summarized her experience with enteral feeding in her 1981 paper "A Rationale for Enteral Feeding as a Preferable Route for Hyperalimentation and Its Consequences."[37]

But we are getting ahead of ourselves. Fraser Gurd was building a reputation in the American Association of the Surgery of Trauma (AAST), where he was recorder and associate editor of the *Journal of Trauma*. He was president in 1968 and, in 1969, was also elected president of the Central Surgical Association. He gave the Scudder Oration in 1979, which his father had given in 1938. His topic was his many contributions to trauma care. To top off this year, a volume of the *Surgical Forum* was dedicated to him. In 1985, he received the Surgeons Award for Service, given jointly by the US National Safety Council, the AAST, and the American College of Surgeons.

Other Surgeons, 1960–75

Alan Thompson, L service chief and second to Fraser Gurd, opened a research laboratory to study diseases of the pancreas. He had spent a year at Ohio State University in Columbus working with Robert Zollinger, a famous surgeon and authority on the pancreas. Many residents spent time in Thompson's lab, including Brian Haig, John Moffat, and Rea Brown, who contributed to the understanding of pancreatic disease. Thompson studied severe pancreatitis for thirty years and has reported his results.

Cam Dickinson and L. Ogilvie were responsible for the ER. Ogilvie also directed undergraduate teaching and eventually took a job as vice-dean of admissions. S.J. Martin and John Palmer ran the tumour clinic for some years until the oncology clinic and department were formed under Michael Thirlwell. Robert Estrada continued his interest in malformations of the gastro-intestinal tract and thyroid and parathyroid diseases. Donald Ruddick had spent a few years as a surgical fellow in the United Kingdom and had brought back a new operative procedure for hiatus herniae (the Hill repair).

Larry Hampson returned from the Lahey Clinic in Boston in 1955 with a new procedure for treatment of severe chirrosis and esophageal varicies. Alan

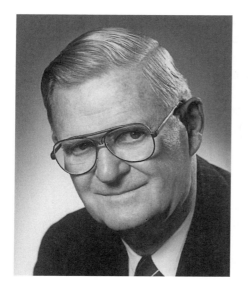

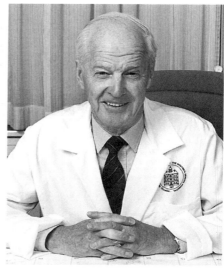

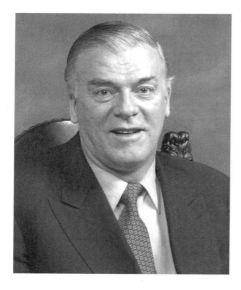

Clockwise from top left
Fig. 19.9 Fraser N. Gurd, surgeon-in-chief, 1962–71
Fig. 19.10 Alan Thompson, surgeon-in-chief, 1971–77
Fig. 19.11 Dave Mulder, surgeon-in-chief, 1977–98

Thompson was appointed surgeon-in-chief at the Queen Mary Veterans Hospital in 1969, so Larry Hampson assumed his position as second to Fraser Gurd. He continued a research career in the Donner Building at McGill in addition to his surgical duties at the MGH. In 1963, he was put in charge of a four-bed surgical intensive care unit on the ninth floor. It was so successful that the MGH built a thirteen-bed unit for intensive care in 1966. The obvious benefit of the unit for all surgery was reported and published by Gurd in 1966.[38] George Wlodek, a research-oriented surgeon, came to the MGH in 1963 and worked in a laboratory on the ninth floor on gastric acid production related to ulcers.

In their research year, Dave Mulder and Rea Brown worked in the University Research Clinic on pancreatitis and presented their work in the *Surgical Forum* in 1965. Mulder, an outstanding student at the University of Saskatchewan, was enticed to come to the MGH by Robertson, who gave a graduation speech in 1962 at Mulder's graduation. He obtained an MS from McGill in 1964 and eventually trained in cardiovascular thoracic surgery (CVT). He was MGH's surgeon-in chief from 1977 to 1998. Rea Brown, after his residency, spent a year in Milwaukee with the famous E. Ellison (Zollinger-Ellison syndrome), an expert on pancreatic tumours. In 1964, he did extra work in anatomy at McGill, working on electron microscopy with C.P Leblond and Yves Clerment.

October 1970 – Politics, Government Health Bills, and the Separatists

Nineteen seventy, a year of social upheaval in Quebec, is remembered for Castonguay's Bill 65, passed on 15 October 1970, which affected the incomes of junior staff at the MGH and required all doctors who wanted to practise in Quebec to accept fee caps. This resulted in a specialists strike on 1 October. The penalties for those who didn't return to work by 1 November was loss of licence and a fine.

This was followed by the violent actions of a militant separatist group, the Front de Liberation du Québec, which kidnapped and murdered Quebec minister of labour Pierre Laport, leading to martial law in Montreal under the Canadian army. When cooler heads prevailed, not surprisingly, ten of McGill's clinical faculty left the province, including surgeons George Wlodek and Arnold Jones.

The original fee schedule for the junior faculty, restricted by Bill 65, was so low that the economic survival of the major teaching hospitals was in jeopardy. A consultant firm concluded that the hospital income would not pay some members of the staff in general surgery. Rea Brown and Andy Hreno realized that they might have to leave if adjustments were not made, and this was a serious threat. Fortunately, after concessions were made, an acceptable fee schedule was accepted. I doubt that anyone realizes how depressing the situation was to those who had spent so many years training just to be treated in this fashion.

Nineteen seventy-one brought new light to the MGH general surgery program, but the Department of Anaesthesia was decimated by the crisis of the past year and took time to recover. All patients were now under Quebec Medicare, so there were no non-paying patients. The old L and M services were changed to M, G, and H services. The chiefs were Palmer for M service 9 West, Hampson for G service 9 East, and Estrada for H service 15 West.

The recovery of general surgery from the 1970 crisis was heartening, but a sad note was sounded in 1971 when, after thirty years at the MGH, F.N. Gurd retired to go Ottawa to the Royal College of Physicians and Surgeons of Canada. The last of the Gurds, he had had a distinguished career and was an able leader. A new chief was sought, and Alan Thompson assumed Gurd's position in December 1971 – to everyone's great relief. He was MGH surgeon-in-chief and, in 1972, McGill chair of surgery. He was well known, popular with the staff, had a research laboratory, and supported the younger surgical staff – Rea Brown, Dave Mulder, John McFarlane, and H. Brown. So the baton was again passed in 1971, and another era of general surgery was to begin at the MGH.

A new face, A. Voitk, appeared in 1971 as a resident working with Hope McArdle, who published a number of papers on the benefits of the elemental diet. A surgical nutrition service was finally established in 1972 to deal with the costly management of patients needing enteral or parenteral ancillary nutrition. In 1971, another resident, Joseph Feller, published a paper on the management of acute severe pancreatitis.

In 1971, Noelle Grace was the first woman to graduate from the general surgical program at the MGH, and she earned her fellowship from the Royal College the same year. Rea Brown thought so much of her ability as a junior that he let her be first surgeon on a gall bladder case while he assisted. It ruffled some of the senior staff, but Brown explained the he considered it part of her training. She went on to the Montreal Children's Hospital (MCH).

Nineteen seventy-seven was a notable year for the MGH surgery program because the separatist Parti Québécois and René Lévesque came to power, and this created uncertainty. Lévesque's Bill 101,[39] which declared that all business in Quebec, including hospital business, be conducted in French and that required a French competency exam for all employees educated outside the province, was another reason for people who could not speak French to leave the province. New financial restrictions were imposed, beds had to be closed, and nursing shortages occurred. Funding for vital areas, such as the ORs and CCUs, was inadequate. However, all the general surgeons remained at the MGH. Money was raised by private donations to help keep vital areas going.

The MGH School of Nursing closed in 1972 after eighty-two years (see section 5), and Livingston Hall was renovated to provide office space for the geographic full-time physicians and surgeons. Surgery was on the ninth floor and 7 East of the main hospital. A new ambulatory surgical centre was opened in 1972 to provide for the growing volume of outpatient surgery, which was becoming more common as techniques and anaesthesia improved.

The University Surgical Research Clinic continued its active programs between 1978 and 1990. Nine residents earned MSc degrees in experimental surgery. L. Rosenberg, MD, CM, earned his PhD for research on pancreatic disease. Four residents won the annual F.N. Gurd Research Prize. David Fleiszer (1979) and Shirley Chou (1981) won the Canadian Association of General Surgical Residents prizes. In 1982, David Sloan won the American Surgical Oncology Residents Prize and a prize awarded by the American Society for Surgery of the Alimentary Tract.

New Faces and Activities in Surgery in the 1980s and 1990s

General surgery at the MGH was given division status in 1983, with John Hinchey as its first director. McGill still did not have a general surgery subdepartment. C.-J. Chiu was director of the University Surgical Clinic, I was director of the Critical Care Trauma Unit and Chief of the M service, while Andy Hreno was chief of the H service.

General surgery at the MGH gradually changed as the staff from the Second World War era began to retire. They were replaced by many new faces in the 1980s and early 1990s, along with subspecialists. For example, L. Rosenberg, who trained at Michigan State University in liver and pancreas transplant techniques, came to the MGH Surgical Research Clinic in 1982. He earned a PhD from McGill and was appointed to the surgical staff in 1987. He organized renal transplantation and performed his first solid organ transplant in 1988. Recognized for his ability, he was appointed surgeon-in chief at the Jewish General Hospital.[40] Judith Trudel, the first female general surgeon in the long history of the MGH, was a specialist in colorectal surgery. Dave Owen and Gerald Pearl came to the MGH when the Reddy Memorial closed in 1985 and joined the trauma team. Robert Salasidis, after a year of training at the University of Alberta, also joined the trauma team. Dave Evans and Tarek Razek returned from a year away in 1983 to became directors of the MGH trauma unit.

In May 1981, D. Mulder, Tony Ty, and I went to Toronto to become the Canadian faculty teaching the new American College of Surgeons Advanced Trauma Life Support (ATLS) Program. This program covered the diagnosis and treatment of trauma victims in the "golden hour" after injury. Brown became region 12 chief of the college's Committee on Trauma, which was in charge of establishing trauma facilities for all universities from Ontario to Newfoundland.

The first course was held at the MGH in 1982, and faculty from the MGH and the University of Montreal were trained. In the following years, courses were conducted and faculty members from the University of Western Ontario, McMaster, Queen's, Ottawa, Sherbrooke, Laval, Dalhousie (and its New Brunswick affiliate), and Memorial were graduates. Approximately one thousand fourth-year students also took the course, which was given only by McGill in Canada and by the Uniformed Services University of Health Sciences in the United States.

For my contribution to this program and the work at the MGH during the University of Montreal shooting rampage in 1989,[41] and "for exceptional meritorious service as a member of the regional committee on trauma," I received the Trauma Achievement Award from the Committee on Trauma of the American College of Surgeons in February 1991.

E.J. Hinchey, a long-time member of the Royal College examining board, was chair from 1981 to 1983 and was elected president of the Canadian Association of General Surgeons in 1986. His presidential address, *The Future of General Surgery in Canada,* published in 1988, highlights the shortage of qualified general surgeons in Canada (partially due to the allure of subspecializations such as CVT or plastic surgery).[42] In 1998, he was able to establish a surgical scientist program at McGill thanks to the FAST Foundation, a family foundation interested in supporting research and education related to oncology.

In 1989, laparoscopic cholecystectomy was a new procedure that offered surgeons a low morbidity way to remove the gall bladder. Gerald Fried and John Hinchey, with financial aid, went to Colonge, Germany, and returned in the spring of 1990 having been trained in this procedure. Fried went on to perfect and study this minimally invasive procedure. In 1992, he published his controlled trial on laparoscopic cholecystectomy in the *Lancet.*[43] He further developed a simulation laboratory for the procedure to teach and evaluate technical skills, publishing his results in 1998 and 2004, respectively.[44] Thanks to L. Feldman and L.S. Mayrand, laparoscopic repair of gastroesophageal reflux disease (GERD) has also been a success. Following in line, a laparoscopic OR was developed and, in 2009, Gerald Fried became chair of surgery at McGill University.

Dave Fleiszer, a computer-oriented surgeon, came to MGH surgery in 1982. When a computer was provided for the Surgical Intensive Care Trauma Unit in 1983, he set out to establish registries for non-trauma and trauma admissions (the first time this had been done in Canada). In a short time, Fleiszer developed statistics on the present treatment of trauma. He was also interested in colon cancer and was made director of a colon cancer unit in 1991.[45] In 1992, he became the first dean of medical informatics and directed the Molson McGill Medical Informatics Laboratory. Roger Tabah followed Dave Sloan as MGH head and neck surgeon and developed modem techniques for thyroid and parathyroid surgery.

Trauma Centre for Montreal

In 1991, Rea Brown replaced John Hinchey as director of the Division of General Surgery. After the massacre of female students at L'École Polytechnique at the University of Montreal in 1989, and the shootings at Concordia University in 1992, the Quebec government wanted to improve trauma care in the province. Many victims were sent to the MGH, and all survived their wounds. New trauma centre designation (Level 1 [comprehensive] to level 4 [limited]) for English and French hospitals was established and announced by Minister of Health Marc Coté in 1993. (In 2006, a third college shooting episode occurred at Dawson College in downtown Montreal, with nineteen wounded and one killed.) This required Level 1 care for victims at the MGH. As a result of this, MGH was designated a Level 1 adult trauma centre in 1997, meaning it was capable of treating multiple traumas in all categories. In 2003, when the Quebec government decide to leave the MGH on Cedar Avenue rather than move it to the MUHC Glen site, it was declared the only Level 1 trauma centre in downtown (Centre Ville) Montreal.

John Sampalis presented his data in "The Outcome of Trauma Center Designation: Initial Impact on Trauma-Related Mortality,"[46] which shows definite improved survival in trauma centres. In 1996, the first H. Rocke Robertson Visiting Professorship in Trauma was held, and Robertson was present for the presentation in the Osler Amphitheatre at the McGill Medical School. He was eighty-four years old at the time, and this was a great tribute to a great man at the MGH and McGill.

Recognizing the unacceptable wait time for patients with breast tumours to get to the breast clinic, Fleiszer organized a coordinated visit in 1996. The patient had a clinical exam, a mammogram, and a needle biopsy all in one visit. A new automatic breast biopsy instrument was marketed at the MGH, and Fleiszer quickly proved that this instrument was accurate, with a low morbidity and cost per procedure – the dream of Medicare.

With people like Francis Shepherd, Thomas Roddick, Arthur Bazin, Fraser B. Gurd, Rocke Robertson, Fraser N. Gurd, Alan Thompson, and Dave Mulder, along with many others who have made notable contributions, it is little wonder that the general surgical program at the MGH has had such an illustrious history.

NOTES

1 H.E. MacDermot, *The History of the Montreal General Hospital* (Montreal: Montreal General Hospital, 1950), 66–7.

2 Ibid., 14–18.

3 A.F. Holmes, "Employment of Chloroform," *British Medical Journal* 3 (1847): 263.

4 C.W. Long, "An Account of the First use of Sulfuric Ether by Inhalation as an Anaesthetic in Surgical Operations," *Southern Medical and Surgical Journal* 5 (1849): 705–13. Although Long first used ether in 1843, the public didn't hear about it until Morton's famous public demonstration in the Ether Dome at the Massachusetts General Hospital in 1848.

5 T.G. Roddick, "Some Remarks on Lister's Antiseptic Method as Practiced in the Montreal General Hospital, in *The MGH Clinical Pathological Reports*, ed. W. Osler, vol. 1, 243–51 (Montreal: Dawson Bros., 1880).

6 J. Hanaway, "Sir Thomas George Roddick," *Dictionary of Canadian Biography*, vol., 15, *1921–30*, 1.

7 W.S. Halsted, *Johns Hopkins Hospital Report* 4 (1894): plate 11. Halsted had Goodyear make arm's-length rubber gloves for his OR nurse, who had an allergy to the antiseptic. He published this information in 1894. It was a Johns Hopkins house officer who first suggested the gloves be used for antiseptic reasons.

8 F.N. Gurd, *The Gurds, the Montreal General, and McGill: A Family Saga* (Montreal: General Store Publishing House, 1996), 17–19.

9 J. Hanaway and R. Cruess, "Sir Thomas George Roddick," *McGill Medicine* 1 (1996): 172–6.

10 H.E. MacDermot, *The History of the School of Nursing of the Montreal General Hospital* (Montreal: Southern Printing Co. Ltd., 1940), 36.

11 Ibid., 47.

12 J. Bell, "Cases of Gunshot Wounds of the Chest," *Canada Medical and Surgical Journal* 15 (1887): 5 ; "Two Cases of Gunshot Wounds of the Testicle," *Canada Medical and Surgical Journal* 14 (1886): 334–7.

13 J. Hanaway, "The Early Years, 1819–1885," chap 2, this volume.

14 Ibid.

15 Hanaway, "Roddick," 1.

16 J. Hanaway and R. Cruess, *History of McGill Medicine: The Second Half Century, 1885–1936* (Montreal and Kingston: McGill-Queen's University Press, 2006), 2:171.

17 Ibid.

18 Ibid.

19 Ibid.

20 C. McBurney, "Experience with Early Operative Interference in Cases of Diseases of the Vermiform Appendix," *New York Medical Journal* 50 (1889): 676–84.

21 T.C. Allbutt, "Medical Thermometry," *British Foreign Medical-Surgical Review* 45 (1870): 429–41.

22 F. Shepherd, *Origin and History of the Montreal General Hospital*, privately published ca. 1925, 30. He mentions that, in 1912, Joseph Wray supplied motor ambulances for the MGH. They were so underpowered that, at times during the winter, the old horse-drawn wagons were used.

23 M. MacLaren, "Dr George Eli Armstrong, 1855–1933," *Canadian Medical Association Journal* (July 1933): 103–4. In 1909, Armstrong went to Paris to the Radium Institute to learn how to use and to purchase radium to be used at the MGH. There is no record or report about its use to be found at the hospital or in the literature.

24 A. Murphy, "James Bell's Appendicitis," *Canadian Journal of Surgery* 15 (November 1872): 335–8. The article fails to mention the date of Bell's illness, but in 1911 he took sick at home and was treated by Frank Shepherd. Both of them knew appendicitis well, but apparently Bell refused surgery for some reason and died within eight days. Shepherd gives no explanation. An out-of-place appendix was found at the autopsy.

25 MacDermot, History, 98.

26 Gurd, *Gurds*, 73.

27 Ibid., 119–20.

28 Ibid., 373.

29 F.B. Gurd, "The Treatment of Gunshot Wounds," *American Journal of Surgery* 55 (1942): 189–209.

30 Gurd, *Gurds*, 19.

31 C.H. Organ, "C.R. Drew: A Doyen of American Surgery," *Bulletin of the American College of Surgeons* 81 (1996): 13–15.

32 Gurd, *Gurds*, 299.

33 R.W. Pound, *Rocke Robertson: Surgeon and Shepherd of Change* (Montreal and Kingston: McGill-Queen's University Press, 2008), 105.

34 Ibid., 120.

35 Ibid., 129–224.

36 Gurd, *Gurds*, 315–16.

37 A.H. McArdle, C. Palmason, L. Morency, and R. Brown, "A Rationale for Enteral Feeding as the Preferable Route to Hyperalimentation," *Surgery* 20, 4 (1981): 616–23.

38 F.N. Gurd, L.G. Hampson, J. Innes, W. Gibson, and D.S. Mulder. "The Value of a Clinical Shock Study Protocol in the Management of Refractory Shock," *Journal of Trauma* 6 (1996): 157–5.

39 Bill 101, 1977 Charter on the French Language at http://en.wikipedia.org/wiki/charter_of_the_french_language.

40 Personal communication with Lawrence Rosenberg.

41 1989 shooting at the University of Montreal. Patients were treated at the MGH.

42 E.J. Hinchey, "The Future of General Surgery in Canada," *Journal of Sirgury* 31, 2 (1988): 94–6.

43 J.S. Barkun, A.N. Barkun, G.M. Fried, et al., "Randomized Controlled Trial of Laparoscopic versus Mini Cholecystectomy," *Lancet* 340 (1992): 1116–19.

44 G.M. Fried, L.S. Feldman., M.C. Vassiliou, S.A. Fraser, et al., "Proving the Value Simulation in Laparoscopic Surgery," *Annals of Surgery* 240 (2004): 518–28.

45 Personal communication with David Fleiszer.

46 J.S. Sampalis, A. Lavoie, B. Steel, et al., "Trauma Center Designation: Initial Impact on Trauma Related Mortality," *Journal of Trama Infection and Critical Care* 39, 2 (1951): 232–9.

20

Cardiovascular Thoracic Surgery

David S. Mulder and Ray C.J. Chiu

David Mulder is a cardiac and thoracic surgeon at the MGH and a former chair of surgery at McGill. C.J. (Ray) Chiu was internationally known for his basic and applied cardiac research.

Introduction

There are excellent books on the historical development of cardiovascular thoracic surgery, both globally and in Canada.[1] This chapter describes the evolution of the exciting changes related to this surgical discipline at the Montreal General Hospital. The specialty grew from general surgery as a result of progress in the surgical management of pulmonary tuberculosis. There were many Canadian trail blazers, including Edward Archibald at the Royal Victoria Hospital[2] and Fraser Baillie Gurd at the MGH.[3] Gallie in Toronto was instrumental in proposing a formalized training program for surgical trainees in every surgical discipline.

To understand the history of this specialty in Canada, it is best to review development at the Royal College of Physicians and Surgeons of Canada.[4] This organization set the educational requirements for all specialty training in Canada. Changes in university hospital structure and function mirrored the Royal College educational requirements. Scientific advances have been the major driving force in shaping clinical, educational, and research progress in the field of cardiovascular and thoracic surgery at the MGM. Such evolution is continuing and, in fact, accelerating.

Dawn of the Art and Science of Thoracic and Cardiovascular Surgery

Thoracic Surgery

The development in the early twentieth century of a system of ventilation with an endotracheal tube to allow oxygenation while the chest was opened ushered in the feasibility of surgical management of thoracic diseases such as pulmonary tuberculosis and bronchogenic carcinoma. Edward Archibald at McGill is known as "the father of thoracic surgery" not only in Canada but also in North America. F. Douglas Ackman (1898–1978) was active in this field, and in 1953 Eric McNaughton was appointed as head of thoracic surgery at the MGH.

William Edward Gallie, chair at the University of Toronto (1929–47), developed an organized training program in thoracic surgery that established the specialty of thoracic surgery, with certification by the Royal College of Physicians and Surgeons of Canada in 1946 (five-year program, one-year rotating internship).

Open Heart Surgery

Although cardiovascular surgical procedures without cardiac bypass (such as those for patent ductus arteriosis, coarctation of the aorta, and closed valvular surgery) had been feasible, the open cardiac procedures became possible only after the advent of cardiopulmonary bypass technologies. The first attempt at open heart surgery in humans under cardiac bypass using pump-oxygenator was carried out in Minneapolis by Clarence Dennis in 1951. The first successful open heart closure of an atrial septal defect was achieved in 1953 by John Gibbon at Jefferson Medical College in Philadelphia. It is of some interest that the two protégés of these two pioneers – Tony Dobell trained under Gibbon and Ray Chiu under Dennis – would later serve as the first and second directors of the CVT Division at McGill University.

In 1967, Rene Favaloro at Cleveland Clinic successfully carried out saphenous vein graft bypass for coronary artery occlusion. Peter Blundell would bring this major breakthrough to the MGH shortly after this milestone achievement.

The Formative Years of CVT Surgery at the MGH

Shortly after the relocation of the MGH to its new facility on Cedar Avenue in 1955, a pivotal development in cardiothoracic surgery occurred. In 1959, H. Rocke Robertson became chair of the Department of Surgery and soon appointed an experienced general surgeon, Harry L. Scott, who was trained at McGill and the Lahey Clinic in Boston, as the head of the Cardiovascular and Thoracic Surgery Service at the MGH site.

He was supported by cardiology colleagues Pat Cronin, Stewart Reid, and (later) John Burgess and others to get this new endeavour off the ground. Fraser Gurd, who succeeded Robertson as chair of the Department of Surgery at the MGH, encouraged the development of a university-based training program, under the direction of A.R.C. Dobell, which was approved by the Royal College of Physicians and Surgeons of Canada as well as the American Board of Thoracic Surgery. Dobell had just returned from training under Gibbon in Philadelphia and was well known for his ability to instill a deep sense of humility and honesty, along with technical excellence and academic devotion.

The first historic open heart surgery at the MGH was carried out successfully on a young woman with congenital atrial septal defect on 30 June 1960 by a team of surgeons under Anthony R.C. Dobell and Harry L. Scott, while cardiac bypass using a disc oxygenator was maintained by the first perfusionist, Mr Roger Samson

In those days, thoracic, cardiac, and peripheral vascular surgeries were under one roof, named the Division of Cardiovascular and Thoracic Surgery. Although the specialty of cardiovascular surgery services was separately established at several sites in the McGill teaching hospitals, which included the MGH, the RVH, and the Montreal Children's Hospital for teaching and training of medical students and residents, it was unified under the umbrella of the McGill Division of CVT Surgery, chaired by Dobell.

The first formally trained CVT surgeon to join the MGH's CVT Service was Peter Blundell, who was a resident under Wilfred Bigelow, a pioneer in hypothermia for cardiac surgery, at the University of Toronto. He received further training at the Mayo Clinic and Great Ormond Street in London, England. He was recruited by Gurd and Scott in 1965 as a staff surgeon at the MGH and was appointed an assistant professor in the McGill Faculty of Medicine. Upon the retirement of Scott in 1988, Associate Professor Blun-

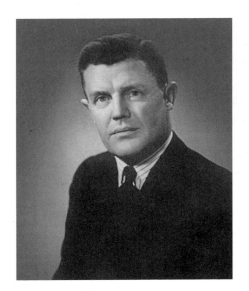
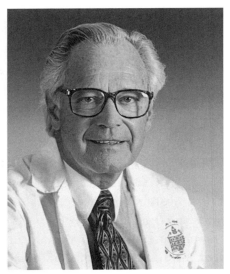
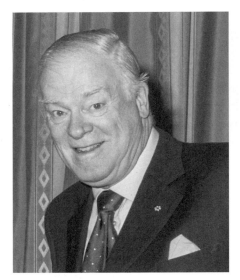
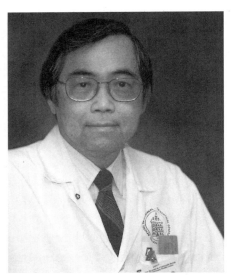

Clockwise from top left
Fig. 20.1 Harry Scott, director, cardiovascular thoracic surgery, 1959–88
Fig. 20.2 Peter Blundell, director, CVT, 1988–98
Fig. 20.3 C.J. Ray Chiu, director, University Surgical Clinic, 1980–97
Fig. 20.4 David Mulder, chair, McGill Department of Surgery, 1982–87, 1993–98; director, general thoracic surgery, 2000–

dell took over as the director of the Division of Cardiovascular and Thoracic Surgery at the MGH. He was an ambidextrous, dedicated, and skilled surgeon, who played a major role in patient care and teaching for over three decades until his retirement in 1998.

David S. Mulder, graduating magna cum laude from the University of Saskatchewan School of Medicine, arrived in Montreal in 1963 to pursue surgical training at McGill. It was in 1964–65 when he conducted research towards an MSc thesis entitled "A Study of Myocardial Function in Hemorrhagic Shock," which stimulated his interest in training for CVT surgery at the MGH. He then spent two years at the University of Iowa under L. Ehrenhaft before returning to MGH as an assistant professor in surgery in 1971. In subsequent years, he rapidly rose to the rank of full professor and served as chair of the Department of Surgery at McGill University from 1982 to 1987, and again from 1993 to 1998. He assumed many national and international surgical leadership roles as well, including the presidencies of the American Association for the Surgery of Trauma (1984–85) and the Central Surgical Association (2000–01), was governor of the American College of Surgeons (1986), and received the honour of the Order of Canada in 1997. He has been the director of the Division of General Thoracic Surgery since 2000.

In 1971, Ray Chu-Jeng Chiu was recruited to the McGill CVT Surgery Division after he received a PhD in experimental surgery from McGill in 1970. He was a graduate of the National Taiwan University College of Medicine. He did his internship at Baltimore City Hospital, which is affiliated with Johns Hopkins University, under Mark Ravitch, and residencies at the Downstate Medical Center in New York (1962–68), where Clarence Dennis, a pioneer in extracorporeal circulation, was the chair of Surgery. In 1980, matured as a surgeon scientist, Chiu was appointed as professor and director of the University Surgical Clinic at the MGH, which had been established by Rocke Robertson to expose surgical trainees to surgical research in the laboratories.

For more than two decades, from the mid-1960s to the late 1980s, this team of Scott, Blundell, Mulder, and Chiu were the working force for patient care, teaching, and research in cardiovascular and thoracic surgery at the MGH.

Stikeman Visiting Professor for Cardiovascular and Thoracic Surgery, McGill University

The Stikeman Endowment Fund for Surgical Advancement was established following the untimely death of Richard Alan Stikeman, who, in August 1965, died of a malignant mesothelioma. The Stikeman and McCall families set up the endowment under the guidance of Mr Stikeman's surgeon, D.D. Munro, who was the surgeon-in-chief at the Royal Edward Chest Hospital (now the Montreal Chest Institute) affiliated with McGill University. The fund was mandated to be "people-oriented," its main objective being to "sharpen people" who are engaged in the practice, training, and research of cardiovascular and thoracic surgery. For more than forty years, this fund has supported the Annual Stikeman Visiting Professorship, in which world leaders in cardiovascular and thoracic surgery were invited to visit McGill, gave lectures, and participated in discussions. Over the years, it evolved into an occasion for the reunion of previous residents in cardiovascular and thoracic surgery at McGill University, providing a forum for professional, scientific, and personal interactions among the alumni, current staff, and trainees. Thus, the Stikeman Visiting Professorship has become an outstanding occasion both for scholarship and friendship, contributing significantly to the development and vitality of cardiovascular and thoracic surgery at McGill University. This professorship has been referred to as the "glue" that holds the McGill division together.

Table 20.1
Stikeman visiting professors

1967	CVT Visiting Professor Dr David P. Boyd Lahey Clinic, Boston	1989	Dr Francis Robicsek Charlotte, NC
1968	Strikeman Visiting Professor Dr Donald Paulson Dallas, TX	1990	Dr Bruce A. Reitz Baltimore, MD
1969	Dr James V. Maloney, Jr. Los Angeles, CA	1991	Dr Delos M. Cosgrove Cleveland, OH
1970	Dr Donald Ross London, England	1992	Dr Anthony R.C. Dobell Montreal, Quebec

1971	Dr Hassan Najafi Chicago, IL	1993	Dr Aldo Castaneda Boston, MA
1972	Mr Charles Drew London, England	1994	Professor Sir Magdi Yacoub London, England
1973	Dr Norman Delarue Toronto, Ontario	1995	Dr Jean Deslauriers Ste-Foy, Quebec
1974	Dr Watts R. Webb New Orleans, LA	1996	Dr Hillel Laks Los Angeles, CA
1975	Dr Frank C. Spencer New York, NY	1997	Dr John a. Waldhausen Hershey, Pennsylvania
1976	Dr Herbert Sloan Ann Arbor, MI	1998	Dr Denton A. Cooley Houston, Texas
1977	Dr Eugene f. Bernstein La Jolla, CA	1999	Dr Davis C. Drinkwater, Jr. Nashville, Tennessee
1978	Dr Johann L. Ehrenhaft Iowa City, IA	2000	Dr William A. Baumgartner Baltimore, Maryland
1979	Mr Mark Braimbridge London, England	2001	Dr Peter K. Smith Durham, North Carolina
1980	Dr Dwight C. McGoon Rochester, MN	2002	Dr Alain Carpentier Paris, France
1981	Dr Thomas B. Ferguson St. Louis, MO	2003	Dr David Craig Miller Stanford, California
1982	Dr Hermes C. Grillo Boston, MA	2004	Dr Vaughn Alden Starnes Los Angeles, California
1983	Dr Norman E. Shumway Palo Alto, CA	2005	Dr W. Randolph Chitwood, Jr. Greenville, NC
1984	Dr F. Griffith Pearson Toronto, Ontario	2006	Dr Douglas J. Mathisen Boston, MA
1985	Dr Andrwew S. Wechsler Richmond, VA	2007	Dr Tirone E. David Toronto, Ontario
1986	Dr Mark B. Orringer Ann Arbor, MI	2008	Dr Eugene H. Blackstone Cleveland, Ohio
1987	Dr Richard R. Lower Richmond, VA	2009	Dr Garrett L. Walsh Houston, Texas
1988	Dr Martin F. McKneally Toronto, Ontario		

Table 20.2
Residents McGill cardiovascular thoracic surgical training program

1965–67	E.J.P. Charette	1982–83	A.K. Jain
1966–67	C. Mercier	1983–85	A.J. Bayes
			L.E. Errett
1966–68	M.S. Chughtai		
	E.F.G. Busse	1984–86	C.L. Tchervenkov
1968–70	J. Asirvatham	1985–87	RJ. Novick
			G.S. Hedderich
			H. Shennib
1969–71	M.A. James Sheverini		
1970–71	G. Malave	1986–88	M.L. Dewar
1970–72	N.L. Poirier	1987–89	D.A. Latter
			J.N.K. Odim
1971–73	G. Lemire		
		1988–90	T.A. Burdon
1972–73	E.D. Foster		G.L. Walsh
1973–75	J.F. Symes	1989–91	B. de Varennes
	R.M. Becker		G. Kochamba
1974–76	J.R. Allard	1990–92	J.B. Riebman
			W.T. Kidd
1975–77	T.A. Salerno		
		1991–93	P. Ergina
1976–78	J.W. Dutton		S. Ratnani
	A.S. Cain		
1977–79	A. Grignon		
1978–80	D. Modry		
	L. Mickleborough		
1979–80	E. Abdulnour		
1980–82	R.W. Long		
1981–83	D.C. Drinkwater		
	F.M. Keith		

Table 20.3
Residents McGill cardiothoracic surgical training program (7 yrs – 5 yrs, general surgery; 2 yrs, cardiothoracic surgery)

1992–94	D. Marelli
	D. Nguyen
1993–95	K. Lachapelle
	d. Shum-Tim
1994–96	G. Baslaim
	F. Ma
1995–97	R. Cecere
	G. Salasidis
1996–98	S. Helmer
	M. Quantz

Table 20.4
Residents McGill cardiac surgery training program (6 yrs, cardiac surgery)

1992–99	J. Tsang (7 yrs)
1993–99	S. Tahta
1994–2000	M. Pelletier
	J. Dorfman (resigned from program)
1995–2001	V. Chu
	N. Roy
1996–2002	S. Korkola
1997–2003	E. Chedrawy
1998–2004	A. Al-Khaldi
	B. Bittira
	P. Bui
	C. Wan
1999–2005	H. al-Sabti
	D. MacDonald
2000–2006	K. Sharma
2001–2007	M. Grenon
	C. Teng
	S. Trop
2002–08	T. Albacker
	R. Atoui
	S. Mohammadi

Evolution of Specialty Training for CVT Surgery in Canada: The Role of Royal College of Physicians and Surgeons of Canada

The CVT Division at the MGH evolved over the past half century with the progress in the art and science of cardiovascular and thoracic surgery, guided by the regulations of the Royal College of Physicians and Surgeons of Canada. This history is listed briefly and chronologically below:

1946: thoracic surgery certification established by the Royal College (mostly related to surgeries for pulmonary tuberculosis and lung cancers).

1958: University Cardiac Surgery Program to train cardiovascular surgeons developed, led by Dr Wilfred Bigelow (University of Toronto).

1961: CVT Surgery Fellowship and Thoracic Surgery Certificate.

1964: General Surgery followed by two to three years training in CVT (as required for the American Board of Thoracic Surgery)

1966: at the University of Toronto, Dr F.E Pearson separated general thoracic surgery from cardiac surgery.

1966–92: explosive expansion in volume and complexity of CVT surgeries.

1976: two approved pathways to general thoracic surgery in Canada (1) five-year program in CVT surgery (2) general surgery (five years) plus two years general thoracic surgery (Certificate of Special Competence).

1980: Certificate of Specialty Competence in Vascular Surgery established. Subsequently, at McGill, vascular surgery was separated from cardiothoracic surgery and became an independent division located at the RVH in 1997.

1992: core surgery and principles of surgery examination. Introduced in the second year of training in any surgical subspecialties.

1994: cardiac, thoracic, and vascular surgeries each became primary specialties.

2003: Harmonization with College des Médecins du Quebec achieved.

Growth and Maturation of Cardiac, Vascular, and Thoracic Surgery at MGH: Patient Care, Clinical Training, and Research

The McGill CVT Division separated out the Vascular Surgery Division in 1997 and then the Thoracic Surgery Division in 2000. As of 2008, both the Cardiac Surgery Division and the Vascular Surgery Division are located at the RVH site of the McGill University Health Centre, while the Thoracic Surgery Division remains at the MGH site.

During the era when A.R.C. Dobell was the McGill University division chair (1964–91), it contained the cardiac, vascular, and thoracic surgery components. By the time Ray Chiu succeeded the chair (1992–2000) vascular surgery had split off, and it consisted of cardiac and thoracic subsections. By the dawn of the twenty-first century, general thoracic surgery became independent, as described above.

In cardiothoracic surgery, many of our own trainees later joined our faculty and contributed much to its continued growth and maturation. Some of them later departed to new locations and institutions. All cardiac surgeons are now located at the RVH since the MUHC Cardiac Surgical Services merged with that site in 2008. The surgeons in our division who were located at the MGH site over the years are discussed below.

Christo Tchervenkov (completed training in 1987) undertook a paediatric cardiac surgery fellowship at Boston Children's Hospital, Harvard University. He is currently professor and chief of paediatric cardiac surgery at the Montreal Children's Hospital and a staff member in adult cardiac surgery at the RVH. Among various other positions, he is the first president of the World Society for Paediatric Cardiac Surgery, of which he was a founding member.

Lee Errett joined the Cardiac Surgery Service at the MGH in 1985. He is currently chair of cardiac surgery at St Michael's Hospital in Toronto and professor of surgery at the University of Toronto.

Hani Shennib (1988–2003) was a professor and the director of the Lung Transplantation Program before his departure from McGill.

Jean-Francois Morin (1989–2002) was site director of the Cardiac Surgery Service at the MGH and is currently at the Jewish General Hospital.

Dao Nguyen (1996–99) was an assistant professor at the MGH for several years, then moved to NIH in Bethesda, Maryland, and is currently at the University of Miami, specializing in general thoracic surgery.

Dominique Shum-Tim (1999–present) did a clinical and experimental fellowship at Boston Children's Hospital, returned to the MGH, and is currently an associate professor at McGill.

Many of our trainees left McGill and contributed significantly to other institutions. A number of them attained a chair in cardiac and thoracic surgery services, such as Tomas Salerno at the University of Miami, Davis Drinkwater at Vanderbilt University, and Richard Novick at the University of Western Ontario. Two alumni, Drinkwater and Garrett Walsh, who is a professor at the M.D. Anderson Cancer Center in Houston, Texas, served as our annual

Stikeman Visiting Professors. Many of our residents and fellows from Canada and abroad are now leaders in their institutions in several countries.

In addition to patient care and resident training, another leg of the tripod for this specialty is research that contributes to the advancement of the science of CVT surgery. Over the years, many clinical scientific papers have been presented and published in national and international meetings and journals. These consist of case reports and series of clinical findings. Many interesting observations and innovations originated in the research laboratory in the University Surgical Clinic on the ninth floor of the MGH.

As described earlier in this chapter, when H. Rocke Robertson returned to the MGH and became chair of the Department of Surgery in 1959, he had the foresight to allocate a wing of the MGH to research and teaching in surgery. This wing was named the "University Surgical Clinic." Surgical residents spent a year or more there to be exposed to laboratory research, and many obtained an MSc or PhD in experimental surgery as an integral part of their surgical training. During the tenure of Fraser Gurd, Ray Chiu was the first recipient of a PhD in this lab, and he was recruited to expand laboratory research and teaching. Residents were taught not only to be well informed and skilled but also to be critical and imaginative. Over the years, a number of new surgical techniques and ideas were developed. In the early 1970s, the technique of "spiral vein graft," which replaced vena cava, was invented. In subsequent clinical applications it has been reported to have a nearly 90 percent patency rate of a ten-year period. Other innovations included procedures like "retrograde cardioplegia" and "dynamic cardiomyoplasty"; and, in 1992, the world's first paper to introduce the concept of "regenerative stem cell therapy" for myocardial repair was published. Explosive advances in this approach are currently undergoing multicentre clinical trials, including those at the RVH.

Future Perspectives

In 2008, the adult cardiac surgery units that were developed separately over the years at both the MGH and the RVH sites were unified and are presently located at the RVH until the "super hospital" at Glen Yards is realized. The General Thoracic Surgery Service is concentrated at the MGH site, while the Vascular Surgery Service has been developed at the RVH site. It is expected that all these divisions will move to the Glen Yards when the project is completed. The MGH will take on a different mission. Nevertheless, McGill CVT surgery will undoubtedly continue to flourish by ensuring that this field of surgical care will benefit future generations of patients in this city, and by advancing our skills and knowledge in order to improve the quality of life for humanity in general.

NOTES

1 R. Hurt, *The History of Cardiothoracic Surgery from Early Times* (New York: Parthenon, 1996); N.C. Delarue, *Thoracic Surgery in Canada* (Toronto: B.C. Decker Inc, 1989); R.M. Pound, *Rocke Robertson: Surgeon and Shepherd of Change* (Montreal and Kingston: McGill-Queen's University Press, 2008).

2 M.A. Entin, *Edward Archibald: Surgeon of the Royal Vic* (Montreal: McGill University Libraries, Fontanus Monograph series, 2004); B.S. Goldman and S. Belanger, *Heart Surgery in Canada: Memoirs, Anecdotes, History and Perspective* (Xlibris Corporation USA, 2004).

3 D. Waugh, *The Gurds, the Montreal General, and McGill: A Family Saga* (Burnstown, ON: General Store Publishing House, 1996).

4 D.A.E. Shephard, The Royal College of Physicians and Surgeons of Canada, 1960–1980. Publication of RCPSC.

21

Neurosurgery

Joseph G. Stratford

Joe Stratford was the first director of the Division of Neurosurgery at the MGH. His manuscript was completed by Garth Bray and Joe Hanaway after his death. His was the first manuscript to be submitted.

Joseph Stratford, the first full-time neurosurgeon at the MGH (1962–92), describes the development of the Department of Neurosurgery starting in 1951 with Harold Elliott, its on/off relationship with neurology, the appointment of three full-time staff and their contributions, and, finally, their transfers and retirements. The department closed in 1999.

Neurosurgery at the MGH may be said to have started in 1859 when the annual report first recorded "trephining" of the skull.[1] It was probably performed by George Fenwick, who was particularly accomplished in carrying out new surgical procedures. Later, in 1865, 1868, and 1881, there were similar reports of trephination.

Brain surgery in the 1870s was limited to trephining for depressed skull fractures,[2] an operation performed about twice a year. Rapid advances were made in the 1880s due, in large part, to the advent of Listerism. The benefit of carbolic acid spray in surgery was first advocated by Joseph Lister in 1865. Francis J. Shepherd observed its being used in Edinburgh in 1874, but it was Thomas Roddick who introduced antisepsis to the MGH in 1877 after he visited Lister in London.[3] There was a special burst of activity about 1886, when many operations were reported for tumour and abscess of the brain as well as for relief of epilepsy by trephining the skull.

When another hospital was planned as a tribute to Queen Victoria 1887, the MGH made a counter-proposal, but neither side would compromise. When it was decided that amalgamation of the MGH and the new hospital could not be arranged, the Royal Victoria Hospital was built and opened in

1893. At the same time, the project of erecting new buildings on the grounds of the MGH was resumed. A new surgical wing was built in 1892, resulting in more than one hundred beds for surgical patients, along with a large new operating theatre.[4]

Early in the twentieth century, a surgeon at the RVH, Edward Archibald, developed a special interest in neurosurgery. In a letter to the Medical Board of the MGH dated 23 November 1907, he requested permission to review the records of all cases of skull fracture at the General.[5] This was granted, and the next year Archibald travelled to England to train with Sir Victor Horsley, the eminent neurological surgeon at the National Hospital, Queen Square, London. In view of his experience with Horsley in London, it is possible that Archibald may have been involved with neurosurgical cases at the MGH, but there is no evidence of this in the reports of the Medical Board. He was interested in head trauma and published a 375-page treatise on the subject in 1908.[6]

There was an important development in 1927, when a letter from Edward Archibald was read to the Medical Board of the MGH regarding "the desirability of securing the services of Wilder Penfield, at present neurological surgeon to the Presbyterian Hospital in New York." After much discussion it was moved by Fred Mackay, head of the Department of Neurology, that "it is the opinion of the Board that every facility should be extended to Penfield to carry on Neurological Pathology and Neurological Surgery in association with the Neurological Department of the Montreal General Hospital."[7] Archibald wanted Penfield to take over his neurosurgical cases and to develop his own practice at the RVH, and this was the primary reason for his appointment: his relationship with the MGH was to be secondary.

In 1928, correspondence from Dean Charles P. Martin to the chairman of the MGH Medical Board, Arthur T. Bazin, referred to the establishment of a surgical neurology clinic and the appointment to be offered to Penfield. A committee of four attending surgeons and the neurologist Fred MacKay was formed to draft recommendations concerning the establishment of a surgical neurological clinic at the MGH.[8] This committee decided that all cases should be operated on at the MGH and that traumatic neurological surgery should remain under the control of the Department of General Surgery. In addition, the committee recommended that William Cone be appointed as an assistant in surgery attached to the neurological surgery clinic and that an appointee of the Medical Board be accepted for training in neurological surgery.[9] The Medical Board then approved the purchase of $1500 worth of surgical equipment for neurosurgery.[10] By the end of 1928, it was decided that Penfield and Cone should be attached to the Department of Neurology and that the chief of neurology "be empowered to arrange the division of work and responsibilities."[11] Neurological cases requiring operation were to be allotted beds on the M surgical service with the senior interne of M service serving as intern for the neurosurgical patients. Within a matter of months this arrangement proved to be unacceptable to Penfield, who insisted on being responsible for his own surgical cases. On 8 May 1929, he submitted a memorandum stating that the management of neurological cases at the MGH was unsatisfactory and that surgical cases not considered suitable for reference to members of the MGH staff should be transferred to the RVH for operation and then, after an appropriate postoperative course, referred back to the MGH with their complete record.[12]

Reluctantly, the MGH medical staff were obliged to transfer patients for operation to the RVH as a temporary measure until a neurosurgeon could be trained for the General's staff.[13] If neither proposal were to be approved, both Cone and Penfield stated that they were ready to withdraw altogether or to help with any proposed plan. Within a few months, it was decided to retain the services of Arthur Elvidge, starting 1 July 1929.[14] Upon completion of his training,[15] Elvidge returned to the staff of the MGH in 1932. In 1933, the MGH Medical Board established neurosurgery as a subdepartment of neurology and surgery,[16] with Elvidge in charge of neurosurgical patients, including all head injuries. Penfield and Cone were appointed consulting neurosurgeons to the MGH.[17]

When the Second World War ended in 1945, Major Harold Elliott (fig. 21.1),[18] who had been the commanding officer of No. 1 Canadian Mobile Neurosurgical Unit and neurosurgeon-in-charge at Basingstoke, returned to Montreal. He was appointed director of Neurosurgery at Queen Mary Veterans Hospital and, in March 1946, was appointed as clinical assistant in surgery.[19]

In 1948, the enlarged Department of Neurology was renamed the Department of Neurology and Neurosurgery,[20] patterned after the arrangement at the Montreal Neurological Institute and at McGill. In 1951, when Preston Robb, a neurologist, was appointed to succeed Francis McNaughton as director of neurology and neurosurgery, severe criticism arose, largely from the surgeons, with the result that Harold Elliott was named to the position instead.[21]

Having made many contacts during the war, Harold Elliott arranged for neurosurgical fellows to come to Montreal from England and Scotland for a year or more at the MGH. The first of these was Rankin Hay in 1953, followed by Alister Paterson in 1954.[22] At this time, the Department of Neurosurgery made an unprecedented request for permission to admit unconscious private patients to the public ward, where better care and supervision was possible.[23] The new MGH – an 850-bed hospital built on the site of the Cross estate on Cedar Avenue,[24] was opened in May 1955. All patients were transferred from the Central and Western divisions over the following two weeks.

Joseph Stratford[25] was appointed as the neurosurgical fellow and, later, junior assistant neurosurgeon at the MGH in January 1955.[26] When Stratford moved to Saskatoon in 1956,[27] Rankin Hay returned to the MGH as neurosurgical fellow.[28]

The appointment of H. Rocke Robertson as surgeon-in-chief at the MGH in 1958 was an important milestone in the history of the hospital.[29] Decisions were made over the next several years that profoundly affected neurosurgery.

When the MGH moved to its new site on Cedar Avenue on 29 May 1955, the Department of Neurology and Neurosurgery was assigned all thirty-five beds on Ward 15-East. These beds were not fully utilized, so neurology and neurosurgery patients were moved to separate wards in 1959. In spite of Harold Elliott's objections, neurosurgery was assigned ten beds on 12 West, the ward of the Traumatic and Reparative Service, which had been created by Rocke Robertson. As neurosurgeon-in-chief, Elliott wrote to the MGH Medical Board in 1960 regarding his dissatisfaction with having neurosurgical beds on a ward shared with the Trauma Service, insisting that the standard of care had dropped, with a significant increase in operative infections.[30] Elliott recommended a return to the previous arrangement on 15 East and stated that the neurological and neurosurgical services must be in the same department, as they were at the MNI, and the responsibility of one person.

Prior to presenting his recommendations to the Medical Board, Elliott had written to neurosurgical colleagues in other centres asking for their opinion as to how neurosurgery should be structured in a teaching hospital. Neurosurgeons contacted included Joseph Pennybacker, Thomas Ballantine, Joseph Evans, Thomas Speakman, John O'Connel, Earl Walker, Rankin Hay, and Joseph Stratford. Most of them responded, and many advised that neurosurgery should be a division of the Department of Surgery. Copies of Harold Elliott's letter and letters from the neurosurgeons were distributed to members of the Medical Board.[31]

The response to Harold Elliott's letter to the Medical Board proved to be crucial in the history of neurosurgery at the MGH. A special committee of the Medical Board, chaired by Douglas Cameron, was asked to make recommendations for a neurosurgical unit in a modern teaching hospital. The committee invited three prominent senior surgeons from other universities (Professors Robert Milnes Walker, Isidor S. Ravdin, and Walter Mackenzie) to come to Montreal to assess the situation. Their opinion was given in a letter from the University Club, dated 4 February 1961, which stated: "We are agreed that a combined Department of Neurology and Neurosurgery is NOT a satisfactory arrangement in an undergraduate teaching hospital."[32] In their report dated 20 February 1961, the Cameron Committee recommended that the Department of Neurology and Neurosurgery be disbanded and that a Division of Neurosurgery be created in the Department of Surgery.[33] These recommendations were strongly endorsed by H. Rocke Robertson, MGH surgeon-in-chief.[34] There was to be a reallocation of beds to provide accommodation for ten neurosurgical patients other than the multiple-injury trauma cases. Of significance was the added recommendation "that private, semi-private and standard ward patients should be nursed together in a segregated area." Among the hospital staff affected by the decision, there was considerable disagreement concerning the dissolution of the hospital Department of Neurology and Neurosurgery.

In 1961, Hugh Samson joined Harold Elliott as a junior assistant in neurosurgery, having just completed his neurosurgical training at the MNI.[35] This appointment was terminated in 1962. Meanwhile, H. Rocke Robertson had been negotiating with Joseph Stratford (fig. 21.2), professor of neurosurgery at the University of Saskatchewan and director of the Division of Neurosurgery at the University Hospital in Saskatoon. As a result, in August 1962, Joseph Stratford was appointed director of the newly created Division of Neurosurgery at the MGH.[36] John Blundell, director of neurosurgery at the Montreal Children's Hospital, was appointed to the staff at the MGH, and Joe Stratford was given a reciprocal appointment at the Children's Hospital so that both hospitals could be covered at all times. Harold Elliott continued his practice of neurosurgery at the MGH and at the Queen Mary Veterans Hospital until he retired.

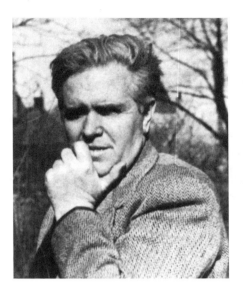 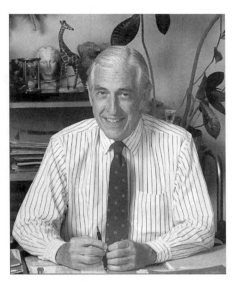

Fig. 21.1 Harold Elliott, director, Department of Neurology/Neurosurgery, 1951–61;
director of Division of Neurosurgery, 1961–62
Fig. 21.2 Joseph Straford, first full-time director of Neurosurgery, 1962–92

Because the close observation of unconscious or disorientated patients was considered essential, Rocke Robertson agreed with Joe Stratford's request that a special intensive care area for seriously ill neurosurgical patients was needed. For this purpose, the wall of a four-bed room on 12 West was opened to facilitate observation of patients from the main nursing station. Furthermore, it was accepted that all categories of patients, public and private, could be admitted to this special observation area. This caused some administrative confusion in the days before Medicare.

In 1963, neurosurgery at the MGH was strengthened by the arrival from Philadelphia of one of Joe Stratford's former University of Saskatchewan colleagues, neurologist Donald Baxter: "The ties of personal and professional respect formed at the University Hospital in Saskatoon were to prove of great benefit in [their] joint undertaking at the Montreal General Hospital and McGill."[37]

In 1965, Robert Ford was appointed as the second geographical full-time neurosurgeon at the MGH.[38] This appointment was well timed as the volume of cases had increased. In addition to being a technically skilled neurosurgeon, Bob brought expertise in the new technique of echoencephalography, which was found to be of inestimable value in neurosurgery in the pre-CT scan era. Bob Ford also initiated the use of the microscope in the operating room and directed the Neuro-Intensive Care Unit, where he supervised the neurotrauma program and perfected the use of intracranial pressure monitors.

In 1966, after several years of negotiation and planning, a joint clinical neurology-neurosurgery unit was built on 7-East Pine in a newly constructed addition to the MGH.[39] It consisted of thirty beds for neurology and neurosurgical patients and included a neuro-intensive care unit that was essential for the close observation of seriously ill patients.

Leslie Stern, a resident in the McGill neurosurgical training program, carried out an extensive research project, supported by a Killam Scholarship, in the surgical laboratory at the MGH in 1971. This culminated in a PhD dissertation entitled "The Role of the Brain in Haemorrhagic Shock."

In 1976, Jules Hardy, senior neurosurgeon at Montreal's Hôpital Notre-Dame, applied to the MGH for permission to admit and operate on patients with pituitary lesions, predominantly tumours. In the preceding decade Hardy had perfected the technique of transphenoidal hypophysectomy at Hôpital Notre-Dame and had become world-renowned, with patients referred to him from many foreign countries for this specialized surgery. His application was accepted, and he became a consulting specialist in neurosurgery. Hardy was already professor of neurosurgery at the Université de Montréal, but it took some time for McGill to appoint him an associate in the Department of Neurology and Neurosurgery. In his first ten years at the MGH (1976 to 1986), Hardy carried out 350 pituitary operations, providing a most valuable experience for neurosurgical residents as well as the Division of Endocrinology. Jules Hardy was awarded the Izaak Walton Killam Memorial Prize in Health Sciences in 1989.

In January 1977, Peter Richardson became the third geographical full-time neurosurgeon at the MGH. A graduate of the University of Toronto in 1967, Peter Richardson completed two years of residency in Montreal at Hôpital Notre-Dame and the RVH before returning to the Toronto neurosurgical training program, which he completed in 1974. In 1975, he gained experience in peripheral nerve research with P.K. Thomas at the Royal Free Hospital, London, England. Subsequently, he did neurosurgical work in Kuala Lumpur, Malaysia, before returning in 1976 to Montreal to be on the neurosurgical staff at Hôpital Sacre-Coeur.

Richardson's appointment at the MGH was arranged so that he would be able to devote half of his time working in the MGH Research Institute. He developed a significant involvement in important basic research, while at the same time carrying his full share of the neurosurgical clinical responsibilities. In 1992, Richardson was promoted to professor of neurosurgery and became the director of the Division of Neurosurgery at the MGH following the resignation of Joseph Stratford, who had held the position for thirty years. In 1993, the Society of Neurological Surgeons awarded Richardson the Grass Prize for "outstanding continuous commitment to research in the neurosciences by a neurological surgeon." Richardson's research activities during the twenty-two years he spent at the MGH are best described in his own words (see note).[40]

In 1997, the University of London offered Richardson an appointment as the chair of Neurosurgery. Negotiations continued until 1999, at which time he accepted the position of professor of neurosurgery and director of the Department of Neurosurgery at the Royal London Hospital in Whitechapel.

Jean-Louis Caron was appointed as the fourth full-time neurosurgeon effective 1 September 1985. A graduate of the University of Ottawa, he completed the McGill neurosurgical training program in 1985 and was granted a leave of absence to spend a year with Charles Drake at the University of Western Ontario to gain experience with cerebrovascular problems and, in particular, intracranial aneurysms. This exceptional year on the internationally renowned neurosurgical service in London, Ontario, was facilitated by a Frank McGill Travelling Fellowship from the MGH.

In January 1987, Caron started neurosurgery at the MGH and was appointed assistant professor in the McGill Department of Neurology and Neurosurgery; later he was promoted to associate professor. In addition, he was made an associate in the Division of Neurosurgery at the Montreal Children's Hospital as well as a consulting surgeon to the Lakeshore General Hospital and the Centre Hospitalier de Valleyfield.

Jean-Louis Caron became an investigator in the North American Symptomatic Carotid Endarterectomy Trial and also participated in the McGill oncology trial, with Luis Souhami and Ervin Podgorsak, involving stereotaxic radiosurgery to treat malignant brain tumours. Another area of special interest developed by Caron was that of percutaneous lumbar discectomy after several years of limited success with chemodiscolysis, which was started earlier in the 1980s by other MGH staff, both neurosurgical and orthopaedic.

In September 1999, coincident with the departure of Peter Richardson for the University of London, Jean-Louis Caron accepted an offer to move to Hôpital Notre-Dame, where he became the co-director of neurovascular surgery with an appointment as associate professor of surgery at the Université de Montréal. Subsequently, in 2004, Caron accepted an offer of professor of neurosurgery at the University of Texas in the Health Sciences Center in San Antonio.

Karen Johnston, a graduate of the University of Toronto and trained in the McGill Neurosurgical Program, took on the role of director of Neurotrauma at the MGH and the MUHC in 1999. Johnston was appointed an assistant professor in the Departments of Neurosurgery and Surgery at McGill but left the MGH in 2003 to become director of the Concussion Program at the McGill Sport Medicine Centre. In 2006, she moved to the University of Toronto.

With the departure from the MGH of Richardson and Caron in 1999, and the retirements of Stratford and Ford earlier in the decade, the previously active neurosurgical service, with four geographical full-time neurosurgeons, ceased to exist. Most of the neurosurgical cases were transferred to the Montreal Neurological Hospital, and only neuro-trauma was covered at the MGH.

NOTES

1 38th Annual Report of the Montreal General Hospital, 1860, 15, MUA.
2 Medical specialization was beginning to develop during this era. In 1876, Frank Buller was the first surgical subspecialist at the MGH when he was appointed "oculist and aurist." In 1880, Thomas Roddick and George Ross were the first to restrict their practices to the specialties of surgery and medicine, respectively (see Medical Board Minutes, vol. 44, 3 November 1880). It was also during this period that William Osler became the first person at the hospital with extensive knowledge of diseases of the nervous system. During the decade from 1874 to 1884, when he was pathologist to the MGH, Osler performed 780 autopsies and reported many of his clinic-pathological correlations to the Montreal Medico-Chirurgical Society and in various publications. A number of these reports concerned neurological problems (see M.E. Abbott, "Osler's Pathological Collections and His Literary Output," *Canadian Medical Association Journal* 42 (1940): 284–8).
3 H.E. MacDermot, *A History of the Montreal General Hospital* (Montreal: Montreal General Hospital, 1950), 67–8.

4 Ibid., 81–2.

5 Medical Board Minutes, 3 December 1907, 307, MUA.

6 E. Archibald, "Surgical Affections and Wounds of the Head," in *American Practice of Surgery*, ed. Bryant and Buck (New York: Wood, 1908), 4:3–378.

7 Medical Board Minutes, vol. 49, 1 November 1927, 246, MUA.

8 Ibid., 7 February 1928.

9 Ibid., 6 March 1928, 258.

10 Ibid., 6 November 1928, 290.

11 Ibid., 18 December 1928, 294.

12 Ibid., vol. 50, 8 May 1929, 21.

13 The reason for Penfield's decision is recorded in his autobiography, *No Man Alone*. He concluded that the lives of patients might be in danger during the hours and days that followed operation after transfer while he and Cone were busy with their patients and in their laboratory at the RVH (see W. Penfield, *No Man Alone* [Boston: Little, Brown and Co., 1977], 364).

14 Board of Management Minutes, vol. 2, 9 May 1929, 198–9, MUA.

15 Arthur Elvidge came to the attention of Penfield as a potential young trainee for neurosurgery at the MGH. Elvidge, a medical graduate from McGill in 1924, earned an MSc in 1925 and a PhD in 1927 for his research on blood coagulation in the Department of Physiology. In 1928, he started training at the RVH under Edward Archibald and obviously was influenced by Penfield and Cone. It was planned that he enter a course of training for three years, with time spent abroad, after which he was to be placed in charge of neurosurgical work at the MGH. In 1932, after his surgical training at the RVH and his exposure to Penfield and Cone, Elvidge gained experience in London at the National Hospital, Queen Square, and in Lisbon, where he worked with Egas Moniz, the Portuguese neurologist who had recently developed cerebral angiography (with thorium dioxide, a gamma-emitting isotope with a four-thousand-year half-life that eventually killed all who had the procedure). He returned to the MGH as a staff member in 1932. At McGill, he was appointed lecturer in neurosurgery and given an appointment on staff at the RVH and (later) the MNI (see letter from Penfield, 5 June 1933, appended to Medical Board Minutes, 7 June 1933). Arthur Elvidge received his FRCS(C) degree in 1939.

16 Medical Board Minutes, vol. 50, 7 June 1933, 220, MUA.

17 Board of Management Minutes, vol. 3, 28 February and 14 March 1934, 467 and 470, respectively.

18 Harold Elliott (fig. 21.1) was born in Cache Bay, Ontario, on 21 December 1907. He graduated in medicine from McGill University in 1936. After an internship at the RVH, he trained at the National Hospital, Queen Square (1937–38); at Barnes Hospital, St Louis (1938–39); and at the MNI (1939–40). Harold Elliott married Doris Gales on 24 July 1937 (personal communication from Bonnie Elliott, 5 October 2007).

Elliott joined the Royal Canadian Army Medical Corps in 1940 and was assigned to the Department of Neurosurgery at No. 1 Canadian General Hospital in Basingstoke, England. From 1942 to 1945, he was the commanding officer of the Mobile Neurosurgical Unit and was attached to the 1st Canadian Army as it pushed across the Rhine and into Germany. Before demobilization in 1945, Major Elliott was in charge of neurosurgery at the Canadian military hospital in Basingstoke and the Montreal Military Hospital.

Harold Elliott was appointed to the staff of the MGH in 1946 and became chair of the hospital's Department of Neurology and Neurosurgery in 1951, a position he held until 1961, when the department was disbanded. He was also in charge of neurosurgery at Queen Mary Veterans Hospital and was an assistant neurosurgeon at the MNI. On 2 October 1961, he was named to the consulting staff of the MGH.

In 1952, Harold Elliott was instrumental in organizing an annual formal event that included the Francis J. Shepherd Memorial Lecture, which was to be given by "an outstanding member of the medical profession" (Medical Board Minutes, vol. 56, 5 November 1952, 132). The first of these lectures was given by Sir Sydney Smith, dean of the Faculty of Medicine, Edinburgh University, on 1 May 1953, the day before the laying of the cornerstone of the new MGH on Cedar Avenue (Medical Board Minutes, vol. 56, 4 February 1953). Subsequent Shepherd Memorial Lecturers were Sir Stewart Duke-Elder (1954); E.P. Scarlett, chancellor of the University of Edmonton (1955); C.P. Martin, dean of the McGill Faculty of Medicine (1956); Professor John Bruce, surgeon from Edinburgh University (1957); O.M. Solandt, vice-president for Research and Development (1958); and, L.J. Witts, Nuffield Professor of Medicine, Oxford University (1959).

Harold Elliott became a strong advocate for the prevention of traffic injuries. He organized an international symposium on the problems of traffic crashes and published an article on the problem in 1956 (see H. Elliott, "Medical Research In Traffic Accidents: A Plan for Studying the Problem through Research Units in Casualty Wards of Teaching Hospitals," *Canadian Medical Association Journal* 74 [1956]: 557–9).

He was also responsible for designing a wheel-chair that could be transformed into a stretcher (the "McGill chair"), a special reflex hammer, and surgical instruments (William Feindel, personal communication, 14 September 2007). Harold Elliott died in Brockville, Ontario, on 29 May 1973 (see *Montreal Gazette*, 31 May 1973).

19 Medical Board Minutes, vol. 54, 26 June 1946, 20, MUA.

20 Ibid., 3 March 1948; Board of Management Minutes, vol. 6, 17 March 1948, 10, MUA.

21 Medical Board Minutes, vol. 56: 4 April and 6 June 1951, MUA.

22 Ibid., vol. 57, 1 April 1953.

23 Ibid., 14 April 1954.

24 Ibid., vol. 55, 2 March 1949.

25 Joseph G. Stratford (fig. 21.2) was born in Brantford, Ontario, where the Stratford family was well known for its philanthropy. He graduated from the McGill Faculty of Medicine in 1947, interned at the MGH, and then began neurosurgical training by doing a year in neurophysiology research with Herbert Jasper at the MNI. This work resulted in an MSc thesis entitled "A Study of Certain Corticothalamic Relationships," in which he presented novel evidence that challenged the prevailing opinion that the thalamus was exclusively a relay station for afferent sensory input.[50] From 1950 to 1951, Joe Stratford spent a year in London, England, at the National Hospital, Queen Square, and as a house-surgeon at the Hammersmith Post-Graduate Medical School. From 1951 to 1954, he completed his training in neurosurgery with Penfield, Cone, and Elvidge at the MNI. Towards the end of his residency, Joe Stratford married Aurelie Forbes, who had been Penfield's secretary (see W. Feindel, "An Appreciation of Joseph Stratford, 1923–2007: Teacher, Neurosurgeon, Humanist," at http://www/mni.mcgill.ca/neuroimage/index.html).

On completing his residency, Joe Stratford became a fellow in neurosurgery at the MGH in July, 1955; in January, 1956, he was appointed as junior assistant neurosurgeon. An event during this period illustrates the integrity that was a hallmark of Joe Stratford's career. In November 1955 he received a five-hundred-dollar grant from the R.P. Campbell Memorial Fund to cover the expenses of a two-week visit to the University of Colorado to study the use of hypothermia in head injuries (see Medical Board Minutes, vol. 58, 9 November 1955) . In January, 1956, the Medical Board received a letter from Joe expressing his appreciation for the grant and returning two hundred dollars because his expenses were only three hundred dollars (see Medical Board Minutes, vol. 58, 6 January 1956).

While at the MGH, Joe Stratford received the offer of an academic appoint-ment at the new University Hospital in Saskatoon from William Feindel, who had gone to Saskatchewan from the MNI some months earlier. Feindel had been a long-time colleague at McGill and the MNI while training in neuro-surgery with Penfield, Cone, and Elvidge. Having decided to accept the Saskatchewan proposal, Stratford resigned from the MGH in May 1956. He and his family arrived in Saskatoon on 2 May 1956 to join the neurology and neurosurgery unit that William Feindel and Allan Bailey were developing in the exciting environment that existed at the University of Saskatchewan.

In 1962, H. Rocke Robertson, chair of the McGill Department of Surgery and surgeon-in-chief at the hospital persuaded Joe Stratford to return to Montreal as director of the Division of Neurosurgery at the MGH. For the next thirty years, he worked tirelessly to build a neurosurgical service whose reputa-tion for excellence was recognized by McGill neurosurgery residents as a key component of their program. Working closely with his friend and colleague, Donald W. Baxter, Joe Stratford developed a neurology-neurosurgery care unit first on 7-East Pine and then on the fourteenth floor of the hospital.

For several years, Joe Stratford was the hospital's only neurosurgeon, gain-ing respite only through cross-coverage with John Blundell at the Montreal Children's Hospital. He gradually expanded the Division of Neurosurgery with the recruitment of Robert Ford (1967), Peter Richardson (1977), and Jean-Louis Caron (1995). In addition to his passion for the growth and maintenance of the MGH neurosurgery service, Stratford had particular interests in the use of hy-pothermia in neurosurgery, spinal cord surgery, isotope brain scanning, and a simple surgical approach to the management of ulnar neuropathy. In the 1970s, he helped to establish a multidisciplinary pain clinic at the MGH. He served on several McGill University committees, was a representative of the Faculty of Medicine at the senate, and was president of the Canadian Neurosurgical Society from 1974 to 1975.

Stratford's other interests and contributions were diverse and generous. He had an ardent passion for Canadian art and the works of early twentieth-century English writers. He was an active member of the Board of Directors of the Victorian Order of Nurses from 1985 until 2007. He died on 22 July 2007 in the south of France while visiting his daughter and her husband. "He will be remembered by his medical colleagues for his deep concern for patients and by his many friends for his unruffled charm – reflecting Osler's 'Aequanimitas'" (see W. Feindel, "An Appreciation of Joseph Stratford, 1923–2007: Teacher, Neu-rosurgeon, Humanist," at http://www/mni.mcgill.ca/neuroimage/index.html).

26 Medical Board Minutes, vol. 57, 1 September and 1 December 1954

27 Ibid., vol. 58, 2 May 1956.

28 Ibid., 4 April 1956.

29 Credentials Committee of the Medical Board of the Montreal General Hospital, Minutes of Meetings, vol. 60, 24 July 1958, MUA.

30 Correspondence of the Medical Board of the Montreal General Hospital, box C407, fol. 00443, letter, 21 November 1960, MUA.

31 Ibid. Letters dated May 1959, 29 March 1960 (x2), 4, 11, 16, 24 April 1960; 23 May 1960; and 2 September 1960.

32 Ibid., letter, 4 February 1961.

33 Ibid., Report of the Special Committee of the Medical Board, 20 February 1961.

34 Ibid., letter, 10 February 1961.

35 Credentials Committee of the Medical Board of the MGH, minutes of meetings, vol. 60, 30 May 1961.

36 Board of Management Minutes, vol. 8, 16 May 1962, 162, MUA.

37 D.W. Baxter and J.G. Stratford, "Neurology and Neurosurgery at the Montreal General Hospital 1960–1980," *Canadian Journal of Neurological Science* 27 (2000): 79–83.

38 Robert Malcolm Ford graduated in medicine from the University of Western Ontario in 1958. He completed a rotating internship and a year as a medical resident at the MGH. On the recommendation of Harold Elliott, he gained considerable neurosurgical experience in Glasgow with Sloane Robertson and in London, England, with Wylie McKissock before completing his training in Montreal at Queen Mary Veterans Hospital and the MNI. In 1964, he was appointed to the staff of the Queen Mary Veterans Hospital and in 1965 to the staff of the MGH. While in England, Ford had worked with James Ambrose perfecting the use of ultrasound to determine intracranial midline shifts. Although he was left-handed, this was not noticeable as he was completely ambidextrous. He was obliged to retire for health reasons in 1997 and died on 6 March 2004.

39 Board of Management Minutes, vol. 9, 17 April 1963, 35, MUA.

40 "I was fortunate to join an exciting neuroscience research environment built up through the efforts of Don Baxter, Albert Aguayo, and others (Doug Cameron, Phil Gold, Garth Bray, Joe Martin). An early project was to revisit studies done by Ramon y Cajal early in the century, which had been neglected and were ripe for investigation with neuroanatomical techniques developed in the 1970s. The results supported Cajal's claims that injured nerve fibres from the central nervous system had potential for regrowth in the favourable

environment provided by Schwann cells. This finding was one of several at the time, which rekindled an interest in the neuroscience world in regeneration in the brain and spinal cord. The research work fitted in well with one of the missions of the Montreal General in trauma, started by Rocke Robertson, Joe Stratford, and others, and reignited by Dave Mulder, Rae Brown, and Bob Ford. The explosion in molecular biology in the 1980s made it opportune to investigate the growth factors, which underlie the ability of Schwann cells to promote axonal growth.

"I was introduced to the field of growth factors by Rick Riopelle and Ted Ebendal in Sweden and tutored in molecular biology by Robert Benoit and Rob Dunn. One of the achievements was to localize receptors for classical nerve growth factor in the brain. Although nerve growth factor may be important in neurodegenerative disease and pain, it has little to do with axonal regeneration. Therefore, studies in the 1990s focused on another class of neurotrophic molecules, including ciliary neurotrophic factor, which seems to initiate the regenerative program in injured neurons. Ray Chiu and I considered ourselves dinosaurs who started our careers early enough to be able to combine surgery with basic laboratory research before the latter became an exclusively full-time occupation" (personal communication from Peter Richardson to J.G. Stratford).

22

Plastic Surgery

H. Bruce Williams

Bruce Williams was director of the Division of Plastic Surgery until he moved to become chief of surgery at the Montreal Children's Hospital.

Introduction

I describe the origins of plastic surgery at the Montreal General Hospital and McGill University up to 1976, when the MGH, the Royal Victoria Hospital, and the Montreal Children's Hospital combined to form a cooperative training program. The success of this venture, along with numerous staff and their contributions to the clinical and research aspects of plastic surgery, are discussed.

The development of plastic surgery at McGill University closely paralleled the rapid expansion of reconstructive surgery in Canada and other countries throughout the world. For the past five decades, McGill has been at the forefront of new developments in plastic surgery teaching, in basic laboratory research, in the care of children with congenital anomalies, in hand surgery, in the care of patients with facial and spinal injuries, in burn treatment, and in the rapidly developing exciting area of microsurgery.

The Early Days of Plastic Surgery

Plastic surgery at McGill was recognized as a definitive specialty in the early 1930s. The first fully trained plastic surgeon was John W. Gerrie, who entered practice in 1935 at the MGH with affiliate appointments at St Mary's Hospital, the Queen Mary Veterans Hospital, and the MCH. Gerrie was a graduate in dentistry from McGill in the early 1920s and in medicine in 1931. His internship at the MGH was completed in 1933, and he then practised for nine months in Cadomin, Alberta. His early interest in plastic surgery stimulated his visits to the few plastic surgery centres at that time in St Louis, Missouri, where he spent three months with Vilray Blair and James Barrett Brown and then spent time with Sir Harold Gillies and Sir Archibald MacIndoe at Bart's Hospital in London. He became an otolaryngology registrar at the Golden Square Hospital in London, and, following his return to Canada, he spent some time with Fulton Risdon, A.W. Farmer, and Stuart Gordon in Toronto. Gerrie was trained in dentistry, otolaryngology, and plastic surgery, and, at that time, there were very few, if any, procedures carried out in the latter as we now know it. The taking of skin grafts was very rare, and cleft lip and cleft palate surgery was performed by Dudley Ross at the MCH and by Ralph Fitzgerald at the MGH. Gerrie brought home the first dermatome from Kansas City in 1936 during one of his visits to that area where he had the opportunity to meet with Earl Padgett. Gerrie continued his long interest in facial surgery, and he became president of the American Society of Maxillofacial Surgeons.

The second plastic surgeon to arrive in Montreal was Hamilton Baxter, who started his practice at the RVH and the MGH in 1937. Baxter trained at Cook County Hospital in Chicago and under an outstanding group in St Louis. He was an enthusiastic, well trained surgeon with many new ideas and techniques for developing the specialty, and he quickly became an influence in plastic surgery in North America, writing several key articles, particularly with regard to burn treatment and in repair of cleft palate defects.

Gerrie and Baxter represented the specialty of plastic surgery for nine or ten years until the end of the Second World War. At that time, Gerrie was actively engaged in a busy practice at the QMVH, where there was a seventy-bed unit, and he was in desperate need of assistance. About this time, Frederick M. Woolhouse accepted a position at the QMVH, moving directly from active service in the navy, and Georges Cloutier, who had trained with Sumner Koch in Chicago, was similarly seconded from the air force. Woolhouse graduated from McGill with an MD, CM in 1936 and, after completing his General Surgical residency, entered the Royal Canadian Navy, serving from 1940 to 1946 as the medical officer on the HMCS *Assiniboine* and then as surgeon at the Royal Canadian Naval Hospital in Halifax. He trained with Farmer in Toronto and then visited plastic surgery clinics at Barnes Hospital in St Louis and the Presbyterian Hospital in Philadelphia. He and Farmer treated a large number of burn patients following a disastrous Knights of Columbus Recreation Hall fire in St John's, Newfoundland, and then he proceeded to further his studies at Basingstoke Neurological and Plastic Surgery Hospital, then at East Grinstead with Sir Archibald MacIndoe, at St Alban's with Rainsford Mowlen, and at Rooksdown House with Sir Harold Gillies at Stoke Mandeville.

He returned to Montreal in February 1946 and became a consultant in plastic surgery at the QMVH, director of plastic surgery at the MCH, and a member of the Plastic Surgery Division at the MGH. Woolhouse was one of the founding members of the Canadian Society of Plastic Surgeons and a past president of the organization. He has had a great influence on the teaching of plastic surgery residents and an annual prize in his name is awarded to the resident who presents the best paper at the annual meeting of the Canadian Society of Plastic Surgeons.

These were the busy years of reconstructive surgery at McGill, with new advances in maxillofacial surgery, in burn treatment, and in local and pedicle flap development. It was common to see many veterans who were undergoing reconstructive surgery at the QMVH with tubed pedicles on various parts of their body during these staged procedures. This rich and rapid development of the specialty stimulated other surgeons to further their training in plastic surgery and to join the staff at McGill, among these were John Drummond, Martin Entin, and Albert M. Cloutier.

John A. Drummond graduated in dentistry from the University of Toronto in 1934 and practised in Sarnia until 1939. When the Second World War broke out, Drummond entered medical school at McGill and graduated in 1943. He served in the navy during the war and joined the staff at the RVH in plastic surgery 1951 and became chief of the subdepartment in 1966. Drummond was a kind and thoughtful surgeon with great consideration for others. He was president of the American Society of Maxillofacial Surgeons and the Quebec Society of Plastic Surgeons. He died in 1970 at the age of fifty-nine after a prolonged battle with heart disease.

Martin Entin graduated from McGill Medical School in 1945 after receiving his BA from Temple University and an MSc from McGill. His postgraduate training in hand surgery (in which he has maintained a life-long interest) was under the tutelage of Sterling Bunnell in San Francisco. After training, he joined the attending staff at the RVH and obtained a consultant's position at the Shriners Hospital.

Entin became the surgeon-in-charge of plastic surgery at the RVH, and his major interest in basic research was devoted to thermal injuries, wringer injuries, and hand surgery. He is a major contributor to the specialized area of congenital anomalies of the upper extremity and has produced many publications in this field, including a landmark paper entitled "The Classification of Congenital Hand Anomalies." He is a past president of the American Society for Surgery of the Hand and continues to be a major influence at the McGill Plastic Surgery Inter-Hospital Rounds and in other aspects of surgical teaching. He received the Distinguished Service Award in November 1994 from the RVH and is the president of the Canadian Authors Association.

Albert M. Cloutier was born in Quebec City and graduated from McGill in 1951. He completed his general surgical residency at the MGH, and then his plastic surgery residency was divided between the MGH and the MCH, and with one year's training at the University of Toronto with Farmer, Gordon, and Robertson. Prior to medical school, Cloutier served as an officer in the Canadian Armoured Corps and had numerous exploits in the frontline battles. He was awarded a McLaughlin Travelling Fellowship, visited centres in England in 1957, and returned to the MCH and the Reddy Memorial Hospital. Cloutier.had always been rich in new and innovative techniques, and he developed his personal operation for repair of hypospadias and for the correction of prominent ears. His contributions to the McGill Inter-Hospital Rounds continue to be legendary.

Frederick V. Nicolle joined the attending staff of the MGH and MCH in 1962. He was a graduate of Cambridge University in 1956, and he completed his plastic surgery residency within the McGill hospitals. His early career involved research into silicone tendon rods and implants for small joint arthrodeses. He and Professor Calnan of England developed a silicone and stainless-steel joint implant for treatment of rheumatoid arthritic deformities in the hand. Within a few years, Nicolle returned to London, England, and he is currently practising in that city.

Cooperative Program at McGill, 1976–

I became director of the Division of Plastic Surgery at McGill in 1976, when I succeeded Frederick M. Woolhouse. At that time, the McGill University training program became a single, completely integrated program with equal rotations through the MGH, the RVH, and the MCH. At present, the teaching faculty in plastic surgery has ten members, including both full-time and

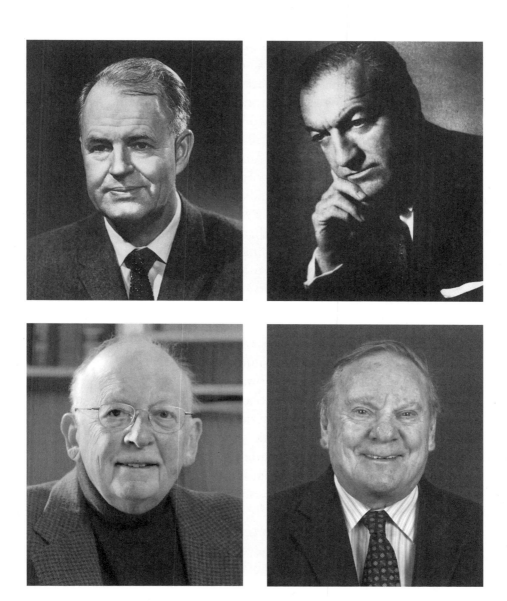

Clockwise from top left
Fig. 22.1 John W. Gerrie, MGH Plastic Surgery, 1936–46
Fig. 22.2 Frederick M. Woolhouse, director, Division of Plastic Surgery, 1946–76
Fig. 22.3 Bruce Williams, director, McGill Integrated Plastic Surgery, 1976–96
Fig. 22.4 Harvey Brown, director, McGill Integrated Plastic Surgery, 1996–2001

part-time teachers. In addition, a number of plastic surgeons from other hospitals within the Montreal area and from neighbouring communities participate actively in the weekly inter-hospital rounds and seminars. The reading lists and tutorials on plastic surgery topics continues to be an important component of the residency program, and the excellent results obtained in the Quebec examinations, in the Royal College of Physicians and Surgeons examinations, and in the American Board of Plastic Surgery examinations likely represents the importance of these teaching components.

I graduated from Acadia University with my BA and from the McGill Faculty of Medicine in 1955. My general surgery and plastic surgery residencies were completed at McGill, along with a one-year residency in pathology in Charlotte, North Carolina. I was awarded a McLaughlin Travelling Fellowship in 1962 and undertook postgraduate studies in England, Sweden, and Russia during this year. I have several major interests, which include basic laboratory research, paediatric plastic surgery, microsurgery, and hand surgery.

I have been a visiting professor to most of the Canadian universities and to over sixty programs in other countries, including the United States, Japan, Brazil, Germany, Mexico, Bermuda, Greece, and Egypt. I have been chair of the Royal College Committee on Plastic Surgery and was the Royal College Lecturer in 1993. I have been the president of a number of medical and surgical societies, which include the Quebec Society of Plastic and Reconstructive Surgeons, the Canadian Society of Plastic Surgeons, the Plastic Surgery Educational Foundation, the American Society of Plastic and Reconstructive Surgeons, the American Society of Reconstructive Microsurgeons, the American Society of Peripheral Nerve, and the International Microsurgical Society and am a past vice-chair of the American Board of Plastic Surgery. I have received the Distinguished Service Award from Acadia University and from the American Society of Plastic and Reconstructive Surgeons as well as the Clinician of the Year Award from the American Association of Plastic Surgeons. I have also received the Lifetime Achievement Award and the ASPS/PSEF Appreciation Award for over twenty-five years of service. In 2006, I received an award from the Canadian Society of Plastic Surgeons, the Medical Award of Excellence from the MCH, and an honorary award from the American Association of Plastic Surgeons, which is the highest honour in the specialty. I am currently the surgeon-in-chief at the MCH.

Plastic Surgery Staff, 1970, MUHC

Harvey C. Brown joined the staff in 1970, and he has contributed greatly to the specialty. His major interest in trauma was recognized recently when he became a member of the Trauma Committee of the American College of Surgeons, and his past offices include presidency of the Canadian Society of Plastic Surgeons. Brown's early participation in basic research in burns and his interest in the research components of the specialty has continued, and he has added Annie Phillip as research director in plastic surgery at the MGH. He has also contributed in the field of hand surgery, particularly in the reconstruction of rheumatoid hand deformities and in rehabilitative surgery for patients with pressure sores related to paraplegia and quadriplegia. His interest in meshed skin grafts for wound closure is another area of interest. Brown was chairman of the McGill plastic surgery program from 1996 to 2001.

Rene J. Crepeau graduated from the University of Sherbrooke and continued in his general surgical residency at that university. He then completed his plastic surgery residency at McGill and spent a one-year fellowship under Paul Tessier in Paris in order to learn the newer techniques in craniofacial surgery. Crepeau then joined the staff at the MCH and the MGH in 1976. He continues to have a major interest in the reconstruction of complex craniomaxillofacial problems and in rehabilitative surgery for cleft lip and cleft palate patients. Recent advances in internal fixation procedures for maxillofacial fractures is also an interest of Crepeau's, and he has a major influence on the teaching of these techniques.

Gaston Schwarz received his high school education in Lima, Peru, and his BA from Syracuse University. He is a graduate in medicine from the University of Ottawa. His general surgery and plastic surgery residencies were completed at McGill, and he then had a fellowship with Ralph Millard at the University of Miami. Schwarz is the past president of the D. Ralph Millard Plastic Surgical Society and the Quebec Board of Specialty Examinations in Plastic Surgery. He is also the past president of the Canadian Society for Aesthetic [Cosmetic] Plastic Surgery. He has been.a visiting professor at the University of San Simon in La Paz, Bolivia, and at the Faculty of Medicine in Lima, Peru. Schwarz joined the faculty in 1972 and he has been an outstanding supporter and contributor to the division. His major interest has been in the development of newer techniques in aesthetic surgery, and he has become widely recognized for his expertise in this field. He is also largely responsible for the development of the *McGill Plastic Surgery Newsletter*.

Carolyn Kerrigan received her BSc and her MD, CM in 1977 from McGill. She was also awarded an MSc in experimental surgery in 1981. Following a Hand Fellowship at the New York University Medical Center, she joined the Plastic Surgery Division in 1984 with a full-time geographic appointment at the RVH. She has presented many papers at meetings across Canada and the United States and succeeded. Rollin K. Daniel as chief of plastic surgery at the RVH in 1987. Kerrigan is exemplary in combining a busy clinical load with a major emphasis on basic laboratory research, along with her ingenious ability to raise five boys in her expanding household. Much of her laboratory investigations are considered a gold standard and the excellent support that she has had from the Medical Research Council and other granting agencies confirms this observation. She was the president of the Canadian Society of Plastic Surgeons, and she is a past associate editor of the *Journal of Plastic and Reconstructive Surgery*. Kerrigan is now the chairman of plastic surgery at Dartmouth University in Hanover, New Hampshire, and she is a major influence on the American Board of Plastic Surgery, the American Society of Plastic Surgeons, and its educational foundation.

Roland Charbonneau joined the staff at the RVH in 1980. He is a 1972 graduate from the University of Montreal in medicine, and he completed his general surgery and plastic surgery residencies at the University of Montreal. Charbonneau was one of the early trainees in microsurgical procedures and he has continued to contribute in this area. His unique appointment at both McGill and the University of Montreal has been a step towards Anglo/French collaboration and added stature to the division. And his activities within the Federation of Medical Specialists, the Regie de L'Assurance Maladie du Québec, and the Association of Plastic Surgeons of Quebec (as its former president) have brought further recognition to the division.

Lucie Lessard joined the staff in 1987. She also completed her training in otolaryngology at McGill, obtained her FRCS(C) in that specialty, and completed a two-year residency in plastic surgery at the Peter Bent Briqharn and Children's Unit in Boston. She has brought back an expertise in craniomaxillofacial abnormalities and in reconstructive surgery of the face and skull. She has a major interest in basic research and continues her investigation of steroid effects in wound healing and leech therapy.

Jeffrey Khoury joined the RVH as an associate in 1992 and has contributed to teaching residents in microvascular techniques and in trauma. Khoury is a graduate of McGill with a BSc in physiology and with an MD from Queen's University as the winner of the Gold Medal in Surgery. He completed general surgery and plastic surgery training at McGill. He participated as a fellow in experimental surgery and obtained his MSc in experimental surgery with some excellent work on the vascularization of free bone grafts using microsurgical techniques. Following his residency, he took further training in microsurgery at the University of Kentucky. Unfortunately, He retired from active practice due to a severe illness.

Daniel Benatar is an MD from the University of Sherbrooke, and he obtained an MSc in experimental surgery in 1978. He completed the McGill Plastic Surgery Program in 1979, and he also had a productive fellowship year in the basic research laboratory with a study of free transplantation of skeletal muscle and further work in bone transplants. His McGill activities were focused at the Jewish General Hospital, but he continued to participate at Inter-Hospital Rounds and with advice on research activities. Benatar unfortunately received a serious hand injury and has not returned to clinical practice. He is living in France.

Ronald G. Zelt joined the staff at the MGH in 1992. Zelt is also a graduate of the McGill program, and he spent an additional year in a fellowship with Ian Taylor at the Royal Melbourne Hospital in Australia. His main interest is in surgical education following one year at the University of Southern California, where he obtained his MEd. Zelt has contributed to curriculum development and in assessment techniques in the Department of Surgery and he has a major interest in both undergraduate and graduate learning experiences. He has added a major contribution to the microsurgical reconstruction of extensive defects following trauma and tumour excision. The rapid increase in microsurgical free fiap procedures were clearly evident since his return to the university.

Teanoosh Zadeh returned to McGill in 1997. He received his FRCS(C) in both general and plastic surgery in 1993 and 1994, respectively. After his residency, he completed a fellowship in hand surgery at the University of Milwaukee and a further six months in tissue engineering at Harvard University. Zadeh's main interests are in hand surgery, microsurgery, and free flap tissue transfers. His inter-specialty collaborative efforts in reconstruction of soft tissue and bony defects with orthopaedics has led to a great advance in the care of malignancies and traumatic defects.

Daniel Durand, who is also a graduate of the McGill program, joined the staff of the MCH with a specific focus on the development of a brachial plexus clinic. He had extensive training in brachial plexus reconstruction during a fellowship year at the University of Southern California, he returned to the MCH with his expertise. A multidisciplinary clinic under Zadeh and Durand's direction, which includes neurologists, neurosurgeons, physiotherapists, occupational therapists, and imaging services, has recently been established and will continue to expand and improve treatment modalities in this difficult area of management.

Chen Lee returned to McGill as chair of plastic surgery in 2002. He is a graduate of the McGill Plastic Surgery Program and took further training in paediatric surgery at the University of Toronto. He was a member of the teaching faculty of the University of California, San Francisco, until his return to McGill. His major interests include craniomaxillofacial procedures and cleft lip and palate problems. His major contributions continue in bony fixation procedures of the face and extremities, particularly those following trauma. Lee is now in private practice in Montreal, and he continues with a large practice at Hôpital Sacre Coeur.

Annie Phillip is the director of plastic surgery research and co-director of surgical research at the MUHC. Her laboratory has become the centre of basic experiments, with several MSc and PhD students working towards their degrees. Her main focus is the influence of TGF beta factor in wound healing and in other aspects of basic research.

External Support for Research and Education

Members of the Plastic Surgery Division at McGill have been very successful in obtaining research grant support for many important laboratory investigations. This support has come from the Medical Research Council, the Educational Foundation, the Cedars Fund, industrial organizations, and from the Quebec Hydro Corporation.

Despite this past success, and related to increasing difficulties in obtaining grant support, we were pleased with the recent establishment of the Neville G. Poy Endowment Fund in Plastic Surgery for the support of research and education. The inauguration was held in the Osler Library at McGill, with all members of Vivienne and Neville Poy's family in attendance. Poy, a popular medical graduate from McGill in 1960, trained in plastic surgery and experimental surgery at McGill, working on skin flap survival. It should be noted that Neville and Vivienne Poy have contributed to many charitable and academic causes in Canada, and we salute them for their philanthropic grace.

Summary

The Plastic Surgery Division at McGill, with its three component parts at the MGH, the RVH, and the MCH, remains strong, having a dynamic influence on the specialty in Canada as well as in other countries. The teaching of plastic surgery, both at the undergraduate and graduate levels, also continues to be strengthened, and the quality of' our graduating residents is a clear indication of success.

SECTION 4

Other Departments

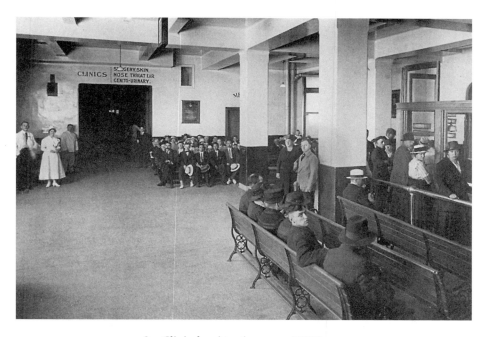

S.4 Clinical registration room MGH 1920

23

Anaesthesiology

John H. Burgess, Richard Robinson, and Ian Metcalf

Ian Metcalf was chief of anaesthesiology at the MGH and Richard Robinson is a staff anaesthesiologist. John Burgess rewrote their manuscripts for this chapter.

The Beginning of Anaesthesia at the Montreal General Hospital

The founding of the Montreal General Hospital in 1821 preceded the advent of surgical anaesthesia by some twenty-five years. The first use of ether anaesthesia was by Crawford W. Long in Jefferson, Georgia, on 10 March 1842. Unfortunately, he did not publish this event until 1849, after he had heard of Morton's claim and following press accounts of the first use of ether in the "ether dome" at the Massachusetts General Hospital in 1846.[1] Within the space of a year surgical anaesthesia with ether had been administered to hundreds of patients in North America, Europe, and elsewhere. Both ether and chloroform were volatile liquids and were vaporized by cautiously allowing drops of it to soak into a multilayered cotton gauze mask that covered the mouth and nose of the spontaneously breathing patient. These "open" methods of inhalation anaesthesia persisted for the next forty to fifty years before machines were finally devised to deliver predictable and adjustable concentrations of the anaesthetic vapour.

Worldwide enthusiasm for surgical anaesthesia was tempered by experience. There were many problems. Risk of upper airway obstruction, vomiting, regurgitation of gastric content, and pulmonary aspiration were ever present. Fatal overdose, particularly with chloroform, was soon reported. The need for sterile instruments and operative field were not understood, and patients died of sepsis after technically satisfactory surgery and administration of anaesthesia. The cumulative risks of anaesthesia and surgery became such that operations were performed in as little time as possible and often undertaken as a last resort. This situation was slow to improve, but by the 1880s ascetic surgery was being widely practised and administrators of surgical anaesthesia were being better trained and becoming more experienced in anticipating and surmounting problems.

The Early Anaesthesiologists

The first anaesthetic was given in Montreal by a Dr Nelson at the Hotel Dieu Hospital. The house surgeons would live in at the hospital for six years. It was their duty to assist the staff surgeons and give the anaesthetic, although they had no specific training in anaesthesia.[2] In 1892, H.P. Carmichael, one of the house surgeons, spent a year training in anaesthesia and was appointed to this service as a full-time job. From then on one house surgeon annually gave all the anaesthetics.[3] By 1913, W.B. Howell was providing all the anaesthetics, but, as he started to develop the first department of anaesthesia, his career was interrupted by the First World War. W.G. Hepburn then became the anaesthetist at the MGH until 1926, when he was succeeded by C.C. Stewart, who developed the first Department of Anaesthesia at the MGH.

Sir William Osler had considered becoming an anaesthetist but then decided on a career in general medicine. The pioneer in anaesthesiology at the MGH was Wesley Bourne, who came from the West Indies in 1907 to study medicine at McGill. After graduation he began surgical training, but he abandoned it in favour of anaesthesia. Bourne joined the Department of Pharmacology at McGill for its laboratory facilities, which enabled him to carry out his experimental work. He became one of the first to apply basic pharmacological and physiological principles to the practice of anaesthesiology. He put anaesthesia on a scientific basis and became world famous for so doing.

Although he was never at the MGH, the other leading McGill anaesthetist at this time was Harold Griffiths, who introduced curare and other muscle relaxants to the practice of anaesthesiology. Both Bourne and Griffiths were world renowned for their contributions but initially received little recognition for them at McGill.

Introduction of Local Anaesthetic Agents

In 1884, cocaine was first used as a local analgesic but was shown to be toxic and highly addictive. It was largely replaced by the synthetic drug procaine in 1904. Soon field blocks, blocks of specific nerves or nerve plexuses, spinal blocks, and epidural blocks were becoming widely practised as relatively safe alternatives to general anaesthesia.

Improvements in Airway Management

Topical anaesthesia of the upper airway made direct laryngoscopy and instrumentation of the upper airway possible. The first use of endotracheal anaesthesia was reported by Sir William MacEwen in London, England, in 1880.[4] In 1911, George Armstrong performed the first endotracheal intubation at the MGH under direct vision.[5] This technique allowed the anaesthetist to better control the upper airway and, later, to assist and control ventilation by intermittent positive pressure.

The Modern Era

The great reductions in surgical infections with aseptic techniques and the advances in anaesthetic agents and muscle relaxants were increasing the MGH anaesthesiology service load even before the Second World War.

Bob Ferguson had joined the department in 1935.[6] He was initially assigned to the Private Patients Pavilion at the Montreal General Hospital (the Western Division of the MGH) on Tupper Street as a resident working for twenty-five dollars per month. He was married in 1939 and joined the army in 1940.

J.J. Kelly remained at the Western Division during the war as there was a severe shortage of trained anaesthesiologists for the service load. This left little time for the continuation of academic work and research that had been begun by Wesley Bourne. Ferguson returned to the MGH in 1946 and shortly thereafter became head of the department. He was soon joined by Bert Robillard and others. With the move to the new MGH site on Cedar Avenue, the provincial medicare system and Blue Cross put the practice of anaesthesia on a more firm financial basis. There was still little university support for academic work.

One of Ferguson's early clinical recollections was the performance of a spinal anaesthetic on a wealthy woman, enabling her to pass a large amount of flatus. More important anaesthetic procedures followed. Obstetrics moved to the Cedar Avenue site, where Asquith introduced patient-administered trilene inhalations during labour and also pudendal blocks. Robillard recalls his first epidural, for which the point was filed off a spinal needle to reduce the potential trauma of insertion.

Robillard visited the Central Division to witness Ferguson deliver the anaesthetic for Harry Scott's first mitral comissurotomy (a closed heart procedure to alleviate a narrowed mitral valve). Until that time the patient's ventilation was managed by hand, but soon machine-assisted ventilation through endotracheal tubes became available. Robillard was frequently the only anaesthesiology resident on call at night. This increased responsibility resulted in his salary being increased to one hundred dollars per month. In the late 1950s, an organized teaching program under Bourne became available, and the resident teaching was more scientifically based.

The New MGH on Cedar Avenue

The new site offered greatly expanded facilities for the Department of Anaesthesiology. The chief, Ferguson, now had his own office, but the ever increasing staff members did not. There was a large workroom and secretary's office, indicating that the staff anaesthetists were not simply at the surgeons' disposal. A private billing group – Ferguson, Kelly, and Associates – was formed, and Larking, Sutherland, and Neilson were added. Later, Boright, Matzko, and Dunkley arrived.

Invasive postoperative monitoring became available for critically ill and postoperative cardiac cases. John Burgess of the Division of Cardiology provided indwelling arterial lines and pulmonary artery catheters. Hypothermia was added for neurology and neurosurgical patients.

Anaesthesiology developed subspecialty interests, with Robillard initially taking over the operative and postoperative care of the open heart cases. He also attended the cardiology and cardiac surgical conferences. Team work in patient care had arrived.

Intensive Care

The increasing volume of cardiac surgery, and the MGH's being named a high-level trauma centre, soon overwhelmed the resources of the recovery room. An intensive care unit was required. The first ICU at the MGH opened under the cardiac surgeon Harry Scott and was initially under the control of surgery; however, by the later 1970s, anaesthesiology became regularly involved. New recruits to anaestheiology, Richard Robinson and Peter Slinger, took a special interest in closed chest trauma. They were the first to use continuous thoracic epidural anaesthesia for flail chests. Robinson took over the postoperative care of the cardiac surgical cases. Andrew Scott and Michael English developed research programs in heat exchange. Holland, Michel Germain and Donald Hickey collaborated with Ronald Melzack of the McGill Department of Psychology in the study of pain.

Chiefs of Anaesthesiology at the MGH

Bob Ferguson became head of anaesthesdiology in 1956, when the MGH moved to its new site on Cedar Avenue. He formed a professional and business partnership of trained anaesthesiologists known as Ferguson, Kelly, and Associates, which came to include Larking, Sutherland, Neilson, Robillard, Boright, Dunkley, and Matzko. This team, which had a heavy service load, was to experience even more service problems when, in the late 1960s, political uncertainty about the future of Quebec, the introduction of universal medicare in the province, and (later) restrictive language policies made it difficult to recruit new staff, while, at the same time, staff members were relocating to other provinces and to the United States. Moreover, graduating residents were electing to work elsewhere.

Ferguson retired in 1970 and was replaced by Tom McCaughey from the University of Manitoba. McCaughey vigorously promoted the concept of employing graduate inhalation therapists as assistants to the anaesthesiology staff. Revolutionary at the time, this concept has become an established feature of contemporary Canadian anaesthesia services. A vigorous recruiting program for clinical and research fellows helped to alleviate staff shortages at this time. Metcalf and Holland, Australian-trained anaesthesiologists, were recruited, followed by Scott and English, both of whom had expertise in research methodology and helped to inspire young trainees to stay on after graduation. Robinson, Slinger, Germain, Hickey, and Gordon were included in this group, all contributing to the academic growth of the department. Robinson and Slinger went on to do innovative work in the field of cardiothoracic anaesthesia. Metcalf became chief of the department in the late 1970s and remained the MGH chief when Franco Carli became the combined MUHC chair.

NOTES

1 C.W. Long, "An Account of the First Use of Sulphuric Ether by Inhalation," *Southern Medical Journal* 5 (1849): 705–13. Although Long first used ether, technically, the credit for publicizing it should go to Morton, who arranged to have it used by John Collins Warren, the great Harvard surgeon, at the leading hospital in the country in front of a large audience.

2 J. Hanaway and R. Cruess, *McGill Medicine: The First Half Century, 1829–1885* (Montreal and Kingston: McGill-Queen's University Press, 1996), 59.

3 H.T. Davenport, ed., *Anaestheia at McGill* (Montreal: privately published by the author, 1966), iii.

4 W. MacEwen, "Clinical Observations on the Introduction of Tracheal Tubes by Mouth Instead of Performing Tracheotomy," *British Medical Journal* 2 (1880): 122–4, 163–5.

5 J. Hanaway, R. Cruess, and J. Darragh, *McGill Medicine, 1885–1936* (Montreal and Kingston: McGill-Queen's University Press, 2006), 161.

6 Davenport, *Anaesthesia at McGill*, 74.

24

The Auxiliary

Lois Hutchison

Lois Hutchison is a past president of the MGH Auxiliary and was involved in its well-known early bird Christmas sales for many years.

Introduction

A truly remarkable story is that of the foundation of the Montreal General Hospital Auxiliary at the Dorchester Street Building and, thanks to enlightened leadership, its continuation on Cedar Avenue and its extraordinary contributions to the functioning of the hospital. The auxiliary, through its varied endeavours – snack bar, hospitality shop, gift shop, library and library wagon, sales events, equipment gifts, fellowship funds, the early bird events, thousands of hours doing things around the hospital, planning for the MUHC challenge, and more – represents a shining example of the MGH mission "to care for the sick" in all ways.

The Women's Auxiliary of the MGH was formally established in 1949. However, as far back as the nineteenth century, volunteers from the Ladies' Benevolent Society were present to help care for the hospital's earliest patients. Today, the work of the auxiliary is impressive. It includes an enormous number of projects and hundreds of thousands of dollars in fundraising, which touch the care of the patients, those who care for them, and many community organizations.

Early Days of the Auxiliary

The true founders of the auxiliary were members of the Tuesday Club. The following is from an address by Barbara Whitley on the occasion of the twentieth anniversary of the auxiliary, in which she paid tribute to the club.

They were 12 friends who met every second Tuesday, to work for the Hospital. They sent bonnets, sweaters, nightgowns, shirts, socks, bloomers and mittens to the children's ward. In addition, they sent Christmas boxes and money to help provide gifts and decorations. Fines of 25 cents were levied on members for non-attendance.

The Club carried on until one day in 1948, when Mrs. Alexander Hutchison went down to the Hospital with the Club's contributions. At that time there was a flu epidemic and the nurses were as busy as can be. There was Miss MacDonald, a white-faced, over-burdened nurse, staring blankly at bags of unwrapped Christmas gifts for patients, sent in by kind friends. It was during this visit that someone, probably Miss Matheson, the Director of Nursing, said, 'If only we had someone to help.' Mrs. Hutchison got the message.

Also from minutes of the Tuesday Club: "There appear to be members who have a fear of having to produce the large sum of 25 cents – and, in order to avoid being fined arrive at the meeting at 4.30 – just in time to take part in the delicious tea."

Helen Hutchison, one of the dynamic members of the club (and whose father, Alexander McCall, was treasurer of the hospital), recognized the need for a formal structure for volunteers. After the Second World War, she had observed that a great number of American women were becoming involved in a blossoming of women's auxiliaries in hospitals. Hutchison's first step was to obtain the approval of the administration of the hospital. In October, along with Mrs Fleming, a meeting was arranged with S.C. Norsworthy, president of the hospital, and B.S. Johnston, the hospital's general superintendent. These gentlemen had no idea why they were meeting with these two formidable women, but they soon realized that the request was to form a women's auxiliary. It was stressed to our founders that the auxiliary was to promote efforts that would contribute, in part, to their own support and that money-raising schemes were to be avoided. The organization of a shop, tea room, and library for the patients was also discussed. Of course, the plan to form the MGH Auxiliary was approved.

At that time, the Joint Hospital Campaign was busy with its goal of a new hospital building. Needless to say, the women of the auxiliary were to play an important role in this campaign. As plans for a new building proceeded, the administrators could foresee the need for influential women to help raise money. In the blink of an eye, I became chair of the Women's Special Names

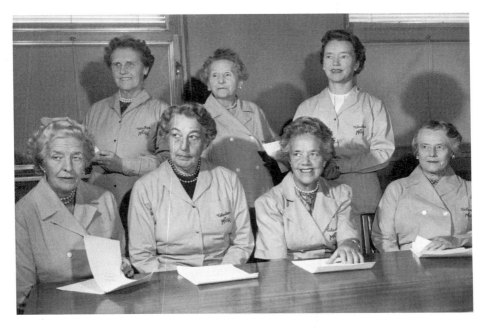

Fig. 24.1 The First Board of the Auxiliary, 1949

Committee and Mrs Fleming was to be responsible for the general canvass-ing of women. The first contribution that Helen obtained was for $25,000. This, remember, was the same Tuesday Club that had objected to those twenty-five-cent fines.

Tremendous community support for the hospital was established during these fledgling years. As Barbara Whitley later reflected: "I always felt that one of the great things that the Auxiliary did was to involve the community. It was sort of a reflection of the early Hospital governors who would go from door to door around the city, collecting money."

In 1949, the Women's Auxiliary was established to:

Promote the Welfare of the Hospital and its patients through:
-Voluntary service within the Hospital
-Fundraising
-Fostering good public relations between the Hospital and the community.

The charter members and past presidents are listed below.

The Auxiliary in the 1950s and After

By 1950, a gift shop and a snack bar organized by volunteers had been opened at the Western Division of the MGH. The first annual report stated that these projects were to provide a service to patients, visitors, and hospital staff. In addition, a travel-wagon brought selections from the shop to the patients' bedside. At the Central Division, volunteers had taken responsibility for the patients' library and instituted a travel-book-wagon, which distributed books and magazines to the patients. With over seventeen hundred auxiliary members in the first year, volunteers undertook the operation of a driving service for patients coming for their clinic appointments.

In the early years, the auxiliary would give a layette to each intern's wife. Members would knit the clothing and then add to the layette until it was complete. The first time the gift was made to one young woman, it was so appreciated that it became a regular project. It should be remembered that, in those days, the interns were not paid.

Shortly after the move to Cedar Avenue in 1955, the auxiliary was asked to assist in two important projects. Doctor Gordon Copping, a great supporter of the auxiliary, asked it to help host a review course for doctors. The MGH wanted doctors without admitting privileges kept up to date on activities at McGill and in the hospital, both medically and technically. The auxiliary sent out the invitations, set up a telephone committee, provided refreshments, and looked after many details. On another occasion, the auxiliary was asked to track patients, who, following their cancer treatment, did not return as directed. This was the type of spot work that volunteers enjoyed. It was clear that the work and capabilities of these women was highly regarded.

In the late 1950s, as the number of volunteers grew substantially, it became clear that there was a need for a professional coordinator. Through meetings with American contacts, Helen had learned a great deal about acquiring and administering volunteers. After an intense search, the hospital's very first director of volunteer services was hired and financially supported by the auxiliary. The director, Flora Baptist, was sent to observe a well established volunteer department in a New York City hospital. Together, Baptist and Helen Hutchison set high standards for MGH volunteers and worked to ensure that these standards were met. Although the MGH Auxiliary was not the first to be established, it was always a leader in establishing new and exciting activities that were emulated by others.

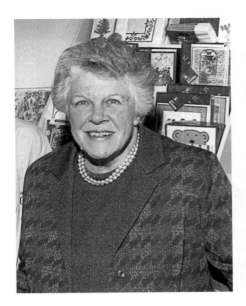
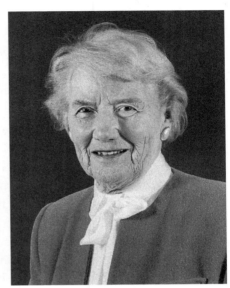

Fig. 24.2 Barbara J. Whitely, president, 1957–60
Fig. 24.3 Lois Hutchison, president, 1993–95

Helen Hutchison was always looking for new ways to develop community interest in the hospital. She established branches of the auxiliary in different areas of the city and, thereby, broadened interest and hospital support. By 1957, there were seven active branches – Chambly, Hampstead, Lake of Two Mountains, Montreal West, Outremont, TMR, and Westmount. Each branch had its own executive and held its own meetings in its community. Speakers from the MGH were invited to meetings to inform members about new developments and plans. Branches raised money by holding community bridges, raffles, house tours, and garden parties. In the Cedar Avenue Building, each branch operated the new hospital shop for a day a week. When members could not volunteer at the hospital, they took part in the activities closer to home. As outlying communities developed, other hospital auxiliaries were formed and our own changed. For instance, as the Lake of Two Mountains area was geographically closer to the newly built Lakeshore General it seemed natural for it to realign itself. This was a sad loss as its chair was the daughter of MGH's F.J. Shepherd.

When the Red Cross suddenly called the director of volunteers for duty in Korea, it was an auxiliary member, Thelma Graham, who temporarily replaced her. It is interesting to note that Graham had originally been recruited by one of the doctors to help in his department. She later became an auxiliary member, then interim director, then auxiliary board member, and, in 1960, president of the Auxiliary. In 1978, under the presidency of Maggie Torrey, the word "Women" in "Women's Auxiliary" was dropped. It was hoped that a flood of men wishing to volunteer would apply. Unfortunately, this did not happen.

As the auxiliary was established to represent the community in the MGH it seemed to follow that a doctor's spouse should not be president. However, it became clear that some of the MGH's most outstanding volunteers were doctors' wives and this rule was abandoned when Marni Blundell, wife of Peter Blundell, became president in 1982.

The auxiliary's work rapidly gained recognition. The first shop, which was only a cupboard, was meant, first, to be a service for patients and staff and, second, a means of raising money. Mrs Frank McGill, a well-loved, hard-working volunteer established the shop and became its first chair. With a thriving business, the little cupboard was soon left behind for more spacious quarters. Since its inception, the MGH Auxiliary has sought to better the lives of patients through volunteer service and raising funds for the purchase of equipment.

The Auxiliary and the MUHC

With the inauguration of the McGill University Health Centre, bringing together five hospitals, including the MGH, it was necessary to standardize the equipment in each hospital and to introduce a central system to oversee and to assess overall equipment needs in order to maximize the use of limited resources.

In 1999, the Equipment Planning Committee was formed under the chairship of Paul Legault, with representatives from the five hospitals, including from the Auxiliary, which the MGH recognized as having played an important role in funding the acquisition of equipment. The committee's initial mandate was the huge task of bringing up to date the individual equipment inventories of the five hospitals and putting them together in a common database. Later, subcommittees were set up to channel requests for equipment. A point system was developed to prioritize needs, whether it be replacing existing equipment, adopting new technology, or recruiting staff.

The auxiliary was now able to purchase equipment specifically needed by the MGH, its primary concern, choosing from a list of the most urgent needs

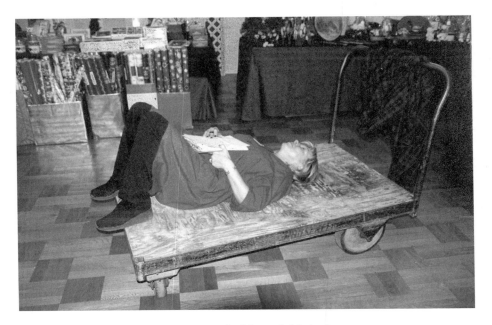

Fig. 24.4 End of the early bird sale

within its price range and, thus, doing the most good with its contribution. Between the years 2000 and 2006, the auxiliary donated equipment to the MGH in the amount of $1.7 million. This amount does not include the cost of renovating the nineteenth-floor surgical west wing, the creation of a family room on the twelfth floor, and the construction of an additional medication room for the fifteenth floor, all of which were funded by the auxiliary. The range of items donated goes from large equipment, such as an ultrasound, a cardiac catheter laboratory physiological monitoring system, an orthopaedic operating table, EKG machines and defibrillators, to items that improve the quality of patient care on a daily basis, such as mattresses, patient controlled anagesia (PCA) infusion pumps, wheelchairs, and patient furniture. Today's Hospitality Corner is the keystone and centrepiece of the organization. It has a paid staff of six and requires the service of over 125 volunteers per week. In the year 2000 a gourmet coffee shop was opened in the Cedar Avenue lobby, and, since then, the Livingston Hall kitchen has been renovated to handle the ever-growing catering service. Plans are under way to open another coffee shop in the ER area. From 1981 to 2006, $497,035 in "tip money" was raised in the snack bar. This money was donated to the Research Institute.

Early bird was the creation of Jean Grout and Dot Martin. Each year, these two volunteers would travel to New York to buy new and unusual gifts at wholesale prices for the Hospitality Corner. On one such trip, as they relaxed back at their hotel, it occurred to them that they needed a special venue to show all these wonderful purchases. Livingston Hall was thought to be the ideal area to display everything. At that time, it was meant to be a show as opposed to a sale. From this came an extremely successful early bird sale that attracts patients, staff ,and the community. Every year, the number of volunteers participating has increased and the funds generated have multiplied. The number of tables varies, along with the products. However, the home baking, frozen foods, and antiques remain at the top of everyone's list. A preview evening, which is open to the community, has been an exciting addition to the sale. It has become a reunion for many who are unable to regularly participate in auxiliary activities.

In the late 1990s, discussions took place with regard to changes in the traditional early bird, which would generate more funds for the hospital. The decision was taken to design a new event, which would focus on a particular piece of equipment and/or department and, in addition, to take the fundraiser out into the community. The 1st Noel initiative continued for two years in Ogilvy's Tudor Hall. Much needed funds were raised, new volunteers were attracted, and the community was sensitized to the work of the MGH Level 1 Trauma Centre. The auxiliary had succeeded in its goal of achieving more visibility and a broader community of support.

One of the very first projects that the auxiliary undertook was one that would become an all-time favourite assignment. Members arranged special Christmas trays with seasonal foods and small gifts for hospitalized patients. This practice continues with the delivery of "Santa bags" to the in-patients.

The Memorial Fund was the creation of the MGH Auxiliary, and it was an important first among auxiliaries. When Colonel Andrew Fleming died, a large sum of money was sent to the auxiliary. This became the foundation of the Memorial Fund. Shortly after, Mr E.A. Whitley died and money was donated to the hospital through this fund. Donations were so well administered that Mr A.H. Westbury, executive director, asked the auxiliary to take over all the memorial donations that were made to the Hospital. Mrs Lank, the first chair of the Memorial Fund, ordered attractive printed thank you cards, which were promptly sent to donors. The Memorial Book, a beautiful ledger donated by Lank in memory of her parents listed the names of all the deceased. The auxiliary was very strict about how this money would be used. Funds were to be for life-sustaining projects and were to be given in memory

of the deceased. In addition, the MGH nursery received a great deal of attention. The isolettes, for example, were a donation from the Memorial Fund.

In 1967, auxiliary president Mary Fowler received a request from the
Bonaventure Hotel asking if the auxiliary would sponsor its opening. The
first night had been promised to the United Nations because it was United
Nations Day at Expo '67. The auxiliary would have the second night. Coin-
cidentally, there was to be a dinner dance for the medical staff during the
same period. The auxiliary convinced the doctors that they should all work
together. The evening was extremely successful and so popular, in fact, that
it was the beginning of the Annual Dinner Dance. The committee ensured
that the orchestra included music that was enjoyed by all generations

Barbara Whitley remembers the turmoil caused by the fact that the
province wished the auxiliary money to now go to general hospital funds.
Thankfully, William Storrar went to Quebec and argued that money from
the shop and other auxiliary undertakings must be left in the hands of the
women. He said: "It's a drop in the bucket; for heaven's sake, let the ladies
have their fun." Whitley summed up the event by saying, "And they did,
and it certainly wasn't a drop in the bucket." Over the past twenty-three
years, the auxiliary has given over $1 million to provide nineteen research
fellowship grants to promising young researchers working at the MGH
Research Institute.

It was important that volunteers to be easily identified by patients and
staff. As the MGH colours are scarlet and silver, it was decided that grey,
the closest to silver available, would be the colour of the first volunteer
smock. After a few years, many volunteers wanted a cheerier colour and so
red was chosen.

The relationship between the Canadian Red Cross and the MGH Auxiliary dates back to 1960. Twice a year, under an Auxiliary chair, a blood donor
clinic was organized. Dozens of volunteers would bake goodies, serve coffee
and juice, hold hands with nervous donors, guide others to the waiting Red
Cross nurses and, in general, make the clinic a pleasant visit. As the clinics
evolved, a drawing of wonderful gifts, such as autographed hockey sticks,
made for a party feeling. The auxiliary still provides volunteers to assist at
blood donor clinics now run by Hema-Quebec.

The auxiliary is now part of a larger institution – the McGill University
Health Centre. It is proud to be linked with four strong entities with similar
roots and history in this city. The auxiliary has been a part of shaping the

vision, structuring linkages, and creating a new environment. Since 1998, the Friends of the MUHC, which is comprised of auxiliary members from the MCH, MCI, MGH, MNH, and RVH, have been meeting to promote inter-action, communication, and cooperation within the MUHC. Its goals are to foster volunteerism and links to the community and to have a common voice at the level of the administration and the board. If the women of the Tues-day Club were alive, they would be astonished and very proud of the work performed by the auxiliary today.

25

Dentistry

Kenneth C. Bentley

Ken Bentley was dental surgeon-in-chief and former dean of dentistry at McGill. Clinical dentistry has been housed at the MGH since the Faculty of Dentistry began.

Introduction

I am an MD, CM, DDS graduate of McGill, and in this chapter I describe the development of dentistry and the MGH dental clinic in the Dorchester Street and Cedar Ave buildings, the struggle to keep the school open at McGill, the expansion in subspecialty dental education, and the beginnings of dental research. A long-standing relationship between the Department of Dentistry of the MGH and the Faculty of Dentistry of McGill University resulted in the clinical teaching facilities of the faculty being housed physically within the department and, as such, the history of the two is inextricably linked.

When I was appointed dean of the Faculty of Dentistry in 1977, I asked Mervyn A. Rogers, former associate dean, to compile a history of the faculty to commemorate the seventy-fifth anniversary of the school, which would take place in 1979. This resulted in the publication of a book entitled *A History of the McGill Dental School*,[1] and much of what is found in this chapter is taken from that publication.

The Beginning

In 1892, the MGH recognized dentistry by appointing a staff dentist, R. Hugh Berwick. This marked the first appointment of a dentist to the staff of a Canadian hospital. His qualifications for the post were unique in that he had indentured with S.J. Andres in Montreal and had received his licentiate in dental surgery, following which he began the study of medicine at McGill, graduating in 1891. He decided to confine his practice to oral surgery and, in doing so, was probably the first specialist in oral surgery among Canadian dentists. Unfortunately, he died from tuberculosis at the early age of twenty-six.

However, the post of staff dentist had been established, and J.S. Ibbotson was appointed to succeed him. Ibbotson had qualified for the LDS in 1886 and was one of a group of twenty-six dentists whom Bishop's had honoured in 1896 by conferring upon them the degree of doctor of dental surgery, ad eundem. He remained at the hospital, but there is no evidence that he joined the staff of the McGill dental school until 1910. In that year he became director of the dental clinic, the first mention there is of this position in the hospital.

Early Dental Education in Quebec

In the 1800s the principal sources of dental education for Canadians were to be found in the United States, either at the Baltimore College of Dentistry, the Harvard University Dental School, the New York College of Dentistry, or the California State University Dental School. It was not until 1875, when the Royal College of Dental Surgeons in Ontario began its school, that Canadians could obtain a dental education in their own country. Prior to this, candidates were required to become indentured to a licensed dentist for a period of four years. Upon the successful completion of this indentureship, the candidate was required to satisfy a board of examiners before being admitted to the profession.[2]

In 1892, the Dental College of the Province of Quebec was established. Teaching was to be in both English and French, and it was hoped that the school would be affiliated with McGill University or Université Laval, or, perhaps, both. This attempt was not successful, but in 1896 an arrangement with the University of Bishop's College in Lennoxville was achieved. At that time Bishop's had a medical school in Montreal.

For eight years, the Bishop's dental school continued until the school was absorbed by McGill in 1905.[3] The school began as a department of the Faculty of Medicine and continued as such until 1920, when it was designated a faculty.

Clinical Facilities Established in MGH, 1908

Initially, the clinical teaching facilities of the McGill school were housed on St Catherine Street at St Lawrence, where Bishop's had moved in 1898. In 1908, the clinical teaching facilities were moved to the MGH. The university announcement of 1908–09 described the new clinic as follows:

> The space devoted to the clinic contains, in addition to the office and a waiting room a large well-lighted operating room furnished with Columbia chairs having fountain cuspidors and operating brackets. Communicating with the operating room is the anaesthetic room equipped with all modem conveniences for the extraction of teeth, including a nitrous-oxide apparatus for gas anaesthesia. There is also a laboratory with complete equipment including electric lathes and a plaster and vulcanizing room.
>
> In addition, each student is provided with a locker for keeping instruments.[4]

No doubt these premises were an improvement over earlier clinics, but it was, in fact, an area that had once been used by the hospital as a morgue. Those who attended classes there described the area as crowded and unpleasant. However, it was the beginning of an association of the McGill dental school with the MGH, an association that continues to the present day to the admitted mutual benefit of both parties. To the hospital it has been the greatest dental department that one could imagine – a luxury enjoyed by few, if any, other hospitals. To the school it has brought the great convenience afforded by the various laboratory and diagnostic services that such a hospital can offer.

The first clinic was used until 1922, but because of increasing enrolment of classes, the existing facilities proved to be entirely inadequate. A new clinic was built as a one-storey annex to the old Central Division of the MGH. It faced onto de la Gauchitière Street at the comer of St Dominique. It was intended only as a temporary clinic, hastily erected to accommodate the growing classes, but it remained in use until the move to the new MGM on Cedar Avenue in 1955. Further expansion of the department came in 1972 when the hospital made available to dentistry that portion of the third floor that had been occupied by the Social Service Department. This entire area was given over to the hospital dental service and to oral and maxillofacial surgery, which was expanding at that time. When this space became available, university authorities were convinced to renovate it and, in addition, to replace and update the equipment in the entire undergraduate clinic. Later, a beautifully equipped lecture room was provided for the first time since the building was occupied in 1955.

Superintendents and Directors of the Dental Clinic, Deans and Dental Surgeons-in-Chief

Details are sketchy with respect to early directors of the dental clinic, or what was otherwise known as the dental infirmary of McGill University at the MGH. The first mention of the post of director was in 1910, when. J.S. Ibbotson was appointed to the position. In 1915, he was succeeded by O.A. Lefebvre, who joined the staff as superintendent of the dental infirmary. He, in turn, was succeeded by C.H.P. Moore in 1918. He held this post for only one year. It was not until 1924 when, Arthur Walsh was appointed director of the dental infirmary, that a line of continuity was established. In 1927, Gordon Leahy was appointed director, and he remained in this position until 1956, a period of twenty-nine years. In 1956, James McCutcheon was appointed dean of the Faculty of Dentistry and also designated dental surgeon-in-chief of the Department of Dentistry and director of the undergraduate teaching clinic. In 1970, when McCutcheon resigned as dean, the position of dean and dental surgeon-in-chief was separated, and Kenneth C. Bentley was appointed dental surgeon-in-chief and Ernie Ambrose was appointed dean.

Peter Brown

It was Peter Brown who guided the Bishop's dental school through its affiliation with McGill, and he remained chair of the Dental Executive until ill health forced his retirement in 1909. He had gone to New York to study dentistry at the New York College of Dentistry, graduating about 1884. Not only was Brown one of the leading dentists of North America, but he was a great researcher and had a keen interest in the development of electrical appliances for use in dentistry. One such development was an ionization machine, and he was one of the first to use the electric motor in preparing teeth. He served as president of the College of Dental Surgeons of the Province of Quebec and was one of the charter members of the Montreal Dental Club.

D.J. Berwick

There is reason to believe that the successor to Brown as chair of the Dental Executive was David James Berwick. He had received his DDS from Bishop's University and was one of those who were instrumental in persuading the Faculty of Medicine at McGill to establish a department of dentistry. The McGill University Calendar of 1910 lists him as professor of operative dentistry and chair of the Dental Executive, a post that he held until 1913.

A.W. Thornton

Alexander Walker Thornton was chair of the Dental Executive from 1913 to 1920 and dean of the Faculty of Dentistry from 1920 to 1927. He had graduated with the degree of DDS from the Royal College of Dental Surgeons, Toronto, in 1890. After practising in rural Ontario, he moved to Toronto in 1906, becoming professor of crown-and-bridge work in the school of the Royal College of Surgeons. He came to McGill in 1913, and, largely due to his efforts, the school became a faculty and he became its first dean. He was a fellow of the American College of Dentists and served as president of the American Association of Dental Schools in 1926.

A.L. Walsh

Arthur Lambert Walsh followed Thornton as dean. He was named acting dean of the faculty in 1927, a post that he held until 1940, when he was appointed dean. Walsh was one of the pioneers in dental education, and he maintained a keen interest in it throughout his lifetime. He was one of the first educators to recognize that dental education must change its emphasis from a technical approach to a science-oriented biological approach. It was largely through his efforts that the Council on Education of the Canadian Dental Association was formed. He served as president of the American Association of Dental Schools, president of the Canadian Dental Association, and president of the Montreal Dental Club. He was a fellow of the American College of Dentists and of the International College of Dentists. He was elected a fellow in Dental Surgery of the Royal College of Surgeons of England and was awarded the degree of DDS, honoris causa, from the Université de Montreal. He was a member of the medical boards of the MGH the Children's Memorial Hospital and the McKay Institute.

Gordon Leahy

Gordon Leahy studied dentistry at McGill, graduated in 1920, and opened an office in Cowansville, Quebec. Very shortly thereafter, he developed health problems requiring complete rest for more than a year. After his recovery he went to see Arthur Walsh, director of the dental clinic at the time. Walsh invited Leahy to assist him at the clinic, believing that this would provide the opportunity he needed to resume his career in dentistry. He came expecting to stay for one year; he remained for thirty-two. When Walsh was appointed acting dean, Leahy became the clinical director, and, from that time until Mowry assumed the deanship in 1948, he was the only full-time member of the faculty. That he endured the years during the Second World War was a miracle! Most of the regular staff was away in the armed services, and he had to deal with every type of situation in whatever way he could. Added to this was the matter of accelerated classes, which brought no end of problems. The personnel at all hospitals without dental services and at nursing and convalescent homes in the area knew him well and loved him. He received calls almost weekly from one of them, where some confined person had developed a dental problem. He would pack a few things in a bag and go on another errand of mercy.

His students loved him, for not only was he kind but he was also always full of surprises. He could be severe if the occasion required it, but usually his sense of humour was not far from the surface. He never sought the limelight in any way, and, strangely enough, few honours came to him. After his retirement he was awarded Canadian dentistry's highest honour – honorary membership in the Canadian Dental Association. He served as clinic director for twenty-nine years.

D.P. Mowry

Succeeding Walsh as dean was Daniel Prescott Mowry. He received his DDS from McGill in 1917. After graduation he became associated in practice with I.S. Dohan and, encouraged by the latter, began the study of periodontia (periodontics), which brought him into contact with some of the noted specialists of the day. While continuing to practice, he became associated with the Faculty of Dentistry, becoming professor and head of periodontics. Upon the resignation of Walsh in 1948, Mowry was appointed dean. He was twice president of the College of Dental Surgeons of the Province of Quebec and president of the Montreal Dental Club. He was a fellow of the American College of Dentists, a member of the American Academy of Periodontics, a member of the

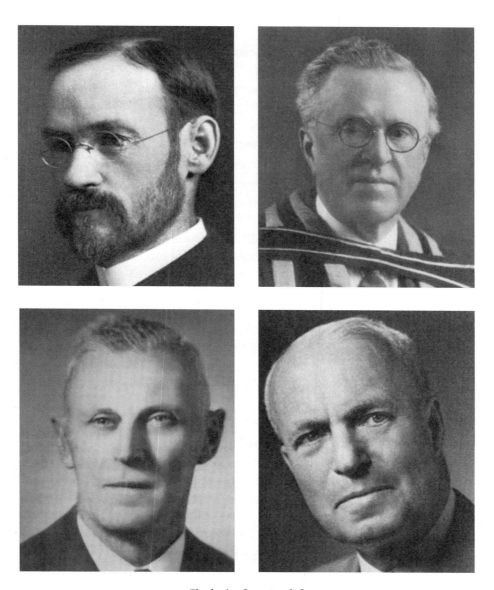

Clockwise from top left

Fig. 25.1 Peter Brown, first chair of the Dental Executive of the
Faculty of Medicine, 1903–09

Fig. 25.2 Alexander W. Thornton, chair, Dental Executive, 1913–20; first dean of the
Faculty of Dentistry, 1920–27

Fig. 25.3 Arthur Walsh, dean, Faculty of Dentistry, 1927–46

Fig. 25.4 Gordon Leahy, director, Dental Clinic, 1927–48

Montreal City Board of Health, and a governor of Sir George Williams College. He was an active member and served as president of the St James Literary Society and read many papers before that group. He received a Fellowship in Dental Surgery of the Royal College of Surgeons of England. It was he who, in January 1953, negotiated the contract that was to ensure the continuing association between the MGH and the McGill Dental School. He became ill in the late days of 1954 and was subsequently hospitalized in the MGH. On that memorable day – 20 May 1955 – when the hospital moved to its new location on Cedar Avenue, he was one of those patients who were transferred from the old hospital. He died shortly thereafter.

James McCutcheon

Upon the death of Dean Mowry, James McCutcheon was appointed acting dean and, in March 1956, was confirmed as dean, a post that he held with distinction for the next fourteen years. Simultaneous with this appointment was his designation as dental surgeon-in-chief of the MGH. He had obtained his DDS in 1945 from McGill. From 1945 go 1946 he served in the US Naval Reserve as a lieutenant in the Dental Corps, following which he entered the University of Michigan as a W.K. Kellogg fellow, obtaining his MSc in prosthodontics in 1948. During his tenure as dean he developed the faculty, increasing the number of full-time teachers from two to thirteen. He was a governor of the College of Dental Surgeons of the Province of Quebec. Active in the Canadian Dental Association, he was chair of its Council on Education. He was a fellow of the American College of Dentists, the International College of Dentists, and the Royal College of Dentists of Canada. He was president of the Canadian Academy of Prosthodontics, and a member of the executive of the Montreal Dental Club. He served on the Board of Health of the City of Montreal, the Child Health Association of Montreal, and as a consultant to the Royal Canadian Dental Corps. McCutcheon left McGill in 1970 to assume the position of dean of the Faculty of Dentistry, University of Alberta.

E.R. Ambrose

Ernest Reynolds Ambrose was appointed dean in 1970. He received his DDS from McGill in 1950, opened a private practice in Montreal, and joined the part-time staff of the faculty. He soon became known as an excellent teacher as well as for his outstanding ability in restorative dentistry. He was very active in organized dentistry and was much sought after internationally as a lecturer. His years as dean were progressive ones. He oversaw the expansion and re-equipment of the dental department at the hospital and was instrumental in establishing research within the faculty. He was awarded fellowships in the American College of Dentists, the International College of Dentists, and the Royal College of Dentists of Canada. He resigned the deanship in 1977 to accept the post of dean of the College of Dentistry, University of Saskatchewan.

K.C. Bentley

I received my DDS from McGill in 1958 and immediately enrolled in the Faculty of Medicine, receiving my MD, CM degree in 1962. Following one year of rotating internship and one year of surgical residency at the MGH, I proceeded to Bellevue Hospital in New York City to do a residency program there in oral and maxillofacial surgery. I returned to McGill and the MGH in 1966 and became head of oral surgery in 1967 and was appointed dental surgeon-in-chief of the hospital in 1970, a post that I retained when appointed dean of the faculty in 1977 – a position I held for ten years. Active in organized dentistry, I served as chair of the Council on Hospital Services, chair of the Council on Education and Accreditation of the Canadian Dental Association, and was chief written examiner of the National Dental Examining Board of Canada. At the hospital level I served as chair of the Medical Advisory Committee; the Council of Physicians, Dentists and Pharmacists; and of its Executive Committee. I was president of the Association of Canadian Faculties of Dentistry and president of the Montreal Dental Club. I was awarded fellowship in the American College of Dentists, the International College of Dentists, the Royal College of Dentists of Canada, the Pierre Fauchard Academy and l'Academie Dentaire du Quebec. I received honorary membership in the Canadian Dental Association. It was I who began the specialty residency training program in oral and maxillofacial surgery and who established the liaison with the Baffin Regional Hospital.

Ralph Y. Barolet

Ralph Y. Barolet succeeded me (K.C. Bentley) as dean of the faculty. After graduating from McGill in chemical engineering and after spending twelve years in the workplace, he pursued his studies in dentistry, obtaining his DDS degree from l'Université de Montreal. He then furthered his education in the science of dental materials, obtaining a master of dental science degree from Indiana University. He was appointed to the staff of l'Univer-

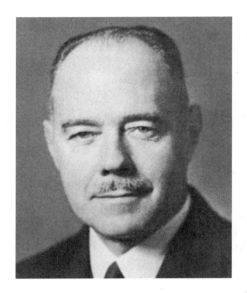

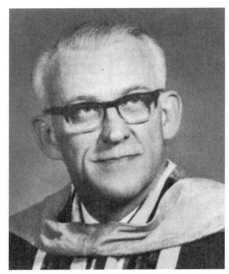

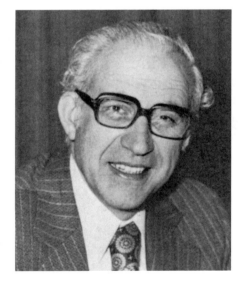

Clockwise from top left
Fig. 25.5 D. Prescott Mowry, dean, Faculty
of Dentistry, 1948–55
Fig. 25.6 James McCutcheon, dean, Faculty
of Dentistry, 1956–70
Fig. 25.7 Ernie Ambrose, dean, Faculty of
Dentistry, 1970–77

sité Laval and was one of the pioneers for the establishment of a new dental school in Quebec City. He was associate dean there when named dean at McGill in 1987.

Barolet was awarded fellowships in the American College of Dentists; the International College of Dentists; the Academy of Dentistry International, of which he served as president; the Pierre Fauchard Academy; and l'Academie Dentaire du Quebec.

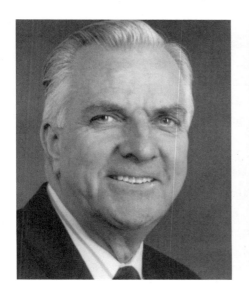

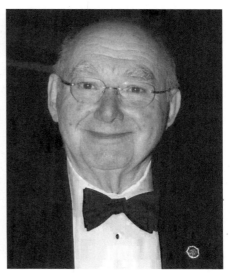

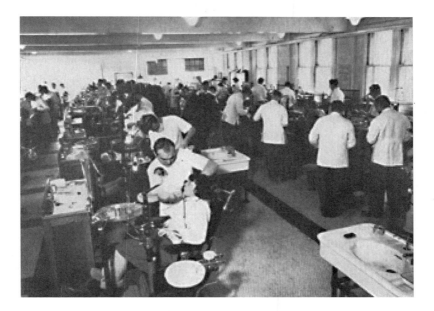

Clockwise from top left
Fig. 25.8 Kenneth Bentley, DDS, MD, CM, dean, Faculty of Dentistry, 1977–87
Fig. 25.9 Ralph Barolet, dean, Faculty of Dentistry, 1987–94
Fig. 25.10 MGH dental clinic in the 1950s

Women in Dentistry

In 1922, another significant event took place respecting the Faculty of Dentistry: it admitted its first female student. This step had not been possible until about 1918. Up until then the Faculty of Medicine had refused to admit women, and since the dental school was a department of that faculty, it was bound by that policy.

The first woman to be admitted was Florence Johnston, who graduated in 1926. She practised general dentistry in Montreal for many years and then limited her practice to children's dentistry. Upon her death in 1970, she bequeathed her entire estate to McGill University. The Board of Governors of the university decided that this bequest should be used for research in the Faculty of Dentistry, and the Florence B. Johnston Fund was established.

For many years it was uncommon for women to study dentistry at McGill. Dora Gordon graduated in 1934, Anita Mendel in 1939, Gwen James in 1943, and Roberta Dundass in 1947. Many years passed before there was more than one woman enrolled at a time. Now the number of women in any given class is about 50 percent.

Development of Internship and Residency Programs

The MGH was one of the first hospitals in Canada to institute dental internships and the first to introduce student internships. Dental interns had existed at the MGH for many years. In 1957, it was thought wise to increase the hospital experience of first-year dental students by appointing them assistants to these interns. Students were appointed for periods of two weeks, during which they would forgo their regular clinical duties. They lived in the hospital for this period, followed the regular interns, and carried out such procedures as the interns and attending staff saw fit to assign. This was the first time that such an experience had been provided for any dental student in Canada; it has been maintained with some modifications.

The general practice residency program was given a boost in 1972, when a designated physical area was assigned to it. Under the capable direction of Harry Rosen, this program flourished. This additional year of experience serves to enhance a dental graduate's preparedness for general practice. In 1972, a specialty residency training program was established in prosthodontics under the directorship of Harry Rosen. This program continued until 1979. In 1971 the specialty residency training program in oral and maxillofacial surgery was inaugurated. This program was under my directorship and continues until this day (2015).

L.E. Francis

This chapter would not be complete without mention of the contribution of Lyman Ellwood Francis. Francis graduated from McGill in 1949. He opened an office and, at the same time, began graduate studies in pharmacology at McGill. He received his MSc degree in pharmacology in 1958. He joined the full-time faculty in 1958 and became the first full-time staff member to devote time to research. Half his day was spent at the hospital, the other half in his laboratory in the Mcintyre Medical Building. Through his efforts the research division of the faculty was developed, and clinical investigative studies in the Department of Dentistry at the hospital began.

Active in organized dentistry, Francis served as chair of the Council on Research of the Canadian Dental Association and as chair of the pharmacology section of the American Association of Dental Schools. He served on the Council of the Royal College of Dentists and was a fellow of the American College of Dentists, the International College of Dentists, and the Royal College of Dentists of Canada.

Space does not permit the inclusion of the names of hundreds of individuals who have contributed to the department and the undergraduate teaching clinic, other than those who served in a full- or half-time position. These are:

Associate Director of the Department
   Mervyn A. Rogers

Prosthodontics and Restorative Dentistry
   Donald Kepron, Harry Rosen, John V. Blomfield, Ed Ostro, Nasser Dibai, Ivan Stangel, Andrew Pullinger, Lindsay Risk, Pierre Lamontagne, Don Henry, Oscar Sykora, and John Townsend

Orthodontics
   Robert Faith, Michael Rennert and Dan Lipke

Oral Medicine
   Martin T. Tyler

Oral Radiology
Marie Dagenais

Oral Pathology
Thomas P. McCrory, Peter I. Chauvin, and Araceli Ortiz

Oral Diagnosis
Gerald Racey and Robert Johnson

Paediatric Dentistry
Gerry G.H. Weinlander and Stephane Schwartz

Periodontics
Jim Kenrick, Robert Harvey, Wessam Al-Joburi, and Louis
Z.G. Touyz

Endodontics
Wilf Johnston

Oral and Maxillofacial Surgery
Eric P. Millar, Timothy W. Head, and David Shapiro

Pharmacology
Howard S. Katz

Quarter-time appointments, Ben Sedlezky and Herb Borsuk, served as directors of Endodontics, and Jack McCarthy and Roger McMahon faithfully served the hospital dental service for many years.

In 1997, the MGH became part of the McGill University Health Centre and, as of that date, no longer exited as a separate entity, though physically it remains on Cedar Avenue and as a campus of the MUHC.

Over the next decade the faculty weathered the storm that ensued when the university threatened its closure. In 1994, Barolet completed his term as dean. John V. Blomfield was appointed acting dean until the appointment of James P. Lund in 1995. In that same year further renovations and re-equipment of the entire department took place. In 1996, the university began renting space at the MGH for its undergraduate teaching clinic, and the teaching facility no longer forms part of the Department of Dentistry. In 1998, I stepped down as director of oral and maxillofacial surgery and was succeeded by Timothy W. Head, who had been coordinator of the graduate program since 1981. In 2000, I retired as dental surgeon-in-chief, after serving for thirty years, and was succeeded by Antoine Chehade, who is dental surgeon-in-chief of the MGH and the RVH components of the MUHC (2015).

NOTES

1 M.A. Rogers, *A History of the McGill Dental School* (Montreal: Faculty of Dentistry, McGill University, 1980).
2 D.W. Gullett, *A History of Dentistry in Canada* (Toronto: University of Toronto Press, 1971).
3 Ibid.
4 E.H. Bensley, "Bishop's Medical College," *Canadian Medical Association Journal* 72 (1955): 463–5.

26

Emergency Department

Michael Churchill-Smith

Michael Churchill-Smith is a former director of the Emergency Room.

This chapter provides an account of the creation of the Emergency Department at the MGH. Starting with the relatively unstructured Emergency Room headed by the popular Lorne Cassidy, the MGH conferred department status on the emergency service in 1987. I discuss the evolution of emergency medicine as a specialty and the need for trained personnel in the modern Emergency Department as well as the 2003 designation of the MGH as the only Level 1, Adult Trauma Centre in Montreal. This acknowledgment of the extraordinary contribution of the Emergency Department to the MGH and the Montreal public was over-due.

In the mid-1980s, the Emergency Department, as it now is known, was then referred to as the Emergency Room (ER) and was simply a service without any formally defined structure within the administration of the hospital. Both the Department of Surgery and the Department of Medicine provided leadership through doctors such as Tony Ty and Lorne E. Cassidy, who would ensure that patients requiring either emergency surgical or medical services would be properly cared for. Residents of all levels would be rotated through the ER as a part of their academic training, coming principally from the internal medicine and general surgery programs.

In those days, the ER was fast becoming a busy and intense place to work, and there were greater numbers of patients with increasing acuity and complexity at our doorstep. A turning point came with the 1961 Quebec Hospital Insurance Plan that mandated hospitalization, and ER services were now free. With the floodgates opened, hallways were regularly clogged with

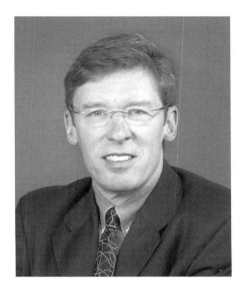

Fig. 26.1 Michael Churchill-Smith, first director, Emergency Department, 1987–98

patients, and it was not unheard of to find patients with serious social issues lying on a stretcher for up to six weeks. The thorny issue of access to our medical system was beginning to rear its ugly head, placing even more emphasis on the importance of the ER to the overall functioning of the hospital itself. In order for us to provide full staffing, we depended on the likes of Alan Barkun, Jean Louis Caron, Françoise Chagnon, Scott Kenick, Louis Fortin, legions of moonlighting medical and surgical residents to chip in and help out. To these individuals, a big thanks; and to those whom I have forgotten, an equally big thanks and please forgive my failing memory.

In July 1987, I became the chief of the service, replacing Lorne Cassidy. Within the next few months, the hospital administration was convinced that the ER should be recognized as a formal department on equal footing with all others. This proved immensely helpful in terms of budget and collaborative interaction with other services, but it also reduced the other departments' sense of commitment to providing clinical coverage on a regular basis. Given the fact that patients were presenting to the ER sicker and with greater co-morbidities, there was less obvious immediate association with either medicine or surgery. As a consequence, regular, permanent staffing for the department was needed quickly, but a complete resolution to this thorny problem would only be achieved a decade later.

Life in the ER at that time can be illustrated by three events. One Monday morning, I was on my way to attend morning rounds when two young women in their early thirties strode past me in the corridor. Both were smoking and both were waiting to be assessed by the psychiatrist on call. Unbeknownst to me, they walked straight past me into the garage and stole an Urgences Santé ambulance, roared down Atwater Street, and were brought back in two ambulances as trauma patients after they had caused multiple car accidents.

During these years, we regularly had forty to fifty patients languishing in the ER. One day, I was examining an eighty-seven-year-old woman who had been brought in from the YWCA, where she had fallen down the stairs. She was unable to give a proper history, and, ultimately, I had to rifle through her purse, where I found an airline ticket – Montreal to Chicago one way – that she was due to be on that day! After several hours, we finally tracked down her son's phone number in Chicago. He was relieved to hear that she had been found but was rather indifferent to the fact that she had come to Montreal on her own. He went on to tell us that she had been "disappearing" all her life, taking buses and planes all over the world, and that it was only last year that he took her passport away when she had been found wandering in France. Her previous travels had taken her as far as Russia and Chile!

The most famous ER story of 1987 took place on a Sunday night, 1 November. At 9:00 PM, I received a phone call from the ER medical resident that René Lévesque was being brought into the hospital from his home. I hurried over and arrived at precisely the same time as the ambulance. As I walked in, the same resident was holding the phone telling me that the *New York Times* was on the line and wanted confirmation that the ex-premier was in the hospital. We went on to learn that, in those days, major newspapers paid people to listen to CB radios in an attempt to get a scoop on breaking news. Later that night, we also learned what it was like to be inundated with media as scores of journalists from all over descended on the hospital. The most poignant moment occurred when scores of interested Quebec citizens, all waiting anxiously outside our Emergency Department doors, collectively burst into tears when the public announcement of Mr Lévesque's death was made. The entire event is still talked about today, now more than twenty-five years later.

Amid the chaos of the late 1980s, when we struggled with medical staffing, our head nurse, Pam Roberts, worked tremendously hard to ensure that the ER had an adequate number of available nurses, all of a high quality. The core of nurses under her leadership was one of the most important factors in our being able to maintain an excellent level of care twenty-four hours a day.

The MGH had long established itself as a hospital ready to treat the province's most serious trauma victims. This tradition dated back to the days of Fraser Gurd and H. Rocke Robertson, and, at that time, the same standard was being actively maintained through the efforts of David Mulder and Rae Brown, two surgeons both hugely admired and respected for their clinical and leadership talents. Their skills were never more evident and necessary than in the late afternoon of 6 December 1989, the day of the massacre at L'École Polytechnique at the University of Montreal. At the time, there was no formal trauma program in place in Quebec, but it was a well established fact that if problems arose on the streets of Montreal, Urgences Santé could count on the MGH to take their patients and get the job done. At the first warning that something major was in progress that fateful afternoon, we leapt into action. The ambulance room was cleared of patients and all eight beds were staffed with a surgical resident, an ER nurse, and an orderly. All service departments were advised, and blood from the blood bank was sent down in advance in ample volumes. As fortune would have it, there were several departmental Christmas parties taking place within the hospital, and this meant that many surgeons were immediately available to help. Rae Brown was the trauma leader in charge; and Valerie Shannon, nursing director; and Tom Harrison, senior administrator; were also on hand to facilitate and to coordinate patient flow as well as and to ensure that the right human resources and equipment were constantly available. Suddenly, six seriously injured students arrived in our ER within a span of twenty minutes (the outcome is now public record). Several of these young people nearly died in the moments after arrival but quick, precise action with steady hands, amazing teamwork, and skilful judgment led to a 100 percent survival.

The ER went from intense to entirely calm in fewer than seventy-five minutes as patients were rapidly sent on for definitive care. Over the ensuing few days, as it became clear that these young people were not only going to survive but likely make near full physical recoveries, a kind of quiet pride emerged amongsall the staff who had participated and helped, each in his or her own way, to bring about this remarkable outcome. This collective sentiment has always been a large part of the MGH culture and continues unabated today. It was witnessed again during the Dawson College shootings of 2006, when a new generation of ER professionals handled an eerily similar situation with the same skill and superb judgment that had been on display seventeen years earlier. The few remaining professionals who participated in both tragedies have uniformly made the same observation. The final comment has to do with how much we learned from the École Polytechnique experience, which only became evident during the Dawson crisis in 2006. The critically decisive behaviour of the police; the rapid availability of Urgences Santé, "scooping and running" with the injured students; the activation of trauma teams, leaders, and system protocols in the ER; and, finally, the psychiatry post-stress teams produced another remarkably successful outcome a generation later. The global management of this near-disaster has been uniformly praised in many circles throughout the world and, in my judgment, now stands as one of the hospital's finest hours – borne of our long history in trauma management and of lessons well learned and applied.

The subsequent five years was a period of mutual adjustment for the hospital and the ER. Slowly, trainees were arriving at our door with Royal College certified emergency medicine certification and/or family medicine training with a specific emergency medicine stream. These two groups would progressively come to represent a new body of doctors who, by the late 1990s, would be the core physicians functioning and running the ER. It was also a period of ongoing construction as we needed to be significantly upgraded and physically reorganized so as to accommodate older, sicker patients. During the same period, the MGH had received Level 1 Trauma designation, which meant that we were one of only four selected hospitals in Quebec responsible for the management of the most serious trauma victims. This required that we install important diagnostic equipment (such as a CT scan) in the department itself. The end result was a significantly larger floor plan with a dedicated trauma room, CT scan, and new or upgraded X-Ray units (both fixed and portable) all to help with rapid diagnosis. In the late 1980s, the ER had experimented with the earliest of digital X-ray units, but neither the equipment nor the physicians were ready to use it on a regular basis. By the end of the century, we were a filmless department in which everyone was using digital imagery – a sea change from a decade earlier.

The Mohawk conflict with the Sureté du Québec in 1994 touched our doors one Saturday. On the Kanesatake Reserve, a native became seriously ill, requiring emergency services. The problem was that no hospital would take this person. And there are a dozen good hospitals between Kanesatake and the MGH, where the patient finally ended up. The Mohawk community insisted that the Canadian Forces ensure his safety, and this led to a stand-off with the Sureté du Québec, who were barred from entering the ER itself with the Canadian Army inside. We were not popular that day, but, in the end, this direct conflict led to a resolution between the two organizations and was an important factor in bringing the crisis to closure.

One afternoon, an ambulance arrived from one hour outside of Montreal transporting an adolescent who had fallen into a portable silo on his parents' farm. The silo was full of grain and, in effect, he had drowned. Fortunately, one of his friends had the presence of mind to open the chute, and he promptly fell out. He immediately stood up and then collapsed. By the time he arrived through our doors, every specialist was waiting for him. Each one had a very specific idea on the best way to manage him. The assistant head nurse, Ann Thomas, brilliant and a very experienced clinician herself, suggested turning the patient upside down. The respirologists were convinced that rigid bronchoscopy was the only approach, while the surgeons wanted to immediately go to the operating room and "crack open" his chest. There were several other theories being knocked around. Finally, after what seemed like an interminable period, the surgeons won the day, and off they went to the OR. While they were preparing the patient on the table, he was placed in the Trendelenberg position (i.e., his head well below his feet), and suddenly all the grain started to pour out of his mouth – to such an extent that the surgeons spent their time extracting single pieces to minimize nitrogen poisoning. Subsequently, there were a lot of pretty smart people "eating humble pie," and an assistant head nurse whose clinical credibility went up another few notches yet again. The patient made a great recovery and was able to return home in the coming days. I tell this story to illustrate the dynamic interplay, between the many levels and types of professionals, that regularly goes on in an academic emergency department, particularly in acute circumstances. This tension invariably produces an excellent outcome for the patient, even when little information is available. However, sometimes we are just plain lucky.

The final few years of my tenure saw the completion of construction in the ER and the emergence of specially trained emergency physicians. Despite an increase in the number of patient visits to approximately forty thousand, the number of patients languishing on stretchers in the corridors was reduced. This continued until more bed closures within the hospital took place.

The year 1998 is best remembered for the massive ice storm, which severely affected all the ERs in the city for a period of one month. The sheer volume of patients was overwhelming, and, as would be expected, the corridors were full of elderly patients suffering primarily from dehydration, pneumonia, and associated medical conditions. The mortality rate was three times the usual January rate. As for the staff, they were simply amazing. Clerks, orderlies, nurses, and devoted physicians were doing double and triple shifts, and, without their remarkable efforts, the impact of the storm would have been far more serious.

In summary, 1987 through 1998 was a period of great change in the Emergency Department. The group of professionals had great camaraderie and were unified by a spirit of cooperation and collaboration. We had adopted the culture of the MGH and did our best to keep the patient front and centre in our practice.

I would like to extend a personal note of thanks to Pam Roberts, Ann Thomas, Audrey McLeod, and Suzanne Dubé, Nicole Garceau, and Robert Primavesi for their untiring support. And to the late Lorne Cassidy, my mentor, and to Barbara Watson, my devoted secretary, words will never be enough to express my gratitude for all that they have done over the years.

Editors' Note

As the author mentions, for many decades emergency care at the MGH was provided in the ER, until, in 1987, the Emergency Department was established. Information about the early years of the ER at the MGH is lacking. The first horse-drawn ambulance wagons were supplied by funeral director Joseph Wray in 1883. These were hearses with a reversible sign that hung on the side of the wagon. Business was so good that Wray constructed special ambulance wagons with "MGH" on the side. There being no screening of patients except by the interns on the wagons, whoever the ambulance picked up was admitted through the front door of the hospital. This is why pictures of Wray's ambulances at the MGH and RVH are at the front door. The Outpatient Department was in the basements of the Reid and Moreland wings, with an entrance on St Dominique, but it had no capacity to care for emergencies.

At the MGH, motor ambulances replaced the horse-drawn wagons in 1912 (this occurred in 1909 at the RVH, also serviced by Wray). Up to the 1950s and early 1960s, each hospital had its own ambulances supplied by contract. Even the Royal Alexandra Communicable Disease Hospital had an ambulance. When called, the MGH ambulances naturally brought the patients back to the MGH, but if the intern in the ambulance thought it should go to a nearer hospital, for the sake of the patient it would do so.

In 1961, the ER was forced to make way for major overcrowding caused by Quebec's Hospital Insurance Plan, which made hospitalization and ER care free. It opened the floodgates, but the degree of the demand from people, many whom had had very little medical care before, was not anticipated. It didn't help that most of the French hospitals closed their ER doors in the early evening, leaving the MGH and RVH, open twenty-four hours a day seven days a week, to cope with a problem that took more than a decade to resolve.

27

Obstetrics and Gynaecology

J. Edwin Coffey

Ed Coffey was a senior obstetrician and gynaecologist for over forty years and a past president of the Quebec Medical Association.

When the newly constructed MGH opened its doors in 1822, pregnant women in Montreal were accustomed to childbirth at home, usually assisted by an experienced female relative or self-trained midwife. Consequently there were no planned accommodations for services dedicated to women, such as maternity, lying-in, or obstetrical services. The speciality of obstetrics and gynaecology (Obs/Gyn), which provides unique specialized medical and surgical services for women, had yet to evolve in North America.

University Lying-In Hospital for Charitable Midwifery/Obstetrics, 1843

By 1841, times had changed, and the private Montreal Lying-in Hospital for women during childbirth was established by William MacNider on Bonaventure Street (later St James and St Jacques). Because MacNider had not been invited to join the staff of the young McGill Medical School, he refused to allow McGill medical students to be taught in his hospital.[1]

Following MacNider's death, McGill's Faculty of Medicine took over the Montreal Lying-in Hospital in 1843, renamed it the University Lying-in Hospital, and established clinical teaching for medical students in midwifery/obstetrics. Another group of civic-minded Montreal women was invited by McGill's Faculty of Medicine to form the "Ladies' Committee for Domestic Management," and a medical board was appointed for the professional management of the hospital. The lecturer on midwifery would be the attending physician, and the matron would be a thoroughly trained midwife, if possible. Their objective at this hospital on St Urbain Street was to provide charitable services and improved obstetrical care by midwives and physician accoucheurs as well as the teaching of medical and nursing students.

University Lying-In Becomes Montreal Maternity Hospital 1887

Before long, it was not only the impoverished women who appreciated the comforts and safety of having their newborns delivered in the University Lying-in Hospital. Pregnant women of all social levels began to share this preference for a hospital delivery. The University Lying-in Hospital's name was changed to University Maternity Hospital in 1884 and, in 1887, to the Montreal Maternity Hospital (MMH).[2] Until the RVH and the MGH opened their full obstetrical services in 1926 and 1944, respectively, general physicians and obstetricians from both hospitals increasingly used the Maternity Hospital for obstetrical deliveries rather than for home deliveries. All obstetrical teaching for medical students, interns, and nurses was conducted at the Maternity Hospital.

The early physicians who attended the MGH and the University Lying-in Hospital included Archibald Hall (1813–68), appointed to the MGH in 1836 and director of the University Lying-in Hospital from 1854 to 1857; Duncan C MacCallum (1824–1904), appointed to MGH in 1856 and director of the University Lying-in Hospital from 1867 to 1883. He held McGill professorships in clinical surgery, 1856–60, clinical medicine 1860–67, and midwifery and diseases of women and children, 1868–83. He became consulting physician at MGH in 1875.

Gynaecology Introduced at the MGH in 1883

Gynaecology (gyn) developed as a speciality in Montreal near the end of the nineteenth century. Before this, very little gynaecologic surgery was performed and was usually done by general surgeons. As described in *Telinde's Operative Gynecology*: "The history of Gynecologic Surgery was closely tied to the history of General Surgery and the obstacles to be overcome the same i.e. infection, haemorrhage, shock and pain – all barriers to any but emergency surgical procedures in days before anaesthesia.[3]

Howard Kelly, a gynaecologist and colleague of Osler's at Philadelphia, was influenced by Osler to move with him to Baltimore as part of the "big four" (Osler, Kelly, Halstead, and Welch) to found the Johns Hopkins Hospital and Medical School. Osler and Kelly shared a common interest in pathology and a conviction that a good knowledge of cellular pathology was essential for a fuller understanding of medical and surgical conditions. As a reflection of this conviction, the traditional residency programs in medicine, surgery, and gynaecology at Johns Hopkins, up to the days of my residency, included six to twelve months of laboratory pathology in their respective specialities. Kelly wrote in 1912: "It was anaesthesia which robbed surgery of its horrors, asepsis which robbed it of its dangers and cellular pathology which came as a godsend to enable the operator to discriminate between malignant and non-malignant growth.[4]

In North America, surgical procedures became widely accepted after the introduction of ether anaesthesia in 1842 (Georgia, US) and 1846 (Boston), the practice of antisepsis with carbolic spray of the operative site (Lister 1865), and asepsis following Semmelweis 1847–48 and 1861, who proved the contagiousness of puerperal fever (later known to be streptococcal infection after childbirth) and its prevention through rigorous cleansing of the hands of surgeons and surgical nurses, scrubbing of operating rooms, and sterilization of surgical instruments, drapes, and clothing.

In 1894, at the Johns Hopkins Hospital, one of Kelly's residents in gynaecology, Hunter Robb, was training with the chief of surgery, William Halstead, and observed that Halstead's operating room nurse and surgical assistants wearing rubber gloves. Halstead had ordered the gloves from the Goodyear Rubber Company, made with long cuffs for covering the forearm to prevent allergic dermatitis of their hands and forearms caused by the strong antiseptic solutions used in preparing the patient's skin at the operative site and for disinfecting the assistants' hands prior to surgery. While Halstead was the first to use rubber gloves in the operating room to prevent dermatitis of the operator and assistants, it was Robb, the gynaecologist, who had a special interest in aseptic techniques and published a book on the subject in 1894, in which he was the first to recommend the regular use of rubber gloves by the operator in order to prevent wound infection.

In 1856, Duncan C. MacCallum (1824–1904), a McGill graduate of 1850 and a demonstrator in anatomy at McGill since 1854, was appointed visiting physician to the MGH. At McGill he also held the positions of professor of clinical surgery, 1856–60; professor of clinical medicine, 1860–67, and professor of midwifery and diseases of women, 1868–83. From 1868 to 1883, as professor of midwifery at McGill, he was also in charge of the University Lying-in Hospital, where most of the MGH physicians who practised midwifery/obstetrics admitted their patients for delivery.

The first specialist in gynaecology at the MGH was William Gardner (1842–1926). In 1883, following his peculiar appointment as gynaecologist at the MGH and professor of gynaecology at McGill with no surgical training, he spent six months in England during 1885 learning abdominal surgery. In 1889, Johnston Alloway was the first assistant gynaecologist to Gardner. In that same year, the MGH governors discussed the possibility of amalgamating with the Royal Victoria Hospital, but nothing came of it. In 1893, William Gardner resigned from the MGH and joined the RVH as gynaecologist-in-chief in 1895.

The first separate listing of gynaecological diseases in the MGH annual reports occurred in 1895. The chief causes of death among patients treated in the Department of Gynaecology were haemorrhage, shock, peritonitis, and septicaemia. In 1898, the amended by-laws of the MGH stated: "no one is eligible to the office of Gynaecologist unless he confines his public and private practice exclusively to his special department of medicine or surgery." Specialization was gradually taking place, and the rules were being laid out.

John D. Cameron (1852–1912) joined the gyn department in 1898. The 1903 annual report shows that 1,172 patients were treated in the gyn outdoor clinic. In 1904, there were seven abdominal hysterectomies and one vaginal hysterectomy. A glance at the 1902 annual report of the MMH shows 209 deliveries and three maternal deaths due to eclampsia, sepsis, and postpartum haemorrhage.

In 1906, Herbert M. Little ("Butch" to his colleagues) was appointed to the gyn service as assistant gynaecologist. He had undergone graduate training with Professor Whitridge Williams at the Johns Hopkins Hospital in Baltimore. Williams was a world-renowned professor of obstetrics and author of a *Textbook of Obstetrics*, which is now in its twenty-first edition and still the gold standard for medical students and obstetrical residents. In 1906, there were fourteen abdominal hysterectomies and one vaginal hysterectomy. In 1907, F.A.L. Lockhart was named gynaecologist, and in 1912 there were 113 gynaecologic operations, including twenty-four dilatations and curettages.

RVH Provided Obstetrics before MGH in New Maternity Pavilion 1926

By 1923, the RVH sensed the medical, educational, and safety advantages of offering full obstetrical services within a general hospital and invited the MMH to amalgamate with it at the RVH site.

In 1926, a new maternity pavilion was constructed and named the Royal Victoria Montreal Maternity Hospital (RVMMH), with one hundred obstetrical and gynaecological teaching beds. To ensure that McGill's medical faculty and medical students would have continued access to obstetric and gynaecologic patients for teaching purposes, and to avoid the earlier situation that had occurred in MacNider's Montreal Lying-in Hospital – namely, a prohibition of McGill students – McGill and the RVH made an amalgamation agreement that the professor of Obs/Gyn at McGill would, ipso facto, be the chief of the RVMMH. This had some political connotations for any future MGH chief of Obs/Gyn who might aspire to the McGill departmental chair. It would force his or her relocation to the RVMMH, or "the Mat," as it was commonly known by medical students and residents. The Mat continues as a major provider of health care services for women and newborns, and as a teaching and research unit of McGill's Department of Obstetrics and Gynaecology. Seang Lin Tan was professor and chair of McGill's Department of Obstetrics and Gynaecology and obstetrician and gynaecologist-in-chief of the RVMMH.

The origins of the MGH were largely initiated by loyal women volunteers whose current successors continue their outstanding volunteer services to the hospital. It is ironic that obstetrics, one of the unique services for women, had not been made available in the MGH until 103 years following its introduction at the Montreal Lying-in Hospital and eighteen years after obstetrical services were introduced at the RVH.

To be fair, there had been a desire and mounting pressure by the medical staff of the MGH for increased accommodations for patients in general. In 1919, following the First World War, the minutes of the Medical Board state: "The Board deplores the lack of financial support from governments and the lack of adequate beds for private and semi-private Patients and suggests the need for a private pavilion at the Western Hospital Site."[5] In 1920, the MGH Board of Management made a decision to amalgamate with the Western Hospital (now the Montreal Children's Hospital) on Atwater Street at Dorchester (now René Lévesque Blvd) and establish a separate medical board at the site. In 1924, the Board of Management renamed the MGH and the Western Hospital as the Central Division of the MGH and the Western Division (the Western) of the MGH, respectively.

Combined McGill University Department of Obstetrics and Gynaecology, 1912

In 1912, McGill's Faculty of Medicine amalgamated the departments of Obs/Gyn under Walter Chipman (1866–1950). He was a graduate of Edinburgh and had done graduate studies there before coming to the RVH. He was also the physician accoucheur of the MMH and had succeeded William Gardner as professor of gynaecology in 1910. The combined university department of Obs/Gyn was a major advance in the teaching program at McGill and raised its status to the level of medicine and surgery. Chipman became one of the great leaders in McGill's medical history.

In 1913, patients were moved into the new section of the MGH. There were 169 gynaecological operations, including nineteen abdominal hysterectomies and one vaginal hysterectomy. Lockhart and Little are listed as specialists. The gyn outpatient clinic treated 1979 patients. D. Patrick was appointed assistant gynaecologist in 1914, and C.C. Birchard as junior assistant gynaecologist in 1915.

With the First World War under way in 1915, thirty-three doctors from the MGH were already enlisted in the armed forces and moved to the front, along with fifty-one graduate nurses and twenty-eight orderlies. That year, 239 gynaecologic operations were recorded. T.H. Lennox and Douglas Gurd were appointed junior assistants in 1916. In 1919, the Medical Board deplored the lack of financial support from governments and the lack of adequate beds for private and semi-private patients.

In 1920, the board next decided to amalgamate the MGH with the Western Hospital. It suggested the need for a private pavilion at the Western site. In 1921, A.D. Campbell and Ivan Patrick were appointed junior assistant gynaecologists. In 1922, G.J. McMurtry was appointed to the same position. In 1923, the amalgamation of the MGH and the Western, as well as their individual schools of nursing, occurred.

In 1925, F.A. Lockhart, the chief gynaecologist at the MGH, died of tetanus after serving the MGH for thirty years. H.M. Little was named gynaecologist-in-chief; Charles C. Gurd FRCS (Edin) gynaecologist; D. Patrick associate gynaecologist; and A.D. Campbell, Ivan Patrick, C.D. Robbins, and

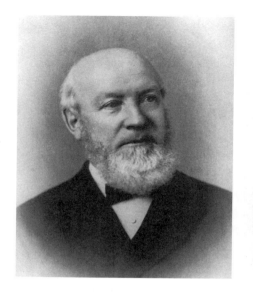
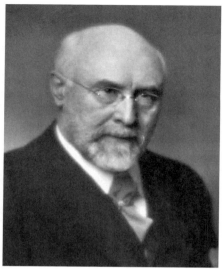
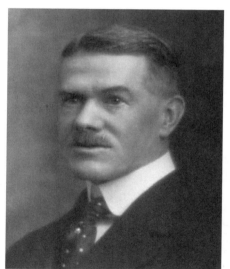
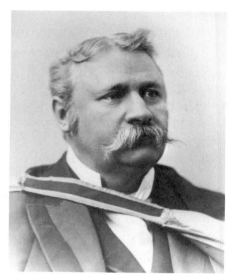

Clockwise from top left
Fig. 27.1 Duncan MacCallum, professor of midwifery and diseases of women, 1868–83
Fig. 27.2 William Gardner, gynaecologist-in-chief, 1883–93
Fig. 27.3 John Galloway, gynaecologist-in-chief, 1893–97
Fig. 27.4 F.A. Lochart

Eleanor Percival assistant gynaecologists. Percival was the first female gynaecologist at the MGH.

In 1926, a joint committee of the MGH, the RVH, and the Board of
Governors of McGill was appointed "to undertake the coordination of the
planning, building, teaching, patient accommodation etc and to assist in
the completion of RVH MMH Pavilion." It was finished in June 1926, adding
to the RVH medical campus. In 1927, the MGH and the RVH established
reciprocal admitting privileges for their attending staffs at the Ross Pavilion
for private patients.

Also in 1927, the Medical Board sent Eleanor Percival, assistant gynaecologist, to Vienna, Paris, and Stockholm for further study in radiotherapy, with
the expenses paid out of the R.G. Campbell Memorial Fund. She was the first
to use radium for treatment of uterine cancer in the hospital in 1928.

In 1928, a motion, directed to the MGH Board of Management, was put
forward at the Medical Board by H.M. Little, chief of gynaecology, expressing the urgent need for a private pavilion at the Western, which made sense
for the MGH staff. The medical staffs of the Central and Western divisions
were finally amalgamated under one Medical Board in 1929. Appointments
in that year were William Gardener to consulting staff and C.D. Robbins
as junior assistant. The year saw 682 gynaecology patients admitted to the
Central Division and 161 to the Western Division.

Friendly Rivalry between MGH and RVH and Medical Politics – A Tradition

The naming of the chairs and heads of clinical departments in McGill's Faculty of Medicine has always been food for speculation regarding whether the
MGH or the RVH chiefs would be favoured. In 1929, when Walter Chipman
stepped down as chair of the Department of Obstetrics and Gynaecology at
McGill and chief at the RVMMH, there was great expectation at the MGH
that Herbert Little, chief at the MGH, would be named as the new McGill
chair. Much to the chagrin of the medical staff at the MGH, the governors
of McGill and the RVH had another preference. John R. Fraser was appointed to succeed Walter Chipman as chair of the McGill Department of
Obstetrics and Gynaecology and chief of the RVMMH. The MGH medical
staff members expressed their sentiments in the following resolution, passed
unanimously by the MGH Medical Board in 1930:

It has been the hope and expectation of this Board that H.M. Little, because of his seniority and conspicuous services to this hospital and the University, would in time succeed to the Chairmanship of the Department of Obs/Gyn in McGill University; and because this Board deplores the decision of the Governors of the University: Be it resolved that the Medical Board reaffirms its full confidence in Little as Gynaecologist to this Hospital and its highest personal regard for him, coupled with the hope that he will continue unabated, his skilful services to his department and his support in the councils of this Board.

It was resolved that this be inscribed in the minutes and a copy transmitted to the Board of Management, which approved the resolution.

The obvious disappointment of Herbert Little and his MGH colleagues, on being bypassed for the McGill University Chair of Obstetrics and Gynaecology would be somewhat assuaged by a subsequent event. Fifty-four years later, in 1983, "Butch" Little's McGill- and Harvard-trained son, Brian Little, was appointed professor and chair of McGill's Department of Obstetrics and Gynaecology and was named obstetrician and gynaecologist-in-chief at the RVH.

In 1931, the MGH Medical Board approved the Report of the Building Committee and recommended the construction of a private pavilion at the Western, estimated cost $1,375,000. Construction began with renovations to the Outpatient Department at the Western. In 1931, the MGH House Committee declared that it was not necessary to undertake liability insurance at $1,500 per year "since any claims against the hospital are invariably unjustified." How times have changed!

The 1932 report of the Radium Therapy Department listed thirty new cases of "Malignant Diseases" of Female Genital Organs treated, forty-six breast and one hundred non-malignant gynaecology cases. A.D. Campbell published a paper in the *Lancet* entitled "Further Study of Anterior Pituitary-like Hormones." A year later, Campbell published papers entitled "Endocrine Therapy in Menstrual Disorders" and "The Damaged Birth Canal and Its Repair."

Private Patient Pavilion Opened at Western Division of the MGH, 1934

On 9 October 1934, the Private Patient Pavilion at the Western Division of the MGH at the Western Division of the MGH was formally opened by Governor General Earl Bessborough and, using the flour completed floors, was opened for patients on 17 October. There was still talk of "the acute dearth of beds for Gynecology and other departments and long waiting lists in the Admitting Office." In October 1934, the Board of Management reported the untimely death, due to a coronary thrombosis, of Herbert M. Little, the chief of the MGH Department of Gynaecology since 1924. Archibald D Campbell, better known to his colleagues as "A.D.," succeeded the late Herb Little as chief of the department in December 1934. In 1934, Kenneth T. MacFarlane joined the department as junior assistant obstetrician–gynaecologist. private and semi-private admitting privileges were finally given to junior assistant and assistant members of the department in their own names.

Limited Obstetrics Opens at the MGH in 1934 under Protest of the RVH

In May 1932, the MGH Medical Board suggested that obstetrical services be included in the plans for the new Private Western Pavilion, with the cost not to exceed nine thousand dollars. This recommendation was promptly approved by the MGH Board of Management the following month. One month later, the superintendent of MGH received a letter from the RVH superintendent regarding the decision to provide facilities for obstetric patients at the Private Patients Pavilion of the MGH Western Division. It read: "The Governors of the RVH deprecated the possible duplication of services and accommodation already provided in the RVH Montreal Maternity Hospital." It should be noted that, over the years, the RVH has repeatedly challenged the MGH's right to develop its own services as a competitive move.

In January 1934, the Joint Hospital Board (MGH, RVH, and McGill) requested a definition of the "cases of complications of pregnancy" as referred to in the MGH recommendation of July 1932. Responding to this letter in February 1934, the MGH Board of Management reassured the RVH and clarified the definition of obstetrical cases to be admitted to the Western as "such cases as are considered by those members of the staff, confining their practice to Gynaecology and Obstetrics, requiring the cooperation of other departments of the hospital for example Nephritis or such cases referred to that department by members of the staff for special co-operation and investigation, for example cardiac disease complicating pregnancy" … [T]his new private facility at the Western was only intended to enable Medical Staff of MGH to bring to a conclusion cases with complications of pregnancy and

there is no intention to compete with the RVH in simple obstetrical cases."
MGH obstetricians, caring for high-risk obstetrical patients also suffering
from diabetes or cardiac, renal, and other diseases complicating pregnancy,
were very happy with this decision, which brought obstetrical and other
specialist consultants under the same roof for improved patient safety and
convenience. Physicians at both sites would have equal rights and privileges
in all the private and semi-private wards of both hospitals. This limited
private obstetrical service at the Western Division was opened in 1934.

Private Gynaecology Introduced at Western Division of the MGH, 1935

In 1935, the ninth floor of the new Private Pavilion at the Western Division
opened for gyn patients. The Final Report from the Building Committee
of the Private Pavilion indicated that there would be thirteen floors, with
ORs on the tenth floor and obstetrics and newborn nurseries on the ninth.
Douglas W. Sparling joined the staff as clinical assistant in 1937, and Eleanor
Percival advanced to associate status. The schedule of private hospital room
charges ranged from $4.50 to twelve dollars per day. There was approval to
hold the annual meeting of the American Gynecological Association at the
MGH facilities in February 1938. In that year, 909 gyn patients were admit-
ted and 6,996 gyn patients treated in the Outpatient Department.

Full Obstetrical Service Opens at Western Division of the MGH, 1944

In 1944, ten years after the MGH Medical Board had recommended that a
full obstetrical service be planned, and in response to strong patient demand,
the MGH Board of Management decided to undertake the construction of
an obstetrical and newborn facility on the ninth floor of the Private Pavilion of the Western.

Consequently, as the Second World War was winding down in 1944, this
eighteen-bed private obstetrical and newborn nursery service was opened
in the Private Patient Pavilion of the Western Division of the MGH. This
marked the beginning of full obstetrical services at the MGH. In 1943, with
30 percent of the MGH attending staff serving in the armed forces, there was
an acute staff shortage. The hospital requested that two surgeons and one
ENT specialist be recalled from the armed forces to serve the hospital.

Colonel Cliff Ward and Major Doug Sparling were recalled from the armed forces to resume duties at the MGH in 1944. K.T. MacFarlane and D. Sparling were each promoted to associate obstetricians and gynaecologists, and D. Gurd and Robbins were promoted to assistant status. A.D. Campbell was appointed chair of the Radium Therapy Committee.

Name Changed to Department of Gynaecology and Obstetrics, 1944

With a full obstetrical service finally available at the Western Division, the Department of Gynaecology changed its name to the Department of Gynaecology and Obstetrics. Obstetrical services had never been provided at the hospital's Central Division.

In 1945, the Joint Hospital Commission recommended a consolidation of the Central Division and the Western Division of the MGH in a new building on a new site. J. Lorne MacArthur was appointed junior assistant gynaecologist and obstetrician. It was also a lucky year for MGH resident staff as the hospital began paying them a stipend of twenty-five dollars per month. Rotating interns were not so lucky as they were excluded from this largesse. W.J. Friesen and James H. Routledge were appointed junior assistant gynaecologist and obstetricians in 1946 and 1947, respectively.

RVH Protests Inclusion of Obstetrics in New MGH on Cedar Ave, 1955

In 1948, the MGH Medical Board and Board of Management discussed a suggestion by the Joint Hospital Commission for a merger of the RVH, the MGH, and the Children's Memorial Hospital at the RVH site, but this was turned down; instead, approval was given to rebuild the MGH on a new site. The Cross Estate on the south side of the mountain was purchased, and a campaign committee was appointed to raise funds. That same year, A.D. Campbell, chief of gynaecology and obstetrics, was awarded five hundred dollars from the Medical Board Research Fund to investigate the value of cytology in the diagnosis of cancer of the female genital tract. C.J. Pattee, an endocrinologist, was appointed as an assistant in the Department of Gynaecology and Obstetrics.

In 1949, there was much debate over the pros and cons of the newly chosen site for a new MGH and over whether the Capital Campaign, an MGH

public fund raising venture, would succeed. The city helped make the decision by expropriating the front sections of the buildings of the old MGH site
in order to widen Dorchester Street (now Blvd. René Lévesque). Thus, the
completely out-of-date central facility, along with the Joint Commission's
suggestion that a new hospital combining the Central and Western divisions
be constructed, made it obvious to all that something had to be done. That
year, 1,591 inpatients and 3,547 outpatients were treated in the gynaecological service.

In 1950, A.D. Campbell stepped down as chief and was appointed as consulting staff. "A.D." left a colourful and impressive history. He always re-
minded people of his rural background, having been raised on an early
pioneer farm in southwest Ontario by his Scottish parents and, later, graduating from McGill Medical School in 1911. He had served overseas in the
First World War with the Canadian General Hospital No. 3, together with his
colleagues Herbert Little and John McCrae (author of "In Flanders Fields").
Campbell published some thirty papers and two books as well as contributing to four other books. He teamed up with J.B. Collip at McGill. Collip was
famous for purifying insulin and was exploring the anterior pituitary-like
hormone in women and placentas. In the 1930s, Campbell delivered most
babies at home, as was customary. His surgical technique for vaginal hysterectomy was widely known. Campbell was elected president of the American Association of Obstetricians and Gynecologist. Clifford Ward succeeded
A.D. Campbell as the new chief of gynaecology and obstetrics in 1950. Peter
R. Blahey was appointed junior assistant that same year.

In 1951, Evan A MacCallum was appointed junior assistant and, after several years in a successful ob/gyn practice, was appointed the director of professional services at MGH in 1968. Also in 1951, several RVH obstetricians
and gynaecologists were appointed to the MGH staff, including: S.S. Henry,
G.C. Melhado, and G.A. Simpson as associates as well as W.R. Foote, George
B. Maughan, Hilary B. Bourne, James R. Dodds, Grace C. Donnelly, Myer
Hendleman, J.P.A. Latour, Harry Oxhorn, Thomas Primrose, F.J. Tweedie,
and M.H. Vincent Young. In 1952, N.W. Philpott from the RVH was appointed a consultant. The Medical Board recommended that all medical staff
of the RVMHl who were not already on the MGH staff be so appointed.

In the summer of 1951, Basil MacLean, a building consultant commenting on the proposed MGH building on Cedar Avenue, stated that he "deprecated the planned duplication of obstetrical facilities already at RVMMH."
At the same time, the RVH president submitted a proposal through the Joint

Hospitals Committee asking "that the plans to include obstetrical services in the new MGH on Cedar Avenue, that would duplicate those at the RVH, be held in abeyance to be discussed at the Joint Hospital Committee."[6] A member of the Joint Committee suggested a reduction of obstetrical beds from thirty-nine to nineteen, and Basil MacLean countered with thirty-nine beds, which would include a certain proportion of public beds. Another resolution from Joint Committee would have all obstetrics and gynaecology in both hospitals relocated to the RVMMH Pavilion. In the end, the MGH Medical Board and the Board of Management elected to protect MGH obstetrics and gynaecology and not to accept the above proposals, which would have eliminated obstetrics. They instructed the MGH Building Committee to proceed on the basis of its original plan for thirty-nine obstetrical beds with some public beds and two nursing units.

In 1952, the Board of Management stated that cost reductions must be made in the planned construction costs of the new hospital to be built on Cedar Avenue but that "the obstetrical unit must be retained." The board also decided that, in view of the RVH decision to start paying the intern and resident staff, the MGH would do likewise and would pay interns twenty-five dollars per month, junior assistants forty dollars, assistant residents sixty dollars, and residents one hundred dollars.

In 1953, Premier Maurice Duplessis laid the cornerstone for the new MGH on the mountain, and A.H. Westbury was appointed executive director and William Storrar medical director.

In 1954, P.N. MacDermot was appointed associated paediatrician in charge of the newborn nursery. That year yielded 678 newborn babies and 2,538 gyn operations. This was the first year that the Department of Obstetrics and Gynaecology presented its own separate report in the MGH annual reports. Papers were published by C.C. Lindsay ("Potassium Permanganate as an Abortifacient"); K.T. MacFarlane ("Uterine Inertia, Toxemia of Pregnancy and Management of Ovarian Tumors"); J.H. Routledge ("The Pelvic Anatomic Nervous System"); and C.V. Ward and R.M. Parsons ("A Five-Year Analysis of Breech Presentations").

Obstetrics and Gynaecology Flourish under One Roof on Cedar Avenue, 1955

On 30 May 1955, the new MGH was finished and ready to be occupied. It was a nine-hundred-bed, twenty-story building on Cedar Avenue on the south side of Mount Royal. Now the Central and Western divisions were consolidated in a modern state-of-the-art facility. Sixty-five patients from the Western Division and 103 from the Central Division were transferred by ambulance and moving vans to the new mountain site "without any untoward incident" all in one week.

That same year D.C. Crawford Lindsay was appointed junior assistant in Obs/ Gyn. In October of that year the president and representatives of the Johns Hopkins Hospital in Baltimore toured the new MGH and renewed their historic link, forged by the most famous son of the MGH and the McGill Medical School, William Osler, who became the founding professor and chief of medicine at Johns Hopkins in 1889.

In 1956, Winnifred Ross was appointed junior assistant and George B. Maughan was appointed as consulting Obs/Gyn. C.V. Ward published "Uterine Prolapse and Procedures for Operative Treatment" and "Carcinoma of the Uterine Corpus," while K.T. Macfarlane published "Ectopic Pregnancy and Obstetrical Problems." There were 2,092 babies delivered and 2,421 patients treated in the gyn outpatient clinic.

In 1958, there were 3,066 in-patients treated in gynaecology and 2,363 outpatients. In January it was reported that the obstetrics service was fully booked for eight months. K.T. MacFarlane was elected honorary treasurer of the Royal College of Physicians and Surgeons of Canada. Doug Sparling served on the Program Committee of the American College of Obstetricians and Gynaecologists, and Eleanor Percival was appointed to honorary attending staff.

In 1959, C.V. Ward retired and Kenneth T. MacFarlane was appointed obstetrician-gynaecologist-in-chief of the MGH, effective 1 September 1959. In 1960, Darryl E. Townsend was appointed junior assistant and Eleanor Percival was named to the consulting staff in addition to the honorary staff.

With the proposed introduction of the Quebec Hospital Insurance Act, the MGH Board met with government officials to obtain details of the new plan, which would pay the full cost of public ward beds. One member of the board "pointed out that this [was] a misnomer since no insurance is involved."

In 1960, the Quebec government enacted the Quebec Hospital Insurance Act, which established the first part of what is informally known as Medicare. This tax-based and government-controlled universal hospital insurance plan entitled all residents of Quebec to standard ward hospital services for medically required services. It also banned alternative, private hospital insurance for services covered by the public plan and prohibited private medical services in hospitals. However, it permitted the purchase of private and semi-private room accommodation. Later that year, the MGH Board noted that "the demand for hospital accommodation had shown a tremendous increase, no doubt influenced by the free government insurance plan."

In 1962, John M. Elder was appointed assistant paediatrician and John S. Henry, L David Rhea, and R. Peter Beck were promoted. The board reported that, since the government hospital insurance plan has been in effect, the hospital deficit has grown to $791,000. J. Edwin Coffey, having completed the four-year residency training program in gynaecology and obstetrics under Professors Eastman, Telinde, and Barnes at the Johns Hopkins Hospital in 1962, was awarded a Hosmer Teaching Fellowship at the MGH. In 1963, he was appointed to the MGH attending staff as junior assistant obstetrician and gynaecologist.

In 1964, there were 1,390 patients on a waiting list for admission to the MGH; 3,159 patients were admitted to the gynaecology and obstetrics services of the hospital, and 2,924 gynaecologic patients were treated in the gynaecology clinic. J.E. Coffey received a research grant worth six hundred dollars, and K.T. MacFarlane was elected president of the Society of Obstetricians and Gynaecologists of Canada.

In 1965, there were 3,205 patients treated in the gynaecology clinic and 3,077 in-patients treated by gynaecologic and obstetric services. In the gynaecologic tumour clinic, directed by P.R. Blahey, 127 new cases were registered. Norman Buka and Jean Blanchet were promoted. As a representative of the Royal College of Physicians and Surgeons of Canada, K.T. MacFarlane presented the new Canadian flag to the American College of Obstetricians and Gynecologists at its annual meeting in San Francisco, and J.E. Coffey was elected and recognized as the ten thousandth fellow of the American College of Obstetricians and Gynecologists.

In 1966, the MGH Board of Management noted an increasing deficit of $2,750,000 owed to the Quebec Hospital Insurance Board: this was an increase of $1,959,000 since 1962. The government refused to cover it. There were 1,559 patients on the hospital's waiting list for admission. There was a plan for opening twenty-two public obstetrical beds on 7 East with a premature newborn bursary to enable most of the care of premature babies to be provided on site. This would reduce the number of transfers of premature babies to the MCH. K.T. MacFarlane indicated that he would be stepping down as chief at the end of 1967. A selection committee was struck, and there was some discussion over the possibility of naming a joint chief of Obs/Gyn for the MGH and the RVH.

In June 1967, the Board of Management announced the appointment of Robert H. Kinch as the new chief of the Department of Obstetrics and Gynaecology, effective 1 January 1968. In the fall of 1967, the new construction on 7 East for the premature nursery and public obstetric beds was costing $100,000. The board met with officials of the Quebec Hospital Insurance Plan concerning the $5.5 million hospital debt and set up a budget control committee. K.T. MacFarlane was named to consulting staff effective January 1968, and John M. Elder was appointed director of neonatal nursery with Brock Dundas as assistant director.

In 1969, Robert J. Seymour completed his residency training in Obs/Gyn at the University of Texas in Galveston and was appointed assistant obstetrician and gynaecologist at the MGH. Evan MacCallum, obstetrician and gynaecologist, was appointed as the MGH Medical director in May 1968. Department statistics for 1968 show 3,172 patients admitted in Obs/Gyn, 4,446 patients treated in the gynaecology clinic, and 1,498 babies born. Robert J. Seymour was associate professor, McGill, Department of Obstetrics and Gynaecology.

In April 1969, the director of nursing, Isobel MacLeod, reported difficulty in keeping new graduates of the Nursing School due to cutbacks in MGH nursing positions. Nursing School education in Quebec would be taken over by the Colleges d'Enseignment Generale et Practiques, starting in 1970. Amendments to the Criminal Code in March 1969 required that each hospital set up a therapeutic abortion committee consisting of three members of the Department of Obstetrics and Gynaecology, of which one should be the chief of Ob/Gyn, one should be from psychiatry, and one from medicine. In 1969, there were 4,975 gyn patients admitted, 1,539 deliveries, and 4,975 patients treated in the gynaecology clinic.

In 1970, Ann Macaulay was appointed as associate paediatrician and research assistant, and Pamela Fitzhrdinge and John Katiela were appointed as assistant paediatricians. During 1970, the Quebec residents and interns carried out a temporary withdrawal of services, asking Quebec's government for salary parity with their Ontario counterparts. In March 1970, the Board of Management appointed J.E. Coffey to the Protocol Committee of the MGH's 150th anniversary (sesquicentennial) committee. In spite of the steadily increasing number of Ob/Gyn admissions to the hospital, the executive of the Medical Board noted "the low admission rate in the Department of Ob/Gyn." In 1968, there were 4,446 gynaecologic patients admitted.

Quebec Health Insurance Act Brings Medicare to Quebec, 1970

The year 1970 saw the enactment of the Quebec Health Insurance Act, being the second part of the public medical and hospital insurance program informally known as Medicare. This popular tax-based program of universal entitlement to government-funded and controlled medical and hospital insurance, for medically required services, had some unusual features. One was the government's prohibition of private medical and hospital insurance and private medical services in hospitals with regard to those services covered by the public medicare insurance but not always accessible to patients. This feature was unique among the OECD countries and would be challenged several decades later and found invalid by the Supreme Court of Canada.

This Medicare legislation created a major dispute with the Federation of Medical Specialists (FMSQ) in Quebec, leading to withdrawal of services in the fall of 1970. Crawford Lindsay, of the MGH Department of Obstetrics and Gynaecology, was a member of the FMSQ executive and played a significant role in the FMSQ's unsuccessful efforts to convince the Bourassa government to withdraw those sections in the pending Quebec Health Insurance Act that prohibited individual choice (by patients and physicians) regarding alternative private funding and insurance of medical and hospital services – a prohibition that they saw as infringing upon their personal freedom and security. All this occurred in the midst of Quebec's 1970 FLQ terrorist crisis, which included the bombing of mailboxes and government buildings, the kidnapping British consul James Cross, and the murder of Quebec labour minister Pierre Laporte.

During the short-lived specialists' dispute, the Ob/Gyn attending staff of the MGH and associated McGill hospitals set up a volunteer roster to successfully handle all obstetrical and gynaecological emergencies. The dispute ended when the provincial government threatened back-to-work legislation. More important, it marked the beginning of an outward migration by many Quebec specialists, who could not handle the province's threats, to other provinces or the United States.

In 1970, Peter Gillett was appointed to the MGH attending staff as assistant Obs/Gyn, Simpson and Foote were appointed consulting specialists, and Oxorn, Latour, Bourne, Dodds, Donnelly, and Hendelman, who were mainly based at the RVH, resigned from the MGH department. Nineteen seventy-one was the year of the MGH's 150th anniversary. The Anniversary Committee, chaired by Ross Hill, issued a call among the hospital community for suggestions for a special project to mark the occasion. The representative on the committee from the Department of Obstetrics and Gynaecology, Edwin Coffey, suggested that the MGHs sixth-floor amphitheatre be refurbished and named "the Osler Amphitheatre." The reasoning behind the suggestion was as follows: During his residency training at the Johns Hopkins Hospital, Coffey was impressed by the way Hopkins had honoured Sir William Osler. As its most famous physician and teacher, and as its founding professor and its chief of medicine in 1889, the hospital later named the Hopkins Medical Service and building in his honour. It seemed fitting that, since the MGH had been the foundation of McGill's medical school, from which Osler graduated, and was the hospital where he first practised as a physician, teacher, and researcher, it should now honour the name of its most illustrious physician. The Anniversary Committee agreed. Joe Stratford, who was in charge of the event, invited Coffey to participate in the dedication ceremony and to welcome another famous physician and McGill neurosurgeon, Wilder Penfield, a graduate of Johns Hopkins Medical School, founder of the Montreal Neurological Institute, and former friend of Sir William Osler. Penfield graciously dedicated the newly named MGH Osler Amphitheatre and cut the ribbon.

On a more serious note, in 1971, as required by provincial law, the board set up a therapeutic abortion committee. This committee had the following members: D. Sparling (chair), K.T. MacFarlane, and C.C. Lindsay as well as one psychiatrist and one internist.

The Medical Board examined the new Quebec's Bill 65, which reorganized all hospitals and hospital boards, prescribing a new structure of governance and taking complete control of hospital function and policy. The board's summary of Bill 65 reads as follows: "It would seem to suffocate any future interest on the part of capable private citizens being on the Board of a hospital, with the Boards becoming simply a protection for the Government, rather than the community."[8] No one had any idea if such a dramatic change of control relating to all aspects of hospital management would ever work, but the choices were either to work with the system or to leave the province.

The director of nursing was alarmed by the shortfall in the number of entering nursing students due to the French language requirements and to the government cuts in the number of staff. These were real problems and seriously affected the recruitment and retention of nurses. Meanwhile, Beverly Murphy, a medical biochemist, was given a dual appointment as assistant Ob/Gyn. Anne MacCaulay, T. Primrose, Irene Simons, F. Tweedie, and M.A.V. Young were appointed to affiliate status, and Chan Yip and A. Cowan were appointed assistant paediatricians.

Storm Clouds Form in 1973: Rationing of Obstetrical Services Planned

In 1971, a Quebec government-appointed committee made a report, with recommendations, on the state of the obstetrical and newborn care and mortality figures in Quebec hospitals providing obstetrical services. The McGill hospitals had two representatives on the committee from the RVH and none from the MGH. The member of the committee compared the perinatal mortality rates (newborn deaths per ten thousand live births) with the number of live births per year in each hospital for the years 1967 to 1969. The fewest newborn deaths occurred in hospitals with 1,501 to two thousand births per year. In hospitals with more than two thousand births, the mortality was slightly higher, as it was in those slightly below 1,501 births. However, in hospitals having fewer than one thousand deliveries, the newborn death rate was considerably higher. The early recommendation suggested that obstetrical units with fewer than one thousand births per year should try to amalgamate with another obstetrical unit. A later recommendation from the Quebec committee suggested that obstetrical units should regroup to attain a unit having two thousand deliveries per year minimum, in spite of the above figures showing that the ideal number of deliveries was between 1,501 and two thousand per year. In 1970, the MGH had 1,469 births – well above the more generally accepted lower benchmark of one thousand births per year.

With the general birthrate in Quebec falling, and the government determined to seek all possible cost-cutting measures in hospitals, the less productive obstetrical units came under pressure from budget administrators (both outside and inside the hospitals) looking for cost-saving measures. Consequently, the next storm cloud to sweep over the MGH in 1973 came in the form of a message from the Ministry of Health to the MGH Board of

Management stating that the number of obstetrical beds in Montreal would be reduced. Specifically: "The Catherine Booth, Queen Elizabeth and Reddy Memorial Obstetrical departments would be closed and when RVH renovations [were] complete the MGH obstetrical unit would move to the RVH; and … St Mary's, the Jewish General and Lakeshore obstetrical units would remain open."

One month later, John Patrick, the most recent Ob/Gyn appointment, requested a leave of absence and moved to Ontario. Needless to say, the morale of nurses, physicians, and other staff in the affected obstetrical units was severely shaken by this master plan of implementing closures without specific time frames and without taking into consideration the likelihood of increased numbers of obstetrical patients flowing to the MGH as the result of the other obstetrical closures nearby.

Ken Rosenfeld was appointed assistant Obs/Gyn and Bob Seymour became a senior Obs/Gyn. Seymour and M. Kirk established a colposcopy service at the MGH to investigate atypical Pap smears for early cervical cancer detection. In the same year, 1,790 babies were delivered and 2,849 gyn surgeries were performed.

In 1972, the report of the Committee of the Outpatients Department, chaired by E.C. Reid, recommended: "In view of medicare legislation the MGH will have only one standard of care for public and private patients and that facilities in Livingston Hall be made to see all patients including Ob/Gyn, Ophthalmology, Urology, etc." Doug Sparling was named to Consulting Staff and John Patrick to assistant Ob/Gyn (contingent on successful Quebec certification). In 1973, the Board of Managenemt noted continued government budget restrictions and nursing shortages that would require bed closures.

In 1975, George Maughan, Ob/Gyn chief at the RVH and chair of the McGill Department of Obstetrics and Gynaecology retired and was replaced by Fred Naftolin. Edwin Coffey was elected vice-chair of the Quebec Division of the American College of Obstetricians and Gynecologists.

Milton Leong was appointed assistant Ob/Gyn and GFT at the MGH and assistant professor at McGill in 1976. He, George Haber, and Ken Rosenfeld formed a high-risk-Perinatal team for consultation and management of high-risk obstetrics. In 1976, the department was divided into a division of obstetrics and a division of gynaecology, with Haber director of obstetrics and Seymour director of gynaecology. Peter Blahey continued to direct gynaecology oncology, and Edwin Coffey was elected president of the North

American Gynecological Society. In this same year there were 2,079 babies delivered and 2,552 gyn operations performed.

In 1977, the Obstetric Division under George Haber established an arrangement with the Jewish General Hospital and A. Papageorgiou, head of the Neonatology Service, to transfer pregnant women delivering prematurely under thirty-two weeks to the JGH for delivery and neonatal care of the infant. The total deliveries in 1977 were 1,973 with the lowest perinatal mortality rate of 8.5 per one thousand live births. In the obstetrics clinic 123 new patients were booked. The gyn clinic received 2,440 patients and 2,535 gyn operations were performed. The gyn tumour clinic under Peter Blahey treated 229 patients.

The usual volume of publications and presentations continued from department members. National and international participation of the department members was robust, with Robert Kinch, treasurer of the Royal College of Physicians and Surgeons of Canada, sitting on the Council of the American Gynecologic Society and Edwin Coffey presiding over the annual meeting the North American Gynecological Society in Washington, DC.

In 1978, Austin Gardiner was appointed assistant Obs/Gyn, along with Kenneth Rosenfeld and Milton Leong. Robert Seymour with Carolyn Freeman from radiation oncology and a medical oncologist began weekly multidisciplinary clinics for the treatment of gyn cancer patients.

The predicted long-term effects of uncertainty, cast on the future of the MGH obstetrical service by the unsubstantiated conclusion and ill-advised announcement of Quebec's Health Ministry in 1973, were now evident. There was no medical indication to recommend the closure of the top-flight MGH obstetrical service, whose perinatal mortality figures were equal to or better than those of the hospitals likely to inherit the MGH patients should the MGH unit be forced to close. The government's parallel project of closing and regrouping very small obstetrical units had some merit but did not apply to the MGH because of its reasonable volume of deliveries above one thousand and usually above fifteen hundred deliveries per year and likely to increase with the smaller obstetrical units closing. There was no financial reason to recommend closure because the MGH obstetrical unit was operating well within its budget.

In 1979, the exodus continued with L. David Rhea and M. Kirk, the pathologist on the colposcopy team, resigning. Gardiner and Viloria, pathologist, joined the colposcopy group. Fortunately, two new attending staff came on board – namely, Normand Brassard, assistant Ob/Gyn with special training in the United Kingdom in perinatology, and Andrew Mok, assistant Ob/Gyn with special training in infertility and endocrinology.

In 1980–81, Mary Halperin left the department to become a fellow in perinatology at Women's College Hospital in Toronto. Kinch, in his annual report, stated: "This brings the Obs/Gyn department to its lowest ebb of 11 attending staff members."

The name of the MGH Board of Management was changed to the Board of Management of the Montreal General Hospital Corporation. The Eleanor Percival Conference Room was opened in 1981 thanks to a bequest from her estate. She was the first woman on the attending staff of the MGH and probably the first trained gynaecological radiotherapist in Canada. One thousand five hundred and twenty babies were delivered in 1980–81.

In 1981–82, Seymour and Austin Gardiner introduced laser technology for the treatment of gyn oncology patients. Kinch wrote in his annual departmental report: "Many old rumors persist that Obstetrics will close at MGH. My department and I reiterate that there is no threat of closure and in fact we intend to expand our delivery capacity to 2,000–2,500 deliveries. We have the facility and staff to carry out this number." Statistics for 1980 show 1,520 births, a 19.6 percent Caesarean section rate, 2,284 gynaecological operations, and 4,598 patients seen in the outpatient department. Family-centred obstetrics continued to gain popularity among patients. Kinch continued to serve on many national and international associations and became president of the Montreal Medico-Chirurgical Society. Peter Gillett was named secretary treasurer of the Canadian Committee for Fertility. Robert Seymour was an honorary member of the Texas Association of Obstetricians and Gynecologists, and Edwin Coffey was appointed to the Committee of Discipline at the Professional Corporation of Physicians and Surgeons Quebec and elected secretary of the Quebec Medical Association, and secretary-treasurer of Council of Physicians and Dentists MGH.

MGH Deficit: Obstetrics within Budget but Takes the Hit and Closes, 1982

In 1981–82, the president of the board reported that "a plan de redressment" (rectification) had been presented to the health minister, without closing beds, and it was turned down. The hospital anticipated a deficit for 1981–82 of $7.3 million, and the government offered $2.5 million to cover it and required a hospital plan indicating how the MGH would reduce costs of one-half of this deficit by the end of 1982.

To help them sort out priorities in the choosing of services to be cut to meet the government's budget demands, the Board of the Hospital Centre appointed a special committee of priorities, chaired by J.H. Burgess, with two other attending staff members, L. Hampton and W. Duguid; H. Barkun from the administration; and John Sharp and Herb McLean from the Board of the Hospital Corporation. The committee's first recommendation for cost cutting included the closure of the Pregnancy Termination Unit, which had been set up as a requirement of government and provided by the Department of Obstetrics and Gynaecology.

The Ministry of Health and Social Services refused to allow closure of the Pregnancy Termination Unit, so the Board of the MGH Hospital Centre considered the Special Committee's second group of priorities, which included closure of the whole MGH obstetrical and newborn service on the seventh floor. The board referred this second proposal to the Council of Physicians and Dentists for their consideration. The Executive Committee of the Council of Physicians and Dentists was not pleased with the idea of closing down obstetrics, but it saw no ready alternative, and, with the threat of trusteeship being imposed on the hospital, the majority of the Executive Committee, with one dissenting, voted to approve the Priority Committee's proposal to close obstetrics and its newborn service. The vice president of the council's executive dissented in the decision, arguing that a matter of this magnitude should at least be taken to a special meeting of the Council of Physicians and Dentists for a full discussion of the ramifications of the proposal and ask for its general approval.

Instead, an information meeting of the Council of Physicians and Dentists was held to inform the attending staff physicians and dentists about the decision taken by their Executive Committee to approve the closure of the Department of Obstetrics and its newborn service at the MGH. The minutes record that approximately 150 physicians and dentists were present. J.W. Sharp, president of the board, and R.L. Cruess, dean of medicine at McGill, were special guests. Sharp presented the board's reason for its reluctant decision, which had been taken only after receiving the approval of the executive of the Council of Physicians and Dentists and the Medical Advisory Committee. Richard Creuss indicated that McGill would have preferred that obstetrics could have been kept at the MGH, and Ken Bentley, chair of the

Medical Advisory Committee, said that his committee had voted nine to six in favour of a slightly altered Priorities Committee recommendation.

Edwin Coffey, vice-chair of the Executive Committee of the Council of Physicians and Dentists was then invited to speak to the information meeting. He explained the reasons for his voting against the proposed closure of obstetrics at the recent meeting of the council's executive and why he had maintained that a matter of such magnitude should have been presented to a special meeting of the Council of Physicians for discussion and approval prior to the council's Executive Committee decision. The minutes recorded a "sustained round of applause" following his speech. In spite of the information status of the meeting, a motion "deploring the decision that the Board was forced to make to close the Obstetrics Service" was made and carried, with all, with the exception of three abstainers, voting in favour of the motion.

Subsequently, the Department of Obstetrics and Gynaecology appealed to the MGH Board of Directors to reconsider the closure decision and to consider an alternative money-saving plan, with closure of the gynaecology beds on 13 East and consolidation of all gynaecologic and obstetric services on the seventh floor. This would free up 13 East for other hospital uses, such as ambulatory diagnostic and surgical facilities that had been suggested as a priority item for development at the MGH. The appeal and suggested alternatives were turned down by the Board of Directors. The obstetrical and newborn units on the 7th floor were closed permanently on 30 June 1982.

Future Viability of Gynaecology and "General Hospital" Status in Jeopardy

With the unique services for women now cut in half by the loss of MGH obstetrics, and with the future of the other half of the Ob/Gyn speciality at the MGH in jeopardy, the legacy of the women of Montreal, who initiated and entrusted the original MGH concept to future generations, was severely affected. The viability of a stand-alone gynaecology department would now depend on the ability of the hospital to provide adequate resources and to recruit well qualified physicians and other professionals in a professional market in which the preference of candidates was for a combined Ob/Gyn department within a truly general hospital. Unfortunately, neither of these attributes had pertained to the MGH since 20 June 1982.

In his annual report, Robert Kinch, chief of the Department of Obstetrics and Gynaecology, decried the closure of obstetrics as follows:

The Board of Governors decided that the least difficult method of achieving the "plan de redressment" demanded by the Minister was to close our Department of Obstetrics entirely. Our department believes that this was an unwise decision and opposed it strongly on the grounds that it would have serious effects on the functioning of our Department of Ob/Gyn and would have a detrimental effect on the hospital as a whole. 1500 young families will have to find allegiance to another hospital. We will have to stop medical school teaching and our intern and resident complement will be halved. We understand there is no possibility of the Department opening again and feel that it is a matter of regret that the MGH is no longer a "general hospital."

The president of the Board of the Hospital Corporation reported that the plan of "redressment" would cut $8.7 million from the $9.1 million deficit and that the largest item would involve the closure of the MGH obstetrical unit. In September 1982, A. Hamilton, president of the Hospital Centre Board, reported that, with the cuts, the deficit would only be $1 million and that employees whose jobs had been cut would receive full pay while staying at home.

At year's end, J. Edwin Coffey was elected chair of the Council of Physicians and Dentists for 1983 and appointed as council's representative on the MGH Corporation. George Haber became chief of gynaecology at the Reddy Memorial Hospital. Robert Kinch assumed the presidency of the Association of Professors of Obstetrics and Gynaecology of Canada, and Peter Gillett continued as secretary treasurer of the Canadian Committee for Fertility Research.

Also in 1982–83, Erica Eason, Diane Provencher, and Dawn Johanson were appointed assistant Ob/Gyns. There were 4,598 gyn outpatients treated in the clinic, and 1,515 gyn operations performed. In September 1983, Barkun confirmed to the MGH Corporation that 8 million had been cut from last year's budget, mostly from the closure of obstetrics. In 1984, Barkun reported on the board's Strategic Planning Committee's recommendation that the first priority should be the renovation of the seventh floor, vacated by the closure of obstetrics, to house ambulatory surgery and diagnostic services and that the Regional Board of Montreal Hospitals had approved the expenditures for the necessary renovations.

Robert Kinch wrote his final annual report for the Department of Obstetrics and Gynaecology in 1984–85 and retired after seventeen years as chief. During his term, he accomplished much, including the academic development of the department, the organization of a foetoscopy research unit, a six-year adolescent gyn clinic at the MGH and the MCH, and a program for intrauterine transfusion for Rh sensitization for the whole of Quebec and Vermont.

Also in 1984–85, Robert Seymour was appointed director of gyn oncology for McGill. This service was, located at MGH with the cooperation of Gerald Stanimir at the RVH. Seymour was also a member of the Council of the Society of Gynaecological Oncology and an examiner in Obs/Gyn for the Royal College of Physicians and Surgeons of Canada.

In 1985, the hospital budget reported a deficit of $1.7 million but $10 million was raised by a capital campaign. The Board of the Hospital Centre indicated that the minister of health and social services would not tolerate hospital budget deficits. The presidents and CEO's of the MGH and the RVH met to study consolidations of services to reduce costs and the Ministry of Health and Social Services was positive. A joint review committee was set up.

In 1985–86, Robert Kinch was appointed professor emeritus in Obs/Gyn by McGill. Milton (Milt) Parsons retired after a long career at the MGH and the Catherine Booth Hospital. Joel Kitzner, with extra training in perinatology, was appointed assistant obstetrician gynaecologist in charge of the gyn clinic. Charmaine Roye was appointed assistant obstetrician gynaecologist. Josée Laplante was in charge of the premenstrual tension clinic. Diane Provencher left for a two-year fellowship in oncology at the University of Miami. Peter Gillett continued as director of the family planning clinic. Beverly Murphy maintained her research and prolific publication schedule in gyn endocrinology, and, in 1986, Edwin Coffey was named chair of the Canadian Medical Association's Special Committee on Professional Liability in Medicine.

In October 1986, Dan Tulchinsky was appointed Obs/Gyn-in-chief of the department. His plans were to set up a unit for in-vitro fertilization and embryo transplantation, expand the infertility and reproductive endocrinology service, and establish an in-depth research unit at the MGH. In 1987, after a few months as chief of the department, Tulchinsky resigned and returned to Boston when it became apparent that the budget constraints at the MGH would not allow for his planned development and expansion. Peter Gillett was named acting chief of the Department of Obstetrics and Gynaecology. He pointed out the department's difficulties in recruiting since the closure of obstetrics in 1982. Peter Blahey retired after a long career and his pursuit of a special interest in the treatment of cancer of the cervix and endometrium, which followed from Eleanor Percival's interest; Josée Laplante resigned and moved to Boston and Kinch went became visiting professor at the University of Texas.

Also in 1987, a menopause clinic was started. In his annual report, Gillett concluded: "When the Obstetrical unit was closed in 1982 and the hospital's Strategic Planning Committee stated that this department would be given the necessary resources to maintain itself in the forefront of its speciality, the department is again at a low point in history." In 1988, Harvey Barkun resigned as director general of the hospital.

New appointments in 1988–89 were Louise Minor as assistant Obs/Gyn and Louies O'Dea, who was appointed with the idea of setting up an in vitro fertilization service. Total gyn surgical procedures this year were 1,115, and 1,438 gyn clinic patients were treated. Several scientific publications were produced by B. Murphy and L. O'Dea.

Appointments in 1989–90 were Robert Hemmings, to run the menopause and reproductive dysfunction clinic; Michel Welt, who returned from northern Quebec; and Paul Fournier and Loretta Marcon. Resignations included Austin Gardiner; Diane Provencher, who moved across the city to Hôpital Notre Dame; and Charmaine Roye, who moved to Brantford, Ontario. There were 1,106 gyn operations and seventy-four gyn oncology patients treated.

Appointments in 1990–91 were Sophia Tchervenkov and Nancy Hughes and Debbie Cohen, pending approval of the Montreal Regional Council, which is the provincial government's agency for rationing medical personnel in Montreal. Resignations were George Haber, who went to practise in Florida, and Normand Brassard.

There were 1,106 gyn operations and 3,655 patients treated in the gyn outpatient clinic. Acting chief of the department Peter Gillett stated in the annual report that "the Department was still hampered by the inability of the MGH and McGill to appoint a Chief for Ob/Gyn." Robert Seymour, P. Bret, M. Atri, L. Guibaud, P. Gillett, and M. Senterman published a multi-authored paper entitled "Transvaginal Alcohol Sclerosis of Ovarian Cysts under Ultrasound Guidance."

Peter Gillett was finally appointed Obs/Gyn chief at MGH in 1992 and reported a period of consolidation and growth for 1991–92. One hundred new cases of invasive gyn malignancy were treated. Residents and students continued to be taught. Clinical research, although still not strongly established, also continued. Debbie Cohen became an active member of attending staff

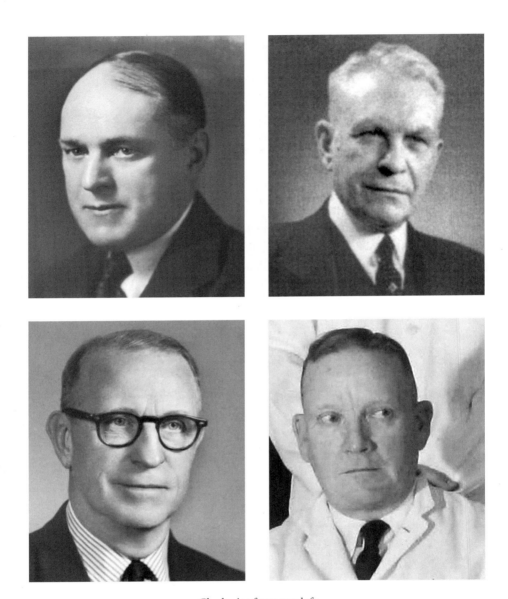

Clockwise from top left
Fig. 27.5 Herbert Little, chief of Obs/Gyn, 1924–34
Fig. 27.6 Archibald Campbell, chief of Obs/Gyn, 1934–50
Fig. 27.7 Clifford Ward, chief of Obs/Gyn, 1950–59
Fig. 27.8 Ken MacFarlane, chief of Obs/Gyn, 1959–67

and Nancy Hughes moved to Toronto. There were 3,991 patients treated in the gyn outpatient clinic. Edwin Coffey was appointed to the Canadian Medical Association's Working Group on Health System Financing in Canada.

J. Lorne Macarthur's death was cited in the 1992 annual report. Macarthur was particularly interested in obstetrics and had a large and loyal obstetrical practice, probably encouraged by his low-key, reassuring, and unhurried approach with patients. He was particularly skilled in the external version of the foetus from a breech presentation to cephalic presentation, in attempting to reduce the need for Caesarean section and/or the risks associated with a breech delivery. For many years he was in charge of the Department of Obstetrics at the Catherine Booth Hospital and, more recently, its gyn service as well. The "Booth," as it was commonly called, was originally established by the Salvation Army as a maternity residence and hospital that provided a safe haven for unwed girls in the later and more dangerous stages of pregnancy, and a safe hospital setting for delivery, with excellent follow-up care. Many of the newborns were given up for adoption. With over fifteen hundred deliveries a year and below average peri-mortality rates, it was closed by the Quebec government in 1973 as part of its cost-cutting, rationing, and centralization of obstetrical services.

In 1992–93, resignations upset the department: Mary Senterman, pathologist, who had worked with the colposcopy team, left for Ottawa; D. Joel Kizner left for Long Beach, California; Louis O'Dea moved to Boston, which resulted in the abandonment of the In-Vitro Fertilization Program at MGH. Erica Eason was chief examiner for Ob/Gyn at the Quebec Corporation of Physicians and Surgeons, and Andrew Mok became president of the Canadian Chinese Medical Society. The department ran a continuing medical education course on office practice in gynaecology and operative laparoscopy. A familial ovarian cancer clinic was started by S. Narod, Aldis, Atri, Reinhold, and Robert Seymour.

From 1992 onwards, the McGill family of teaching hospitals proceeded to discuss the proposed integration of the hospitals into the new McGill University Health Centre. In 1993–94, laparoscopic surgery was initiated in the gyn department, and Tomasso Falcone, with extra training in laparoscopy, restarted the reproductive dysfunction clinic vacated by O'Dea.

Edwin Coffey continued to serve on the Board of Directors of the Canadian Medical Association. and Louise Minor continued to serve as an examiner for the Quebec certification exam in Ob/Gyn. Erica Eason was on leave of absence, doing her master's degree in clinical epidemiology at Harvard.

In 1994, S.L. Tan was appointed Obs/Gyn-in-chief at the RVH and chair of the McGill Department of Obstetrics and Gynaecology. In 1993–94, there were 878 gyn operations, eighty patients treated for gyn malignancies, and 2,490 patients treated in the gyn clinic.

Unique Services for Women Eventually Left to the RVH

In 1994–95, closure of the Department of Gynaecology at the MGH and its merger with the Department of Obstetrics and Gynaecology at the RVH was proposed as a pilot project. At year's end, Gillett reported that serious consideration continued regarding this proposed merger at the RVH site. He was appointed director of undergraduate teaching in the Department of Obstetrics and Gynaecology at McGill.

Edwin Coffey was elected president of the Quebec Medical Association in 1994 after serving on the executive committee for several years and on the QMA Board of Directors for fifteen years. Erica Eason returned from Harvard with her MSc in clinical epidemiology and became involved with clinical research in the department.

Brian Little stepped down as chair of the Department of Obstetrics and Gynaecology at McGill and chief of Obs/Gyn at the RVH. He will be remembered for lending his support, during the early days of his McGill appointment, to the members of the MGH Department of Obstetrics and Gynaecology who, in 1984, along with a large majority of MGH physicians and surgeons, made a second unsuccessful attempt to resuscitate and preserve Obs/Gyn at the MGH.

Appointments in 1994 were Cleve Ziegler, who joined the attending staff, and Kelly Pagi, who was appointed director of the infertility program after completing a subspecialty fellowship. Resignations were John Fernandes, who left for Thunder Bay, Ontario, and Tom Falcone, who accepted a position at the Cleveland Clinic.

Outpatient gyn clinics continued to run at the MGH, with three in general gynaecology, two in colposcopy, one in reproductive dysfunction, and one in the management of vulvar disease (with Judith Cameron, dermatologist). Collaborative studies of the genetic aspects of ovarian cancer continued under the direction of R. Seymour at the MGH, and Diane Provencher and Anne-Marie Mes-Masson at Notre Dame Hospital. There were 904 gynaecological operations, 440 of them in day surgery; seventy-five

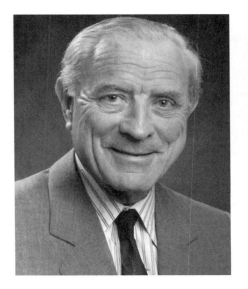

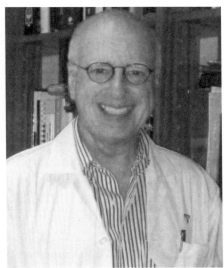

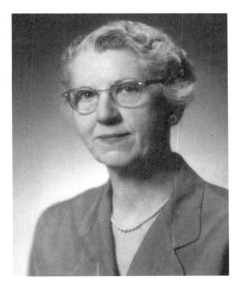

Clockwise from top left

Fig. 27.9 R.H. Kinch, chief of Obs/Gyn, 1968–86

Fig. 27.10 Peter Gillett, acting chief of Obs/Gyn, 1987–92; chief of Obs/Gyn, 1992–97

Fig. 27.11 Eleanor Percival, first woman on MGH attending staff and first gyn radio-therapist in Canada, 1925–59, when she was on the honorary staff. The Elenore Percival Conference Room opened in 1981.

patients with gynaecologic malignancies were treated, and 2,829 patients were seen in the general gyn clinic in 1994–95.

In 1996, after thirty-three years on the attending staff of the MGH, J. Edwin Coffey retired and resigned his appointments as senior Obs/Gyn at the MGH and the RVH as well as his appointment as associate professor of Obs/Gyn in the Faculty of Medicine at McGill University. He had been active in many medical organizations beyond the walls of the hospital, including the QMA, where he served on the board and Executive Committee for seventeen years and of which he was president in 1994–95. He served on the Board of Directors of the Canadian Medical Association for five years and was a Quebec delegate to the annual meeting of the CMA's General Council (the "Parliament of Canadian Medicine") from 1981 to 1997, where he promoted health system reform with greater freedom for individuals to choose alternative models of private or mixed public and private medical and hospital insurance and services.

In 1997, the MGH Board of Management approved a resolution to integrate the McGill teaching hospitals into the McGill University Health Centre, which plans to construct a "super hospital" in the Glen Yards at the foot of Decarie Boulevard. In 1998, the MGH Board reported progress in integrating the clinical departments within the MUHC.

NOTES

1 J. Hanaway and R. Cruess, *McGill Medicine*, vol. 1, *The First Half Century 1829–1885* (Montreal: McGill-Queen's University Press, 1996), 6.

2 C.V. Barrett and John R. Fraser, *The Royal Victoria Montreal Maternity Hospital 1943: The Hundredth Anniversary of the Founding of the Hospital* (Montreal: Privately published, 1943).

3 R.F. Mattingly, ed., *Telinde's Operative Gynecology* (Philadelphia: J.B. Lippencott Co., 1977), 8.

4 Montreal General Hospital, annual reports, 1857 to 1958, MUA, container 352, McLennan Library, McGill University.

5 Montreal General Hospital, Board of Management, minutes, July 1919 to March 2000, MGH Archives, MGH Board of Governors Office.

6 Montreal General Hospital, annual reports, Department of Obstetrics and Gynaecology, 1975–95, PG Gillett Office, MGH.

7 Montreal General Hospital, Board of Management, minutes (unless otherwise indicated, the following quotes are from this source).

8 Montreal General Hospital, annual reports (unless otherwise indicated following quotes are from this source).

28

Ophthalmology

Sean B. Murphy and Duncan Cowie

Sean Murphy was ophthalmologist-in-chief at the MGH and chair of the department at McGill. Duncan Cowie, a master's student in English literature, helped him with the writing of this chapter. The author, the grandson of Frank Buller, the first eye specialist in Lower Canada, gives the reader the history of MGH ophthalmology from his unique point of view. In a series of biographical sketches of the various chairs and academic leaders, the readers see how ophthalmology evolved as a clinical service interested in ocular pathology and research.

Frank Buller, 1844–1905

Although the MGH and McGill's Faculty of Medicine were established in 1819 and 1829, it was not until 1876, some forty-seven years later, that ophthalmology came to the MGH and McGill. Frank Buller, McGill's first surgical specialist, was also the first ophthalmologist at the university, and he brought with him the latest developments from Europe. Recognizing the importance of the specialty and of Buller's unique knowledge, McGill appointed him the first chair of the new Department of Ophthalmology and laryngology in 1883 – without a salary.

Born in Campbellford, Ontario, in 1844, Buller graduated from Rolfe's Medical School in Toronto (later the University of Toronto, School of Medicine). His postgraduate training was in Europe, where, for seven years, he focused on ophthalmology and laryngology. Travelling first to Berlin, he joined Von Graefe's clinic. Von Graefe had established one of Europe's leading eye clinics in 1850 and was a professor of ophthalmology at the University of Berlin.

In Germany during the Franco-Prussian War (1870–71), Buller worked as a volunteer in a German military hospital. When the war was over, he was appointed to the staff of the Graefe-Ever Hospital in Berlin and studied under pathologist Rudolf (Carl) Virchow as well as physiologic optics under Hermann Von Helmoltz, the philosopher, scientist, and inventor of the ophthalmoscope.

In 1872, Buller left for London to continue his studies, passing the Royal College of Surgeons exams and being appointed junior house surgeon at the Royal London Ophthalmic Hospital (Moorfield's). At Moorfield's, Buller's mentors were the leading ophthalmologists Sir William Bowman, George Critchett, Sir Jonathan Hutchinson, Edward Nettleship, and Marcus Gunn. He acquired an in-depth knowledge of all aspects of operative and postoperative treatment from these great men.

While in London, at age twenty-eight, he taught the use of the instruments and treatments he learned in Germany. Having learned modem ophthalmoscopy, Buller taught its use to colleagues at Moorfield's. He also developed the "Buller Shield," used to protect the good eye when treating conjunctivitis. The infection could easily spread to the uninfected eye. Buller's device – a watch glass surrounded by rubber and fixed in place with adhesive tape – isolated the infected eye. A small piece of rubber tubing was inserted at the temporal comer of the shield to prevent the glass from steaming up and to allow the ophthalmologist to view the eye.

In 1876, Buller moved to Montreal, where the governors of the MGH recognized his specialized training and appointed him oculist and aurist for the ensuing year. It was a time when most physicians were not specialized in a particular area of medicine but, rather, had a general medical knowledge and looked after all types of patients. As William Osler recalled in 1914: "I still shudder at the remembrance of the 'good old days' at the MGH, when cases of pneumonia, fractured legs, and cataracts were jumbled in the same ward, under the care of the same man; and it was not without qualms of conscience that the staff consented to the appointment of an ophthalmic surgeon, my friend, the late Dr Buller."[1]

Being the first ophthalmologist at the MGH, there were certain duties Buller was expected to perform:

1   The oculist and aurist shall attend the Outdoor room on such days and at such hours as shall be determined by the Medical Board.
2   He shall have the right to admit to two beds in the male public ward and two in the female public Ward, patients suffering from ophthalmic or aural problems.

3 He shall have the privilege of admitting to one private ward when the same happens to be vacant but shall at no time claim the use of more than one private ward.

4 He shall keep a register and case book, including all cases coming under his department. He shall not be ex officio member of the Medical Board.[2]

Buller, with the support of Osler and Shepherd, established the first ophthalmic clinic at the MGH in 1877. The clinic was central to his required medical teaching duties. Prior to his appointment, all clinical teaching of ophthalmology to McGill medical students had been done by lecturers in medicine and surgery. With his appointment, all teaching was his responsibility, and, as a result of his knowledge and teaching abilities, the importance of ophthalmology as a specialty rapidly became evident. McGill recognized this in 1883 when it appointed Buller to the first chair of ophthalmology.

Buller at first encountered some opposition from other non-specialized physicians who were wary about a new specialist who purported to know more about a particular field than his fellow doctors, many of whom had many more years of medical experience. Given this situation, the senior physicians were, at first, unwilling to give up their ophthalmic patients to the new specialist. However, as Buller's superior training and knowledge became generally accepted, all such patients were assigned to his care. He convinced his colleagues that specialization was essential in the medical and surgical care of diseases of the eye.

Frank Buller and Sir William Osler

Throughout the 1880s, Buller's eye and ear department continued to grow. It was noted in the MGH Medical Board records that ophthalmology had too many patients, and, in 1881, it was suggested that a second oculist and aurist be appointed. Initially, Buller disagreed. However, by 1889, realizing that he required assistance, and recognizing that there was no available second-in-command, he began training three physicians as clinical assistants who were looked upon as senior house staff.

Eighteen eighty-nine also marked the beginning of a debate over the union of the MGH and the still-to-be-built RVH into one institution. These concerns were precipitated by Lord Strathcona and his cousin's plans for the erection of the RVH as a tribute to Queen Victoria on her Jubilee year on the Pine Avenue site. It was noted in the MGH annual reports of that year that Buller felt strongly that the two hospitals should be united. He was not alone in this belief. Many others who felt the same way wrote anonymous letters to the editor of the *Montreal Gazette,* and some joined together to form the Friends of the Union of the Montreal General and Royal Victoria Hospitals.

The RVH supporters had the money and were not going to compromise the project to build the new hospital. For his part, although never seeing the merger of the two hospitals, Buller eventually had second thoughts and, in 1896, chose to accept an appointment at the RVH to start a new department.

Moving to the new hospital, Buller became a member of the Medical Board as well as being the hospital's first ophthalmologist and otologist. Thus, once one department had taken root at one hospital, he proceeded to start up a second, parallel department at the other. The department he had begun at the MGH was part of a growing trend towards specialization at the Montreal hospitals. When Buller left for the RVH in 1896, most medicine at the MGH was still being practised in the "traditional" manner, with two disciplines – medicine and surgery – although the dividing line was not always clear. With the growing specialization at McGill, such as at the MGH's eye and ear department, the dividing lines between medicine, surgery, and the specialties gradually became more sharply defined.

While the MGH's eye and ear department thrived after Buller's move to the RVH, his departure did raise concerns among some MGH staff. Some were concerned that the chiefs of a few departments, such as Buller, were leaving to take up similar positions at the RVH, thereby reducing department staff and expertise at the MGH. This was true, and Roddick in surgery, Stewart in medicine, Gardner in gynaecology, and Birkett in ear, nose, and throat all moved to the RVH to head departments. Considering those left at the MGH, a reasonable balance was accomplished in all the departments.

Throughout his years at the RVH's Department of Ophthalmology until his death in 1905, Buller maintained his affiliation with the MGH and was considered part of its "consulting staff." The continued vitality of the MGH department was also assured in 1890 when Herbert Birkett became Buller's assistant. In later years, Birkett remarked that he had been given much of the work of the department, attending to most of the refractions and generally being assigned older patients, while Buller reserved the younger and better-looking patients for himself! In 1893, the department office was reorganized, with Birkett attending to nose and throat cases and Buller the eye and ear cases. Eventually, Buller limited himself to ophthalmology. Birkett went on to a distinguished military career (1915–18) and was appointed dean of the McGill Faculty of Medicine (1914–21).

After Buller left the MGH in 1896, his position as oculist and aurist was assumed by John J. Gardner, with A. Proudfoot as his assistant. The number of eye and ear cases seen at the MGH continued to grow to over twelve hundred "out-door" patients. By the turn of the century, there was mention in the annual reports of operations and "in-door" patients.

In 1898, J.W. Stirling, a graduate of the University of Edinburgh, succeeded Proudfoot as the assistant to Gardner, while Buller retained his positions as chief at the RVH and at McGill as well as his consulting staff appointment with the MGH until his death, in 1905, of pernicious anaemia.

In the early days, when no trained nurses or assistants were available, it was not unusual for Buller to stay up all night nursing patients who were threatened with loss of vision, including cases in which vitreous was lost and frequent changes of cold compresses were required during the night. Buller was also at his best when treating difficult cases and those that others had abandoned.

Frank Buller was a prolific author and produced seventy-six publications, most of which concerned teaching and clinical practice. His papers may be grouped into three distinct groups. The first group attested to his being the first exponent on this continent (according to Birkett) of the new ophthalmology of Von Graefe, Von Helmholtz, and the Dutch ophthalmologist Frans Cornelis Donders. The second group includes clinical writings. Among these are "Anomalies in the Function of the Extrinsic Ocular Muscles" and his last paper, "Methyl Alcohol Blindness," written in collaboration with Casey Wood. The latter paper was described by the American ophthalmologist George Edmund de Schweinitz as "by far the most important contribution to the subject, and one to which too high praise cannot be given."[3] The third group may be described as practical efforts to improve ophthalmic practice. Included are papers on skin grafting, suturing the canaliculi, the Buller Shield, an improved trial frame, and the modification of Critchett's idea of slitting the lateral canthus in gonorrhoeal ophthalmia in order to apply silver nitrate to the everted conjunctiva. It is remarkable that he was able to direct the department, attend to a large practice, and author this wealth of papers, all long before full-time positions existed at either of the teaching hospitals.

Outside of his medical career, Buller delighted in family life, having three daughters and one son who were devoted to him. When his second daughter, at age eighteen, told him she wanted to study art in Paris, he readily agreed and encouraged her – a broad-minded decision for the time and one that enabled her to go on to a most distinguished career. Respecting her father's profession, she later made use of her artistic talent and education by learning to use the ophthalmoscope and painting a number of fundus pictures. Her son, Sean Murphy (me), became an ophthalmologist and, following his grandfather's example, joined the McGill Department of Ophthalmology in 1955.

John William Stirling, 1859–1923

One of Buller's successors was John Stirling. Born in Halifax, Nova Scotia, in 1859, he completed high school and then proceeded to the University of Edinburgh to study medicine. Graduating in 1884 with an MD, CM, he went on to study ophthalmology and became house surgeon at the Royal Edinburgh Infirmary under Argyll Robertson and house physician under T. Granger Stewart. Leaving Edinburgh, he spent two years in clinics in Vienna, Heidelberg, and Berlin, later returning to England, where he became assistant to Marcus Gunn at the Royal Ophthalmological Hospital in London.

In 1887, Stirling moved to Montreal, where he established a medical practice and was appointed professor of ophthalmology at Bishop's Medical College in 1893.[4] In 1894, Bishop's Medical Faculty sent out a circular to the governors of the MGH recommending Stirling and two other staff members for three vacancies at the hospital. The MGH Board of Governors would not elect these men unless they agreed to resign from Bishop's. This matter caused a considerable dispute between the medical faculties of McGill and Bishop's. In 1899, Stirling decided to take the offer from the MGH and resigned from Bishop's. He became assistant oculist and aurist to Gardner at the MGH, and, following Buller's move to the RVH, J.J. Gardner became the second ophthalmologist-in-chief at the MGH. In 1904, Bishop's Medical College was absorbed into the McGill Faculty of Medicine.

With the death of Buller in 1905, Stirling was considered his successor at the RVH. However, Stirling was at the MGH, and there was already a very promising and gifted young ophthalmologist at the RVH – W. Gordon Byers.

In many ways, Byers was the logical successor to Buller at the RVH and at McGill, and he likely would have expected to be named to both positions. Thus, it must have been a disappointment to him when Stirling was chosen as McGill chair and head of the Department of Ophthalmology at the RVH. It is likely that Stirling's appointment was connected with the problem of McGill's absorbing and properly recognizing the seniority of the faculty members coming to it either directly or indirectly from the now defunct Bishop's. The appointment of Stirling in 1906 led to a certain tension in the Department of Ophthalmology at McGill, which persisted for some time to follow. He retired in 1920 and died three years later.

George H. Mathewson, 1905–31

While Sterling was chief of ophthalmology at the RVH, Mathewson was the third ophthalmologist and aurist-in-chief at the MGH between 1905 and 1931. He had been educated at Montreal High School and McGill, graduating in medicine in 1894. Following a year of medical training in Prague and Vienna, he returned to Montreal in 1895 and became clinical assistant to Buller. Mathewson spent the next four years at the RVH, after which he was appointed chief of ophthalmology at the Western Division of the MGH. He also held the position of professor of ophthalmology at Bishop's College following Stirling's resignation in 1899.

In 1905, Mathewson returned to Europe for a further year of study at Prague and Vienna. Later that same year, on returning to Montreal, he was appointed ophthalmologist and aurist-in-chief at the Central Division of the MGH. Soon after this he decided to confer his practice and interests to ophthalmology. He became an associate professor at McGill until his retirement in 1931.

Throughout Mathewson's years as chief of ophthalmology at the MGH, Hanford McKee, the assistant oculist and aurist, was pathologist to the department. He would prepare an annual "Eye and Ear Pathological Report," which detailed the number and kinds of cases seen by the department and could be used to track changes in the numbers of patients and varieties of disorders diagnosed and treated. The annual editions of the report show that the number of consultations continued to rise from year to year.

In 1914, Mathewson remained chief of service, McKee became associate ophthalmologist, and A. Bramley-Moore was assistant ophthalmologist. That year also saw the introduction of the first junior assistants. These new posts were held by L.G. Pearce and W.G. Ricker. The additional personnel helped deal with the more than seven thousand outpatient consultations attended to that year. Between 1918 and 1921, the number of patients dropped by a couple thousand, and so there were no junior assistants hired during these years. By 1922, the outdoor department was again handling about seven thousand patients, and two new junior assistants were appointed: S.O. McMurtry and G.S. Ramsey.

With so many patients being consulted by the department, arrangements were made with the opticians Messrs. R.N. Taylor and Company in 1921 to have a representative of their firm attend the eye clinic. The physicians felt that the prescriptions for eye-glasses given to patients were not always filled to the patients' best advantage, and it was hoped that relying upon a single consistent optical firm would obviate the problem. This proved to be successful.

The year 1925 marked almost half a century of ophthalmology at the MGH. The Ophthalmology and Otology Department had grown considerably, and there were over two hundred indoor and nine thousand outdoor cases annually. All of this growth did not occur at one location. Between 1925 and 1955 the work of the department was split between two locations. This physical division of the department was the result of the partial move of the MGH from the original Central Division on Dorchester Street East to the new Western Division on Dorchester and Essex Avenue. The Central Division of the department handled the majority of the indoor cases and approximately two-thirds of the outdoor cases.

In 1927, a third junior assistant ophthalmologist, J.O.S. Gilhooly, was appointed to the Central Division, and, in 1928, A. Bramley-Moore and S.O. McMurtry, who remained at the Western Division, were joined by junior assistant E.L.O. Walcott.

In 1929, the second consulting staff member appointed to the MGH's Department of Ophthalmology and Otology, J.L. Gardner, died. Gardner had held this position since the death of Buller in 1905. Following Gardner's death, A. Bramley-Moore and G.S. Ramsey joined S.H. McKee as associate ophthalmologists, and McMurtry became assistant ophthalmologist. In 1929, Mathewson filled the void left by Gardner, assuming the post of consulting staff.

S. Hanford McKee, 1875–1942

Born in Fredericton, New Brunswick, McKee obtained his BA at the University of New Brunswick in 1896. In 1900, he graduated MD, CM from McGill and, for several years, was a house officer at the RVH under Frank Buller, after which he studied in Freiburg, Germany. In 1906, having returned from Europe, he was appointed assistant oculist and aurist at the MGH and assistant demonstrator in ophthalmology at McGill. In the same year, he prepared the MGH's departmental pathology report and continued to do so for many years.

Throughout his career, McKee was the official ophthalmic pathologist of the ophthalmology department and had an "active interest in the lab aspect of Ophthalmology ... [ever] since his graduation in Medicine."[5] His main areas of research were: disorders of the retina, the pathology of tumours of the eye, and the bacteriology of the conjunctiva. He also carried on some experiments concerning the effect of certain vitamins upon the metabolism of the eye.

During the First World War, McKee, by then associate ophthalmologist at the MGH, joined the Medical Corps in the 1st Canadian Contingent. He saw service in France and later in Salonika, Greece, and was twice mentioned in dispatches (a noteworthy honour for any British [or colonial] rank or officer, usually for exceptional work in some field). He returned to England and was given command of the Canadian Eye Hospital at Shomcliffe with the rank of colonel and awarded the CMG (Companion of the Order of St Michael and St George) for distinguished services. For his service during the Great War, his name was placed on the MGH Roll of Honour in 1917.

After the war, McKee returned to Montreal and the MGH. Of his work in the hospital before the 1930s, the MGH annual reports from 1928 to 1930 note: "Dr McKee has consistently done research work in the eye. Besides collecting a very fine teaching collection, he has a number of rare and especially interesting specimens."[6] Furthermore, it reads: "S. Hanford McKee has, as in the past, not only taken an active interest in the lab aspect of his specialty, but he has continued to do constructive work as well and published his work."[7]

In 1930, for his academic contributions, McKee was appointed the fourth ophthalmologist-in-chief at the MGH, a position that he retained until his retirement in 1941. In 1931, he was also elected president of the American Academy of Ophthalmology and Otolaryngology – a significant honour for a Canadian. That same year he contributed chapters to two textbooks: "Diseases of the Conjunctiva" published in Sajou's *Cyclopedia of Medicine*, vol. 4; and "Diseases of the Conjunctiva, except Trachoma," which was to be published in the Textbook of Ophthalmology by Saunders and Co., 1931. In 1932, he gained further international recognition as vice-president of the Pan American Congress and presented the Presidential Address at the meeting of the American Academy of Ophthalmology and Oto-Laryngology, which he hosted in Montreal.

Throughout McKee's tenure as ophthalmologist-in-chief at the MGH (1931–41), the hospital in general and the Department of Ophthalmology in particular were undergoing changes. He led his department during a period of advances, and he contributed to and encouraged clinical research. During the 1930s, the number of patients attending the ophthalmology outpatient clinics continued to grow, surpassing ten thousand per year and even reaching fifteen thousand in some years. In addition, the number of indoor patients almost doubled to nearly four hundred. Alexander was promoted to assistant ophthalmologist in 1934, and, in 1935, McMurtry, Ramsey, and Alexander were promoted to associate ophthalmologists. R.J. Viger was the new junior assistant, and, with a grant, he contributed to the establishment of a glaucoma clinic. In 1937, Mathewson and Bramley-Moore were the consulting staff. Mathewson retired in 1941.

Over the years McKee acquired a reputation for his research, and throughout the 1930s he continued to publish an average of four to five papers a year. He was considered a world authority on bacterial conjunctivitis. Being interested in various eye conditions, his writings ranged from observations on syphilis in the eye to hypertensive retinitis and neuromyelitis optica. In 1932, he published a paper entitled "Blindness from Methyl Alcohol Successfully Treated by Lumbar Puncture," carrying on the tradition of Frank Buller and Casey Wood. In 1933, McKee presented "Observations of the Fundus Oculi in Diabetes Mellitus" to the American College of Physicians – a report based on the study of 1,272 cases – and in 1936 his work on eye tumours was reported to the American Academy.

There was no definite residency training program in the 1930s at McGill. Occasionally, a one-year ophthalmology training position was offered. The first MGH residents graduated in 1935. Graduations were sporadic until the mid-1950s, when the program was well established with yearly entrants who applied directly to the MGH. Then, in 1970, all residency training programs were taken over by the Medical School and applicants applied to McGill

University rather than directly to the hospitals. By the mid-1990s, approximately ninety-five residents had finished their training in the MGH and McGill program.

McKee received numerous honours at home and abroad in recognition of his work. In 1938, he was secretary of the MGH Medical Board, becoming chair the following year. He was promoted to professor of ophthalmology by McGill and was on staff at the Children's Memorial and Alexandra hospitals. McKee was a popular speaker and authored numerous contributions in journals and books. At the 1940 Pan American Congress of Ophthalmology (he was vice-president), he described a new method of detecting hardening of the arteries in diabetics.

Nineteen forty-one marked McKee's last year at the MGH. He, Bramley-Moore, and McMurtry formed the Department of Ophthalmology's consulting staff. Ramsey was promoted to ophthalmologist and Alexander was the sole associate ophthalmologist since Viger was away on active military service. In September 1941 McKee retired, dying just over a year later on 25 November 1942. McKee was a forerunner of the clinical scientists of the 1980s and 1990s, and it is remarkable that he accomplished so much academically while keeping up a large practice outside the hospital, receiving no salary or remuneration from McGill or the MGH.

G. Stuart Ramsey, 1887–1982

Born in Levis, Quebec, Ramsey graduated from McGill University with a BA in 1908 and an MD, CM in 1912. Following graduation, he travelled to China and worked for a year at the Canton Missionary Hospital, returning to Montreal in 1913. Next he interned at the MGH, where he began a year of pathology. With the start of the First World War Ramsey was on his way to England by late October 1914. In the war he served with the Black Watch Highlanders and, toward the end of the conflict, was transferred to the Indian Medical Services, where he served for five years. While in India, he married Juliette Pelletier of Quebec City.

After marrying Juliette, Ramsey became concerned about the potential problems of bringing up a family in a foreign country. As well, he noticed that the senior medical officers of the service had developed a distinct lack of zeal. These factors, in addition to a persistent, chronic sinus condition, which was not improving with his stay on the subcontinent, led him to resign from the Indian Medical Services in 1921. Having decided to pursue a

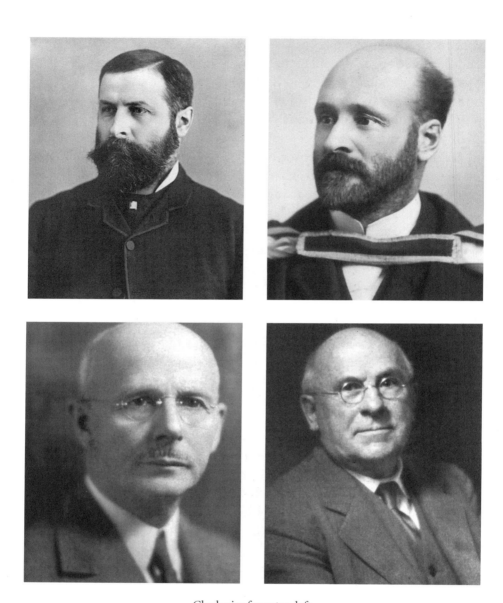

Clockwise from top left
Fig. 28.1 Francis Buller, oculist and aurist at the MGH, 1877–96
Fig. 28.2 John J. Gardner, oculist and aurist, 1896–1905
Fig. 28.3 George H. Mathewson, ophthalmologist and aurist-in-chief, 1905–31
Fig. 28.4 S. Hanford McKee, ophthalmologist-in-chief, 1931–41

career in ophthalmology in the United States, he left India with his family that year. His choice of ophthalmology was in large measure related to his experiences in China and India, where he saw many avoidable and treatable eye conditions.

Following a residency at the Manhattan Eye, Ear, Nose and Throat Hospital between 1921 and 1923, Ramsey was appointed assistant ophthalmologist at the MGH and demonstrator at McGill University. While based in Montreal, he continued to visit ophthalmic centres in London, Paris, and Vienna. As a skilled ophthalmologist who would remain in Montreal for the rest of his career, Ramsey advanced at the MGH, becoming the fifth ophthalmologist-in-chief in 1941, a position that he held for ten years. From 1947 to 1950, he was chairman of the McGill Department of Ophthalmology and in 1949 was appointed professor. Retiring from practice in 1969, he was named emeritus professor in 1971.

In 1951, Ramsey was elected president of the Canadian Ophthalmological Society, and, in the early 1950s, he served as Canada's representative on the International Council of Ophthalmology. This council is the organizing body of the International Congress of Ophthalmology, which meets every four years, and, as a member in 1954, Ramsey was central to overcoming a significant Cold War challenge. That year the Congress was held simultaneously in two cities for the first time: New York City and Montreal. This awkward arrangement was necessary because, during the Cold War, visitors from Iron Curtain countries were not welcome in the United States. As the representative from Canada, which imposed less stringent Cold War restrictions upon Soviet visitors than did the United States, Ramsey organized a second international council, which met in Montreal on very short notice and was a great success.

G. Stuart Ramsey was eventually succeeded by his son, Bruce Ramsey, who also trained in ophthalmology and joined the Department of Ophthalmology at the MGH and McGill in 1954, where he went on to a distinguished career in ophthalmic plastic surgery.[8]

Benjamin Alexander, 1902–88

Like his predecessor, Alexander was a graduate of McGill, having grown up in Montreal and obtained his MD, CM in 1925. He spent the next two years at the MGH as an intern. Then, in 1927, having decided on a career in ophthalmology, he left Montreal for London, where he studied at Moorfield's Eye

Hospital. After two years he obtained the diploma of ophthalmic medicine and surgery from the Royal College. This was followed by two years additional specialized training: one year at the Royal Eye Hospital in Manchester and another in ophthalmic pathology at the University of Vienna.

In 1931, he returned to Montreal, where he established a large practice and was associated with the MGH. He was a clinical leader. At times, patients found him gruff, but they also knew him to be a conscientious, caring, competent ophthalmologist. "Benny," as he was called, exuded energy, which was obvious when talking to him and watching him in action. He was appointed the sixth chief of ophthalmology at the MGH in 1952 and held that position until 1963. His abilities were further recognized in 1961, when he was elected president of the Canadian Ophthalmological Society. He retired in 1972.

Samuel T. Adams, 1919–75

Another McGill undergraduate, Samuel Adams graduated in medicine at McGill in 1943. At that time the standard four-year medical course was compressed into three because of the demand for doctors caused by the Second World War. Adams interned at the MGH while serving as a captain in the Royal Canadian Army Medical Corps from 1944 to 1946. He next accepted a position as a senior intern in ophthalmology at the MGH in 1947–48, a decision that can be partially attributed to Stuart Ramsey, who, as a friend and mentor to Adams, was instrumental in his decision to enter ophthalmology.

In 1948, Adams began a three-year training program at the Massachusetts Eye and Ear Infirmary. There followed an unplanned extension of six months studying and operating with Charles Schepens, a Belgian who had fled to England during the war years, eventually coming to Boston. Schepens had become well known for his contributions to retinal surgery, including devising buckling procedures and developing binocular indirect ophthalmoscopy. In addition, he demonstrated that patients operated on for retinal detachment, instead of lying prone for several weeks with head steadied by sandbags, should be expected to get out of bed the day after surgery.

He returned to the Eye Department of the MGH in 1952, where he was the first surgeon in Eastern Canada to perform buckling operations. As such, he was swamped with patients referred from all over Quebec, the Maritimes, and New England. Since such surgeries had to be performed as soon as possible, his patient load was extremely heavy for two or three years, during which time others were trained to perform the procedure. Adams also found time to establish the first retina clinic in Montreal at the MGH in the 1950s. Indeed, at this time life was gruelling for both Adams and his family, but his actions show that he had a major influence upon the development of up-to-date retinal surgery at McGill.

In 1959, Adams was appointed ophthalmologist-in-chief at the MCH. He remained in this position until 1964, when he was appointed the seventh ophthalmologist-in-chief at the MGH – a position that he held until 1975. He was one of the first faculty members to recognize the importance of geographic full-time ophthalmologists in the Faculty of Medicine. Appointments to these full-time positions had been made earlier in other McGill departments, at the MGH, and the RVH. As the first GFT ophthalmologist at McGill, Adams helped to create additional GFT positions in the ophthalmology departments at both McGill and the MGH. That appointments to full-time positions in ophthalmology lagged behind full-time appointments in other departments was a source of considerable frustration for the ophthalmology staff of both hospitals. It also reflected the weakness of the university's commitment to ophthalmology. As the years went by, it became clear that the GFT staff played a vital role in the development of the departments at McGill. These full-time ophthalmologists worked with Adams's part-time staff as a team, and, under his leadership, the department functioned effectively. A similar development would occur at the RVH.

In 1971, Adams was appointed professor and chair of the McGill Department of Ophthalmology. Very much a university person, Adams believed in McGill and was dedicated to developing a first-rate department. To him, achieving that goal did not exclude consolidation, and, as chief at the MGH and chair at McGill, he started working to bring the hospital ophthalmology departments closer, expressing the hope that one day they might be housed together. When, in 1970, Sean Murphy was appointed ophthalmologist-in-chief at the RVH, the two established an excellent working relationship, meeting frequently to discuss the affairs of the university and hospital departments. Adams also went out of his way to make himself available to discuss problems with department members and residents. A significant decision was getting Dario Lorenzetti (MD, CM, 1960) a GTF appointment. Dario was an excellent student and a first-rate organizer with a specialty in external eye disease (more about Dario later). Other GFT appointments made by Adams at the time included John Little and Sze-Kong Luke.

Also on staff at the time were Arthur Leith, Panos Capombassis, Graham Little, Roland Viger, Bruce Ramsey, Esmond Gordon, and Ken Adams. In subsequent years, a number of the staff left. Alfred McKinna moved to the University of Western Ontario, Sze-Kong Luke to Ontario, Ken Adams to New York, Roland Viger to Virginia, and Graham Little to Belleville. To fill these vacancies at the MGH, Adams recruited Raymond Leblanc in glaucoma and Howard Tannenbaum in retinal diseases. Later, Tannenbaum became chief at the Jewish General Hospital. Mourad Khalil was recruited to work in pathology at the MGH.

During these years the clinics at the MGH were quite large and the residents spent most of their first two years working in them. The partitions between the lanes in the clinic allowed the residents to talk back and forth and furthered the development of a constructive esprit de corps between them. Later, more didactic instruction by subspecialists was introduced into the program. According to Frank Buffam, a resident at the time, starting in the era of Adams's chair at the MGH, McGill had become a leader in promoting resident research, sponsoring annual clinical days, attracting basic scientists, and integrating the hospital departments into a cohesive unit.

Outside of McGill Adams was active in many professional organizations. He was a founding member, and later president, of the Retina Society (United States) as well as a member of the European Retina Society, "Club Jules Gonin," for three years (1962 to 1965). He served as an associate editor of the American Medical Association Archives of Ophthalmology, onetime chair of the MGH Medical Advisory Committee, a past president of the Montreal Ophthalmological Society, a former vice-president of the Association of Ophthalmologists of Quebec, a member of the examining committee and nucleus committee of the Royal College of Physicians and Surgeons of Canada, and a former member of the Council of the Canadian Ophthalmological Society, where he served as chair of the Committee on Indians and Eskimos.

Following his chairmanship at McGill, Adams took a six-month sabbatical in Montpellier, France. There he brought the current techniques of modem retinal detachment surgery to the region and established an excellent liaison with the local ophthalmologists. Significantly, he demonstrated to his French colleagues that it was no longer necessary to keep patients flat in bed for days but that, when treated using the techniques that he had learned with the renowned Schepens in Boston in the early 1950s, they could safely get up only one day after surgery.

After his death in 1975, and with the perspective of time, it is clear that Adams played a significant role in the development of ophthalmology at

McGill and in Canada. He is remembered fondly, and, in tribute to him and his work, the ophthalmological library at the MGH was named the Samuel Adams Library.

The McGill Department of Ophthalmology in Northern Canada, Arthur Leith

The connection between McGill's Department of Ophthalmology and the North began in 1970, when the Faculty of Medicine of McGill was presented with an exciting challenge by the federal Department of Health and Welfare (now Health Canada). The government requested that the university provide medical specialist services to the thirteen Inuit communities in the Baffin Region of the eastern Northwest Territories (NWT). These communities ranged from Grise Fiord on Ellesmere Island to Lake Harbour and Cape Dorset on the south coast of Baffin Island – thus, the area involved was quite extensive, encompassing most of Franklin Territory. No accurate census figures were available at that time, but it was estimated that there were perhaps twenty thousand Inuit in Canada of which forty lived in the Baffin Region.

Ottawa decided that the best way of providing northern Inuit communities access to medical specialists was to call upon Canadian medical schools to provide specialists to the areas that were north of their location. McGill was given the eastern NWT, or Baffin Region, and its specialists were to visit the northern communities under its charge, by air. McGill's most remote village was Grise Fiord, on Ellesmere Island, the northernmost community in the western hemisphere and a little over four thousand kilometres (twenty-four hundred miles) from Montreal by plane.

The overall McGill program in the North was directed by Douglas Cameron, chief of medicine at the MGH. To carry out the project Inuit interpreters, funds for equipment transport, and accommodation of specialist teams and patients were provided under the terms of the McGill Baffin Project contract. In the case of ophthalmology, Samuel Adams was responsible for providing ophthalmologists for the program. When he became ill a few years later, the direction of northern ophthalmology passed to Arthur Leith.

The first McGill ophthalmologists to go north arrived on Baffin Island in the fall of 1970. Peter Rosenbaum worked in Frobisher Bay for a week, while Esmond Gordon went to Pangnirtung. In January 1971, Leith and Nabil

Saheb went to Frobisher Bay and conducted a survey of three hundred randomly selected members of the population. Similar surveys were carried out in other centres by the other universities involved in the NWT. The purpose of these surveys was to find out if the prevalence of ocular conditions was significantly different from that in the south.

Normally the McGill northern eye team consisted of two ophthalmologists and an optician. For the first few years of the program the optician was a volunteer from Montreal. However, the NWT government wanted this work to be done by an Inuit, so they sent a young man to Montreal for some very basic training in frame fitting, and he became the team "optician." After a few years the ophthalmologist in Yellowknife began training excellent ophthalmic technicians, and one of them would go with the optician and visit all of the communities regularly, with the ophthalmologist coming along a few weeks later. The technicians would screen all of the patients and do all of the refracting. They rarely missed a diagnosis. Their participation greatly reduced the workload for the ophthalmologists, such that, beginning in the 1980s, visits to the North required only one ophthalmologist, who could concentrate on medical problems.

Throughout the 1970s, a steady supply of specialists volunteered to participate in these northern medical missions, allowing the program to work well. It worked so well that it attracted the attention of groups in other areas, and the McGill bailiwick in the North kept expanding. At its peak, the McGill northern empire consisted of thirty-eight communities spread over an area measuring twenty-seven hundred kilometres from north to south and fourteen hundred kilometres from east to west. A few years ago Quebec set up a system that formally obliges Quebec's four medical faculties to provide tertiary-level care to defined areas of Quebec. Under this scheme, McGill looks after all of Nunavik and the James Bay area. The Baffin Region is now taken care of by the University of Ottawa.

During the 1970s, transport was often a problem. Only limited scheduled airline service was available, with infrequent flights, especially to the smaller communities. This made it impossible to construct efficient tours of four or five communities. During the 1970s, the doctors were largely dependent on charter aircraft, which stayed with them as they went from village to village. This was efficient but costly.

Accommodation could also be a problem in the 1970s and 1980s. Only the larger communities, such as Resolute or Frobisher Bay, had hotels. In theory, the clinic nurse in each community was responsible for accommodations, but at times the nurse would be unable to find rooms for the visiting doctors. They were sometimes obliged to bring sleeping bags, hoping that there was at least a sofa on which to sleep. Very often, they ended up on the floor, and sometimes in a building without heat.

Another complication with the early northern ophthalmology trips was one of weight. Ophthalmologists require a lot of instruments to do their work, and in the early days of the northern program the bulk and weight of the equipment was often a problem. This even led to doctors sometimes being rejected from boarding a flight because their equipment weighed too much.

As might be suspected in a population with so much angle closure, there was a high prevalence of hypermetropia. However, when the northern program's refraction statistics were studied an interesting discovery was made. In the Inuit about twenty-five years old or older, there was a large amount of hypermetropia and almost no myopia. In patients under twenty, the opposite was true. Ultrasound and keratometry showed that this myopia was axial. Something had happened to the population in the 1950s that had resulted in a marked change in refraction. There was a great change in the Inuit way of life at that time, and it seems almost certain that this change was related to the shift in refraction.

Prior to 1950, the Inuit were largely nomadic, living entirely by hunting and fishing, often following migrating herds of caribou. Their diet consisted of fat and protein as no carbohydrates grow in the Arctic. In the 1950s, the federal government was anxious to provide the Inuit with health care and education, which was impossible so long as they were nomadic. They were enticed off the land and into villages by offers of free houses with heat and electricity. By the end of the 1950s, the great majority of Inuit had moved into the villages. In those villages, they had daily access to refined carbohydrates, for which they developed a great fondness. The quantities of soft drinks and candy that they consumed were enormous. It seems possible that this major change in diet may have affected collagen synthesis, with reduction in tensile strength of the sclera.

A second theory is that, with the Inuit's move into villages, all of the children began to attend school, where they learned to read. Thus, the rise in myopia could be explained by prolonged accommodation, which can induce the condition. However, although traditionally Inuit men had spent all of their days outdoors hunting, the women had dedicated much of their time to preparing hides, sewing garments, and cooking, all activities that made considerable use of accommodation. According to the reading theory, the women who were involved in traditional activities should have been myopic and the men not. Yet, this was not the case.

Many McGill ophthalmologists have supported the university's commitment to the North and found the experience very rewarding. It is to be hoped that future generations will continue to meet the challenge of northern ophthalmology.

Mourad Khalil, 1929–

Mourad Khalil was born in Port Said, Egypt, in 1929 and graduated from Cairo University Medical School, later obtaining a diploma in ophthalmology. Despite limited resources, he first practised ophthalmology in small and remote Egyptian villages. Coming to Canada in 1967, Khalil was accepted for a three-year residency in ophthalmology by S.T. Adams at the MGH. During his time, he developed a friendship and respect for Adams, who invited him to make his first trip to the North to the Baffin Region in December 1970.

Despite his extensive experience and knowledge, Khalil worked well with his fellow residents at the MGH. There he became interested in ocular pathology and, after residency, decided to become an expert. He accomplished this the hard way, with almost no financial support and through self-teaching, while conducting a very busy ophthalmic practice. He also started publishing scientific papers and became a member of several ocular pathology societies. At the meetings of these societies he would give excellent presentations and eventually became well known to leaders in the field. He built up an extensive collection of ocular pathology that McGill residents were able to see and from which they were able to learn.

Dario Lorenzetti, 1936–1994

Following Adams's retirement from the MGH and McGill in 1975 because of illness, the hospital appointed Dario Lorenzetti the eighth ophthalmologist-in-chief, while McGill promoted him to associate professor of ophthalmology. A McGill MD, CM in 1960, Lorenzetti completed the ophthalmology residency at the MGH in 1964, followed by a fellowship in external disease with Herbert Kaufman at the University of Florida, Gainsville. In 1967, he returned to the MGH and was appointed a GFT ophthalmologist by S.T. Adams.

As a researcher, teacher, and physician, Lorenzetti's contributions to ophthalmology were important because, in the 1960s, little ophthalmological research was being conducted at McGill. He was the one exception, continuing his research in external disease, which he started in Miami. At the MGH he conducted research with several fellows and also supervised corneal research. His work, supported by grants, was important as it signalled the era of clinical scientists to come and furthered the research projects and initiatives previously begun by classmate Peter Davis at the RVH.

Lorenzetti was a valued member of the McGill departmental executive committee (ophthalmologists from the MGH, the RVH, the JGH, and the MCH) and often came up with better ways of doing things, especially regarding the complex scheduling of resident rotations among the teaching hospitals. One could always count on him: if he said he would do something it always was done. His administrative and organizing skills were reflected in his involvement with the MGH project to secure new facilities for the hospital's ophthalmology department and clinic on the 4th floor of Livingston Hall. It was a major, totally new design and a project that involved many people, especially Arthur Mildon.

Although not an ophthalmologist but, rather, a technician and dispensing optician, Mildon made a unique contribution to the functioning of the McGill Department of Ophthalmology in the 1950s, 1960s, and 1970s. While on military service in the Second World War he received training in naval optical devices and also came in contact with MGH ophthalmologist Roland Viger. After the war he continued his career as a dispensing optician, but his wartime training had made him much more than that. Using his planning, optical, electrical and cabinet-making skills, he designed, built, and installed the examining room desks at which ophthalmologists sat and with which they controlled the instruments they used. Over a period of three decades he carried out such installations at all four of the McGill teaching hospitals and in dozens of private offices as well. After installation, his skills were required for the complicated repair and maintenance of ophthalmic instruments. Mildon was prepared to dig into the innards of such disparate equipment as slit-lamps (optics) and patient chairs (hydraulics). For many years he would come to the MGH clinic every week to deal with anything requiring his attention. Arthur Mildon's rare combination of technical knowledge and varied capabilities kept the department's clinical facilities functioning at a high level of efficiency. Since his departure it has not been possible to find his equal.

The carefully planned design for the new Department of Ophthalmology at the MGH included a new clinic, excellent GFT doctors' offices, a photographer's office, the Samuel Adams Library, a conference room, and administrative offices. Finally, all outpatient ophthalmological activities were together. A great celebration took place for the official inauguration on 14 June 1979 when ophthalmologists and guests came from all over the city and province to view the superb new facilities that allowed patients to be examined with their dignity intact. No longer were patients ushered into rooms and alleys where every word of their examination could be overheard.

Beyond his research and teaching duties, as well as his official administrative functions, Lorenzetti held a number of university and non-university positions. At McGill, he was chair of the Postgraduate Committee, dealing with resident training, and was succeeded in 1987 by Duncan Anderson. In 1967, formal instruction for the residents took place during regular working hours – a positive change from the traditional time following afternoon clinics when fatigue had often set in. Also in 1987, Lorenzetti became a member of the external disease group, composed of himself and Bruce Jackson and Joel Rosen. The group was trying to obtain greater subspecialty amalgamation between the hospitals. They met for external disease clinics regularly at the MGH and the other teaching hospitals, where patients were examined and discussed. Lorenzetti was appointed chief examiner for the Royal College of Physicians and Surgeons in 1981. He chaired the Canadian Ophthalmological Society's Continuing Medical Education Committee for several years. He was elected president of the Canadian Ophthalmological Society in 1990. Always logical, and a skilled debater, he fought hard for what he believed. Understandably, both the hospital and the university community were greatly saddened by his premature death in 1994, as were his friends and numerous patients. In his honour, the Canadian Ophthalmological Society launched the annual Dario Lorenzetti Lecture. Similarly, the McGill Department of Ophthalmology also established an annual lecture in his honour.

Bruce Ramsey, 1924–2000

Bruce Ramsey was the son of Stuart Ramsey (1887–1982), a former ophthalmologist-in-chief of the MGH (1941 to 1951). He was a colleague of Lorenzetti at the MGH and the first ophthalmic plastic surgeon at the MGH and McGill. He was trained by Byron Smith and Alston Callahan, well known authorities in the field. He was a meticulous surgeon who enjoyed his specialty and solving problems. Following Ramsey, McGill saw the arrival of two ophthalmic plastic surgeons – Francois Codere in 1982 at the RVH and Brian Arthurs in 1986 at the MGH.

Arthur Leith, 1931–

A 1955 McGill MD, CM, Arthur Leith was accepted in the MGH ophthalmology program in 1956 by Ben Alexander, the department chief. His residency training included a Harvard basic science course and a research project at Tufts University, which involved looking at the induction of cataract by microwave in rabbits. Following completion of his residency in 1959, Leith spent two years at the Institute of Ophthalmology in London, where he became familiar with research procedures, including setting up protocols. While in London, he also had the good fortune to be associated with two great leaders in British ophthalmology: Sir Stewart Duke Elder and Norman Ashton. In 1961, he returned to Montreal and was awarded a teaching fellowship at the MGH, supported by a Dominion provincial grant to the glaucoma clinic, which had been founded by Roland Viger in 1954 and was the first of its kind to be supported by the Government of Canada. He brought to the MGH and its glaucoma clinic his knowledge of applanation tonometry, which he gained in London. In 1962, he was appointed to the MGH and the MCH and was appointed consulting ophthalmologist to Ayerst Research Laboratories, followed by an appointment to Bio-Research Laboratories. At Bio-Research he was involved for twenty-five years in the field of ocular toxicology.

Leith worked in the Glaucoma Clinic from 1961 until 1996. His next appointment was as a teaching fellow at the MCH. At this time, S.T. Adams was in charge of ophthalmology at the MCH and among the staff was Wyatt Laws, who performed corneal transplants. Next, Leith joined Stuart and Bruce Ramsey in their downtown office until 1964, when he went into full-time practice and became a staff member at the MGH. At the hospital he joined other progressive ophthalmologists, such as Robert Pearman, who, in the late 1950s, performed a number of Ridley intraocular lens implants. These were probably the first examples of the procedure in Canada, and his results were similar to Ridley's: there were multiple complications.

At the MGH, general ophthalmologists were valued, in particular, Allan Bourne. He worked with Adams in the glaucoma clinic up until the mid-1960s. He was a well trained surgeon and had good results with corneal transplants and retinal surgery. All his colleagues were greatly saddened at his premature death in 1970.

The McGill department was aware of the importance of general ophthalmologists such as Bourne, and efforts were made to ensure they were always represented on the staff of both the RVH and the MGH. Their teaching in the clinics and operating rooms was a valuable contribution, as was their referral of patients to the hospitals. Since they received no remuneration, they were less affected by budget cuts than the GFT ophthalmologists, who relied upon university and hospital funding.

At the same time Leith joined the MGH staff, Adams, the newly appointed ophthalmologist-in-chief, was recruiting a number of GFT staff. These new recruits included John Little, Dario Lorenzetti, Howard Tannenbaum, Szekong Luke, and Ray Leblanc. Leblanc came to the MGH from the University of Sherbrooke in 1972. He worked in the glaucoma clinic with Arthur Leith and Nabil Saheb. He commented on the strength of the glaucoma group and the high quality of the teaching program as well as on the fellowship throughout the department. From 1979 to 2003 he was department head at Dalhousie University, where he became well known for his important contributions to glaucoma research.

During the first years of Leith's work at the MGH, in the mid- to late 1960s, when Adams was chief and Locke was McGill chair and chief at the RVH, relations between the two hospitals' ophthalmology departments were often tense. Fortunately, this situation slowly improved, and, by the early 1970s, inter-hospital relations were becoming noticeably more cordial.

One area in which the ophthalmologists of the MGH and the RVH worked together in the 1970s was in northern ophthalmology. In the early to mid-1970s, when Adams's health began to fail, Leith was asked to take over the organization of McGill's Arctic ophthalmology program. As the leader, Leith arranged for staff members from different hospitals to take turns looking after patients in the North, to everyone's great satisfaction.

A well trained surgeon in 1979, Leith was the first surgeon at the MGH to implant intraocular lenses and to perform phacoemulsification. Earlier, he spent a week in Holland with Binkhorst, one of the pioneers in the field, and thereafter began using iris-mounted lenses.

Nabil Elias Saheb, 1939–

Another MGH co-worker of Leith's during the 1960s, 1970s, and 1980s was Nabil Saheb. Born in Egypt, of a Lebanese family, he graduated from the University of Cairo and came to Canada in 1964, where he completed a one-year internship followed by a year in pathology at the Hôpital Maisonneuve Rosemont.

He was then accepted by Adams for a three-year residency in ophthalmology at the MGH in 1966. In the 1960s, a noticeably strong bond was often formed between the residents, one which was not limited to the hospital but extended to their social lives. Among his fellow residents Saheb, along with Robert Kelly and Rand Simpson, were known as "the three musketeers." The kinship the three residents formed was lasting, with all three now distinguished doctors and maintaining their friendship to this day.

After his residency Saheb worked at the MCH as a clinical fellow for a year and a half. Then, in 1971–72, he obtained a glaucoma fellowship with Stephen Drance in Vancouver. In the Montreal hospitals, at the time, a mechanistic view of glaucoma prevailed, a position that stressed things like aqueous outflow, water drinking tests, and pressure. Drance had developed a new outlook and understanding of glaucoma as well as the means to do a visual field for a specific disease. In his approach, obtaining a proper assessment of the optic nerve was important.

Drance, Armaly, and Anderson, all of whom were recognized for their experience in glaucoma, changed the prevailing understanding of glaucoma treatment from one that focused upon pressure to one that posed the question: "Why is it happening?" Gordon Balazi, from McGill, went to Vancouver after Saheb and similarly benefited from a glaucoma fellowship with Drance. Back in Montreal in 1972, Saheb introduced trabeculectomy, laser glaucoma surgery, automated perimetry, and stereo disc photos to McGill ophthalmology, while also combining McGill glaucoma rounds between the hospitals.

When I was appointed chair of the McGill Department of Ophthalmology in 1975, it was clear that subspecialization was the future for university ophthalmology. There was an urgent need to recruit and find promising candidates for GFT positions if the department was to move ahead. Since McGill lacked sufficient resources to fund Nabil Saheb and Bruce Jackson as GFT ophthalmologists, funds for half their salaries were raised in the private sector, which persuaded McGill to match these amounts. Sometime later, McGill and the hospitals provided funds for the two doctors' full salaries.

In 1972, Saheb received appointments to McGill, the MGH, and the MCH. Over the years, he devoted most of his energies to the study of glaucoma, becoming expert in the field. In recognition of his ability and important contributions to both McGill and its hospitals, Saheb obtained tenure in 1981. In 1984, he was elected president of the Quebec Association of Ophthalmologists to 1986.

Such social events were indicative of the strong "esprit du corps" and camaraderie that prevailed at the MGH in Saheb's days due to the influence of Dario Lorenzetti. Three yearly social events were particularly anticipated: the Christmas party, the Chez Vito's party, and the residents' farewell party. His talent for teaching was recognized by the residents who voted him the first Buller Teaching Award in 1990–91, an award given by the residents for excellence in teaching.

Esmond Gordon, 1928–2008

He graduated from the University of Geneva Medical School in 1955, followed by a year of pathology at the Connecticut Meriden Hospital. In 1958, he began a residency at the MGH in ophthalmology; completed in 1961. The next year was spent in ophthalmic pathology at the Armed Forces Institute of Pathology under Lorenz Zimmerman, a great friend of McGill ophthalmology, who had trained several McGill residents. Then, in 1963, Gordon received appointments at McGill and the MGH.

At McGill, Gordon made important contributions to pathology, organizing the first meeting of the Eastern Ophthalmology Pathology Society at the university in 1968 held in the McIntyre Medical Building. He also contributed to teaching pathology at the university. His teaching method was to project pathological slides and ask students and residents to comment on them. In the late 1960s, he was able to share his teaching responsibilities when he was joined at the MGH by another pathologist, Mourad Khalil. Gordon

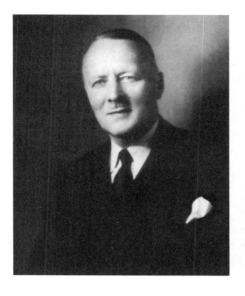
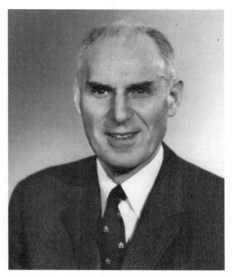
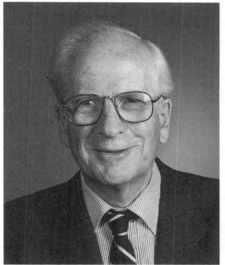
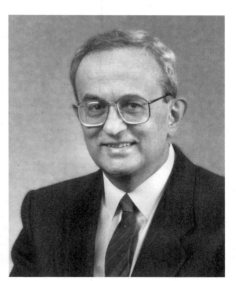

Clockwise from top left
Fig. 28.5 Stuart Ramsey, chief of ophthalmology, 1941–51
Fig. 28.6 Sam Adams, chief of ophthalmology, 1964–75 (Benjamin Alexander was chief
of ophthalmology, 1952–63)
Fig. 28.7 Dario Lorenzetti, chief of ophthalmology, 1975–94
Fig. 28.8 Sean Murphy (Frank Buller's grandson) chief of McGill ophthalmology, 1975,
worked to combine efforts of departments at the RVH, the MGH, the MCH,
and the JGH before the MUHC in 1997.

remained active in teaching pathology for some ten years, eventually gradually reducing his teaching load.

Sean Murphy (the author), 1924–

A 1943 graduate of Harvard, I received my MD, CM from McGill in 1947. From 1952 to 1955 I served in the Royal Canadian Air Force as chief of ophthalmological services. In 1955, I joined the McGill Department of Ophthalmology and the staff of the RVH. In 1970, I became ophthalmologist-in-chief of the RVH and in 1975 professor and chair of ophthalmology at McGill – a GFT position. In forming the executive committee of McGill's Department of Ophthalmology I played a major role in uniting the four hospital departments at the MGH, the RVH, the JGH, and the MCH before the MUHC and as a result of Royal College suggestions. I promoted the training and recruitment of subspecialists and GFT staff and felt it was a priority to send graduating residents away for further specialized training and, wherever possible, to offer them GFT positions on their return. I emphasized the importance of basic research in the department; helped develop a McGill ocular pathology unit with Mourad Khalil, Esmond Gordon, and Seymour Brownstein; and encouraged the development of the Low Vision Clinic.

I became president of the Canadian Ophthalmological Society, president of the Quebec Association of Ophthalmologists, chief examiner for the Royal College for two years, and chair of the Royal College Committee for four. I was awarded the Order of Canada in 1976, the medal of the Canadian Ophthalmological Society in 1987, and was given the society's Lifetime Achievement Award in 2007. In 1989, the Department of Ophthalmology established an annual lecture in my honour.

The introduction of universal medical insurance in 1970 with its restrictions on specialist's income led many doctors to leave the province. At the same time, the Front de liberation du Québec (FLQ) was demanding independence, and, in 1970, responding to their violent tactics of bombing public buildings, kidnapping, and even murder, the federal Liberal government of Pierre Trudeau imposed the War Measures Act, establishing martial law in Quebec for three months. With such events occurring in Quebec it became difficult to attract residents to train in the province.

Despite these difficulties, great advances occurred in ophthalmology in the 1970s. Among these were the widespread use of the operating microscope (with this, cataract surgery was changing from the intracapsular method to

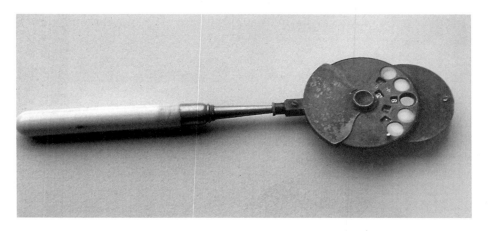

Fig. 28.9 Frank Buller's original ophthalmoscope brought from England and Germany in 1876. The mirror reflects light from behind the patient into the eye, which is examined by the doctor through lenses.

the extracapsular method) and the introduction of intraocular lens implantation. Lasers, ultrasound, and a better understanding of glaucoma were further developments. In addition, retinal surgery saw many developments, including vitreous surgery (several cases previously considered inoperable could now be helped). It should be noted that many of these advances were the result of the increasingly widespread use of computers in the hospitals, including in the departments of ophthalmology.

Brian Younge

His residency in ophthalmology (1969–72) preceded three years in the Canadian Armed Forces in which he was stationed in Germany. As a resident at the time of the introduction of the first soft contact lenses, Younge was one of the first "fitters" of the new Griffin lens. With the introduction of these lenses a large group of myopes and aphakes came for treatment. As the fitter, Younge encountered complications, and one of his first patients presented with a pseudomonas corneal ulcer.

Following his residency and a year at the Mayo Clinic, he returned to Montreal in 1973 and began work at the MNI as a neuro-opthalmologist. As the first neuro-ophthalmologist at the MNI he was received with enthusiasm by Rasmussan (chief of the MNI), Cosgrove (MS interest), and, of course, Sean Murphy who had persuaded him to take the job at the MNI.

He also worked with Francis McNaughton (St Francis to his colleagues), a remarkable neurologist who was at the institute in its early years.

Younge in a letter to me about his career, stated that he and Alf McKinna had the greatest influence on him and that both had remarkable knowledge of the subject before it became a subspecialty.

Duncan Anderson

A graduate of the McGill medical faculty in 1969, Duncan Anderson completed his residency in ophthalmology at the MGH between 1970 and 1973. From 1973 to 1974 he was in Boston at the Massachusetts Eye and Ear Hospital working with David Cogan and Shirley Wray in neuro-ophthalmology. Then, in 1975, he joined the MGH staff and received a GFT McGill appointment.

In charge of neuro-ophthalmology at the MGH from 1975 to 1991, Anderson was the first full-time neuro-ophthalmologist based at the MGH. Donald Baxter, chief of neurology, recognized the importance of neuro-ophthalmology and Anderson's ability back in 1975, and he was able to secure him an office and a secretary in the hospital.

Being a "hands-on" neuro-ophthalmologist, Anderson took the advice of his Boston chief, David Cogan, who suggested that he examine cases in the intensive care, neurology, and neurosurgery areas. His rounds led him from the sixth floor to the eighteenth and down again, seeing patients on the way. He would also refuse to wait for the elevator on this trek, instead preferring to take the stairs, forcing the residents who accompanied him to do the same. He would spend one four-hour morning each week on such rounds seeing neuro-ophthalmology patients. Residents and colleagues alike found that he always had the ability to keep you interested and was able to explain complex problems with clarity.

He was in charge of medical student undergraduate teaching that same year. In 1976, he instituted a series of ten lectures for the medical students covering all aspects of ophthalmology – each one given by a different staff ophthalmologist who had a special interest in the topic under discussion. In addition, Anderson oversaw expansion of early morning teaching sessions at all four McGill hospitals.

In 1988, Anderson became director of McGill's Residency Training Program, a university-based program that represented an important shift from hospital-based programs. Development of this new program had been encouraged by significant pressure from the Royal College. The college wanted to integrate residency training programs across all the McGill hospitals by putting the control of the departments in the Medical School and taking them out of the hospitals, a development that helped equalize rotations to these hospitals. At first there was some resistance to this when it came to the senior year as staff and residents felt that residents' surgical experience would suffer if they were not based at a single hospital for the whole year. However, with the introduction of the program, this was found not to be the case. In 1991, Anderson accepted an appointment at the University of British Columbia.

Mark Gans, 1955–

Mark Gans, a 1981 McGill medical graduate, was a McGill resident in ophthalmology based mainly at the MGH (1982–85). Following his residency, he accepted a position at the Bascom Palmer Institute in Miami, Florida (1985–86) under two well known authorities in neuro-ophthalmology – Joel Glaser and Lawton Smith. The worlds of advanced magnetic resonance neuro-imaging and desktop computers were just emerging, and it was an exciting time to be concurrently exposed to new technology.

Following his fellowship, Gans returned to McGill as a GFT ophthalmologist at the JGH. His practice involved neuro-ophthalmology, managing an electroretinography and visual-evoked response laboratory, and general ophthalmology. He also joined Jack Wise to run the JGH neuro-ophthalmology service for six years. In 1991, Gans accepted an offer to move to the MGH, where he would continue as a GFT neuro-ophthalmologist.

At the MGH, Gans examined patients in his office and at the bedside. In his teaching he combined practical, clinical, and academic issues. In addition to his clinical pursuits at McGill (the MGH, the MNI, and the JGH), his academic work, and his participation in the Canadian Ophthalmological Society, the American Academy of Ophthalmology, and the North American Neuro-ophthalmology Society, Gans has proven himself to be an accomplished administrator as director of undergraduate studies and director of the McGill Residency Training Program. He also assumed the position of clinical director at the MGH and the RVH. In 2008, he was appointed interim chair of the McGill Department of Ophthalmology.

Alf McKinna, 1921–2003

Alf McKinna, a 1952 McGill medical graduate, was a resident in ophthalmology at the MGH from 1957 to 1959. As a resident, he was on call every other night and every other weekend. Like other residents at the time, McKinna lived in the hospital when on call and was paid forty dollars per month. Members of the staff were on call about one in three nights and were expected to be called by the resident for all emergency cases. As staff ophthalmologists they attended at least two and sometime three clinics per week. These clinics were free.

Following his residency, McKinna accepted a fellowship in ophthalmology at the University of California, San Francisco, in 1959–60. In 1960–61 he was a fellow in neuro-ophthalmology at Johns Hopkins Wilmer Institute, Baltimore. There he worked with the great authority in the field, Frank B. Walsh, a Canadian from Saskatchewan who wrote the first comprehensive neuro-ophthalmology textbook, *Clinical Neuro-Ophthalmology* – a work all residents studied.

Returning to Montreal in 1961, McKinna was appointed a teaching fellow at the MCH while also working in neuro-ophthalmology at the MGH. In 1964, he became an assistant professor at McGill and director of the ophthalmology subdepartment at the MCH, succeeding S.T. Adams. During McKinna's period as director, his colleagues who rotated through the clinics were H. Wyatt Laws, Bruce Ramsey, Allan Bourne, Arnold Katz, and John Little. McKinna continued as the director until 1972, when he left to work in neuro-ophthalmology at the recently opened University Hospital of the University of Western Ontario.

John Little, 1938–

John Little, a McGill MD, CM in 1961, completed a three-year eye residency from 1963 to 1966. Little joined the MGH Department of Ophthalmology following several years at the University of Florida's ophthalmology department. While his primary interest was paediatric ophthalmology, while at the MGH it was the management of retinal detachments, including surgical repair by scleral buckling. In addition, he held weekly retina clinics. These activities at the MGH continued after he was appointed head of paediatric ophthalmology and physically moved his office to the MCH in 1975. During his twenty-two years at the MCH he continued as the primary retinal detachment surgeon at the MGH until new members joined the staff.

Susan Lindley

Susan Lindley, a 1980 McGill medical graduate, completed a three-year eye residency (with fellow resident Marie-Louise Lapointe) based primarily at the MGH. She became a staff ophthalmologist in 1985 at the MGH and McGill, practising with Bruce Ramsey, until 1992 when Lorenzetti persuaded her to move up to the MGH as a GFT instead of moving to Vancouver as she had planned.

Lindley continued to practice from her full-time office at the MGH after 1992. In 1987, she started to develop expertise in ophthalmic ultrasound, training with Sandra Frazier Byrne at the Bascom Palmer Eye Institute in Miami, and she has been the resident echographer since then. She progressed from assistant to senior ophthalmologist during that time, and her McGill appointment progressed from lecturer to associate professor.

Lindley branched out into service with the McGill Northern Eye Program (under Leith), travelling to the Inuit and Cree communities of Hudson Bay and James Bay. She has also worked for twenty years with the CNIB eye van outreach program in northern Ontario. She was clinical director of ophthalmology at the MGH from 1995 to 2000, when she was elected president of the Canadian Ophthalmological Society for a two-year term. She became acting chief of ophthalmology at St Mary's Hospital from 2004 to 2006.

Michael Flanders, 1945–

Michael Flanders graduated from McGill, MD, CM, in 1970. From 1972 to 1975 he took part in the McGill integrated program in ophthalmology at the MGH. He was fortunate that, at this time, new staff ophthalmologists were returning from first-class fellowships and setting up offices at the MGH. In 1976, he accepted a position for one year as a visiting ophthalmologist in Abidjan, Ivory Coast, and in 1977 he received appointments to the MGH and the MCH. In addition to his Montreal work, he also worked in a clinic in Ste-Agathe. The Ste-Agathe clinic provided fascinating clinical cases for the MGH Department of Ophthalmology.

In 1980–81, Flanders did a six-month Strabismus Fellowship with Philip Knapp at the Harkness Institute, Columbia Presbyterian, in New York. This launched his career in strabismus and paediatric ophthalmology, with an appointment to the MCH as a GFT in ophthalmology. As was traditional in those years, he continued his adult-related activities at the MGH, which included an active cataract practice and a rapidly growing adult strabismus practice using adjustable sutures. He also nurtured an interest in paediatric ophthalmology.

Flanders's academic activities included clinical research projects in strabismus and neurostrabismus, Botulinum toxin, nystagmus, cataract surgery. and paediatric ophthalmology. He was a member of the eye team in the Arctic Ophthalmology Program on twelve different occasions between 1977 and 1995.

Bryan Arthurs, 1952–

Bryan Arthurs graduated with an MD from the University of Western Ontario in 1979. He entered the McGill ophthalmic program in 1982. Residents at this time rotated through two of the three adult hospitals as well as the Montreal Children's Hospital, with twelve-hour days being the norm and first call every third night as well as second call every other night for the senior resident.

After residency in 1985, Arthurs trained in ophthalmic plastic and reconstructive surgery in New York. at the Manhattan Eye, Ear and Throat Hospital under the legendary Byron Smith, Richard Lisman, and Murray Meltzer. He also spent time with Robert Della Rocca and John Simonton at the New York Eye and Ear Infirmary.

In 1987, Arthurs took a GFT position in MGH ophthalmology. Although his main focus was at the MGH, he devoted one full day of service to the Jewish General Hospital and made sorties to the northern Inuit communities with Susan Lindle.

Miguel Burnier, 1951–

Miguel Burnier, a specialist in ocular pathology, came to McGill from Brazil through the National Institutes of Health and Armed Forces Institute of Pathology (Washington), becoming chair of the university's Department of Ophthalmology in 1993 for the MUHC. He established the Dario Lorenzetti

Lecture in 1995 to be given as an annual event at McGill. In 1993, he created an ophthalmology pathology laboratory, which developed an international reputation attracting trainees and PhD students from different countries. His influence led to a marked improvement in research in the McGill department. In 2008, Burnier completed sixteen years as chair of McGill's Department of Ophthalmology and various clinical directorships.

NOTES

1 Harvey Cushing, *The Life of William Osler* (London: Oxford University Press, 1940), 919.
2 Taken from the minutes of the Montreal General Hospital Board of Governors meeting, 8 March 1876, "Annual Reports, 1851–1965," MUA, RG 96, Montreal General Hospital.
3 Herbert S. Birkett, "Buller, the Ophthalmologist, Politzer, the Otologist, and Lefferts, the Laryngologist," Reprinted from *Transactions of the American Academy of Ophthalmology and Oto-Laryngology* (n.p. 1927), 4.
4 Bishop's was the first medical school in Quebec to accept women, 1890–1900, for ten years only. Maude Abbott, a Bishop's graduate of 1894, became a world famous pathologist, interested in congenital heart disease. And, in 1891, Octavio Ritchie was the first woman graduate in medicine in Quebec. She went on to be a formidable advocate for women's higher education in Canada.
5 Hanford McKee, *Murphy's Portraits of Ophthalmology at McGill University, 1876–1990* (Montreal: published by the author, 1990), 41–5.
6 A.K. Haywood, "Report of the Department of Pathology for the year ended December 31st 1928," in *107th Annual Report: The Montreal General Hospital, and Report of the Training School for Nurses,* 1928 (Montreal: Southam Press, 1929), 73.
7 Ibid., "Report of the Department of Pathology for the year ended December 31st 1929," in *107th Annual Report: The Montreal General Hospital, and Report of the Training School for Nurses,* 1929 Montreal: Southam Press, Ltd., 1930, 78.
8 Most information on the individuals discussed, from Stuart Ramsey on, was taken from private discussions, interviews, and correspondence between Sean Murphy, the individuals mentioned, and other colleagues.

29

Orthopaedic Surgery

Eric Lenczner, Emerson Brooks, Larry Conochie, and Ross Murphy

Emerson Brooks was chief of orthopaedic surgery at the MGH. Eric Lenczner, Larry Conochie, and Ross Murphy, all senior members of the division, had equal shares in the writing of this chapter.

Orthopaedics began in Montreal with Alexander MacKenzie Torrence Forbes (1874–1929), who graduated MD, CM from McGill with honours in 1898. After a trip to the Grenfel Mission in St Anthony's on the Labrador, where he saw many untreated paediatric orthopaedic abnormalities, he trained in orthopaedics in New York at the Hospital for the Ruptured and Crippled. Returning to Montreal in 1902 with no hospital admitting or operating privileges, he and Francis Shepherd (1851–1929), Alex Blackader (1847–1932), Harold Cushing (1873–1947), and Tait McKenzie (1867–1938) founded the Children's Memorial Hospital of Montreal as an orthopaedics centre. It opened in 1904. He was given MGH inpatient privileges in 1906 where he did all his adult work. He was appointed the first chief of orthopaedics at the MGH in 1911. Recognizing the educational problems for disabled children in Montreal who couldn't get to school and who needed special facilities, Forbes cofounded the Crippled Children's School on Cedar Avenue in 1916 and was its director for life. Children were picked up by ambulances and transported to and from the school. He was a lecturer in orthopaedics at McGill, chief of orthopaedics at the MGH, and, finally, a clinical professor in 1922.

Orthopaedics in Montreal attracted the National Shrine organization, which built its tenth Shriners Hospital on Cedar Avenue in 1925, with Forbes as chief of surgery opened in 2015.

A list of his operations at the MGH and the MCH in the early days included club feet, scoliosis, spina bifida, Tbc of the spine, bowed legs, cleft pallet, trauma and fractures of all kinds, Volkmans, tendon transplants, hip fractures, defects from osteomyelitis and polio, and birth defects (unspecified) of the arms and legs. He died in 1929, having left quite a legacy of paediatric and adult orthopaedic surgery.

When the MGH moved to its present location on Cedar Avenue in 1955, the Department of Orthopaedic Surgery located the large walk-in clinics on the first floor adjacent to the Emergency Department. These clinics served a large population, but they were cumbersome, difficult to control, and were located in a very small space.[1] The arrival and foresight of Jo Miller saw their relocation to the second floor, with more space, an organized appointment system, and office space for four geographic full-time staff. An adjacent library and teaching room completed the area. This concept eventuated in a defined department area resulting in better organized clinics and the later development of subspecialty clinics. At present, the Orthopaedic Department area is located on the second floor and still remains true to the original concept of clinic space and office space for the attending staff.[2]

The clinical service was located on the twelfth floor and was divided into an east service headed by E.C. Percy and a west service under the direction of J.G. Shannon; private admissions went to the nineteenth floor. The introduction of medicare eliminated the "private" patient concept, but the nineteenth floor continued to be utilized by the department. This distribution was maintained over the years, with various staff members heading up the two services.[3]

The 1960s and 1970s saw many changes in the management of orthopaedic conditions.[4] Fracture management had long been a priority in the department, and closed reduction was the accepted treatment method. Laird Wilson, however, challenged this concept and began carrying out open reductions on tibia and ankle fractures. This raised considerable controversy and resulted in "the great debate" at a special rounds between Wilson and Holland, a general surgeon who had been treating ski fractures for many years in the lower Laurentians and had significant expertise in fracture management.[5] The result of the debate did not change the manner in which fractures were managed; however, it did set the stage for change as Wilson continued to increase his indications for open reduction.[6] In the 1970s, Emerson Brooks and David Burke felt that the AO approach of open reduction with rigid internal fixation and early mobilization was an important advancement in fracture management. They attended a week-long course in Davos, Switzerland, and instituted this protocol at the MGH. At the request of Brooks, Synthes Canada supplied equipment and audiovisual tapes to set up an annual AO basic course in fracture fixation for the MGH residents, with instruction supplied by Brooks, Burke, and Conochie.[7] This method of fracture management improved patient care and continued to grow in importance, and, under the leadership of M. Aebi, a member of the AO group, resulted in the development of a formal and internationally recognized trauma unit at the MGH as well as the development of a large spine unit staffed by fellowship-trained orthopaedic surgeons. The trauma unit was designated level 1 – one of only three hospitals in the entire province with this designation.[8]

The management of arthritic joint disease underwent parallel change with the introduction of total joint replacement. Hip replacement evolved from cemented to uncemented fixation as more and more pressure was applied to replace joints in younger individuals. Knee replacement saw one of the first joint implants, which as Shier's prosthesis, a hinge type of device. This was replaced by a series of more anatomical prostheses over the next few years. The appointment of Jo Miller resulted in the development of a research laboratory dedicated to the evaluation and development of total joint prosthesis.

Two significant events occurred during this period. Miller, in conjunction with Jorge Galante, developed a knee prosthesis that was utilized throughout the world, and Dennis Bobyn, PhD, was recruited as director of the research program. Their collaboration was extremely productive and resulted in many awards – indeed, they were often the recipients of the Aufranc Award from the Hip Society of the American Academy of Orthopaedic Surgeons. Miller was elected as president of this prestigious society in recognition of his contributions to this area of research. K.C. Chan, an orthopaedic surgeon with engineering background, joined this research team and, among his many accomplishments, was instrumental in developing a vacuum cement delivery system still used around the world.

Following the untimely passing of Miller in 1990, the laboratory area was physically renovated and named the Jo Miller Laboratory for Orthopaedic Research. Bobyn, Tanzer, and others continued to be extremely productive and to receive international recognition.

Teaching of residents took on a more formal tone with the arrival of Miller in 1965. In addition to weekly rounds, evening sessions were organized with a set curriculum for the residents to follow. This curriculum was moved to the Shriners Hospital in order to encompass all residents in the

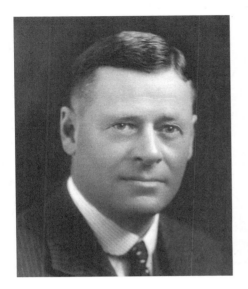 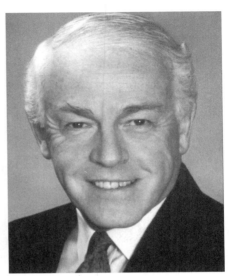

Fig. 29.1 A. MacKenzie Forbes, first chief of orthopaedic surgery, 1911–29
Fig. 29.2 Jo Miller, chief of orthopaedics, 1966–90

training program on Thursday mornings and remains there in 2015. Post-graduate residency education was directed by Brooks and subsequently by Tanzer, after his return from fellowship training in Boston.

The teaching of basic science as it relates to the musculoskeletal system was of interest to Brooks, and he published a book containing references to this topic. Tom Smallman, in Ottawa, was also interested in this subject, as was the Canadian Orthopaedic Association. The latter organization was interested in developing a course on the basic science of the musculoskeletal system for Canadian orthopaedic residents, and this task was assigned to Brooks and Smallman. Their collaboration resulted in the development of the Basic Science Course for Orthopaedic Residents. Residents from all Canadian training programs attend this course, which runs for a full week and consists of lectures by basic scientists, pathologists, and radiologists.

Larry Conochie also had a major interest in education. He produced a series of videos on the examination of the musculoskeletal system, and these videos were promoted by the American Academy of Orthopaedic Surgeons and became the standard teaching tool for most medical schools in North America and beyond. Ross Murphy introduced knee arthroscopy as an improved method of managing with intra-articular injuries. He initially utilized direct telescopic assessment and later introduced camera and monitor visualization. This was to have a profound effect on the future management of knee injuries. Over the course of time Murphy expanded his interest to include other joints, most notably the shoulder. This evolution was of significant importance in the development of the sports medicine specialty.

The MGH had a long association with the professional athletic teams in Montreal – namely, the Montreal Canadiens and the Montreal Alouettes – as well McGill athletic teams. This consisted of a multidisciplinary team of physicians, including E.C. Percy, who was interested in sports medicine as a distinct entity. The departure of Percy and Greenwood for the United States produced a significant void, which was temporarily filled by Emerson Brooks and David Burke. In 1983, Eric Lenczner was recruited to develop a formal sports medicine program. Under the leadership of Lenczner, the Sports Medicine Program now consists of four fellowship-trained surgeons, is a popular training rotation, and attracts postgraduate fellows to a formal fellowship program for an additional year of specialization.

The development of large medical and radiological oncology clinics at the MGH resulted in an increasing number of referrals for musculoskeletal metastases, either with impending or pathological fractures. In order to provide comprehensive care Brooks established a multidisciplinary musculoskeletal oncology clinic with the participation of medical and radiological oncologists as well as a pathologist and a dedicated bone radiologist. In order to manage primary bone tumours Ken Brown was added to the clinic staff and, after his departure to Vancouver, Robert Turcotte was recruited to take his place. This clinic provided overall patient care and also proved to be an excellent educational tool for resident training. Turcotte, after the departure of Aebi, became chair of the department and consolidated his widely based referral practice entirely at the MGH.

The residency training program was international in flavour, incorporating residents not only from English and French Canada but also from around the United States as well as from several Middle Eastern countries – namely, Saudi Arabia, Kuwait, Bahrein, and Oman. The success rate of candidates at the fellowship examination of the Royal College was excellent.

Currently, the orthopaedic department comprises ten full-time surgeons, including several who are exceptionally talented and who have raised the standard of care to a very high level. These include Edward Harvey (trauma and upper extremity surgery), Rudy Reindl (trauma and spine surgery), Gregg Berry (trauma and foot surgery), and Marc Burman and Paul Martineau (sports medicine surgery).

Arthroplasty surgery is currently performed by William Fisher, Michael Tanzer, and Eric Lenczner. The spine unit consists of Jean Ouellet from the MCH, Peter Jarzem from the JGH, and Rudy Reindl from the trauma group at the MGH. A recent addition to the department comprises Canadian army surgeons when they are between overseas deployments – namely, Major Cournoyer and Captain Talbot and their cadre of support personnel.

In summary, the Orthopaedics Department continues to grow in size and scope, reflecting the ever-expanding place of musculoskeletal pathology in our society. An aging and active population have high expectations of life-long mobility and comfort, and the MGH Orthopaedics Department is well positioned to contribute fully to this.

NOTES

1 H.E. MacDermot, *The Years of Changes, 1945–1970* (Montreal: Montreal General Hospital, 1970), 8.

1 J.G. Shannon, Montreal General Hospital, annual report, 1960, 74, MUA.

1 Ibid., 1960, 76.

1 Ibid., 1965, 86.

1 Jo Miller, Department of Orthopaedic Surgery, Montreal General Hospital, annual report, 1969, 68–70, MUA.

1 Ibid., Montreal General Hospital, annual report, 1968, 63–4, MUA.

1 Ibid., Department of Orthopaedic Surgery, Montreal General Hospital, annual report, 1979–80, MUA; ibid., 1980–81, 63.

1 Max Aebi, Division of Orthopaedic Surgery, McGill University Health Centre, annual report, 1996–97, MUA.

30

Otolaryngology

James D. Baxter and John H. Burgess

Jim Baxter was the first combined otolaryngologist-in-chief at both the MGH and the RVH and chair of the McGill department. He wrote a history of Canadian otolaryngology, from which John Burgess extracted this chapter.

Frank Buller (1844–1905) was primarily an ophthalmologist who also trained in laryngology and otology. He was the first specialist appointed to the Montreal General Hospital staff in 1876. His title was oculist and aurist. For the fifty years prior to this, MGH attending staff were listed only as either consulting or attending physicians. Buller had trained in Berlin and London and was convinced by Francis J. Shepherd and William Osler to return to Montreal. Immediately upon his return, the attending staff at the MGH reserved the right to treat eye and ear patients themselves, but Buller's superior training convinced them to transfer such cases to his care. He is listed in the sixtieth MGH annual report as a "specialist" – oculist and aurist.[1] His clinical and teaching expertise was recognized by his appointment to the first chair of ophthalmology at McGill University in 1883.[2] In 1895 he moved his practice to the Royal Victoria Hospital when he was appointed director of its eye clinic.

George Major (1851–1923), a McGill MD, CM (1871), trained in Europe in diseases of the ear, nose, and windpipe. He was appointed laryngologist to the MGH in 1882, the first to dedicate his training to laryngology. It is not certain whether he saw eye patients as well. He retired in 1893 and moved to London, England, in 1894 and died in 1923. He was never a chief.

Herbert Stanley Birkett (1864–1942), Holmes medalist class of 1886, trained in ENT in Europe and returned to the MGH and McGill in 1881. He was appointed MGH chief of laryngology in 1892 and moved to the RVH in 1898 as director of the RVH Deptartment of Laryngology. He became McGill chief of otolaryngology in 1906. Birkett was a very clever doctor. He did a little eye work, as they all had to do. That is where EENT comes from: eye, ear, nose and throat.

Birkett and Buller shared offices and a both saw eye and nose patients until the late 1890s, when Bullar saw only eye and Birkett only ENT patients. On Buller's death in 1905, Birkett formed the McGill Department of Otolaryngology in 1906.[3]

Buller was succeeded by H.D. Hamilton, who was laryngologist-in-charge from 1898 until 1919 and otolaryngologist-in-chief from 1919 until 1928.[4] Otolaryngology became a department under him and was listed separately in the hospital annual reports. The attending staff were all part-time, having offices outside the hospital.

George E. Hodge became otolaryngologist-in-chief from 1928 to 1948. His main contribution was the establishment of research as well as an increase in clinical service, audiology, and speech therapy. The MGH became the leader of ear research in Canada.

Percy B. Wright, associate laryngologist, led research on the treatment of deafness and arranged for the construction of a soundproof room for his studies. Professor E. Godfrey Burr of electrical engineering at McGill and Hector Mortimer from biochemistry collaborated on this project. Mortimer was a British-trained obstetrician and gynaecologist who became interested in endocrinology, atrophic rhinitis, and otosclerosis – the leading cause of deafness. He developed the first audiograms at the MGH and was the first in Canada to publish his research in this field.

E.E. (Ernie) Scharfe joined the staff in 1913, bringing an interest in speech therapy as ancillary treatment for cleft palate and other congenital conditions. He took charge of speech therapy at the Montreal Children's Hospital. This service was initially part of the Physiotherapy Department at the MGH as it was considered a "treatment without medicine."[5] Guy Fisk, director of the Physiotherapy Department, supervised the treatment of these patients, but, in the mid-1940s, Hodge had these patients transferred to his department and established the Division of Speech and Hearing. Hodge had rheumatic valvular heart disease and died at an early age a few years after his retirement in 1948.[6] Scharfe succeeded him as otolaryngologist-in-chief in 1948 and continued as head until 1963.

During Scharfe's leadership, fenestration and stapes surgery (a mobilization of the bones in the middle ear necessary for the transmission of sound) were introduced for otosclerosis. In 1948, Arnold Grossman was appointed

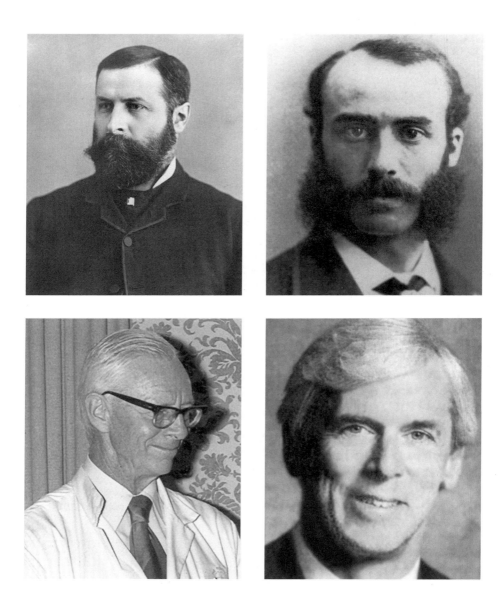

Clockwise from top left

Fig. 30.1 Francis Buller, oculist and aurist, MGH , 1877–1905

Fig. 30.2 George Major, laryngologist, 1882–93.

Fig. 30.3 H.D. Hamilton, laryngologist in charge, 1898–1918, otolaryngologist-in-chief, 1919–28

Fig. 30.4 E.J. Smith, director of Division of Otolaryngology, 1963–77

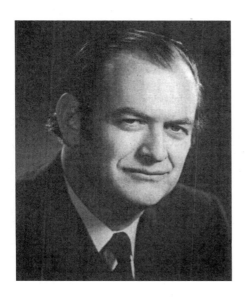

Fig. 30.5 James Baxter, first full-time chief of otolaryngology at the MGH, the RVH, and McGill, 1977–90

to the attending staff. He had graduated in medicine from McGill, served overseas during the war, and subsequently took his graduate training at the University of Illinois. He introduced endoscopy for diseases of the larynx, and his interest in childhood deafness led to the creation of the Iona School for the Deaf. He became associate director of the department in 1965, during E.J. Smith's time as director, and was the first otolaryngologist at the MGH to be awarded emeritus status. An annual lecture is given in his name. Scharfe retired in 1963 and was succeeded by E. John Smith.[7]

Following Royal College suggestions in the 1970s, departments in the hospitals combined activities for better postgraduate (resident) training. During Smith's tenure otolaryngology became a division in the Department of Surgery as it was thought that this would increase its influence in the hospital and university. Smith had a national reputation and was president of the Canadian Otolaryngological Society in 1970.

E. Attia joined the division in 1972 as the first geographical full-time surgeon. He had been trained in head and neck surgery at both McGill and the University of Florida. Until his appointment cancers such as tumours of the larynx were dealt by both otolaryngologists and general surgeons – an unsatisfactory and competitive arrangement. Attia was soon performing 90 percent of these surgeries. He was named associate director until he resigned in 1987 to become chair at Dalhousie University in Halifax.

Smith retired in 1977. When he was succeeded by James D. Baxter, who was chair of the McGill department and chief at the Royal Victoria Hospital,

MGH otolaryngology regained its status as a department. Baxter was the first full-time chief at the MGH and the first to be cross-appointed in the history of the two hospitals. This was twenty years before the creation of the McGill University Health Centre (MUHC 1997). His appointment coincided with major changes in the practice of medicine following the stormy introduction of Medicare in the Province of Quebec. The government assumed control of the budget and played a major role in the appointment and training of specialty residents. Under Baxter the attending staff in otolaryngology received dual appointments at both the RVH and the MGH but usually practised at one or the other hospital. The outpatient area was remodelled with new space for audiology and speech pathology and with offices for full-time surgeons. Space was provided for F. Chagnon for a voice lab oratory. She became chief when Baxter retired in 1990.

Baxter initiated the outreach role of the department in the delivery of health care to the Baffin Region of the Northwest Territories and northern Quebec. He made important contributions to clinical research, particularly the cause of chronic middle ear infections in Canadian Aboriginal people. He published extensively on this subject, gaining international recognition. He was the founding director of SEVEC (Society for Educational Visits and Exchanges in Canada), a national organization developing and coordinating educational visits for Canadian youth between Canada's two founding peoples.

Baxter was president of the Canadian Otolaryngology Society in 1975, vice-president of the American Laryngology Association in 1972, vice-president of the American Broncho-Esophageal Association in 1979, and vice-president of the Pan-American Association of Oto-Rhino-Laryngology and Broncho-Esophogology from 1974 to 1976. He served as examiner in otolaryngology for the Royal College of Physicians and Surgeons of Canada and for the American Board of Otolaryngology.

MGH OTOLARYNGOLOGIST-IN-CHIEF

Aurist to the MGH
1883–95   F. Buller

Laryngologist to the MGH
1882–93   G.W. Major

Laryngologist in Chief
1892–98   H.S. Birkett
1898–1918 H.D. Hamilton

Otolaryngologist-in-Chief
1919–28   H.D. Hamilton
1928–48   G.E. Hodge
1948–63   E.E. Scharfe
1963–77   E.J. Smith, director of the Division Otolaryngology,
           Department of Surgery
1977–90   J.D. Baxter
1990–   F. Chagnon

NOTES

1 J. Hanaway and R. Cruess, *McGill Medicine: The First Half Century, 1829–1885* (Montreal and Kingston: McGill-Queen's University Press, 1996), 170 and 186.

2 J. Hanaway and R. Cruess, *McGill Medicine: The Second Half Century, 1885–1936* (Montreal and Kingston: McGill-Queen's University Press, 2006), 185; Hanaway and Cruess, *McGill Medicine: The First Half Century*, 170–1.

3 MGH, annual reports, 1859–1964, MUA.

4 MGH, Department of Otolaryngology, annual reports, 1964–90, MUA.

5 F.J. Shepherd, *Origin and History of the Montreal General Hospital* (Montreal: Gazette Printing Co. Ltd., 1925).

6 H.E. MacDermot, *History of the Montreal General Hospital* (Montreal: Montreal General Hospital, 1950).

7 H.E. MacDermot, *Years of Change, 1945–1970* (Montreal: Montreal General Hospital, 1970), 21.

31

Pathology

John Richardson

John Richardson was a senior pathologist at the MGH and Strathcona Chair
of Pathology at McGill.

Introduction

To determine the role of pathology at the Montreal General Hospital, the
annual reports, stored in the McGill University Archives, were read. There
was no mention of autopsies or pathology until 1858, when, as a consequence
of a body theft by twelve medical students, a new "dead house" was to be
erected to protect the hospital from scandal.[1] In 1867, there was an increase
in the number of patients with smallpox and dysentery, a separate building
was built as a fever hospital, and mention is made of fifty-seven cases of
smallpox being in this house.[2] Several years later it is stated that "a very much
needed and thorough alteration of the dead house" be made,[3] and this is the
only mention of deaths in the hospital, which, in, 1872–74, had 232 cases of
smallpox, of which thirty-three died. The hospital at this date was con-
structing the Morland Wing for children, with thirty beds, and installing hot
water heating and ventilation.[4] In 1875, Osler was placed in charge of the
smallpox hospital as Simpson had resigned.[5] In this year there were 170 cases
of smallpox, and the hospital board requested that the city build a separate
city hospital as the current General Hospital facilities, with the large number of smallpox patients it was housing, was dangerous for the other patients.
In 1876, the smallpox hospital was closed as the city opened a separate hospital for smallpox and the old building was disinfected and rebuilt as a
twenty-four-bed ward.[6] The basement was repaired with brick walls, ren-
dering it proof against damp, foul emanations and vermin,"[7] and there was

hope that a modern hospital would be built when, prosperity warrants it."[8] There is no mention of Osler in the annual reports until 1878, when he is listed as an attending physician, although he performed most of the autopsies in the hospital.[9] Certain improvements were made to the hospital, but it was clear that a new, modern hospital was needed, and land was purchased for the new site in 1884,[10] with the new hospital being completed in 1892.[11] Despite the fact that a department of pathology was not established in the hospital until 1882, numerous autopsies were performed and their records indexed. These records formed a basis for Osler's medical text. Regular mention of the activities of the Department of Pathology did not appear in the hospital annual reports until 1896.[12]

Many physicians in Europe and Asia had demonstrated the value of the autopsy in medical practice. Some physicians performed thousands of autopsies and correlated the findings with the clinical state of the patients. An excellent example of this is provided by Marie Francois Xavier Bichat who, at the age of twenty-eight, performed over six hundred autopsies in fewer than six months.[13] Bichat introduced the term "tissue," wrote the text *Traite d'Anatomie descriptive*, and is considered the father of modern histology.

In England and Scotland the attending physicians performed autopsies on their patients to either confirm the diagnosis or possibly to learn something new. There were no particular experts, and the techniques were those learned by observation and from the few texts available. The state of pathology in North America in the nineteenth century was behind that of Europe and, in particular, that of Germany. Many North American students, Osler included, were to discover this lack of knowledge of pathology and education when they visited the large clinics in Berlin or Vienna. A review of the recommended textbooks of the McGill University medical school at the period of Osler's student days contains a textbook by Samuel D. Gross entitled *Elements of Pathological Anatomy*,[14] which was first published in 1839 (with the third edition appearing in 1857). This very readable text contains both practical and philosophical observations on disease, and it deals with such problems as distinguishing benign from malignant tissue through the use of histology. The text also contains many microscopic drawings of lesions by J.M. Da Costa, a colleague of Gross's. The use of the microscope was not a feature of either the practice of pathology or the training of medical students at McGill University, but its use was soon introduced by Osler. Gross wrote many other texts that rivalled those coming out of Germany and Austria. Virchow himself complimented Gross on

Elements of Pathological Anatomy at a dinner given to honour Gross in 1868. Karl Rokitansky's *Handbook of Pathological Anatomy* was written between 1842 and 1846,[15] and Rudolph Virchow's concept of cellular pathology was announced in 1855.[16] The insights of Gross and the thorough descriptions of diseased organs in his text provided students with material lacking in their medical school training. This text, however, was unusual for the period for its insights and reasoning.

The germ theory of disease and the work of Louis Pasteur between 1860 and 1864 were not yet accepted, and the bacillus, as the cause of tuberculosis, was demonstrated by Robert Koch only in 1882.[17] Disease, before the era of bacteriology, was thought to arise from spontaneous generation rather than the "life only from life" theory of Pasteur. Some of these theories on the cause of disease are to be found in another textbook from McGill University at the time of Osler's training: *Principles of Medicine: An Elementary View* by Charles J.B. Williams, MD, FRS.[18] This text was revised from the London edition of 1857 and, in discussing epidemics, states: "The cause of these diseases is supposed to be something in the atmosphere: for the atmosphere is the only thing that is common to all places to which the affection extends; but the nature of the epidemic poison is just as mysterious as the epidemic." Elsewhere, on respiratory problems: "The amount of mischief arising from defective respiration varies according to the sudden or the gradual supervention of the evil." The entire text is both fuzzy and philosophical and quite the opposite of the practical, observation-based text of Gross. The curriculum of the Medical School and the practice in the hospital were thus not current with the new ideas of Europe, and the role of William Osler in changing this situation at McGill University was considerable.

The lack of progress in medicine also existed in the United States. And hospitals such as the Massachusetts General Hospital, founded in 1811, performed limited autopsies conducted by physicians and surgeons until the establishment of a clinico-pathologic laboratory in 1896 with the recruitment of James Homer Wright.[19] Prior to the appointment of Wright, a microscopist, in 1847 John Barnard Sweet Jackson was on the staff of the Massachusetts General Hospital, and he became the first professor of pathological anatomy in the United States at Harvard University. But this had little influence on the general practice of pathology. At a later date, Calvin W. Ellis made significant advances in the use of the microscope to evaluate specimens. The practice and teaching of pathology and other specialities in North America was behind that in Europe, and those who wished to change

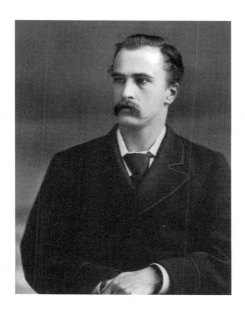

Fig. 31.1 Sir William Osler, pathologist to the MGH, 1877–84

this situation had to leave and study either in Germany or Great Britain and then come back home to introduce these new ideas to the hospitals and universities on their continent. Osler was instrumental in the introduction of modern medical practice to Canada.

Osler Years

Osler entered Trinity College in Toronto in 1867 and was much influenced by Bovell, who was trained in London and Edinburgh and had an MD from Glasgow.[20] Bovell and Hodder organized the medical department of Trinity College into the Upper Canada School of Medicine. Another person who influenced Osler was W.A. Johnson, a clergyman with a consuming interest in nature and who was much disturbed by Charles Darwin's recent publication of *The Origin of Species*, which caused much turmoil in the church. Osler mounted microscopic slides for Johnson, was introduced to the *Microscopical Journal*, and began collecting entozoa. Although he entered the arts program at the college he changed after one year to medicine, much to the delight of Bovell. In medical school he spent most of his time in the dissecting room and used Bovell's microscope to look at cells and became, at the age of nineteen, an accomplished microscopist. During the winter of 1869–70, Osler lived with Bovell and had access to the latter's large and extensive library, which was filled with many classical texts, a fact that aroused Osler's interest in books. Bovell recommended that Osler move to McGill, where there were more clinical opportunities, and gave him his microscope as a gift. Osler and a fellow student, Harry Wright, were taken up by Palmer Howard who introduced them to morbid anatomy and made available texts by Virchow, Rokitansky, Wilks, and Moxon in addition to the *Transactions of the Pathological Society*. Howard continued to practise with Bovell, which allowed Osler continued access to the latter's extensive library. In 1870–71, Osler clerked at the Montreal General Hospital and attended the autopsies, very much influenced by Howard's strong interest in morbid anatomy. The medical school was changing during these years, with new staff and the introduction of the Lister ritual by Roddick, who brought the procedure from London. The introduction of antiseptic procedures greatly improved surgery in the hospital and, together with anaesthesia, allowed more complicated techniques to be utilized. Upon his graduation, Osler was awarded a prize for a thesis that contained thirty-three microscopic and other preparations of morbid structure. A sentence in the thesis indicates the philosophy that guided him in the future: "To investigate the causes of death, to examine carefully the condition of the organs, after such changes have gone in them as to render existence impossible and to apply such knowledge to the prevention and treatment of disease, is one of the highest objects of the Physician."[21] This sentence captures the teaching of Gross, Professor Virchow, and Samuel Wilks, all of whom Osler greatly admired.

In 1872, Osler left Montreal for London, where he worked with Burton Sanderson in the Physiology Laboratory of University College in physiology and histology.[22] Histology at this time was quite separate from anatomy, but E. Klein also worked in this laboratory and had learned embryology and pathological histology in Vienna and so was able to instruct Osler in these fields. In addition, Osler was exposed to the findings of Virchow, Pasteur, Koch, and Lister and thus obtained an excellent knowledge of the latest in physiology and histology. This extensive training helped him in his future career as he was soon offered a position at McGill as professor of the Institutes of Medicine, which encompassed physiology, pathology, and histology. One drawback was the salary offered, which was insufficient to live on without having an additional medical practice. Indeed, the dean at the time, Campbell, told Osler: "A young married couple might as reasonably expect to live upon love as a medical man to live upon pure science in this most practical country." This statement of reality, in addition to the fact that Bovell had failed to live on just physiology, prompted Osler to refuse the offer and to take further studies in Germany and Austria. In October of 1873, he and Stephen Mackenzie left London for Germany, where they visited clinics in Berlin and then later in Vienna. Such travel to Germany and Austria was common for North American graduates in medicine as the training in the specialities was far superior in these countries than in North America. Vienna was usually preferred, but Osler admired the "mastermind of Virchow" and the teaching at the Institute of Berlin, where 140 students were present and microscopes circulated on a small tramway to demonstrate the histology while the results of ten to twelve autopsies were discussed at great length.[23] Over three months, Osler took extensive notes on Virchow's painstaking autopsies and then left for Vienna at the end of December 1873. In Vienna he attended the Krankenhaus, with its two thousand patients and the daily lectures given in medicine. He spent five months in Vienna and was not impressed by the autopsy techniques, complaining: "After having seen Virchow it is absolutely painful to attend postmortems here, they are performed in so slovenly a manner and so little use is made of the material.[24] He left Vienna in April 1874 and returned to London and then to Canada.

Osler learned microscopy during his early education and realized the importance of this instrument in the study of disease. The microscope had been invented in the 1600s and allowed important observations, such as Malpighi's of the circulation of blood in capillaries in 1664 and Hooke's observation of cells in 1665. Little further study appears to have been done, and the microscope became a toy.[25] Morgagni and Bichat saw no need for its use, though their observations and writings are the basis for modern pathology. Despite attempts to interest scientists in the use of the microscope, little was done until the father of Lord Lister perfected the achromatic objective lens in 1830.[26] Microscopical demonstrations began at Oxford in 1845, and students used microscopes on small railways interspersed with trays of coffee, a demonstration technique that Osler was to see in Berlin with Virchow.[27] Despite these early demonstrations, the use of the microscope in universities, let alone hospitals, was exceedingly slow. One principal problem was the resolution of the microscopes and the viewer's fear that what he or she saw might be artefact. This problem is well discussed in the excellent and informative review of the microscope by Guido Majno and Isabelle Joris, who obtained a microscope from this early period and photographed various preparations of fresh, intact adipose tissue that clearly showed some of the serious limiting features of the apparatus.[28] Despite these problems Osler ordered twelve new microscopes from Hartnack in Paris and paid for them with his own salary, even though the use of the microscopes was intended for students. In addition to the problems of microscopic lens, pathologists of Osler's time were limited by the lack of fixatives and stains. Formaldehyde was discovered in 1868 and produced by A.W. Hofmann. Formalin was introduced as a fixative by Alfredo Kanthack in the late 1890s at Cambridge.[29] Thus this common, and very useful, fixative was not available during these years. Seventy percent ethyl alcohol had been used for many years and was introduced by Boyle in the seventeenth century.[30] It was a common fixative at the time (Nelson was returned to England in a casket filled with rum). Various other fixatives had been developed in Europe, mainly by methods taken from the tanning industry. Osler used the fixative of Giacomini in Turin for the fixation of the brain. This fixative contained 50 percent zinc chloride as the initial ten-day treatment then a further ten days in 70 percent alcohol followed by immersion in glycerine with 1 percent carbolic acid followed by a final drying and coating of varnish.[31]

The next problem was staining tissue to obtain good differentiation between its parts. The utilization of aniline dyes and hematoxylin had just started. Carmine had been previously used for nuclear staining, and it was used in various forms to delineate structures in a variety of tissues. Perkins in London discovered aniline dyes in 1856 as a derivative of coal tar. These dyes were perfected by the German synthetic dye industry for textiles and were soon applied to histology. The most dramatic utilization of aniline was by Koch, who found a dye with an affinity for the TB bacillus. One last problem faced by Osler at this time was the lack of a microtome to cut sections. Klebs had introduced paraffin embedding in 1869, and this refined the prior technique of merely coating the alcohol-fixed tissue in wax and then cutting it by free hand. The only microtome available to Osler was one at McGill, and when he required sections he had to have them cut there and then examined at the hospital. These difficulties of technique explain the few mentions of histological details in the pathology reports of these years, and it was some time before standard histological techniques were developed and used in the hospital.

The MGH had a long history of each member of the medical staff performing autopsies on his own patients, but, in 1876, a new position was created for a pathologist, and this of course went to Osler.[32] He now controlled the postmortem room and performed most of the autopsies until his departure from the hospital. This allowed him to give both practical pathological demonstrations in the postmortem room and a course in practical histology. In the medical school curriculum for the year 1879–80 there is a listing for pathological demonstrations on Saturday at 11 AM. In the listing is the following statement: "This course is based upon, and conducted, as far as possible, in the same way as that of Prof. Virchow at the Berlin Pathological Institute." In the year 1876–77, one hundred autopsy cases were written up and presented in book form, and these reports were the first serious pathological reports in North America. Osler's demonstrations were modelled on those of Virchow in Berlin, whereby facts elicited from the autopsy were carefully correlated with clinical histories, and this approach was soon to become standard practice in North America. These reports and the collection of interesting specimens of heart disease and other entities formed the basis of McGill's Osler collection. The MGH was thus one of the first hospitals in North America to adopt the European methods of pathology and teaching, and, under Osler, this was the basis of the future development of experimental medicine and research in the hospital – a process that required many more years.

Just prior to his move from Montreal to Philadelphia, Osler had established a physiology laboratory in the medical building. In this laboratory he had eleven of the twelve microscopes, three microtomes, and a kymograghm but his expertise was mainly with the microscopes. In 1881, he read a paper on ulcerative endocarditis before the New York Pathological Society, and, in the vegetations, he saw micrococci but did not grasp their significance. The field of microbiology was not one of his strong points as he was still under the influence of Bastian, who was a proponent of spontaneous production of disease in tissue and the formation of organisms from the heterogenesis of tissues. Koch's 1881 demonstration of the bacillus in tuberculosis changed this, and, in the next year, Osler demonstrated to a class the presence of the bacilli in the lung of a man who died from the disease. The initial publication of the autopsy cases in 1877 prompted the board of governors to pass a by law in 1881, stipulating "that a history of all the cases treated in the hospital be in books provided for the purpose. This is a most valuable work alike in the interest of medical science and the sanitary history of the country."[33]

In 1885, Osler had moved, and the annual report for that year stated: "[We] regard it as highly complimentary to this institution, in which he for several years cultivated those talents for clinical instruction and scientific investigation which has given him a high reputation outside of his native land."[34] Wyatt Johnston, a resident medical officer, assumed these duties, but there is no mention of this in the annual report of the hospital for that year.

However, Johnston is mentioned in the curriculum of the university, in which it is stated that autopsies at the hospital would be done following the method of Virchow.

Post-Osler Years

Wyatt Galt Johnston was born in Sherbrooke, Quebec, in 1863 and graduated in medicine from McGill in 1884. He assumed the duties of Osler as pathologist for the hospital until his death in 1902 following an infection.[35] Johnston was also a demonstrator in pathology at McGill, was associated with bacteriology during these years, and developed a quick method for culturing the diphtheria bacillus and a dried blood method for the Widal test, which improved its availability.[36] He was very active in medico-legal cases in the city, was considered an expert in this field, and, indeed, became the first medical expert in autopsies in the coroner's cases in Montreal and probably also in Quebec. Johnston, along with MacTaggart, produced the third volume of pathological reports for the hospital. The autopsy form was reorganized according to organ weight, clinical history, and anatomical diagnosis. In these reports there was often a long description of the body and the organs and this markedly differed from previous report, which might just note "deep red colour, resembling raw beef." These forms allowed for better record keeping and provided useful information as to the state of the organ and the diagnosis. Further improvement involved the use of stamps for each organ for record keeping. The diagnosis on each case was obtained by gross examination, with only a few notes on the microscopic features (if they were examined at all). In the autopsy reports for 1893–94, however, there is a great deal of detail, with chemical analysis of iron in the liver and a note that states that blood protein was low. The clinical histories were often on separate paper and were pasted onto the reports. In some cases microscopic examination was also added, and a printed diagram of the body was used to demonstrate lesions. The collected reports, therefore, were far more informative than were the records kept from the autopsy, and these reports were the ones used in the teaching of staff and students. Johnston was very involved in the collection of these reports and in the completeness of the autopsy records. Maude Abbott, who was instrumental in founding the International Academy of Pathology, credits Wyatt Johnston with the idea for an association of medical museums as the basis of the proposed academy.[37] Johnston proposed this idea in 1899 to the staff of the Army Medical Museum,

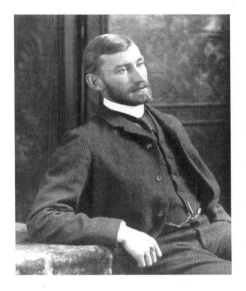

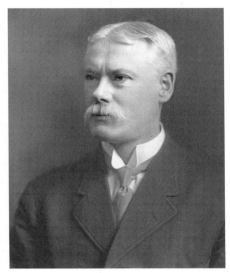

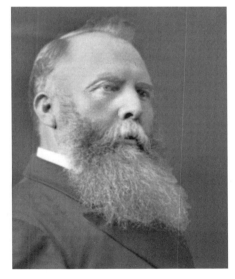

Clockwise from top left
Fig. 31.2 Wyatt Galt Johnston, pathologist
to the MGH, 1884–1902
Fig. 31.3 D.D. MacTaggart, pathologist to
the MGH, 1903–04
Fig. 31.4 B.D. Gillies, pathologist, 1904–06

but nothing was done until D.S. Lamb of said museum repeated the suggestion in 1905 to the curator, Major James Carroll. The academy was founded in 1906 by Maude Abbott. Johnston maintained the meticulous autopsy techniques of Virchow in addition to organizing the records and utilizing the material from the autopsies for teaching. It was thought that he was the equal of Osler in pathology, and his early death was a tragedy for both the hospital and pathology.

John McCrae, the resident assistant pathologist, assumed direction of the department upon the death of Johnson. McCrae was from Toronto, had a BA and an MB, and was said to have a brilliant personality. He continued with the teaching of pathology with clinical correlations and, in addition, contributed some poetic lines to the pathology texts of the hospital. McCrae worked with MacTaggart and, between them, they published four manuscripts on such subjects as typhoid, inflammatory disease, and an analysis of 486 cases of acute lobar pneumonia with one hundred autopsies. In 1904, McCrae resigned and B.D. Gillies became the director, with R. Gibson and D.D. MacTaggart as assistants. In this year, the entire index of autopsies, from 1896 to 1902, was published, thus continuing the practice of Osler and Johnson.

In 1906, C.W. Duval became the director, with D.D. MacTaggart, F.B. Gurd as assistants. The annual report for this year mentions that bacteriological examinations were performed about one thousand times.[38] Von Eberts installed equipment purchased from Sir A.E. Wright of London for the purpose of bacterial inoculation. This was the first laboratory in North America to have and to use this equipment. Almroth Wright was professor of pathology at the Army Medical Hospital at Netly, in England. He is noted for his insistence on the importance of laboratory testing in medical practice and for popularizing preventive vaccination against typhoid, an exceedingly difficult task at the time. Wright is also known for the characterization of opsonins – antibodies that mediate phagocytic responses. He developed an elaborate theory for the treatment of infectious diseases based on the principle of vaccine therapy, in which the patient would be subject to a course of vaccine inoculations made from cultures of the infecting organism. The course of treatment was monitored by measuring the opsonic index, something that proved to be very difficult when applied to patients. The treatment was widely applied but gradually fell out of use. Wright was best known for his fundamental work on antityphoid inoculation and the treatment of war wounds. At the end of the First World War, Lord Kitchener decreed that no soldier would be sent abroad uninoculated, which surely confirmed Wright's original theory. Wright influenced many students of the period, including Sir Alexander Fleming and Sir W.B. Leishman.[39] This treatment was used at the MGH for various diseases, and the results are not noted in the annual reports. The year 1906 also saw the installation of a freezing microtome, along with a trained micromitist who could now cut, stain, and preserve samples of the autopsy tissue.

In 1907, the department increased its work in bacteriology. with the number of autopsies and surgical remaining steady. Twenty-six publications are listed for the year. In 1908, Duval ended his term and G.B. Wolbach became the director. Bacteriology continued to increase, and the autopsy rate is listed in the annual report as 81.2 percent. This is a period of development for both the hospital and the pathology department, and there were plans for a new pathology building to deal with the department's increased workload.[40] The new building was said to be the best in connection with any hospital on this continent. In 1910, L.J. Rhea became the director of the department. In May 1911, the new pathology laboratory was opened and occupied. The aims of the department were: (1) to assist staff, (2) to teach, and (3) to conduct research. The laboratory made vaccines by applying the Wright system and, in particular, ensuring the staff had access to anti-typhoid vaccine. This year the annual report listed 714 surgical specimens, 180 autopsies, and twenty-tow publications. Alex Burgess became the director in 1912, assisted by D.D. MacTaggart and J.J. Ower, and there was no annual report form the Department of Pathology listed in the hospital records. Rhea returned the next year, and Burgess remained the director until 1914, when Rhea assumed this responsibility. Bacteriology was a major part of the work in the laboratory with both cultures and Wasserman blood tests. A rapid microscopic test for the diagnosis of diphtheria, developed by Wyatt Johnson, was employed with success in the identification of patients with the disease. The years 1914 to 1917 were very difficult for the hospital and the laboratory as the First World War resulted in many of the hospital staff going overseas. Rhea was absent for the year 1916 and MacTaggart was responsible for the laboratory.

In 1919, Rhea returned as director of the laboratory and remained as director until 1949. Under Rhea's direction the laboratory flourished with the introduction of clinical chemistry under I. Rabinowitch and parasitology under J.L. Todd. In 1919, the department gave regular weekly CPCs with emphasis on clinico-pathological correlation rather than the previous simple or "casual inspection," of which Rhea did not approve. The annual report of the Department of Pathology in 1920 states that the very high percentage of autopsies ranks among the first on the continent due to "little short of insistence on the part of the staff."[41] The museum was improved and better equipped for the medical students who were taught in the laboratory. Rhea encouraged research and stressed the importance of biochemical tests as well as the establishment of a diabetic clinic. These activities continued for the next year, which Rhea, in his excellent and detailed annual reports, states was the busiest year to date. He also stressed the very close relationship between the clinicians and the staff of the laboratory, and this remained an important element of his directorship throughout the next twenty years. The laboratory planned to extend its services to the outpatient department as Rhea felt there was no reason why these patients should not receive the "benefit" of the laboratory. He also felt that the laboratory must be more involved in the hospital's daily functions and not remain an area of mystery. This year photographic equipment was installed to augment the work of artists who had previously illustrated the records of pathological specimens. The report of the following year, 1922, again stresses clinico-pathological correlation and mentions the introduction of the teaching of normal anatomy and histology so that the abnormal could be appreciated. The course on pathology, bacteriology, and chemistry was improved and lengthened, and more space and equipment were requested.

In 1923, Rhea submitted a very long and detailed report on the Department of Pathology, stating that the past year had been the most active in the history of the department with regard to routine work and research. The main object of the work, that upon which the policy of the laboratory was based, "[was] to be of the greatest possible assistance to the patients that [were] in our Hospital or come to the Outpatient Department on any one day."[42] This excellent report gives a very clear indication of the interaction between the clinical staff and the laboratory and the importance that both found in the regular conferences, at which clear clinical histories were given and detailed pathology discussed. Rhea stressed the great importance of the physicians and surgeons at these conferences. The report also lists the needs of the department, such as the replacement of equipment that had not been changed since the war, the need for more lecture space (adequate for fifty-seven people), and an increase in the number of lectures from four per week to ten.

In 1924, the biochemical laboratory was "furnished and equipped and put into action." This laboratory was under the direction of I. Rabinowitch. This year also saw the amalgamation of the Western Division laboratory and that of the MGH. Further improvements in report filing, the photography department, and the museum are also listed. The next year saw further expansion in teaching, with the lecture room used nearly every day for students and nurses and with Rhea being responsible for the teaching. There is a plea for more staff and for more investigation into disease and not just the examination of material. The number of intraoperative diagnoses of tumours continued to increase, and this carried on over the next few years. Rhea was ill during the year 1926 but returned in 1927, and J.E. Pritchard joined the staff. Pritchard was trained at the University of Manitoba by William Boyd and was a welcome addition to the laboratory.

In 1928-29, the laboratory continued to enlarge and teaching, service and research expanded. Rhea was assisted in the Department of Pathology by Pritchard and Rabinowitch. The status of the laboratory, in the view of the superintendent of the hospital, A.K. Haywood, is stated in the superintendent's report to Lieutenant-Colonel Herbert Molson, the president of the hospital:

> This branch of the hospital's activities, speaking of pathology, is one of those departments behind the scenes so necessary and yet so unremunerative from the dollars and cents point of view that one finds it in cramped quarters, understaffed and poorly equipped and almost invariably under these conditions the result is unnecessary surgery, questionable diagnoses and a lack of clinical consciousness on the part of the hospital staff. We are proud of our Pathology laboratory. We can point with pride to, and exhibit to our visitors a laboratory imbued with a spirit of service to the patient and a most creditable record in the field of research and investigation.[43]

This perfectly summarizes the state of the laboratory and the philosophy of its director, L.J. Rhea.

Teaching was a major component of the laboratory work, and lantern slides and microphotograghs of common lesions were prepared with a new microphotographic machine purchased in 1929. In addition, colour photography was introduced for both microscopic photos and grass anatomical photos. The artist continued to paint both patients and gross lesions for these teaching sessions. Alan Ross joined the laboratory staff but soon left for Boston to train in paediatrics. The diabetic clinic under Rabinowitch continued to enlarge, with 2,876 patients on the list versus thirty-nine in 1920, and Rabinowitch followed Rhea's dictum: it is not enough to merely perform the laboratory work but one must also advance both the knowledge of the techniques and the treatment. With the services of the diabetic laboratory the death rate for diabetics was now equal to that for non-diabetics. In 1930, the lantern slide collection consisted of fifteen hundred slides, all indexed and covering all of the common as well as the rare diseases. A new microtome was purchased from France, and this apparatus allowed the cutting of larger sections of tissue.

The 1930s, under the direction of Rhea, showed continuing growth in the teaching collections and in the introduction of further services. In 1933, T.E. Roy joined as full-time bacteriologist but was unable to continue. A method for the identification of pneumococcus in ten minutes was introduced to the laboratory work, and this service increased. F.W. Wiglesworth joined in 1933 as a resident but left in 1934 to work at the Children's Memorial Hospital. Staffing was a problem, and, in his annual report, Rhea refers to "these trying times," in which enlargement of the staff seemed impossible. In 1937, Rhea stressed the need for a trained bacteriologist and stated that the current staff was just able to perform the day's work. There was some relief in the following years, with Mary Gzowski joining as medical illustrator and Frances Prissick appointed as full-time assistant for bacteriology. The Second World War had just started, and Rhea recognized the transfusion service with improved storage of blood and plasma. Due to the demands of the war the laboratory staff was incomplete and equipment very difficult to obtain. Bacteriology was expanded and a new room was devoted to the preparation of culture media. The laboratory continued to make all of the intravenous solutions for the hospital and to train technicians, many of whom left for war duty. In 1943, the department was renamed the Department of Pathology and Bacteriology and, as stated by Rhea, it was "conducted in such a way that the interest and welfare of the patients should come first." Rhea died in 1944 and Pritchard became the director. Rhea had succeeded in forming a department that provided the finest of diagnostic techniques in North America, and he followed a philosophy similar to that of Osler, of whom he wrote: "Sir William did a great deal for and with the pathology of his time, and pathology did a great deal for Sir William. He, more than any man whom I have known, had the ability to look beyond the gross [features] and even the detail of pathological lesions and apply them to the living."[44]

The annual report for 1949 showed the department to be as busy as before, with a marked increase in the number of surgical cases to 5,282, autopsies at 379, and bacteriological examinations at 6,288. The department was also responsible for the collection of blood for transfusion, with twenty-five hundred donors offering their services and twenty-three hundred transfusions being performed. This year the Red Cross assumed responsibility for the transfusion and collection of blood. Cytology was introduced, with the cooperation of the Department of Gynaecology, for the diagnosis of cervical cancer. Roger Reed was appointed as bacteriologist in the department and there were discussions about the formation of a separate department of bacteriology in the MGH with Reed as the director. Also in the department were W.H. Mathews and Howard Root, both of whom taught undergraduate and graduate students and were responsible for the clinic-pathological conferences of the department. F. Green conducted the serological examination, and consultants to the department from McGill University were E.G.D. Murray (professor of bacteriology) and Lyman Duff (professor of pathology).

The late 1940s were a time when the MGH began to consider expanding and building a new, larger hospital and school for nursing. After very extensive discussion and an external consultation on the future of the teaching hospitals of McGill, a site grouping of the teaching units was felt to offer the most practical solution for the integration of medical service, teaching, and research. Some consideration was given to building the new hospital adjacent to the Royal Victoria Hospital and the university, but this was rejected: "Our conclusion was that all things considered, its advantages were considerably outweighed by the disadvantages." Land was available further west and consisted of 32,220 square metres, which was very adequate for a 600- to 750-bed hospital, and the site was purchased from the Judge Cross Estate in 1948. The area far exceeded the previous hospital area of about 5,760 square metres and was praised for the increased parking space, the access by streetcar, and the grounds around the hospital.[45]

From 1950 to 1954 (the year the new hospital was completed), routine work continued under the direction of Pritchard, Mathews, and Root. Miller Fisher joined the department staff as neuropathologist, Reed left for Dalhousie University, and Green retired. In 1951, Joan deVreis joined as an assistant in bacteriology. In 1954, the new hospital building was completed with the nurses' residence being completed in the following year, and the hospital opened to patients in May 1955. The director of the pathology department was Pritchard, with the assistance of Mathews and Root. Miller Fisher departed for Harvard and the Massachusetts General Hospital and was replaced by David Howell. De Vreis directed the bacteriology service, and Elizabeth Marshall was the director of medical illustrating.

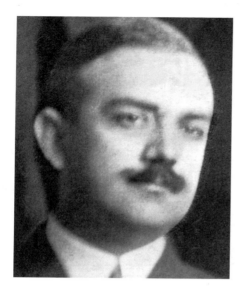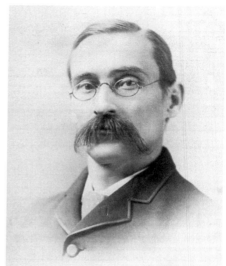
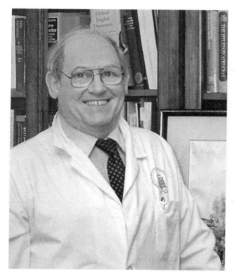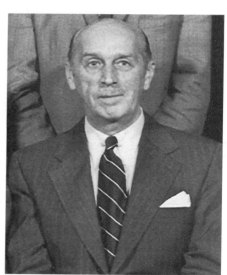

Clockwise from top left
Fig. 31.5 C.W. Duval, chief of pathology, 1906–08
Fig. 31.6 Alex Burgess, chief of pathology, 1912–14
Fig. 31.7 William Mathews, chief of pathology, 1959–71
Fig. 31.8 W.P. Duguid, chief of pathology, 1971–2000

Last Years in the New Hospital

In 1959, Mathews became the director assisted by H. Root, Sean Moore and David Howell. Residents from the McGill Department of Pathology could now spend six months in clinical pathology with bacteriology and toxicology. This pattern continued for the next few years and, in 1962, an autopsy resident was introduced in addition to residents in surgical pathology. These residents were taken from the training program of the McGill University Department of Pathology. In 1964, Root retired and F. Gomes joined as a special fellow, and, in 1965, M.H. Finlayson joined as neuropathologist. The department now dealt with 9,980 surgical specimens and 444 autopsies per year. Over the next few years the department slowly enlarged, with more residents and staff, but essentially functioned as a service department with teaching but little research.

In 1970, William Duguid joined the staff and the next year, upon the retirement of W. Mathews, became the director of the department. Duguid was trained at the Glasgow Royal Infirmary in pathology, and, after a stint in the army, he joined Sir Tom Symington in the Department of Pathology at that institution. There he established an international reputation in endocrine and renal pathology and spent several additional years in the Department of Physiology of the Western Reserve University in Cleveland. Following these two years in Cleveland he became a senior lecturer in pathology at the University of Glasgow and then, in 1970, came to Montreal and the MGH as a senior pathologist. He was much influenced by Sir Thomas Symington to establish a department based on basic research and diagnostic pathology, with the research aimed at understanding basic biological processes involved in disease. He had little use for the simple categorizing of lesions, which was then popular in pathology, and insisted on understanding the importance of the mechanisms of how the lesion developed. He was a founding director of the MGH Research Institute and also chaired the hospital's Medical Advisory Committee for many years. He was able to establish a strong research unit within the hospital and allowed researchers free time away from the diagnostic service of the department. He himself conducted a basic research program in diabetes and demonstrated stem cell differentiation in the pancreas and the production of insulin-secreting cells from these stem cells. In addition to research, the department during these years was very active in university affairs, in teaching, research, and the introduction and

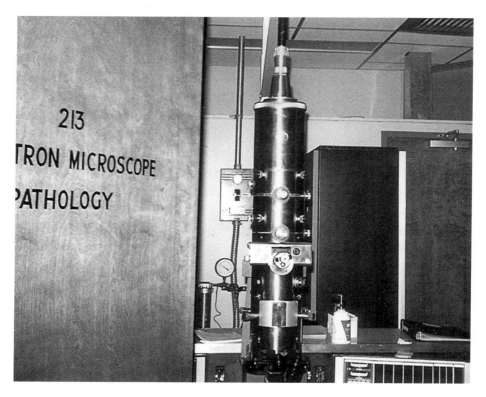

Fig. 31.9 Electron microscope in pathology

development of new clinical techniques. The department under the direction of Duguid resembled the active and productive years of Rhea, when pathology played a vital role in the functioning of the hospital. Both Duguid and Rhea shared a belief in the importance of clarity of ideas and the need for research and understanding of disease processes for the advancement of medicine. Duguid died in 2000, and the department, now part of larger amalgamated collection of hospitals, reverted to a mainly diagnostic unit with no activity in the hospital's Research Institute.

The Department of Pathology at the MGH had an enormous influence on the role of pathology in North America. The early work of the department far exceeded that of the university with regard to teaching, introduction of methodology, and correlation of morphological lesions with the clinical state of the patients. While Osler was instrumental in the founding of the department, those who followed him carried on with the high standards of technique and teaching that he had encountered in Germany and elsewhere in Europe. This importation of ideas and knowledge propelled the medical profession to advance from the backward state in which it found itself when Osler attended medical school. This forward-looking attitude was carried on throughout subsequent years, assuring that the Department of Pathology played an important, influential, and educational role in the MGH and McGill throughout their over one hundred years of existence.

NOTES

1 Montreal General Hospital, annual report, Pathology, 1858, MUA.

2 Ibid., 1868.

3 Ibid., 1869.

4 Ibid., 1873.

5 Ibid., 1875.

6 Ibid., 1876.

7 Ibid., 1877.

8 Ibid., 1876

9 Ibid., 1878.

10 Ibid., 1884.

11 Ibid., 1892.

12 Ibid., 1896.

13 M.F. Xavier Bichat, *Traite d'Anatomie descriptive* (Paris: Chez Brosson libraire, 1771–1802).

14 S.D. Gross, *Elements of Pathological Anatomy*, 3rd ed. (Philadelphia: Blanchard & Lea, 1857).

15 Karl Rokitansky, *Lehrbuch der pathologischen anatomie* (Wien: W. Braumuller, 1855–61).

16 Rudolf Virchow, *Die Cellularpathologie* (Berlin: Verlag von August Hirschwald, 1858).

17 R. Koch, "Demonstration of tuberculosis bacillus," 24 March 1882.

18 C.J.B. Williams, *Principals of Medicine: An Elementary View* (1857). Textbook used by Osler.

19 J.H. Wright, *History of Pathology at the Massachusetts General Hospital* (Boston: MGH Pathology Services, 2006).

20 H. Cushing, *The Life of William Osler*, vol. 1 (Oxford: Oxford University Press, 1925), 47–69.

21 Ibid., 85.

22 Ibid., 91–107.

23 Ibid., 106–11.

24 Ibid., 113.

20 Howard Burchell, "Osler: In Quest of the Gnostic Grail in Morbid Anatomy," *British Journal of the History of Medicine* (July 1975): 235–49.

25 G. Majno and I.G. Joris, "The Microscope in the History of Pathology," *Virchows Arch Abt. A. Path.Anat.* 360 (1973): 273–86.

26 Ibid.

27 Cushing, *Life of William Osler*, 110.

28 Ibid.

29 Pathology at Cambridge, History of the Department, University of Cambridge, http://www.path.cam.ac.uk.

30 F. Marte, et al. "The Stability of Natural History Specimens in Fluid-Preserved Collections," Smithsonian Center for Materials Research and Education.

31 W. Osler, "Normal Histology for Laboratory and Class Use, 1882," McGill Library. This is Osler's histology lab manual for the histology course at McGill.

32 Cushing, *Life of William Osler*, 145.

32 Ibid., 185.

33 Montreal General Hospital, annual report, 1882.

34 Wyatt Galt Johnston Collection, Osler Library Archive Collections, Montreal, MUA.

36 H.E. MacDermot, *History of the Montreal General Hospital* (Montreal: Montreal General Hospital, 1950), 74–5.

37 K.M. Earle, *A History of the IAP: The First Seventy-Five Years, 1906–1981* (Palm Springs, CA: International Academy of Pathology News Centre, 1981).

38 Montreal General Hospital, annual report, 1906.

39 A Silverstein, "The Plato of Praed Street: The Life and Times of Almroth Wright," *Bulletin of the History of Medicine* 76, 1 (2002): 158–60.

40 Montreal General Hospital, annual report, 1908.

41 Ibid., 1920.

42 Ibid., 1923.

43 Ibid., 1929.

44 H. Burchell, "Osler: the Quest for the Gnostic Grail in Morbid Anatomy," *British Journal of the History of Medicine* (July 1975): 239.

45 Montreal General Hospital, annual report, 1949.

32

Pharmacy

Lyson T. Haccoun and John H. Burgess

Lyson Haccoun was a senior MGH pharmacist for many years. John Burgess edited her manuscript for this chapter.

One of the first duties of the pharmacist is to educate the masses
not to take medicine.

When the Montreal General Hospital opened in 1822, an apothecary shop was put in the main lobby to act as the pharmacy. The apothecary era was characterized by high ceilings and numerous wickets, wooden brown narrow sliding cabinets, and black lacquered counters. Arrangements were made to hire someone trained to do the job of compounding medicines, but few persons had the necessary expertise. In 1827, E.B. O'Callaghan was contracted to do the job, but he had no licence. He apparently subsequently got one, but employment at the MGH was tenuous because of constant financial problems. He was let go and the house surgeon was given the job. The house officer lived in the hospital and was also responsible for patient admissions and care as well as drug dispensing. This arrangement persisted until an official pharmacy was created.

The 1823 Rules and Regulations for the MGH apothecary were as follows:

1 No person shall be eligible to the office of Apothecary unless he has attained the age of twenty-one years before he has laid before the Governors satisfactory testimonials of his moral character and of his having been examined and approved by the Medical Board.

2 He shall compound and make up all the medicines required by the hospital, according to the formulae from time to time prescribed by the Medical Board.

3   He shall deliver [no] medicines [that are not] … ordered by the medical officers attending, [nor] shall [he] permit any medicines to be taken out of the hospital except by out patients.

4   He shall make up the different medicines for the wards, and annex to them labels containing the names of the patients and the directions for taking, and shall send the medicines to the different wards by the orderly man, who shall deliver the same to their respective nurses.

5   He shall regularly attend the shop, and never be absent without permission. He shall keep the shop[,] and everything appertaining thereto, clean and in Proper Order, he shall also observe strict economy in all and everything related to his Department, and shall be particularly careful in the delivery of medicines to the Patients.

6   He shall not allow patients under any pretence whatsoever to enter the shop.

7   The Apothecary shall give a bond in the penalty of one hundred pounds currencies a security for the faithful performance of the duties of his office and shall not cease to perform the said duties without giving to the Governors two months' notice of his intention to leave his employment.

8   The funds of the hospital not being at present sufficient to pay a house physician, a house surgeon or apothecary, the duties are in the meantime to be performed by the doctor residing in the MGH.[1]

In the early days of the MGH, pharmaceuticals available for treatment were few in number. Alcohol, in the form of beer, wine, and spirits, was much prescribed. Every patient admitted was given a choice of wine, beer, and at times champagne, in a bottle at the bedside. Moderation was the rule, and drunkenness resulted in discharge from the hospital.

There was no apothecary training in Canada in the nineteenty century except by apprenticeship, mostly with practising doctors who taught them how to compound medicine. According to the 1823 Rules and Regulations (above), a candidate for the apothecary position had to prove to members of the Medical Board that he knew how to compound medicines for hospital patients. The standards in practice were not too high because house officers or volunteer doctors who lived in the hospital did the job. The most common orders, other than purchased medications such as Dover's Powders or Glauber's Salts (to mention two), he had to be able to compound lineaments (alcohol or vinegar and mustard or ammonia), poultices (which were pieces of cloth soaked in hot linseed oil and mustard or camphor), tinctures (alcohol and iodine, laudanum or opium, to be used as drops in water), extracts that were evaporated alcohol extracts from bark (Chincona), digitalis leaves or hemp leaves, and pastes made of sugar and gum with camphor, mustard, or ammonia mixed to be placed somewhere on the body.

Opium and its derivatives were used for the alleviation of pain and discomfort. Sometimes a combination of alcohol and opium were used for added effects, bearing seductive names such as laudanum, paregoric, chloranodyne, along with various tinctures and bitters. It was considered preferable, but not necessary, that the hospital's earliest apothecaries have some medical training. Not even training in pharmacy was considered a criterion.

In 1917, a new pharmacy program was begun at McGill University within the Faculty of Medicine. It was headed by B. Moore, who was the first trained pharmacist at the MGH and became its first chief pharmacist.[2] He had his own special preparation called Golden Glow, which he served at meetings, thus hastening their discussions. A similar product was developed by his successor.

However, the real pioneer of MGH pharmacy was Frank Zahalan (1909–87), who served this institution for forty years, thirty-five of them as chief pharmacist.[3] Frank Zahalan was born in New Liskeard, Ontario, in 1909. His father had immigrated to Canada a few years before Frank's birth and moved to northern Ontario, where he amassed a fortune in silver mining and then lost it all in bad real estate investments. Douglas G. Cameron stated in his eulogy for Frank Zahalan in 1987: "Frank's early tinselled memories of childhood as a young princeling in this booming, raucous, brawling frontier were quickly succeeded by the harsh reality of the severe economic stringencies in Montreal."[4]

Frank graduated from high school in 1927. He was determined to go to university but had to work for the next two years to save money for his tuition fees. He chose pharmacy at the University of Montreal because it was the only program that permitted students to undertake full course work and, at the same time, be employed as apprentices. He got a job in Albert's Drug Store at the corner of Dorchester and Main. His salary was five dollars per week.

In 1934, Frank Zahalan received his degree in pharmacy and, taking his diploma across the street, joined the staff of the MGH. In 1939, he was appointed chief pharmacist and quickly became recognized as the dean of hospital pharmacists in Quebec and one of the pioneers of hospital pharmacy in Canada.

In 1940, Frank was recruited by the Canadian Armed Forces to set up a pharmacy for the No. 14 Canadian General Hospital. The sulpha emulsion that he had developed at the MGH became a standard treatment for burns throughout the armed forces. An sixty-thousand-dollar award was given for the production of a film illustrating its use, and, as a result, a considerable amount of money flowed into the hospital.

In 1961, Frank was appointed a lecturer at the University of Montreal and established a postgraduate course in pharmacy. He published many papers in French and English. He became a founding member of the Canadian Society of Hospital Pharmacists, was president of the Quebec branch, and, in 1952, represented Canada at the first World Congress of Hospital Pharmacists.

Frank Zahalan was renowned not only for developing new medicines but also for originating an alcoholic beverage named "purple passion," which he dispensed to a large number of hospital staff, particularly on Christmas Day. This greatly enhanced the festivities, encouraging many to visit the pharmacy that morning. It was traditional for a member of the resident staff to play Santa. Frank would arrange for him to be suitably primed before he started his rounds on the nineteenth floor and worked his way down. One year Santa stumbled on a top stairwell, giving himself a head wound. This had to be stitched in the emergency room and a stand-in was quickly recruited to resume distributing presents.

Frank was involved with the hospital residency program in its early stages. He welcomed students, innovation, and specialization such as radiopharmacy. He was well respected by physicians, hospital staff, peers, and industry. After his retirement in 1974, he worked as a consultant to industry and created the Frank Zahalan Foundation, which provides bursaries for students.

After the move to Pine Avenue, the MGH pharmacy was lodged on the first-floor Pine entrance. Outpatients awaiting their medications were seated along the hallway benches. The pharmacy dispensing area, with glass wickets, communicated with the front office, and further down was the manufacturing and medication stock area. Tools were limited – three typewriters, ten pharmacists/shift, five technicians, one storekeeper, and one secretary.

Nathan Fox succeeded Frank Zahalan as chief pharmacist from 1974 until 1985. After the introduction of Medicare in Quebec in the early 1970s, control of health care costs and quality control were high on his agenda. His objectives were to extend clinical pharmacy services and to improve drug

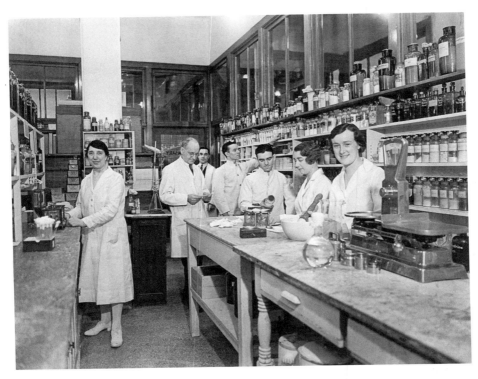

Fig. 32.1 B. Moore, first trained pharmacist, MGH, 1917–39

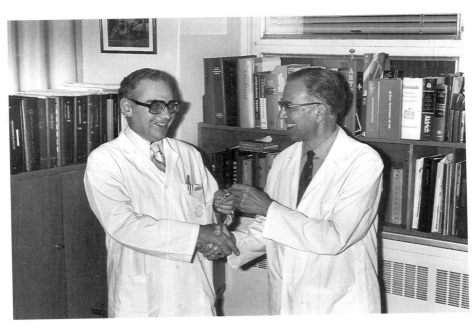

Fig. 32.2 Frank Zahalan, chief pharmacist, MGH, 1939–74 (right); Nathan Fox, chief pharmacist, MGH, 1974–85

utilization control. Fox encouraged the clinical role of the hospital pharmacist by instituting visits to the hospital wards. He also started an adverse drug reaction program and reporting to the Health Protection Board of Canada. Fox and his staff regularly attended weekly clinical pharmacology conferences and journal clubs. Pharmacists gave lectures on drugs to nurses and medical residents. During his tenure as chief pharmacist his department officially became part of the MGH Council of Physicians, Dentists and Pharmacists. He retired in 1985.

Lyson Tobaly-Haccoun became interim chief pharmacist in 1985. She had served as a pharmacist since 1996. Together with Zahalan and Fox she initiated various projects to consolidate basic tools within the pharmacy. She updated the MGH formulary and organized ward visits. She updated cardiac arrest trays (with John Burgess) and created a new design for pharmacy prescription forms. Haccoun then assisted the new chief pharmacist, Marie Pineault, with new projects, acting as a buffer between older and newer staff.

The last MGH chief pharmacist before the MGH became part of the newly founded McGill University Health Centre was Marie Pineault (1985–96).[5] She had previously worked at the Royal Victoria Hospital and brought extensive experience to her new position. She forged close ties with the Faculty of Pharmacy at the University of Montreal and established structures to ensure that all staff pharmacists remained at the leading edge of their profession.

Marie Pineault was a very dynamic, multi-tasking person, well known by her peers and eager to move ahead the pharmacy profession at large. She was a fellow of the American and Canadian Hospital Pharmacists Association and was awarded the distinctive Louis-Hebert Prize from the Order of Pharmacists of Quebec. She served on various government boards: the Advisory Council of Pharmacology, the Review Committee of Senior Management of Health Canada, and the Order of Pharmacists of Quebec.

All MGH pharmacy directors have worked fiercely to overcome difficult challenges and to satisfy essential objectives and high standards of practice. Their relentless efforts, vast experience, and vision have resulted in establishing today's Department of Pharmacy Department within the MUHC as an equal partner of the medical health team.

NOTES

1 Rules and Regulations of the MGH, 1823, regarding the apothecary, in Minute Book of the Committee of Management, 1823, MUA.

2 J. Collin and D. Belliveau, *Histoire de la Pharmacie au Québec* (Sabex : Musee de la Pharmacie du Québec, 1994); J.F. Bussieres and N. Maranda, *De L'Apothecaire au Specialiste: Histoire de la Pharmacie hospitaliere au Québec* (Montreal: Association des pharmaciens des établissements de santé Québec, 2011).

3 Dentistry and Pharmacy report on history of both departments and F. Zahalan, MGH, MUA; L. Legault, editorial, "La Fondation Francis Zahalan," *Quebec Pharmacie* 35 (1988): 127; Honouring F. Zahalan at retirement, Council of Physicians and Dentists, 1974, MGH, MUA, Palmer and Cameron and Chairman Peck.

4 D.G. Cameron, Eulogy – Frank Zahalan, MGH News, 7 December 1986, MGH Library.

5 Marie Pineault, director of pharmacy, pharmacy reorganization update, report, December 1987, MGH Archives 1987.

33

Physical Medicine

Jacqueline Harvey

Jacqueline Harvey was a senior physiotherapist at the MGH.

The Early Years

The first physiotherapist on staff at the Montreal General Hospital was Esther Aspler, a member of the British Chartered Society of Remedial Gymnastics, sometime around 1912. She gained her position by approaching Mackenzie Forbes, an orthopaedic surgeon, and demonstrating her treatment techniques to him. Prior to her appointment, physiotherapists treated patients privately outside the hospital setting. Aspler soon built up a busy clinic, before leaving in 1916 to take up a position at the Montreal Children's Hospital.

In his *History of the Montreal General Hospital*, MacDermott quoted the 1921 annual report, which indicated that there was a Department of Physiotherapy, albeit in poor condition. The department was staffed by foreign-trained therapists, maids, and orderlies until the mid-1940s, when, due to an increased demand for therapists brought about by wounded people returning from the Second World War, a school of physiotherapy was created at McGill University in 1943.

The school was started by Guy Fisk, a physiatrist at the MGH, and Margaret Fletcher, a British-trained physiotherapist. An occupational therapy program was introduced in 1950. From having one therapist in 1912, the MGH had gone on to have a staff of direct referrals (i.e., staff were called and patients referred directly to one person rather than to the department).

Prior to 1985, before receiving any intervention from a therapist, all patients were examined, and treatment modalities were prescribed by physiatrists Fisk or Jesus Silva, the latter having taken up his appointment in 1965. Following Fisk's retirement in 1985, patients referred from the divisions of neurology, neurosurgery, orthopaedics, and rheumatology were referred directly to the therapists, who, based on their assessments, planned and carried out appropriate programs of treatment. Silva retired in the early 1990s, after which time all inpatients and outpatients were referred directly to the therapist. These changes placed greater responsibilities on individual therapists who, with or without some direction from the referring physician or surgeon, planned and carried out treatment programs and then participated in discharge planning.

Specialization

Physiotherapy and occupational therapy services are offered to all the hospital's wards as well as to the busy outpatient department. In the earlier years, therapists rotated through (each of) the various services every three to four months. As therapists took advantage of the increasing number of postgraduate courses and gained expertise in specific areas, this practice was gradually phased out.

Therapists now practise in an area in which they have specialized. There is still opportunity to change services as positions become available, which permits those junior therapists, should they so choose, to gain experience in a number of different areas. The opportunity to specialize resulted in therapists assuming major roles in the hospital's various programs.

Since its creation by Ronald Melzack, Mary-Ellen Jeans, and Joseph Stratford, the pain clinic team has included a physiotherapist. Lois Finch, the first physiotherapist appointed to the pain clinic, participated in research projects on the management of chronic pain. The results of her study on comparing transcutaneous electrical nerve stimulation with transcutaneous electrical nerve stimulation and massage was published in the journal *Physical Therapy* in 1983.

A large area of the outpatient department is devoted to the rehabilitation of patients with hand injuries referred from the departments of plastic and orthopaedic surgeries. Irene Kinach was the occupational therapist who first gained expertise in this area. Rekha Toomey and Rhonda Grief-Schwartz, physiotherapists practising in the Hand Centre, were awarded the Silver Quill Award by the Canadian Physiotherapy Association for their research project entitled "Clinical Evaluation of Whirlpool on Patients with Colles Fracture."

The Hand Centre continues to be a busy area, where physiotherapists and occupational therapists work closely together. It is staffed by therapists with many years of experience and a great deal of expertise (as is required in the management of patients who often present with complex and potentially disabling injuries).

After attending postgraduate courses in Vancouver and Toronto on the management of rheumatic diseases, Jackie Harvey took responsibility for patients referred from the Division of Rheumatology. Together with June Williams of McGill University and Tannenbaum, she conducted a pilot study on the use of superficial heat versus ice for the rheumatoid arthritic shoulder, the results of which were presented at a poster session of the Northeastern Regional Meeting of the Arthritis Foundation, which took place in Toronto in 1984. Their work in this area was published in *Physiotherapy Canada* in 1988.

Both physiotherapists and occupational therapists are important members of the team that manages traumatic brain injuries. Rehabilitation is started soon after admission to the ward, with the aim of getting patients mobilized early on and so the decreasing the length of their hospital stay. Therapists then participate in appropriate plans for patients' discharge from hospital.

There are therapists with the requisite expertise practising on the medical, surgical, orthopaedic, geriatric, neurology, and neurosurgery wards as well as in the outpatient departments and the emergency room. Physiotherapy services, although decreased at weekends and holidays, are offered every day throughout the year.

Education

At its beginning, the School of Physiotherapy at McGill University offered a two-year diploma program, followed by an internship. The program has since evolved to offer a three-year bachelor of science degree in either physiotherapy or occupational therapy; qualifications currently required to practise in the Province of Quebec.

During each year of the three-year program students undergo several weeks of clinical training at various health-care institutions. Senior therapists at the MGH teach, supervise, and evaluate a number of students at all levels of their training. In addition, some therapists add to their busy schedule by teaching clinical courses at the School of Physiotherapy.

The education of patients plays a large role in achieving successful outcomes for treatment programs: As well as teaching patients exercise programs to perform at home on days when they are not attending therapy, there is an increased need to educate patients on correct posture, aimed at minimizing abnormal stresses and strains on the musculoskeletal system. This is not only appropriate for manual labourers but also for those who spend their workdays sitting at desks, working at computers, or other such sedentary occupations.

Changes

As services offered at the MGH have changed, so has the scope of physio and occupational therapy. The transfer of all obstetrics eliminated prenatal and postnatal exercise programs. Patients with severe burns, who were once admitted to the isolation ward and who received exercise programs and splinting to maintain mobility and prevent deformities, are now treated at Sacre Coeur Hospital. The amputee program, with prosthetic clinics headed by J. Silva, no longer exists as changes in management of patients with peripheral vascular disease and the transfer of the vascular service to the RVH has eliminated the need for it.

The transfer of all orthopaedic services from the RVH to the MGH had a big impact on physiotherapy. As many orthopaedic surgeries are performed in day surgery, the bigger impact was felt in the outpatient department. The waiting time for therapy for patients with les acute conditions increased, and the management of the waiting list was an ongoing challenge. This was addressed in 2002 when Antoinette Di Re was appointed manager of the adult sites of the McGill University Health Centre. She arranged for patients, who so chose, to receive physiotherapy at the RVH, thus reducing the waiting list at the MGH.

The designation of the MGH as a level-1 trauma centre has resulted in the admission of larger numbers of patients with varying degrees of injuries.

Therapists play a vital role in the management of these patients. The opinions of the therapist regarding the patient's ability to mobilize, the provision of appropriate walking aids, and recommendations regarding post-discharge care is greatly valued. Early mobilization has proven to prevent complications, aid recovery, and decrease length of hospital stays. This has resulted in therapists being consulted far more often now than was previously the case when patients are acutely sick.

34

Psychiatry

Alan C. Mann, Joseph Hanaway, and Garth Bray

Alan Mann was the second chief of psychiatry at the MGH. Joseph Hanaway and Garth Bray completed this chapter when Alan became ill.

Editors' Note and Introduction

Because of illness, Alan Mann was unable to complete this manuscript prior to his death on 17 November 2011. The format of this chapter is more auto-biographical than are others in this volume. However, Alan Mann's story offers an insightful history of psychiatry at the MGH because he joined the department in 1950, four years after it was formed, and retired as its chair in 1990. The following introductory paragraphs are written by the editors.

Alan Mann was asked to write this chapter on psychiatry at the MGH, as he personally experienced it, between 1950 and 1990 and as chair from 1971 to 1990. The Department of Psychiatry started as a consult service in the old Dorchester Street and Western Division of the MGH, a day centre in 1951 and a night centre in 1954, the first in Canada. Electro-convulsive therapy (ECT) and insulin treatments were performed in these centres. The MGH moved to Cedar Avenue in 1955. With the 1961 Quebec Hospital Insurance Plan,[1] major overcrowding of the hospital occurred, particularly with regard to psychiatric cases. It was a major problem for the psychiatric service for decades and required additional space, new drugs, and more psychiatrists to resolve it. Mann describes the rolls of Ewen Cameron (Allen Memorial) and Heinze Lehman (Verdun Protestant Hospital) at McGill as well as ECT, lobotomy, the effect of the *Diagnostic and Statistical Manual* (*DSM*), and the ill-conceived sectorization of Montreal (1973) in the hope that this would enable it to distribute patient populations more evenly. It did not.

The origins of neurology and psychiatry at the MGH are described in chapter 14. The neurologists F.H. and A.A. MacKay and, particularly, Norman Viner treated psychiatric diseases in the 1920s and 1930s.

During the Second World War, psychiatric disease was better understood and recognized. McGill University opened its Department of Psychiatry in 1943 under Ewen Cameron at the Allen Memorial Institute (AMI), which is associated with the Royal Victoria Hospital. Cameron, a powerful academic politician, had total control of psychiatry at McGill and in all the hospitals. He wanted a department at the MGH and so had Albert Moll appointed its first chief in 1946. A resident training program started at the MGH in 1950, which brings us to Alan Mann and his story as told in his own words.

Alan Mann's Early Interest in Psychiatry

I attended McGill University as an undergraduate from 1941 to 1943. As an undergraduate student, I considered a career in psychiatry after taking a few psychology courses and doing a lot a reading. I then joined the Royal Canadian Navy as a volunteer reserve.

After the war, I went to the McGill Medical School from 1945 to 1949. At that time, there was little psychiatric training in the McGill Faculty of Medicine outside the Allen Memorial Institute. All graduating students in Canada were required to do a rotating internship,[2] which consisted of four-month rotations in medicine, surgery, and obstetrics, which I did at the RVH. As part of my medicine rotation, I was able to spend two months at the Verdun Protestant Hospital (VPH).[3] During that rotation, I came under the influence of the impressive chief of psychiatry, Heinz Lehmann, who became famous for his work with chlorpromazine. Thus, when I finished my internship, I chose a psychiatry residency at the VPH. As a courtesy, I went to see Ewen Cameron, chair of the McGill Department of Psychiatry and director of the Allan Memorial Institute, to inform him that I was starting at Verdun. He was sceptical about the training under Lehmann, over whom he had no control.

The house staff at the VPH in 1950–51 consisted of two rotating interns (from medicine) plus the full-time resident. Patients were admitted to the medical ward and then sent to one of the pavilions. Lehmann, a dynamic European-trained psychiatrist, insisted on daily conferences at 11:30 AM that were mandatory for all staff, including attendings. He gave out a list of patients to the house staff, which indicated what each patient needed. He would later question them about the list and what findings were made regarding the patients. There was often a case presented when a patient was ready for discharge or had an interesting problem. Everyone would participate in these discussions.

I felt that I had an excellent experience at the VPH because there were many patients to be seen and Lehmann was an outstanding teacher. I left Verdun in 1951 for further training at the MGH, where a department of psychiatry had been created in 1946, with Albert Moll the first chief,[4] and where a training program had started in 1950.

I was a resident at the MGH from 1951 to 1953, seeing inpatients and clinic patients. In the spring of 1953, I passed the certification examination given by the Royal College of Physicians and Surgeons of Canada. I thus obtained a CRCP. To prepare for the fellowship examination (FRCP), a booklet was issued by the Royal College that stated that the qualifications for a fellowship included four years of resident training and the examination. The exam, which everyone took because there were no specialty exams, was in general medicine. Of the nine candidates from Montreal – all fully trained in psychiatry – only two passed. One joined the staff at the MGH and the other was trained as a general practitioner. The other seven, who did not pass, were quite upset, as was Ewen Cameron. The Royal College required candidates to have one year in medicine to be eligible for the fellowship examination. I showed this to Cameron, who complained to Oliver Stolkes, professor of psychiatry at the University of Toronto. With enough protest from McGill, Toronto, and Dalhousie universities, this clause was eventually removed from the booklet of qualifications: a rotating internship was deemed to be an adequate prerequisite for psychiatry.

One year later, I went on to paediatric psychiatry at the Montreal Children's Hospital. The program was thought to be "loose," with Taylor Statten as its full-time director. A fellow classmate, John Stanley, and I claimed we taught Statten psychiatry because he focused more on general paediatrics. Caplan was a part-time staff member. Child psychiatry at the MCH was more organized than adult psychiatry at the MGH. The department had a number of social workers and psychologists (for testing) who backed up the program. These services would eventually be available at the MGH.

The Beginning of MGH Psychiatry

Officially, the Department of Psychiatry at the MGH on Dorchester Street started in 1946.[5] There were no beds or wards specifically set aside for psychiatric services; instead, the department offered a consultation service and a clinic and had to share quarters, which consisted of one outpatient room, with the Department of Obstetrics and Gynaecology. Psychiatric outpatients were seen Monday afternoons after the obstetrics/gynaecology clinic was finished.

The only full-time senior staff member at the MGH in 1950 was Albert Moll. Travis Dancey,[6] who helped share the duties, was also chief at the Queen Mary Veterans Hospital and was a well known psychiatrist. Other part-time staff members were Rich Hamilton, who was also on staff at the veterans hospital in St. Anne de Bellevue, and Manuel Straicker, who was a prolific contributor to the literature. Both attended in the clinic half a day a week.

In 1949–50, the twenty-two-bed open children's ward at the MGH was turned into a psychiatric ward for women only. There were no restraints or private rooms, so patients with syphilis or any other psychotic illness could not be admitted and were sent to the VPH. Our patients suffered mostly from mild to severe depression, rarely true bipolar disorder, and serious anxiety neuroses. These patients were referred from outside doctors or came through the Emergency Room.

In the summer of 1954, I finished my residency at the MCH and joined the staff at the MGH. In 1955, the hospital moved from Dorchester Street to Cedar Avenue. The new Department of Psychiatry consisted of twenty rooms for inpatients, a day centre, and some offices but no dedicated clinic area; psychiatry shared clinic space with ENT.

Record keeping at the MGH was a terrible problem because of the concern about the privacy of ward charts. Doctors wrote their own notes on patients and kept them from the patients' charts. The idea was that every doctor had to keep his or her own notes because confidential records did not go in the main chart. This policy made record keeping difficult for follow-up care. Years later, a huge locker was found completely stuffed with notes anywhere from two to ten years old. The only way to destroy these records was to burn them. Patients were seen in the hospital or as consultations on the medical and surgical wards by the residents and staff. The confidentiality of medical records was finally accepted, so the patients' histories were recorded in the ward charts.

The Day Centre

In October 1951, the MGH started the first Adult Day Centre in a general hospital in Canada in a building attached to the Western Division of the MGH.[7] The centre's specific criteria for patients to be seen included a diagnosis of depression or anxiety. Patients came to the centre at 8:30 AM, were treated, and went home at 4:30 PM. The idea was to treat patients who did not need hospitalization but did need special treatment and who could go home daily to be with their families. The demand for more patient care was met at a lower cost. The unit could also be a step-down for patients getting ready for discharge. Psychotic, psychopathic, and mentally retarded patients in any form were sent to the VPH. There were no private rooms, but private patients paid and did not complain about sharing rooms with public patients. Electric shock therapy and insulin sub-coma therapy were performed in the day centre as well as occupational therapy. The average daily census was about twenty.

Analysis was frowned upon by Ewen Cameron, who controlled psychiatry at all the hospitals. Therefore Moll, who was analytically oriented, did not promote analysis at the MGH. The residents, however, were frequently analyzed during and after training, but this was a personal choice for personal insight but did not mean these doctors practised analysis.

The Night Clinic

In October 1954, a night clinic was established that used the beds of the Day Centre patients after 4:30 PM.[8] Patients would leave the day clinic and be replaced by others spending the night getting therapy. These were patients who could go to work but who could get along better during the day if they received treatment during the night, thereby avoiding admission. Thus, the same beds could be used by day patients for insulin sub-coma therapy in the morning, for electro-convulsive therapy in the afternoon, and by night patients after 4:30 PM. This unit operated five days per week and could accommodate up to forty-five patients per day if fully utilized. Eventually, the night clinic closed because an observation unit was more urgently needed.

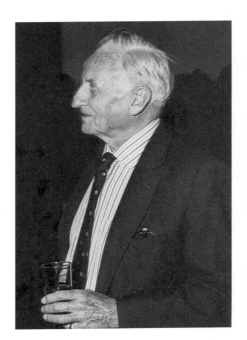 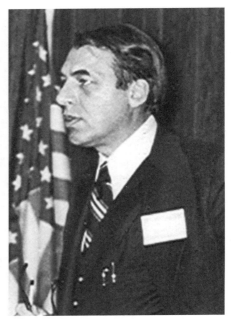

Fig. 34.1 Bert Moll, first chief of MGH psychiatry, 1946–70
Fig. 34.2 Alan Mann, chief of MGH psychiatry, 1971–90

The unit became an acute observation ward with nine beds for patients who usually came through the ER.

Treatment in the 1950s–70s

The various types of treatment included individual or group interview therapy (psychotherapy), occupational therapy, ECT, and insulin sub-coma, which had been used for years. The Inpatient Division and the Adult Day Centre both used ECT. In the early 1950s, anti-depressants had not been developed except for sodium amytal and other barbiturates that were available for manic-depressive illnesses and anxiety.

The ECT routine was six to nine treatments for depression of average severity. ECT's were performed at 1:00 PM. Three treatments were performed per week: on Monday, Wednesday, and Friday. Patients with recurrent depression only need six treatments. By 1957, the amount of ECT being administered was a problem: patients were losing their short-term memory, thus requiring more time as inpatients. The memory loss was usually temporary but could be permanent if too many treatments were given.

The rationale for insulin coma therapy was questioned, but it seemed to work.[9] It continued to be used at the VPH, although there was concern that too much insulin would cause serious hypoglycemia and result in brain dysfunction. For coma therapy, interns would administer insulin at doses of up to 150 units. Patients would fall into insulin coma for many hours but could be aroused by glucose administered either by nasogastric tube or intravenously. A lesser dose of only ten to fifteen units was effective as sub-coma treatment for anxiety and depression; this lower dose produced less hypoglycemia and was much safer than coma therapy, which was not used at the MGH.

After roughly thirty years, by the early 1970s, both ECT and insulin therapy were replaced by better drugs for depression, anxiety, and psychosis. Chlorpromazine, first used as thorazine in the mid-1950s, proved to be very effective in chronic psychotic diseases and began to open the doors of large institutions such as the VPH.[10]

Lobotomy

Lobotomy,[11] or prefrontal leucotomy (developed by Portuguese neurologist Egas Moniz in 1936 and winning him a Nobel Prize in 1949), was performed at the VPH up to the 1960s. A surgeon would come from the Montreal Neurological Institute and perform lobotomies mainly on schizophrenic or severely depressed patients. The procedure, performed through small frontal twist drill holes with a long knife blade called a leukotome, effectively disconnected the frontal lobes from the rest of the brain. Harold Elliot, a neurosurgeon from the MGH, performed one such procedure on a patient at the MGH; the patient did not respond to the treatment so it was never repeated at this hospital. Such poor results were common, and patients that did not respond often remained in the hospital for an excessive amount of time with serious personality changes that at times were worse than the disease being treated. In retrospect, lobotomy was a bad procedure, created by a person of great reputation who had little knowledge of the anatomy and physiology of thalamo-cortical relationships in human beings.[12] It worked in subhuman primates but not in humans, who merely had one condition converted into another. In the mid-1960s, a stereotaxic approach to frontal lobotomy was developed for more precision.

The target was a tract from the anterior thalamus to the frontal lobes. Instead of surgically interrupting all the pathways to the frontal lobes from the diencephalons and the rest of the cortex, only one was interrupted. Due to well known stereotaxic imprecision,[13] frequently the target was never affected. The results were variable, not what was expected, so the procedure was eventually abandoned.[14] In the early 1970s, a house near the MGH, called Birks House, was given to the hospital for patients who were difficult to place. It was used for patients who were not sick enough for hospital but were not mentally well or capable of living outside an institution. The disposition of chronic patients was a serious situation; because there was no facility for post-psychiatric care until after the 1980s, the inpatient psychiatric service gradually expanded, filling with chronic patients who had no place to go.

The *Diagnostic and Statistical Manual* (DSM)

As psychiatry evolved in Europe and North America in the analytical and non-analytical fields, with no standards, the variety of diagnoses got out of control. The *DSM* (which had been planned for years) had a great influence and officially standardized psychiatric diagnoses. Each acceptable diagnosis was given a number, much like the ICD-9 (the International Classification of Disease), which came many years later for all medical diagnoses. A problem with the *DSM* was the change in the numbers denoting each diagnosis with each update. The *DSM* first appeared in 1952 and was revised in 1969, 1987, and 1994, and it has to be considered a great advance in clinical psychiatry. A controversial update was published in 2013 but has not been universally accepted.[15]

Psychiatry Nurses

There were two well known psychiatric nurses at the MGH, Diane Moreau and Inga Schamborski, who attracted students from the McGill School of Nursing.[16] Evelyn Malowany was involved in teaching for ten years and had a distinguished career after leaving the MGH. She made nursing in the psychiatry ward interesting and helped to promote the need for specialty-trained nurses. Such training was eventually to be offered in many specialties.

Resident Training

By 1960, there were up to five residents who could spend three years at the MGH. Under supervision, they were responsible for thirty inpatients, consultations, a handful of day patients, and a small OPD clinic. If psychotic patients came to the MGH, they were still sent to the VPH. This changed dramatically by the mid-1960s, with the downsizing of the VPH and the province's reduced spending on chronic psychiatric disease. After the mid-1970s, the MGH had to take care of its own psychotic and acute chemical-dependent patients, mainly because the VPH made it more and more difficult to transfer them. The doors of the VPH were being closed due not only to the development of better medications but also to financial constraints. So the MGH had to have restricted rooms or locked wards to handle patients previously transferred to the VPH.

Ewen Cameron was still chair of the McGill Department of Psychiatry in 1955, but he rarely came to the MGH.[17] He advertized widely for training at McGill. The applications came to him, and he decided who went where in the program. A committee was established to read the applications for training, but Cameron still had control over MGH and MCH staff to the point at which he would be upset when things did not go his way.

New MGH, 1955–97

When the new MGH opened in 1955, there was no psychiatry clinic and even the inpatient ward was small. Psychiatry initially had a shared clinic with ENT and eventually adopted Birks House on the MGH grounds for outpatient care in the 1960s.

The 1965 staff in the Department of Psychiatry consisted of twelve attendings, and residents varied in number from nine to fifteen, depending on the year. By this time, Moll was not as much of an advocate for the teaching program. He withdrew and delegated responsibility for everything in the department to his assistants. Many of the staff were part-time. By 1967, there were seventeen residents. Besides the resident program, there was a McGill diploma program requiring attendance at a lecture series at the Allan Memorial Institute. In 1978, there were about fifty inpatients.

Expansion of Services

The major problem for psychiatrists from 1960 to 1980 was the enormous increase in requests for psychiatric treatment: it was as if a floodgate that opened in 1961, when Quebec assumed all hospital costs.[18] So the department had to invent ways to increase the use of psychiatric services as the demand increased. A day centre was opened in 1950 and a night centre in 1954; group psychotherapy sessions were developed so that one member of the staff could advise a group of patients with similar problems. A twenty-four-hour walk-in psychiatric service was provided and by 1960 seven hundred patients were seen in one year. As the waiting list in the general psychiatric clinic lengthened and patients had to wait longer and longer to be seen, the number seen by the emergency service increased to 959 in 1967 and to over one thousand in 1970. A short-stay service for up to seventy-two hours was opened in 1968. The patients who were admitted to this unit needed to be started on new medications but were expected to be released for home care. The approach worked and helped clinic staff make decisions to let patients who could be treated with new medications go home without requiring admission. At times, this put a burden on patients' relatives, but there was no alternative when hospital beds were full.

A home care service was also developed in the 1970s to follow up on patients discharged from the hospital or the clinic. This attempt to begin community involvement in psychiatric care would involve public health, the Victorian Order of Nurses, and even the police. It was a broad, long-term project that would take years to accomplish.[19]

Sectorization of Psychiatric Care in Montreal and Its Effect on the MGH

It became evident by 1963 that the situation with regard to psychiatric emergencies was not being handled well. None of the psychiatric units in general hospitals such as the RVH, the MGH, the JGH, and their counterparts on the francophone side had been designed for the heavy load of emergency psychiatric patients wanting care after the 1961 Quebec hospitalization plan.

This situation coincided with Lehmann's development of chlorpromazine and its widespread use on chronic psychotic patients, at first at the VPH and then elsewhere. This resulted in an exodus from both the VPH and the francophone mental hospitals, and it coincided with the big push in the United

States to "free the mentally ill." The result was that thousands of people were released because of the efficacy of the new drugs as well as the more liberal attitude towards mental illness.

Only later was it realized that many of these patients needed a great deal of after-care, housing, financial assistance, and clinic follow-up and that compliance was to become a problem. This being the first time anyone had experienced such a situation, no one had anticipated that these needs would be on such a large scale.

As far as the MGH was concerned, no one anticipated the huge number of emergency and outpatient visits that would come from one specialty. The move to increase outpatient care for all specialties did not occur until the 1990s, except in psychiatry, which had unique problems created by the closure of the chronic mental institutions. As the cost of running these institutions increased, the solution to this problem was to discharge the patients and to let others provide their care.

The emptying of the mental hospitals was in full progress by the mid-1960s. Many patients showed up at the ER, and we did the best we could to admit them but found we were being overwhelmed. The other anglophone hospitals were in more or less the same position and the francophone hospitals were no better off. One difference, however, was that most of the francophone hospital ERs closed their doors at 5:30 or 6:00 o'clock in the evening. This meant what those who needed attention after 6:00 PM could not get it at these hospitals, and if the same people showed up in the daytime, they would be turned away after a very brief evaluation in the ER because it was not the policy of these institutions to accommodate people so seriously ill.

The Quebec government's solution was to establish regional psychiatric directors who were supposed to coordinate psychiatric treatment as best they could and to establish government policy for the disposition of psychiatric care. There was one anglophone and about three francophone directors, and nothing was done to alleviate the MGH problem

In 1963, One of these regional directors, Denis Lazure,[20] a child psychiatrist at Hôpital St. Justine, called a meeting of representatives (chairs) of all the major hospitals in the city having any kind of psychiatric facility. We sat around a table at his house for about three hours discussing the imbalance in ER care of psychiatric patients. The problem was that the hospitals that stayed open (e.g., the MGH) and received emergencies after 5:00 PM were taking on an extra load. Lazure was very concerned about those who closed their doors to emergency psychiatric patients overnight, but agreement for all the ERs to stay open for psychiatric patients 24/7 was never reached.

During this meeting, we all looked at a map of Greater Montreal, including the South Shore regions, which then had only one hospital. We informally divided up the map so that each hospital would take primary responsibility for the psychiatric care of people in a certain area. These were known as "sectors," and the concept of sectorization became an article of faith to which we adhered as strongly as if it were law. This task was accomplished in one evening, with little thought of the populations involved or the problems with the decision.

The sectorization scheme was very much an ad hoc distribution. At the MGH, we found ourselves with a considerable segment of the population and some weird geographic features. For example, if you lived on the west side of Atwater Avenue, you could *not* come to our ER and be evaluated or admitted to our in-patient service, but if you lived on the east side, you were in the MGH sector. This anomaly was not unique to the MGH, and it resulted in bad public relations. Some hospitals had special missions. For example, the Jewish General said that Jewish patients from any sector would have priority. Some similar arrangements were set up elsewhere but only in a limited way.

After the infamous meeting that created the sectors, we all returned to our respective hospitals. Suggestions were eventually given as to how to improve the sectorization map. At the MGH, we found we were left with a large area that had not been assigned and had fallen to us by default. The area was Lachine, where, according to our emergency psychiatric director, there was a high prevalence of mental illness. Then, a would-be epidemiologist among us decided that we should have a larger English-speaking area to balance the very large French-speaking population. At the time, we had Lachine and some downtown regions going as far as Pointe St Charles. This epidemiologist was to do comparative research on the prevalence of psychiatric diagnoses from the different regions, but he never did.

We took responsibility for about twenty-five thousand or more people from the South Shore region to give us the required balance. This was probably a bad decision, but it was not much worse than the whole idea itself, which should have been thought out in more detail before drawing lines on the map. As far as I was concerned, the decision to assume responsibility for the South Shore worked out rather poorly for us. It put even more pressure on us and nobody did the research that was supposed to have been carried out.

As a consequence of this division of duties, the MGH was gradually getting overwhelmed with psychiatric emergences. In the 1970s and 1980s, it became a common sight to see beds lined up in the ER and to have people waiting for a week or ten days or even longer to get from that ER bed up to our inpatient department for treatment. Some patients were, in fact, diagnosed, treated, and discharged from the ER after anywhere from twenty-four hours to several weeks.

The division of responsibilities according to sector both helped and hindered us. We were overloaded with difficult patients, but it did prevent some of the "bad" emergency departments from "dumping" their more demanding patients on us. In the long run, it would have been better had everybody agreed to keep their emergency rooms open twenty-four hours per day. At that particular moment in 1963, however, because we were the newest hospital with a reputation for both proficiency and modernity, we at the MGH were ecstatic over any help we could receive.

In retrospect, I believe that sectorization was a poor and inflexible arrangement. I thought it was the worst possible arrangement, and I made whatever limited exceptions I could. Unfortunately, there was no way to explain that the long list of patients already in the ER had priority. Without more beds, we had no capacity to accommodate special patients. Eventually, more beds became available and there were better medications with which to treat patients who did not need admission. Sectorization persists today.

Alan Mann's Chairmanship, 1971–1990

When I was appointed chairman of the Department of Psychiatry at the MGH in 1971, I was also promoted to full professor at McGill University. The McGill chair of psychiatry was R.L. Cleghorn at the AMI.

I inherited major problems as chair, the main one being the overwhelming number of patients coming to the new MGH for psychiatric care. The reasons are described above. By 1971, the situation was far from being settled. My advantage was that I had lived and learned from the clinical problem and had some idea of how to cope with it. More space, nurses, and house officers, all of which were needed, were eventually provided. The home care system provided by the community took much longer to achieve.

A break came when, in the 1960s, the Birks family donated a large mansion adjacent to the MGH for the expansion of the Department of Psychiatry. Birks House was renovated for in-patients and outpatients use but was soon inadequate. In the 1970s, the McConnell family donated an adjacent indoor tennis court which was renovated for outpatient use.[21] Both facilities are still in use.

The psychiatry department at the MGH was vulnerable because we had a new hospital (opened in 1955), and its ER was open twenty-four hours per day, seven days per week, and we had a twenty-four-hour psychiatry service. Once this became widely known, people came, not having any idea of the logistical problems this created. We had to solve the problem not by turning people away, which other hospitals did, but by being innovative with the resources we had.

Help came from the pharmaceutical industry, which saw the opportunity to develop medications for the large outpatient population. New drugs were produced for other than psychotic disorders (Thorazine and Stelazine). Manic-depressive disease (now called unipolar and bipolar affective disorders) and anxiety neuroses, including panic disorder and adolescent hyperactive disorders (now called attention deficit disorder), were all addressed. The development of Meprobamate in the 1950s,[22] and the diazepams in the 1960s, helped control the anxiety states, particularly panic disorders. In the 1950s and 1960s, the tricyclic antidepressants (Elavil and Tofranil) were an enormous help in dealing with the affective disorders. Benzadrine and Dexadrine allowed many patients with attention deficit disorders to live normal lives outside of hospitals.

We still used ECT in the 1970s in the Day Centre and for inpatients. It was gradually phased out because of the newer medications and the unfortunate long-term morbidity of repeated ECT. A "hemishock" procedure was developed to reduce morbidity, but it was not as effective and never caught on at the MGH.

Clinical psychologists, psychiatric social workers, and nurses for the adult psychiatric population were not as well developed as they should have been until the 1980s and 1990s.

I was beholden to the "sectorization scheme," as were all the MGH staff. We bent the rules and would see patients outside our sector for a few consultations, but they would eventually have to go back to the psychiatrists in their own sectors. Admission of such patients was very difficult because of the number of patients waiting in the ER for admission.

Another problem that I had to deal with was the compensation for psychiatric services, which was controlled by the Quebec government. In the 1970s, the Quebec Ministry of Health decided to reduce all doctors' incomes as a cost-control measure. Many physicians who were fed up with the province's inability to deal with the cost of medical care left Quebec for other parts of Canada or took long vacations to wait out the situation. In a draconian move, the Ministry of Health threatened doctors' licences and imposed fines on those who maintained a Quebec licence but did not come back to practise. This affected all specialties, not only psychiatry. Many young, newly appointed staff members would have had insufficient income to survive. When it became apparent through negotiations that this approach was not going to work in Quebec, reason prevailed and the problem was resolved.

Another great concern of mine was the gradual closing of the VPH, by this time renamed, the Douglas Hospital. No longer could we call and send a psychotic patient from the ER by ambulance. By the 1980s, its past open-door policy was ended as Quebec reduced the funding for large mental hospitals such as the VPH, which, in the 1960s, had a patient population of up to fifteen hundred. Forensic psychiatry was not an interest at the MGH at the time, mainly because of the absence of contingency statutes in Canada and the relatively small need for legal experts on mental disease.

When I retired from the chairmanship in 1990, many of the problems that had existed, when I started in 1961, had improved. The development of specialty-trained nurses and a greater number of practising psychiatrists in the Montreal area, together with the new medications, all helped our situation. In 1970, Quebec Medicare created compensation problems for all MGH physicians,[23] but these were resolved. When I look back at my sixty years in psychiatry, I think that we at the MGH confronted the challenges of helping people in *the most politically charged period in Canadian medical history* and we prevailed. As "we pass and are forgotten," as the old Yale song says,[24] I have no regrets.

NOTES

1 Quebec's 1961 version of the 1957 Federal Health Insurance and Diagnostic Services Act paid for all hospitalization and ER care. It opened the door to Montreal citizens for hospital care at the new MGH and people flocked to the hospital. http://en.wikipedia.org/wiki/healthinsuranceDiagnosticServicesAct.

2 Rotating internships were developed in the 1920s to provide all the graduates with some hospital experience and, by 1934 up through the Second World War, were required in order to obtain a licence. Most of the graduates were going to become GPs. By 1960 specialization training required straight medicine or surgery internships and the rotating internship ceased to be practical.

3 The Protestant Hospital for the Insane was founded in Verdun in 1881 by Alfred Perry and a group of Protestant clergy and Montreal citizens. The hospital became known as the Verdun Protestant Hospital for the Insane, abbreviated as VPH. In 1965, the hospital was named the Douglas Hospital in honour of James Douglas, MD, a former director, and his family, who were generous supporters of the hospital.

4 MGH Medical Board Minutes, vol. 53, p. 194, 3 April 1946; vol. 54, p. 27, 26 June 26 1946, MUA.

5 Ibid.

6 Dancey's first appointment at the MGH was in the Department Neurology from 1942 until 1947, when his appointment was transferred to psychiatry.

7 H. MacDermot, *Years of Change, 1945–70* (Montreal: Montreal General Hospital, 1970), 31.

8 Ibid.

9 Insulin shock therapy, https://en.wikipedia.org/wiki/insulin_shock_therapy, twenty-one references.

10 Chlorpromazine, https://en.wikipedia.org/wiki/chlorpromazine, forty-three references. Heinz Lehman, director of the VPH, pioneered the use of chlorpromazine in Canada in a large mental hospital where the doors were opened to allowr patients to go outside. An important advance in the treatment of psychotic diseases.

11 Egaz Moniz, a Portuguese neurosurgeon (1874–1955), first described the prefrontal leucotomy (lobotomy) in 1936. He published one book on the subject in 1936 and shared a Nobel Prize for his work in 1949. The truth is that Moniz was an inadequately trained neurosurgeon who developed two disastrous procedures: (1) the lobotomy and (2) the angiogram. He used a radio active substance (gamma emitter) known as Thoratrast, with a four-thousand-year half life, that could not be excreted from the body and that eventually killed anyone who had been subjected to it. He won his Nobel Prize before anyone knew what harm he had done.

12 P. Brodal, *The Central Nervous System: Structure and Function*, 3rd ed. (Oxford: Oxford University Press, 2004), 443–6.

13 H. Hamlin, P. Rakic, P Yakovlev "Stereotactic Imprecision," *Confinia Neurologica* 28 (1965): 426–36.

14 The mental side effects and law suits and better psychoactive drugs teamed up to bring an end to ECT in the 1970s.

15 *DSM V* https://en.wikipedia.org/wiki/DSM, seventy-three references. The idea behind the *DSM*, which was to categorize psychiatric disease and standardize diagnoses, was useful; however, it has fallen short of its goals in *DSM V*.

16 Names provided by Valerie Shannon and Evelyn Malowany

17 Ewen Cameron established psychiatry at McGill in 1943 and made an international name for the department for twenty years. Unfortunately, he got involved in an NIH funded project on brain function called "depatterning" (multiple ECTs). With little knowledge of brain physiology, this destroyed many patients' memory function, did nothing to advance psychiatry, and was eventually abandoned by the CIA as of no value. A project that would never make it past a Human Rights Committee today. See D. Gillmor, *I Swear by Apollo* (Montreal: Eden Press, 1987).

18 With the 1961 Quebec Hospital Insurance Plan funded by the 1957 federal Health and Diagnostic Services Act, all hospitalization and ER care was free.

19 MacDermot, *Years of Change*, 32

20 Lazure, an ardent separatist since the earliest days of that movement, was subsequently elected to the Quebec National Assembly and became minister of health in the Parti Québécois government.

21 In the 1960s, A large house adjacent to the MGH property owned by the Birks family was given to the MGH and converted for use by the department of psychiatry. Later, an indoor tennis court owned by J.W. McConnell (of the *Montreal Star*), also adjacent to the MGH property, was donated to the hospital for use by psychiatry, and the owner paid for the rennovations.

22 In 1955, meprobamate (Milltown) became the first tranquilizer produced. See https://en.wikipedia.org/wiki/meprobamate, twenty-four references.

23 Claude Castonguay's "Bill 65," the Quebec Medical Care Act, 1970, provided "universal" health care for the Québécois. Overshadowed in October 1970 by the FLQ Crisis and the specialists strike, it still got passed. Part of Bill 65 was a plan to reduce costs by cutting doctors' income.

24 The Yale "Wiffenpoof Song," the theme of the Wiffenpoofs, the oldest acapella singing group in the United States (associated with Yale University, founded in 1909). The line is: "We will serenade our Louie, while life and voice shall last, then we'll pass and be forgotten with the rest."

35

Radiology and Nuclear Medicine

Leonard Rosenthall and John Gibson

Len Rosenthall was chief of nuclear medicine from its inception. He wrote this chapter on radiology, using John Gibson's previous manuscript, when no other radiologist was available.

After Röentgen announced his discovery of a "new kind of ray" in the closing days of 1895, the "X-ray" caught the public imagination, if not its understanding, almost at once, and physicists, inventors, and engineers were at work within days to confirm his findings and to attempt to find practical applications. The possibility of medical usefulness was recognized at once, and the first verified North American medical radiograph, a fractured ulna, was made at Dartmouth, New Hampshire, on 3 February 1896, just over five weeks from the date of Professor Röentgen' s publication in December 1895.

In Montreal, four days later, Robert Kirkpatrick, a surgeon at the Montreal General Hospital, took a patient with a healed, but still troublesome, gunshot wound in the leg to Professor John Cox of McGill University's Department of Physics, who had been working with radiographic images. They succeeded in producing an image that satisfactorily localized the position of the bullet, thereby facilitating its removal and thus becoming the first example of clinically applied radiology in Canada. In a subsequent legal action it became the first radiograph to be accepted in a court of law. In their rush to get the article about this case published, the authors forgot to mention which leg was shot.

Professor Cox did not maintain his interest in radiography for very long, but Gilbert P. Girdwood (1832–1917), professor of chemistry in the McGill medical faculty and consultant physician to the MGH and the Royal Victoria Hospitals, promptly obtained the necessary apparatus and began providing radiological services to the staffs of both institutions. It is not clear when the MGH first acquired its own equipment, but Shepherd dates the founding of the X-ray department in September 1898. Mention of the "Radiographic Department" first appeared in the annual report of the MGM for 1898–99, which stated that 574 cases were "skiagraphed" (radiographed) and 307 fluoroscopic examinations were made to 30 April 1899.

W.P. Watson, an apothecary to the hospital since 1889, was placed in charge of the service and, after 1900, was listed as "Apothecary and Radiographer" until March 1908. Thereafter, the title of "Radiographer" was passed to Walter A. Wilkins, the first physician to specialize in radiology at the MGH. Watson continued as apothecary until May 1910.

The Wilkins Years

The department that Wilkins took over was probably well equipped for its time, but few details are available. It was reported to the Board of Governors in 1901 that "the new x-ray apparatus was installed in September 1901," in 1903 that "work is at present being carried on to establish a first-class x-ray laboratory," and in 1904 that the "X-ray Department has been completely equipped." Under Wilkins in 1908, the department registered 1,508 skiagraphic examinations and 207 treatments but only ninety-eight fluoroscopies. The type of treatments were not reported but presumably were limited largely to skin conditions.

Initially the work was predominantly fractures, dislocations, and foreign bodies, plus a few non-traumatic bone afflictions. In 1910, three "bismuth meals" are reported, indicating that gastrointestinal radiology was undertaken for the first time.

Wilkins carried on as the sole "radiographer" (after 1913 he is listed as "roentgenologist") until 1918, with a steadily increasing workload: in 1918, there were 11,104 skiagrams and 622 fluoroscopies. The following year, A. Stanley Kirkwood joined Wilkins as a junior assistant, having returned from three years overseas as an X-ray officer in the First World War. Prior to that, he had been a houseman in medicine and surgery at the MGH four years. His stay was brief, however, for in 1922 he departed to become the first full-time radiologist in St John, New Brunswick, where he had a distinguished career.

Wilkins was then alone until W.R. Harwood joined his staff in 1924, but this also appears to have been a brief appointment. Wilkins resigned as director of the department in April 1925 and moved to the consulting staff. His reports for the years 1920 to 1925 document the gradually but steadily increasing volume and complexity of diagnostic work, and increasing frustration with limitations of space, personnel, and equipment. His department was administering ultraviolet (quartz lamp) treatments as well as X-ray therapy, training technicians, and teaching nurses and medical students. In addition, he provided darkroom facilities for dental department X-rays, electrocardiogaphy, and medical photography. The latter was performed by amateur volunteers as there was then no official hospital photographer.

The Ritchie Years

In April 1925, W. Lloyd Ritchie replaced Wilkins as director of the Department of Roentgenology, and major changes were made. These were economic boom times, and his report for that year lists the names of twelve generous benefactors through whom a complete renovation of the service was made possible:

Col. Herbert Molson	Mr. A.E. Oglivie
Mr. J. W. McConnell	Lt.-Col. G.R. Hooper
Mr. C.W. Lindsay	Mr. R. Adair
Mr. W.J. McCall	Mr. Geo. Hogg
Mr. W.J. Morrice	Miss Alice Ogilvie
Mr. and Mrs. Gavin Ogilvie	

Five new machines were installed, including a shock-proof dental unit and a two hundred kilovoltage peak (kVp) water-cooled therapy machine, the first of its type in Canada. In addition, there were new overhead tube mounts, new tables, and improvements to the darkroom, film storage, and patient reception areas. The number of patient changing-rooms was increased and the whole department was redecorated. All this was accomplished without suspending a continuing increase in the volume of service demanded. The quartz lamp treatments were transferred to the physiotherapy department at this time.

Ritchie sounded very self-satisfied when he reported "we now have the most complete X-ray Department in Canada and it is a most happy feeling that everything at present known in the way of x-ray diagnosis and treatment can be done here." He was not inclined to remain complacent, however, as in the next year, despite the acquisition of more equipment (like a film changer designed to permit stereoscopic images to be made), he was agitating for replacement and upgrading of the gastrointestinal table, increased work space and more dressing cubicles, and the employment of a full-time photographer.

Ritchie's workload had jumped again: in 1926 there were 11,249 patients seen, an increase of 22.6 percent from the previous year, with over thirty thousand radiographs taken, twenty-two hundred fluoroscopies carried out, and 729 treatments given. This could probably not have been handled without additional technical staff, but in February 1927 Ritchie was joined by Joseph W. McKay, who became his long-term colleague and eventual successor.

Ritchie's 1928 annual report was considerably less euphoric than were those submitted earlier. While the appearance of the department had been improved by complete repainting, the extensive changes trumpeted previously are now described as "only such as should have been made years before" and "sufficient for the present needs at the time." There was some justification for his petulant tone as he notes that his workload increased by nearly 100 percent over three and a half years (36,915 radiographs taken in 1928 versus 18,422 in 1924). The 1929 report was more sanguine, as he states that nearly all of his previously ignored requests had been met and that he himself "felt much elated" by the possibility of the further expansion of his overcrowded department.

The amalgamation of the MGH and the Western Division became official on 1 January 1924, but their X-ray departments merged only on 15 November 1929 after Colin Ross, who was in charge at the Western Division, resigned. The annual reports of the Western Division are less detailed than are those of the Central Division but seem to mirror the latter's experience on a smaller scale – that is, a busy service with ever-increasing demands on it, even to the imposition of quartz therapy when it became popular and no other hospital department had space for it. The X-ray facility at the Western Division had been considerably refurbished in 1926, and the superintendent, A. Lorne C. Gilday, stated: "We are very proud of our X-ray Department, as we consider it a model for a 100 bed hospital." With the departure of Ross, Ritchie became director of both departments, and a third radiologist, E.M. Crawford, was added to the staff.

The 1929 report makes reference to "the terrible catastrophy [sic] which occurred in one of the large American hospitals" that year to justify the decision "made some five years ago" to change from the "quick burning" film (cellulose nitrate base) to the "slow burning" film (cellulose acetate base).

The catastrophe alluded to was the disastrous Cleveland Hospital fire, with 125 deaths.

Among staff changes in 1929, a Miss Noseworthy, who had charge of the dark room, resigned, and "Miss A. Muirhead was engaged to take charge of this work and she proved very satisfactory," remaining a valued member of the department staff for thirty years.

The period from 1930 to 1939, the "hungry thirties," saw less rapid change as money became tight and those who had jobs and housing tended not to disturb the status quo. Ritchie, McKay, and Crawford were staff radiologists for the entire time, and other staff changes were few, although the ever-increasing requests for service led to the hiring of some additional personnel after 1934. Funds apparently did not dry up entirely as the Western Division acquired new equipment to bring it up to what Ritchie deemed an acceptable standard, and, in 1934, the new Private Patient's Pavilion of the Western Division was opened, boasting a modern fully equipped X-ray facility. This accelerated a trend already noted to increase work in the Western Division and decrease it in the Central Division (although the decrease in the latter was not as much as had been anticipated). In 1935 and 1936, there were alterations to the Central Division building, which added two new rooms, including a rebuilt and newly equipped therapy room, solely for therapy, which Richie had advocated for years. Largely due to a generous benefactor, Colonel Molson, it was possible to acquire a considerable amount of other new equipment in the middle of these Depression years.

Despite all this, shortage of space in the Central Division remained a recurring theme, but to solve that problem it would have been necessary to add another floor to the West Wing. Technical developments continued during the 1930s. References to new equipment show rotating-anode tubes replacing obsolescent older types, "shock-proof" apparatus becoming standard, a spot-film changer provided for gastrointestinal fluoroscopic units (installed in the Western Division, advocated for the Central Division), and improved film-drying and film identification methods. In 1939, 15,365 patients were seen at the Central Division and 37,004 radiographs taken, and another 10,518 patients and 26,339 radiographs at the Western Division. Compared to 1930, the Central Division saw almost the same number of patients – 15,201 – and performed a somewhat greater number of radiographs – 42,509 – compared to 4,414 patients and 10, 591 radiographs at the Western Division. The increased burden on essentially the same staff, and the westward shift of patients from the strained-to-capacity Central Division are apparent.

The War Years

The early months of the Second World War, in 1939, do not appear to have affected the department greatly, but the director refers to a possible "depletion of our staff" and adds: "at the present time I would not know where to turn should it become necessary to secure a well trained Radiologist to our staff."

In the next year two darkroom technicians were lost to the armed forces, and three radiologists spent several Sundays commuting to Ottawa to review radiographs of troops slated to be shipped overseas. They also undertook to service the Montreal Children's Hospital after Arthur Childe, who had been radiologist there, was posted overseas. The department agreed to accept four technician trainees supplied by the army.

In 1941, the departure of Crawford, to be chief at the Homeopathic Hospital in Montreal, made it necessary to discontinue the service to the MCH, but this was alleviated to some degree by the promotion to staff of Beaton, who had been in training in the department for two years, and the addition of someone named Taylor as a new trainee. Despite wartime shortages some new equipment was obtained and a few structural alterations were made at the Central Division to improve efficiency.

Taylor was lost to the military in 1941, but another trainee, Thorliefson, was acquired. Wartime restrictions were beginning to be felt in the availability of supplies, and it was therefore decided to upgrade the older equipment so that all machines were shock-proof and equipped with X-ray tubes of the limited number of types still being manufactured (and thus replaceable). Film and chemicals were still available but not from Britain and at a considerably higher cost. Shortages were noted, particularly in metal goods such as film holders.

Beaton left to become chief at a Sherbrooke hospital in 1943, and Thorliefson departed for Toronto in 1944, leaving the team of Ritchie and McKay as the only radiologists for a busy department spread over two widely separated divisions that, ideally, should have had at least two full-time people each. The case load had been roughly constant from 1940 to 1942, but it began increasing again, even though services were at times curtailed by interruptions in the film supply. Ritchie reports that he and McKay were near exhaustion when they greeted Thorliefson "with open arms" when he returned in 1945. His stay was only for one year, but soon after he left yet again W.B. Taylor returned from active service to join the staff. The war years had been successfully weathered, but the wartime problems of shortages and delays did not cease immediately, and the chronic problems of aging technology, limited space, and barely adequate personnel persisted.

New equipment had been ordered and, in 1946, was delivered to the Western Division, but the Central Division had to wait another year. Personnel remained stretched as Norman Brown was added to the staff in 1947 and Taylor departed. It was recorded at the time that the working area had not changed in twelve years at both locations and that both patients and referring physicians were growing dissatisfied with prolonged wait times.

Major professional staff changes occurred in 1948. Ritchie retired at the end of September; McKay and Brown were joined by Everett Crutchlow, who was previously awarded the OBE for his service in the Royal Navy and held an appointment at the Herbert Reddy Memorial Hospital; and army veteran Archibald Edington came over from Queen Mary Veterans Hospital. Two radiology interns were added – Marvin Lougheed and Darius Albert – and a two-year technician course was instituted. This was in response to a need for expanded staff as twenty-four-hour technical service had apparently not been made available up to that time and was deemed necessary. Both hospital divisions were operating at the limit of their capacities.

The retiring director, William Lloyd Ritchie, had served the hospital for twenty-three years and, as well as building up the Department of Radiology in the hospital, he was also a major force in establishing a corresponding department in the McGill University Faculty of Medicine in 1941, becoming its first chair. An Ontario native and Toronto medical graduate, he had studied radiology in New York after engaging in general practice in western Canada. He was a radiologist at the Toronto General Hospital and then chief radiologist at the Ottawa Civic Hospital before coming to Montreal. He became a fellow of the Royal College of Physicians of Canada and, in 1937, was a founding member of the Canadian Association of Radiologists. He found time to teach residents, medical students, technicians, and junior colleagues as well as to write papers while carrying a prodigious workload, often under less than ideal conditions.

Joseph McKay, his associate through almost the entire period, succeeded Richie as chief, and, in 1949, extensive physical alterations were made to both departments, in offices and filing areas, and in the radiographic rooms. Some of these rooms were re-equipped with more powerful machines permitting high-kilovoltage radiography and photo-timed spot-filming. At about this time, the Department Neurology and Neurosurgery was founded, and this incurred a greater demand for complex and time-consuming X-ray procedures such as pneumoencephalography and angiography. This constant demand for space, funds, and staff throughout the radiology history of the MGH was influenced by the rapid advances in medical X-ray machine development, which expanded its field of clinical application and resulted in increased demand for health care.

The major weaknesses in 1950 were the therapy machines, which had not kept pace in the general upgrading, and staff size (after Edington left). Three new radiology interns and seven technicians were subsequently taken on, and new therapy apparatus arrived. Lougheed, after an additional year of training at the Swedish Institute in Seattle, Washington, returned to join the staff in 1953 to take charge of radiation therapy. A number of radioisotopes had come into use in the hospital by this time and, as of 1952, were the responsibility of an interdepartmental committee chaired by McKay. In 1954, Brown opted for private practice, leaving only two staff radiologists when four were required. The arrival of D.J. Sieniewicz relieved some of the strain.

In 1955, the long-awaited move to the new hospital building on Cedar Avenue took place, and, while the integration of the two divisions, which had in effect been separate hospitals, caused some problems, the director reported: "For the first time the Montreal General Hospital has a Department of Radiology worthy of the institution." There was more space, and four new fluoroscopic units (two General Electric "Imperials" and two Picker "Constellations") in air-conditioned rooms, and a Picker "Craniograph" and Schönander film changer for carotid and cardiac angiography were installed. The Department of Urology was located adjacent to radiology, permitting close cooperation; two of four urology tables were X-ray equipped, and a separate darkroom for their film development was provided. Nearly all of the equipment from the former divisions was moved to the new quarters.

On the therapy side, a very generous donation by J.W. McConnell funded the acquisition of a Canadian-developed high energy treatment device using a radioactive cobalt source. The advantage of the high-energy gamma rays emitted by cobalt over the previously available X-ray machines was their ability to deliver an effective radiation treatment dose to deep tissues with relatively little skin and bone damage.

Edward Epp, PhD, a radiation physicist, was added to the staff, but there were still only three staff diagnostic radiologists and one radiation therapist, with Sieniewicz serving as a therapist when needed for backup.

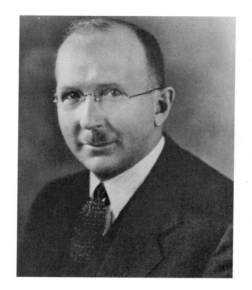

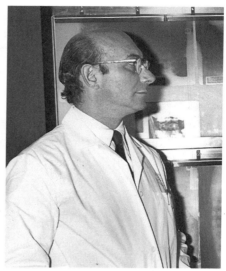

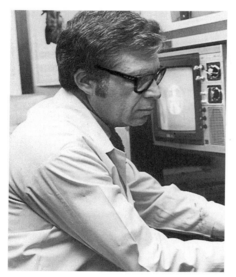

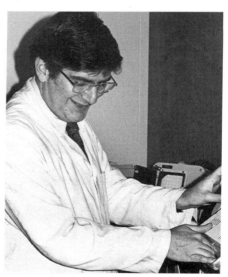

Clockwise from top left
Fig. 35.1 Lloyd Ritchie, 1927–48
Fig. 35.2 Jacob Fabricant, 1975–78
Fig. 35.3 Fred Winsberg, 1978–85
Fig. 35.4 Leonard Rosenthall, 1968–2007

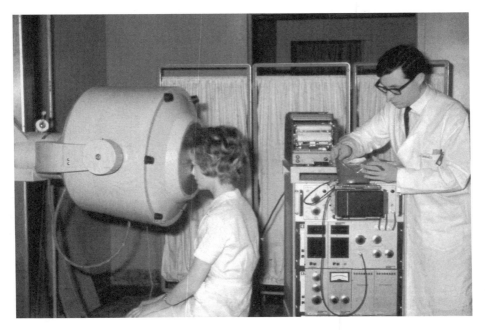

Fig. 35.5 Nuclear medicine scanner

A photofluorographic chest screening unit was put in the admission area on the first floor. "Portable" machines, which served the operating rooms and all other radiological services, were concentrated on the fifth floor. The workload diminished slightly over the transition period

In 1956, the radiology demands rose again, and the director noted that the equipment salvaged from the old divisions was deteriorating and in need of replacement. He also lamented that there was no time for his limited staff to engage in academic pursuits as there were eight residents in training who had to be actively taught and not exploited plus the usual escalating service responsibilities to be tended. This situation was improved somewhat in 1957 when T.F. Philips, a former resident, joined the staff, and later J.A. Liver was taken on as a teaching fellow. However, McKay states succinctly: "In the original planning of this department we thought that the space allotted would be adequate for some time to come. That is not the case." There were also complaints that the X-ray service was not offered on a twenty-four-hour basis. and this was remedied by initiating a rotating on-call service for emergency technician coverage on weekends and at night.

The hospital physicist, Epp, resigned and moved to New York in 1957. The cobalt unit had become the mainstay of the radiation therapy section, but, because of the 5.27 year half-life of the radionuclide cobalt-60, the treatment sessions got progressively longer with age and thereby decreased patient throughput. This necessitated replacing the cobalt-60 source periodically in order to maintain efficiency.

In 1958, two more radiologists – Flemming McConnell and J.A. Liver – and a physicist, Rene Beique, replacing Epp, were added to the staff. Mc-Connell, who had spent a year in Sweden after his initial radiology training in Boston, introduced catheter angiography to the hospital and began training radiologists who would ultimately succeed him. The technician training program was expanded and some old equipment replaced, but the major event for the department was the resignation from the staff of McKay on 30 September, his having reached the age of sixty-five. Joseph William McKay was from Nova Scotia and had received his medical degree from Dalhousie University in 1918, after having interrupted his medical training to serve in the First World War from 1914 on. He took graduate training in radiology first at the MGH, then in London, England, and finally in radiotherapy at the Memorial Hospital in New York. He joined the staff in 1926 and stayed on for thirty-two years, the last ten of which he was chief of the department. He was a founding member and past president of the Canadian Association of Radiologist and a prominent figure in his specialty in Canada.

Siieniewicz succeeded him as chief and, in 1959, engaged a firm of management consultants to review the administrative and patient-handling functions of the department in order to improve the efficiency of non-technical aspects of radiologic practice. There were no immediate major changes under him, but an additional radiologist, G.H. Maguire, was added and the number of technician trainees further increased. In radiotherapy the old decaying radiocobalt source was clinically spent and replaced with a new one. A cesium-137 therapy unit, designed by Lougheed and Beique in association with the Aviation Electric Company, was ordered.

Major changes took place in 1960, notably the installation of the department's first automatic film processor, which developed, fixed, and dried films in eight minutes rather than in an hour or more. Integrated with this were rearrangements in the film storage areas and, throughout the hospital, the change of film filing from using a sequential numbering system to using the patients' medical record number. A grant was obtained to permit outfitting of a "special procedures" room to house a biplane film changer and the hospital's first image intensifier.

It was at this time that the Quebec Hospital Insurance Scheme ("Medicare") took effect, and, in 1961, after its first year, the anticipated increase in workload occurred. It consisted of a greater number of patients and an increase in the average number of examinations per patient, but preparations for this proved adequate.

The special procedures room was now complete and functioning, but it was found that the demands of angiocardiography occupied it almost constantly, with the result that there remained a need for space and equipment for other special procedures.

It was felt desirable to have an X-ray facility in "casualty" (as the emergency department was then known, following British usage), but this conflicted with the department policy of centralizing all services on the fifth floor. A workable compromise was reached by installing an X-ray machine in, and assigning a technician to, the emergency area, but using a pneumatic tube system to transport the exposed film to the fifth floor for processing and interpretation.

Dr Maguire moved to St Mary's Hospital at this time, but the staff was augmented in July 1961 by the addition of J.D. Gibson in diagnosis and R.O. Hill to the therapy staff. Leonard Rosenthall was also appointed to the therapy side at this time, but with major responsibility for the development of the relatively new area of diagnostic imaging employing radioactive test agents. A slight decrease in demand for radiation therapy was registered, and it was attributed to the growing use of chemotherapy in treating malignant disease.

By the next year it was clear that demand for services was increasing in all areas as the range covered by government insurance expanded. In just seven years after moving to the new hospital, space limitations were again becoming a problem and equipment was working to its capacity. Under Rosenthall, the radioisotope laboratory was enlarged in scope from predominately thyroid and haematological tests to include a variety of renal, brain, hepatic, and bone functional and anatomical studies; additional equipment was installed and the work volume doubled.

In 1963, department concerns were related almost entirely the problems of maintaining patient care at a satisfactory level in the face of changing modes of medical practice, with ever greater reliance on hospital for first contact and primary care, and a corresponding increased demand for radiological and laboratory assessment. The department staff was augmented with the return of Maguire, and Douglas MacEwen was taken on and given the additional responsibility of the resident training program. A research associate in radiology was added for the first time, and she, Shirley Lehnert, worked largely in the facilities provided by the University Surgical Clinic.

In 1964, the total patient visits to the department approached 100,000. There were no major changes except for the addition to the staff of former residents Martha Grymaloski and Jozsef Kiss. Expansion of the Pine Avenue wing of the hospital was being planned and change was held back, to be integrated with the availability of new space. The radioisotope unit continued to expand in terms of patient throughput, range of procedures, and clinical research as the number of new organ-specific radiopharmaceuticals became available. Beique and Maguire developed techniques for imaging the larynx and trachea by using selective filtration and high kilovoltage. These worked well and became locally popular. Staff members produced several papers and exhibits and delivered a number of lectures outside of the department.

More staff changes ensued in 1965 as McConnell departed in October to take the chair the Department of Radiology at the University of Alberta, and MacEwen, at the year's end, left to achieve the same status at the University of Manitoba. These major losses were partially offset by the acquisition of M.J. Herba and F.R.J. Racine.

The radioisotope unit became the Division of Nuclear Medicine, with Rosenthall as its director, and continued to be the area of most rapid growth and greatest interest. The acquisition of one of the first Anger gamma cameras in Canada through a Hartford Foundation grant enabled the performance of both static and dynamic organ function with the short-lived technetium radionuclide (Tc-99m). Rosenthall undertook some pioneering work, which contributed to his growing reputation as an international authority in this new field of medicine. He no longer had the time to do radiotherapy, and since other trained therapists were moving to exclusively diagnostic work, Lougheed needed help, and this was provided by the arrival of C.J. Powell-Smith, a full-time radiation oncologist.

In 1966, a physical restructuring of the department was carried out, and radiology was officially divided into three divisions: diagnosis, radiotherapy, and nuclear medicine. Also, a second medical physicist, Daniel Rotenberg, joined the group. The workload in radiotherapy and nuclear medicine continued to increase, as did the academic output of papers, lectures, and exhibits.

The following year, remembered as Expo year and the Centennial of Canada, was one of turmoil for radiology as disputes between Quebec provincial government agencies and the professional associations of the medical staff led to mass resignations of radiologists and the physical departure of many from the province. Only emergency radiology services were provided in the Quebec hospitals during the ten weeks of the walkout. When the work stoppage was settled by a legislated return to full services, with some points gained and some lost from the viewpoint of the radiologists, the department suffered significant losses as three physicians elected, for various reasons, to pursue their careers elsewhere. Only nuclear medicine continued to grow in demand and provision of services during this year.

In 1968, with the establishment of Colleges d'Enseignment Generale et Practiques, a two-year, postsecondary, pre-university college program, the government removed technician training in radiology from the hospitals. Students continued to work in hospitals in a more limited basis in order to gain practical experience, but the reduction in hours onsite, and the loss of some technicians to teaching positions, aggravated the shortage of technicians. There were other major changes that year that also affected the department. Sieniewicz resigned as chief of radiology and left for Sweden on a sabbatical year, and Lougheed resigned from the Division of Radiotherapy and moved to Hopital Notre-Dame accompanied by the physicist R. Beique. Maguire became acting chief, and the staff was bolstered by the acquisition of Catherine Cole and two experienced teaching fellows – neuroradiologist Jack Chan and Francis Boston – in the diagnostic area. The ever-expanding Division of Nuclear Medicine was given approval to take on two residents.

W. Paul Butt was appointed director of the department in 1970. He felt its effectiveness could be increased without incurring increased cost by emphasizing consultation and by integrating radiological study more closely with clinical management as well as by reducing or eliminating routine and screening procedures that consumed a lot of resources but yielded few useful results. He found himself embattled on many fronts, fighting government agencies that were slow to listen to requests for newer and more reliable equipment to replace obsolescent units and fighting colleagues who found his proposed changes in established methods of practice and remuneration too difficult to accept and too rapidly introduced. He made some progress by deliberately reducing the number of total examinations performed while maintaining the levels of patient care and teaching. He added Fred Winsberg. an experienced diagnostic ultrasonographer, to the staff, and Michael O'Donovan, a teaching fellow. The Women's Auxiliary of the hospital financed the provision of ultrasound equipment for Winsberg and an up-to-date mammographic unit, of which Cole took control. An integrated resident teaching program for all McGill hospitals was developed, involving subspecialization and a complex system of rotations. The department now had a total staff of thirteen radiologists, twenty residents (including two in nuclear medicine), and 127 other personnel.

In the early 1980s the angiography division grew in terms of the number of patients examined and in terms of the number of new interventional procedures performed. This entailed an expansion of the existing facilities. The era of computerized tomography (CT) began at the MGH with the installation of the EMI 7070 scanner in 1980. A second unit was acquired in 1984. Because of the rapid improvement in the technology, these two units became dated and were replaced by two Toshiba 900 S/X scanners in 1990. These scanners were situated in the Department of Radiology area on the fifth floor, but they were supplemented by a third scanner in the ER area on the first floor in 1996 in the interests of patient convenience and because of the waxing workload. Magnetic resonance imaging (MRI) was introduced with the acquisition of the General Electric device in 1990.

36

Radiation Oncology

Carolyn Freeman and Ervin Podgorsak

Carolyn Freeman is chief of radiation oncology at the MGH and subsequent MUHC. She also worked under two previous chairs. Ervin Podgorsak was a radiation physicist.

X-rays were reported by Wilhelm Reöntgen in November 1895, natural radioactivity by Henri Becquerel in 1896, and radium by Pierre and Marie Curie in 1898, spawning, at the end of the nineteenth century, the birth of the disciplines of diagnostic radiology, radiation oncology, and medical physics. During the twentieth century all three disciplines underwent tremendous growth in sophistication, technological development, and importance to medicine.

The news of the discovery of X-rays spread very rapidly around the world. In January 1896, reports of the use of X-rays for medical purposes appeared in the scientific and medical literature. The first reported use of X-rays in Canadian medicine took place in early February 1896 in Montreal as a result of a collaboration between Robert Kirkpatrick, a Montreal General Hospital surgeon, and Professor John Cox of the McGill Department of Physics. Much has changed at the MGH since then, but one can state that, for most of the intervening years, the hospital remained at the forefront of technological developments in radiation medicine, at times barely and at other times, most notably since the 1970s, in an internationally recognized leadership position.

It is remarkable that by the turn of the century X-rays were already being used for treatment of cancer at the MGH, the annual report for 1901 speaking of the installation of new X-ray equipment and some "250 exposures for therapeutic purposes."[1]

By 1922, operation of the X-Ray Department was said to be hampered by lack of space, outdated equipment, and lack of technicians. By this time, too, the properties and potential usefulness of radium were becoming better understood and concern was being expressed about the lack of radium – and this meant turning away patients.[2] In 1925, a new 200,000-volt treatment machine with water-cooled X-ray tube equipment was installed, making the X-Ray Department "the most complete ... in Canada."[3] Radium, in the form of needles and plaques, was finally purchased in 1928 as a result of what was at the time a very generous gift of $50,000, and Eleanor Percival, a gynaecologist with special training in radiotherapy, visited clinics abroad to learn how to use it.[4]

The next major advance in radiotherapy at the MGH was the installation of a cobalt unit, also the result of a generous private donation, in the new hospital on Cedar Avenue in 1955. Chapter 36 traces the history of radiotherapy and medical physics at the MGH through the early years of the twentieth century and up to the late 1960s, during which time radiotherapy practice was closely aligned with that of diagnostic radiology.

The situation in radiotherapy at the MGH at the end of the 1960s was far from satisfactory. The equipment was "as backward as any 3rd world country," according to Julio Guerra, who had been recruited along with Ted Roman to staff the department following the abrupt departure of the previous staff radiation oncologists, Marvin Lougheed (who had moved to Montreal's Notre Dame Hospital) and Cyril Powell-Smith (who had moved to the United States). There were only three treatment units: a cobalt unit whose source was now so old that treatment times were extremely long, a cesium unit in a very dilapidated state, and a superficial X-ray unit of very limited usefulness in the new megavoltage era. All requests to hospital management to replace or at least upgrade the equipment had met with failure. The workload was very heavy and morale maintained, according to Guerra, only as a result of the organizational and personal skills of the chief therapist, Agnes Hoffmann, a long-standing and very capable member of the staff.

The 1970s were then a time of great change for radiation oncology and medical physics at the MGH. Under the leadership of John Webster, a radiation oncologist who was recruited from the well known Roswell Park Memorial Cancer Center in Buffalo, New York, the radiation oncology service separated from the Department of Radiology and a major reorganization of radiotherapy services at the McGill hospitals took place. A small department at the Queen Elizabeth Hospital, which had operated with only a single cobalt unit, closed, and the Department of Radiotherapy at the MGH was completely rebuilt in new space under the driveway and parking spaces to the north of the west wing of the hospital. When it opened in 1974, the new Department of Radiation Oncology had the very latest equipment for treating patients, including the first linear accelerators to be installed in Quebec. New recruits included Montague Cohen as chief of medical physics, Taik Kim and Pierre Del Vecchio as radiation oncologists, joining Julio Guerra and Ted Roman, and Ervin Podgorsak and Fadel Behman as staff medical physicists.

The department worked in close collaboration with the radiation oncology departments at the Royal Victoria Hospital and Jewish General Hospital, where Webster also served as radiation oncologist-in-chief. The overall concept was that services required by only a subset of patients would not be duplicated and that the medical and medical physics staff, as well as some of the senior radiation therapists (technologists) and the manager for the department, would work at all three sites. The department began taking residents into a newly created radiation oncology postgraduate training program and radiation therapy (technology) students into a college-level program jointly sponsored by Dawson College and the McGill teaching hospitals that, for the first time, offered training exclusively in radiation therapy in order to meet the knowledge and skill needs required to practise in an increasingly complex field.

In 1979, Webster returned to the United States. Carolyn Freeman, who had received part of her training in the United Kingdom and part at McGill, took over as radiation oncologist-in-chief, and Podgorsak took over as head of medical physics. The following decade was a time of tremendous growth for both the radiation oncology and medical physics departments, and one that saw the development of some highly novel and sophisticated cancer treatment techniques as a result of extremely productive close collaborations between the staff of these departments. These included an isocentric breast irradiation technique (1980), total body irradiation with a sweeping beam (1982), a rotational total skin electron beam irradiation technique (1983), electron arc irradiation (1985), and a dynamic radiosurgery technique (1986) that was a first in North America and a precursor of the technology used in modern linear accelerators (linacs) today.

In 1994, the hospital foundation supported the purchase and installation of the first CT simulator in Canada, leading into the era of 3D conformal radiotherapy. Later in the same year one of the low-energy linacs was replaced with the first high-energy multi-modal linear accelerator in Quebec. Such equipment rapidly became the norm for treatment, and the staff worked long hours until very late at night in order to accommodate all of the patients benefitting from the improved dosimetry that such a unit provided. Lack of a high-energy linac at the RVH and the impossibility of installing one, given the physical constraints there, led to a decision in 1997 to close the department at that hospital and to consolidate all activities in radiation oncology and medical physics at the MGH. This was finally accomplished in 2001 in a completely renovated, upgraded, expanded and still, a decade later, very functional facility at the MGH.

Notable Successes, 1970–96

A Leadership Role in Professional Societies

MGH staff played leadership roles in numerous provincial, national, and international professional and scientific organizations. Moreover, their vision and active involvement at many levels led to the creation of several new organizations that have been central to the further development of the specialties of radiation oncology and medical physics, including the Canadian Association of Radiation Oncologists in 1986, the Canadian College of Physicists in Medicine in 1980, the International Stereotactic Radiosurgery Society in 1991, and, later still, in 2005, the International Paediatric Radiation Oncology Society. Staff members served these new and many other already established professional organizations in numerous capacities, most notably as president of CARO, president of CCPM, chair of the Specialty Committee of the Royal College of Physicians and Surgeons of Canada, and chair of the CCPM Certification Examination Committee. They also made important contributions in many other areas, for example, as members of editorial boards of the most prestigious journals in radiation oncology and medical physics, as authors of textbooks, as book editors, and as chairs of professional committees and national and international task groups.

A Leadership Role in Education and Training in Radiation Oncology and Medical Physics

Arguably one of the greatest successes of the MGH radiation oncology and medical physics programs, the specialty teaching and training programs in radiation oncology and medical physics have been enormously important to the development of the two fields in Quebec as well as nationally and internationally.

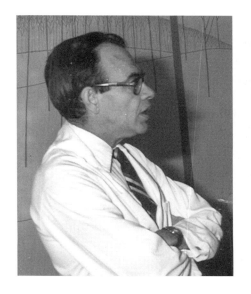
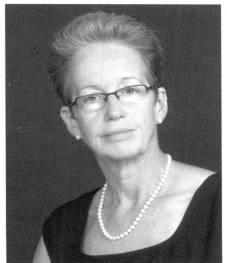
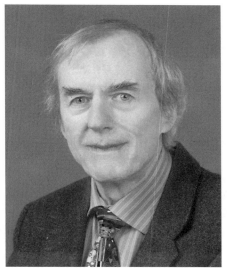
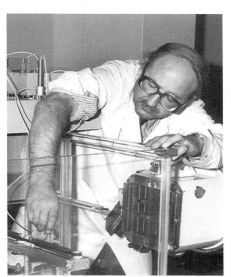

Clockwise from top left
Fig. 36.1 John Webster, director, radiation oncology, 1971–79
Fig. 36.2 Carolyn Freeman, radiation oncologist in chief, 1979–97
Fig. 36.3 Montague Cohen, director of medical physics, 1980–91
Fig. 36.4 Ervin Podgorsak, co-author, director of medical physics since 1991

From a very small program with only a single trainee in the 1970s, the McGill postgraduate program in radiation oncology developed over the next two decades into an extremely strong, academically oriented program, and graduates of the McGill program are to be found in academic positions in many other Canadian centres as well as in some very prestigious US institutions. The medical physics MSc and PhD programs based at the MGH were inaugurated in 1980 under the leadership of Professor M. Cohen, who remained in charge of the programs until his retirement in 1991, at which time Podgorsak was given the responsibility for the two academic programs in addition to his leadership of the MGH Department of Medical Physics. The McGill academic programs in medical physics were first accredited in 1993, at which time McGill was, and remained for ten years, the only Canadian university to have such accreditation and one of only a few in North America. McGill also led the way in the development of a medical physics residency program in that, a few years later, in 2000, McGill was the first Canadian university to obtain accreditation for its residency program in this field. For most of the 2000s, until the development of programs in other centres, McGill graduates accounted for half of all medical physicists practising in Quebec, and approximately one-third of all medical physicists working in Canada were trained wholly or partly at McGill.

A Leadership Role in Clinical Practice and Clinical Trials in Oncology
From the mid-1970s onwards, MGH radiation oncologists pioneered and supported multidisciplinary care, working with colleagues in ENT (Elhami Attia) and in gynaecology (Robert Seymour) to set up some of the first multidisciplinary clinics at McGill hospitals and, indeed, in Quebec. By the 1990s, such practice, which ensured the best possible care for patients, was the norm, requiring identification of space outside the Department of Radiation Oncology.

In addition to in-house developmental work and a growing reputation for excellence in clinical care, MGH staff members made numerous important contributions to national and international clinical trials groups, such as the National Cancer Institute of Canada and the NIH-supported Radiotherapy Oncology Group and Children's Oncology Group, among others, over the years accruing large numbers of patients as well as contributing to the science of the groups, pioneering and testing new treatment approaches, and playing active roles in quality assurance efforts and administration.

NOTES

1 Montreal General Hospital, annual report, 1901, MGH Archives, MUA.
2 H.E. MacDermott, *History of the Montreal General Hospital* (Montreal: Montreal General Hospital, 1950), 105–6.
3 Montreal General Hospital, annual report, 1925.
4 MacDermott, *History*, 36, 110.

37

Research Institute

Samuel O. Freedman

Freedman has had a remarkable career at McGill as chair of allergy and clinical immunology, dean of medicine (1977–81), and vice-principal of McGill University, 1981–91.

Introduction

Scientific research is not new to the Montreal General Hospital. The world-renowned pathologist and physician, William Osler, first introduced research and bedside observation to medical students at this hospital in 1879. From that time until the end of Second World War, most hospital-based research took place in clinical laboratories within the hospital. In 1947, Judah Quastel, a highly regarded biochemist from Great Britain, accepted the position of assistant director of the newly founded McGill University-Montreal General Hospital Research Institute on University Street.[1] The reason for this location was that it was adjacent to both the Department of Biochemistry in the biology building and the Montreal Neurological Institute. Quastel excelled in several research areas, but neurobiochemistry was his primary interest when he was appointed to the institute. One year after his arrival, Quastel was appointed director of the institute and brought to this position his own management style. The institute was located in a two-story mansion that had been converted to contain several laboratories on each floor. Quastel, who was a "control freak" in today's terminology, often stood on the stair landing between the two floors and shouted instructions to each investigator in the building. The collaboration with the MGH, which was then located on Dorchester Street, was largely confined to clinical studies on patients with neurological and psychiatric disorders. During his nineteen years as director, Quastel supervised seventy PhD candidates, and the institute published over three hundred scientific papers on topics that included neu-robiochemistry, neurotropic drugs, anaesthesia, cancer biochemistry, and enzyme inhibition. In 1966, when he reached the McGill University manda-tory retirement age of sixty-five, Quastel accepted a professorship in neuro-chemistry at the Department of Biochemistry at the University of British Columbia. Without his leadership, the productivity of the institute was greatly diminished and it was closed three years later, with the tenured staff relocated to several other departments at McGill.

Research at the MGH

Despite many outstanding scientific contributions, the McGill University-MGH Research Institute had very little collaboration with the hospital. When Douglas G. Cameron was appointed physician-in-chief in 1957, one of his first priorities was to establish the University Medical Clinic in order to introduce some structure and a scientific approach to clinical medicine in his department. Cameron was the director, but the scientific leadership was provided by a succession of distinguished deputy-directors: Arnold Burgen, Francis Chinard, and Charles Hollenberg. Because several other hos-pital departments had first-class research programs, a joint planning com-mittee of the hospital board of directors and the medical staff was struck in 1968 to consider the establishment of a research institute that would include all departments. The Honourable Mr Justice G. Miller Hyde and Samuel Freedman played key roles in this endeavour. In 1973, a new five-storey re-search building was completed adjacent to Livingston Hall at a cost of over $2 million: 50 percent of this amount was contributed by private donors and 50 percent by the Health Resources Fund of Canada. L.G. Elliott served as executive director from 1976 to 1981. He was a pharmacist who was the re-tired co-founder of a successful generic drug company and was well known to the medical and scientific staff for both his administrative and intraper-sonal skills. Joseph Shuster, a clinician-scientist in the Division of Allergy and Clinical Immunology, succeeded him with the title of scientific director from 1984 to 1996.

Another important priority for Cameron concerned recruiting neurolo-gists with outstanding research programs to the Department of Medicine. Although the Montreal Neurological Institute was firmly opposed to this policy, both the MGH and the Jewish General Hospital felt that the term "general" meant that all medical and surgical specialities should exist in their

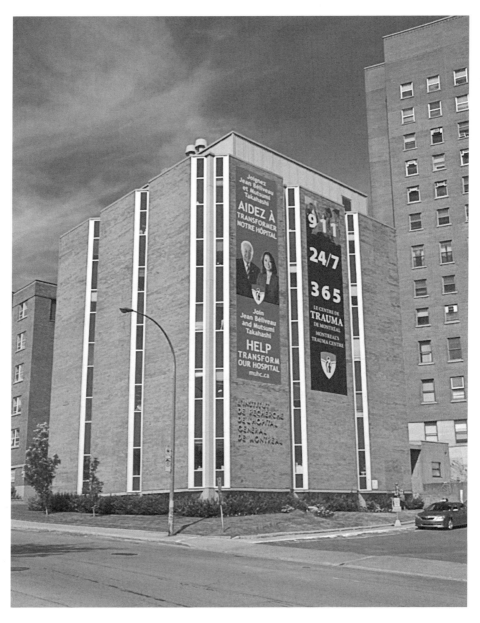

Fig. 37.1 MGH Research Institute from Pine Ave., 1973. This facility made the MGH the leading clinical research centre at McGill.

institutions. The most outstanding scientist recruited for neurology was Albert Aguayo, who was the founding director of the Centre for Research in Neuroscience at the MGH Research Institute. Aguayo made a fundamental breakthrough in the understanding of the nervous system when he demonstrated that damaged nerve cells in the mammalian brain do not die immediately but can regenerate under certain conditions.[2] This funding completely changed one of the most basic paradigms in neuroscience and generated a stream of promising research on regeneration in the nervous system. Joseph Martin began his distinguished career in neuroscience when he was appointed to the Department of Neurology and Neurosurgery at the MGH in 1971. His research was focused on the hypothalamic regulation of pituitary hormone secretion and on the application of neurochemical and molecular genetics to better understand the causes for Alzheimer's and other neurodegenerative diseases. He became chair of the McGill Department of Neurology and Neurosurgery in 1977, but the university failed to appoint him director of the Montreal Neurological Institute despite a positive recommendation from a search committee chaired by the dean of medicine. As a result, he accepted a position as the Bullard Professor of Neurology at Harvard University in 1978. He subsequently was appointed dean of medicine at the University of California, San Francisco, from 1989 to 1994. He then served as chancellor of that university for four years before returning to Boston as dean of the Harvard Medical School from 1997 to 2007. Thus, the world-renowned excellence in neuroscience that characterized the findings of Quastel at the first MGH Research Institute was continued by Aguayo, Martin, and their many talented colleagues.

Phil Gold and Samuel Freedman

Phil Gold and I were the co-discoverers of the carcinoembryonic antigen (CEA) test for colon cancer.[3] This finding was reported in the *Journal of Experimental Medicine* in 1965 and was subsequently found to be the first clinically useful biomarker for colon cancer. The finding of a tumour-specific antigen for a human cancer attracted worldwide attention in scientific journals and the news media. The *Toronto Star* had a red headline splashed across its front page following my presentation to the National Cancer Institute of Canada, and photographs of Gold and myself appeared on the covers of Life magazine and Cancer Research journal. After several years, it became apparent that measurement of CEA levels was not a reliable diagnostic test for

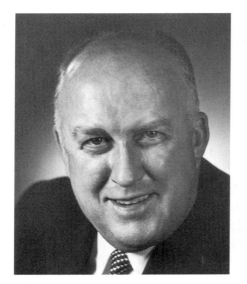

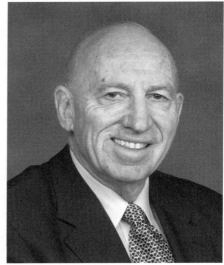

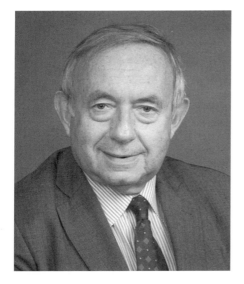

Clockwise from top left
Fig. 37.2 L.G. Elliot, executive director of research, 1976–81
Fig. 37.3 Joseph Shuster, scientific director of research, 1984–96
Fig. 37.4 Emil Skamene, McGill Centre for the Study of Host Resistance, 1988

colon cancer in most patients but that it was a valuable indicator of tumour recurrence after surgery. For example, a rise in the level of CEA postoperatively might indicate the need for adjuvant chemotherapy or "second look surgery." The serum assay for CEA remains the most frequently used test for tumour markers on a worldwide basis. John Krupey, a chemist, made a major contribution to the development of the radioimmunoassay of CEA by devising a method for linking radioactive iodine to the antigen. Three other members of the Division of Allergy and Clinical Immunology had a significant impact on the CEA project: David Thomson, Joseph Shuster, and Abraham Fuks. Charles Hollenberg joined the University Medical Clinic in 1960 as a clinician-scientist with a major interest in fat metabolism. In addition to his many scientific contributions, he served as a role model to students and professional colleagues alike for his integrity and straightforward approach to both his research and his clinical activities. At that time, the University Medical Clinic was located on the tenth floor of the hospital, with several large open laboratories on the tenth floor centre wing. This space was later incorporated into the MGH Research Institute. When Burgen returned to Cambridge University in 1962, Hollenberg succeeded him as deputy-director. In 1970, Hollenberg was appointed Lady Eaton Professor and chair of the Department of Medicine at the University of Toronto, where he led the Faculty of Medicine to a position of international significance.

Carl Goresky was a superb clinical investigator whose principal interest was the study of human liver function in both health and disease. In addition, he collaborated extensively with his colleague and friend, Harry Goldsmith, in the detailed study of blood flow through small blood vessels.[4] The latter project is of great importance in the study of vascular events leading to coronary artery disease or strokes. Unfortunately, a brilliant career was terminated at a relatively early age when Goresky was stricken with an incurable and painful malignancy. In this situation, he displayed remarkable courage by continuing research on a daily basis and refusing opioids so that his mind would remain clear at all times. He died in 1996, leaving a legacy of first-class research for others to emulate.

Emil Skamene was appointed to the Division of Allergy and Clinical Immunology in 1973. His major interests included infectious diseases and immunity in both adults and children. In this context he founded the McGill Centre for the Study of Host Resistance in 1988. The centre is one of the most important research groups at both McGill University and the MGH Research Institute. The centre's most important contributions to scientific medicine include the identification of genes controlling susceptibility to infectious diseases such as tuberculosis, leprosy, and malarias. His research models have been applied on a worldwide basis to several other infectious and genetic diseases.[5] A long-standing collaboration with Philippe Gros, a professor in the McGill Department of Biochemistry, was highly productive for Skamene and other members of the centre. In addition, an unusually large number of graduate students received high-quality training in infectious diseases and host resistance.

Research in Other Areas

In addition to the research projects outlined above as examples of what can be accomplished by hospital-based research, the MGH Research Institute was also responsible for the creation of many other outstanding medical research groups. In this respect, the Institute was fortunate to be located in Quebec, where generous infrastructure and salary support was provided by les Fonds de la Recherche en Santé du Québec. Funding of this type was available only in Quebec and Alberta, much to the dismay of the other Canadian provinces.

In 1997, the MGH, the RVH, the MCH, and the Montreal Neurological Institute as well as their research institutes were merged to form the McGill University Health Centre,[6] to be located in newly constructed buildings. Emil Skamene was appointed as the first scientific director of the MUHC in 1998 in recognition of his many scientific and administrative achievements. Over the last fifty years hospital-based biomedical research, which combines basic science and clinical studies, has become an increasingly important source of major Canadian discoveries in the understanding, prevention, and cure of human diseases. The Canadian Institutes for Health Research has estimated that hospital-based research facilities account for about 75 percent of Canadian medical research funding. In this context, the MGH Research Institute served as an outstanding example of the scientific excellence that can be achieved when there is strong institutional support for "bench-to-bedside" research.

NOTES

1 MGH Annual Report, 1947.
2 A. Aguayo, G.M. Bray, et al., "Prolonged Delivery of Brain-Derived Neurotrophic Factor by Adenovirus-Infected Muller Cells Temporarily Rescues Injured Retinal Ganglion Cells," *Proceedings of the National Academy of Sciences* 95, 7 (1998): 3978–83.

3 D.M.P. Thomson, J. Drupey, S.O. Freedman, and P. Gold, "The Radioimmunoassay of Circulating Antigens of the Human Digestive System," *Proceedings of the National Academy of Sciences* 64 (1969): 161–7.
4 C.A. Goresky, "A linear Method for Determining Liver Sinusoidal and
   Extravascular Volumes," *American Journal of Physics* 19, 3 (1963) : 144–8.
5 E. Skamene, P. Gos, A. Forget, et al., "Genetic Regulation of Resistance to
   Intracellular Pathogens," *Nature* 197 (1982): 506–10.
6 MGH Annual Report, 1997, MUA.

38

Social Services

Constance Lechman

Constance Lechman was director of social services during its modern development.

The Beginning: 1910

The story of organized social services in Montreal begins with the establishment of the Montreal General Hospital itself. In 1818, before there was a formal MGH, a group of socially conscious women mobilized to help local refugees of the One Hundred Years War. Their public appeal succeeded in raising funds, which were entrusted to the Ladies' Benevolent Society – an organization that established soup kitchens and schools for the benefit of those in need.

Before long, the Ladies' Benevolent Society found that many immigrants who sought its help suffered from medical illnesses. This drove the group to raise additional funds to establish a "House of Recovery." The initiative was so successful that, by 1819, enough money was raised to purchase a house on Craig Street and equip it with twenty-four beds. Ultimately, the House of Recovery was christened "the Montreal General Hospital."[1]

In 1910, Montreal was struck by a massive typhoid epidemic. Hospitals were overflowing and volunteers were taken on to help the overburdened staff. Helen Reid was in charge of these volunteers.[2] After the epidemic abated, many volunteers, still eager to be of assistance, visited patients at home and organized a Christmas tree party with gifts for the children. Reid became a strong advocate for the volunteers, arguing that they could be of help to patients in hospital. She wrote: "The Montreal General Hospital offers a special opportunity ... as its clientele includes hundreds of people who are affected with the awful diseases of ignorance and poverty which the trained social worker is better fitted to cope with than the busy doctor."[3]

Reid met a like-minded collaborator in Reverend John Lochhead, a Presbyterian minister of the Melville Church in Westmount. Lochhead had done an apprenticeship in social service in the Glasgow University Settlement in Scotland. His first encounter with a medical social service department prior to his arrival in Montreal from Scotland in 1909. Before coming to Montreal he spent the winter in New York City, where he visited the newly created Social Service Department in the Presbyterian Hospital. This experience left such an impression, that Lochhead "felt that a west-end church should develop a social outlook."[4] To this end, he began studying social service developments in the medical field. Among those whom Lochhead studied was Richard Cabot, a senior physician at the Massachusetts General Hospital, and a pioneer in establishing hospital-based social service programs. Cabot had learned about hospital social service in London.[5] On his return to Boston, Cabot was responsible for establishing the first structured hospital social services department in North America in 1905 and for hiring the hospital's first social worker, Ida Maude Cannon.[6]

Inspired by Cabot's work, Reverend Lochhead decided to limit his volunteers to the hospital closest to his congregation – namely, the Western Hospital, as it was known then. He arranged to see the matron, but: "I got the impression that she regarded me as a sentimental, hair-brained faddist, although she was too polite to say so."[7] He therefore approached the MGH in 1910, which was under the administration of Nora Livingston, "a very formidable old lady and delightful in her crabbed way." He was met with a similar detached attitude. "Even the General, the reported gathering place of all outcasts, failed to satisfy our appetite for cases"[8] It is interesting to note that Livingston Hall, a pavilion of the current MGH building, is named after Livingston. It houses the current MGH Social Service Department. Reverend Lochhead finally gained the support of MGH surgeon L.M. Elder, which allowed him to focus his efforts on the MGH: "I cannot express too strongly my respect and love for Dr Elder ... The impression he always gave me was that in a large sense he thoroughly approved of hospital social service.Reverend Lochhead started in the winter of 1910–11 by sending volunteer visitors to the wards of the hospital. The first annual report of 1910–11 noted that 119 cases were served: "We had learned the lesson that we must work from the inside. We therefore took the step of offering to the hospital a salaried whole-time social worker." The funds for her salary were financed through the Thanksgiving collection at the Melville Church: "The Montreal General had accepted our gift of a Social Worker with resignation but no elation; no sense of pride in being probably the first hospital in Canada to possess so up-to-date a gadget.

The First MGH Social Worker: 1912

It took time to find the right candidate, but finally Emma J. Foulis, a former nurse, was hired in January 1912. According to Reverend Lochhead, "She had no experience of hospital social service ... and only dimly understood what she was being asked to do." She persevered and "did try her best, conscientiously and perseveringly, in what was to prove a discouraging and lonely road. She had to find her own way and walk in unassisted." Later she was sent to visit Ida Cannon at the Massachusetts General in November 1912 for a two-week period of apprenticeship. According to Reverend Lochhead, "She returned a different person ... full of new ideas."

Emma Foulis wasn't given an office and was largely ignored by the rest of the staff. But she had the freedom to walk around the MGH and talk to patients. "It was as if an elevator had been installed, but everyone continued to climb the stairs ... She had simply to dig out work for herself, any bits and scraps she could find."[9] Foulis received her first real recognition when it was found that she could help "rid the hospital of some of its chronic cases. Every ward was congested with them."[10] Word soon spread that Foulis might be able to find places for them in the community. The hospital began to see that she was saving them hundreds of dollars and easing the pressure for beds.

In 1912, the office-bearers for the MGH Social Service were:

• J.M. Elder, honorary president
• Reverend John Lochhead, president
• Elsie Williamson and Grace Waterston, secretaries
• Grant Sclater and Roberstson Gibb, treasurers.

In addition to Emma Foulis, the salaried social worker, there were twelve volunteer visitors:

• H.M. Batnes

- L.C. Cole
- Ethel Hanna
- Elizabeth Harold
- Annie Harrower
- Margaret Hendry
- Gertrude Jarvis
- Frank Jarvis
- R.H. McNaught
- Gordon Morrison
- Jessie Munro
- Lillian Murray

In his 1912 annual report, Reverend Lochhead described the following cases that were serviced by Emma Foulis:

- "Man in hospital with abscess in lung. Wife with two baby children at home. Eldest child, 2 years old, has finger crushed and has to be taken to outpatient department for dressings. Visitor assists mother with car tickets, food, moving expenses, etc., and gets other societies to help. After two months the man is discharged from hospital, but still needs five weeks care and nourishment. Thereafter returns to work feeling perfectly fit."
- "English woman mortally ill with cancer. A widow, no friends, was twice in hospital and could not be readmitted. Social worker visited and found indescribable condition of filth, starvation and neglect. Had transferred to Incurable Home where her last days are now being cheered by our friendly visitors."
- " Man three weeks in hospital with acute rheumatism and unable to work for considerable time after. Patient a widower with two daughters. Visitor found house bare of furniture saving one mattress on the floor. Supplied with stove, bed, clothing and necessities until father was able to return to work. Very grateful and now doing well."
- "Case from Out-patient Department. Man had hand crushed in Angus Shops after being three months out of work. Wife and six children. Family found in extreme destitution. During period of visitation mother taken to hospital with pneumonia and one child sick. After mother's recovery found it necessary to take her to oculist to procure glasses. Family now on their feet."

The twelve volunteer visitors completed visits to ninety-seven patients in their homes. The department handled a total of 491 cases that year. Emma Foulis's salary for eleven months was $550. The total budget was $1,185.40 and was described as follows:

Disbursements.

Spent on cases through Mrs. Foulis	$206.02
Spent on cases through volunteer workers	286.79
Salary, eleven months	550.00
Telephone	18.50
Sundries	41.15
Balance	82.94
	$1,185.40

Reverend Lochhead started his 1912 annual report by saying: "While some at first wondered what a salaried worker would find to do, these persons now recognize that there is room for several." However, since there was only one worker, Emma Foulis concentrated her time on the inpatient wards. She helped move patients who needed to be transferred to other institutions. She visited all of the charitable institutions in Montreal to learn their mandates and resources to assist her in dealing with poor and homeless patients. In the first year, Foulis transferred seventy-six patients to other institutions. Reverend Lochhead also noted that she accompanied convalescent sailors "to the dock and [saw] to the securing of their baggage and arrears of pay."

In 1911, the Melville Church congregation gave a residence situated on the summit of Westmount Hill to the MGH to use as a convalescent home for several months.[11] This was the precursor to the Montreal Convalescent Hospital. The MGH also later contributed money to help establish the Convalescent Hospital.

About a year later a new hospital superintendent, James Fyshe, a grandson of Anna Leonowens of Siam, came to the MGH via the United States. While in the United States he was impressed by the work of hospital social services departments. According to Reverend Lochhead, he was the first medical person at the MGH to really understand the value of social service: "When he came across Mrs. Foulis and learned what she stood for, he was thunderstruck. 'A social worker in the Montreal General! How in the devil's name did you ever get her?'" Under his leadership Foulis was given a small office and allowed to interview all patients who were admitted. "It was not long till the hospital assumed responsibility for the worker's salary. Social Service had come to stay. Its expansion henceforth was only a matter of-time."[12] The third annual report of the Social Service Department documented 769 cases dealt with from 1 January to 31 December 1913.[13] The transfer of patients from the hospital to incurable homes and convalescent homes was noted as a vital part of the social worker's job. The report notes: "Anyone who has tried to get a person into a charitable institution knows the amount of resistance and red tape that have frequently to be encountered … It is here that the Social Worker comes in with her special knowledge and experience." In 1914, 198 such cases were transferred by the social worker. The report details the cost per day of each case as two dollars and therefore notes the financial saving to the MGH. In fact, that year the social worker was on holiday for a month and cases needing transfer piled up. This led to her being affectionately known as "the Exporter."

The third annual report goes on to document that the social worker played an important role in ensuring that charitable agencies were being utilized. For example, once Emma Foulis learned of the Protestant Orphan Asylum she referred many women and children to it, to the point at which the MGH accounted for "one fourth of all the transferred cases in 1913 … to this institution." To quote Reverend Lochhead: "She is a sort of director of traffic in the philanthropic world guiding people into the proper channels of help." He also noted that, in addition to the transfer of cases, Foulis arranged for an MGH doctor to visit the asylum to treat and discharge patients.

Some very touching cases were documented at the end of the third annual report. Three of these are listed below:

[1] A pathetic case was that of a mother with two children, aged nine and three, who was traveling from Saskatchewan to England to undergo an operation. She arrived in Montreal in so exhausted a condition that she had to be removed from the train to the hospital. The poor woman was greatly troubled about her children thus left like waifs in a strange city; but the Social Worker was able to allay all her anxieties. She handed over the children to kind friends who took them into their own home. She then stopped the baggage, which had gone on to Quebec, and finally when the mother's case appeared hopeless, telegraphed to her

husband in the West. He came through at once, but owing to the train being late, his wife died a few hours before his arrival.

[2] A similar case was that of a mother and young daughter who arrived in Montreal on their way to England. The mother had to be removed to the hospital where she died. The daughter was cared for by the Social Worker, the funeral arranged, the two steerage tickets exchanged for one second-class, and the girl put under the care of the stewardess on her sad and lonely voyage.

[3] One family as a result of sickness lost all its furniture and was boarding under indescribable conditions. A pulpit appeal for household necessaries brought a generous response, and two cartloads of things were taken to a little house which one of the volunteer workers had secured for them. The goods contributed completely furnished the new home, and the family, very grateful for the unexpected assistance, has since been doing very well.

Emma Foulis continued in charge of social services at the MGH for eight years and was followed by H.B. Broderick and then Mildred Forbes.

Expansion of the Department, 1917–39

In 1917, Ada Davison was appointed as the director of the Social Service Department. She remained as director for twenty-two years. She reported that the department's activities for 1935 included seeing 2,744 new patients.[14] In her 1935 annual report she mentioned the use of a special fund raised by the Westmount Operatic Society to help indigent patients. She also reported that, when the Soldiers' Wives League discontinued its charitable work in June of 1931, it donated one thousand dollars to the department to use "for the benefit of the wives, widows, and families of Canadian soldiers or ex-soldiers who are in difficulty or distress." With this money the department was able to help 153 families with dental treatment, spectacles, clothing, braces, taxis, and artificial eyes.

In 1935, the sixty-sixth annual meeting of the National Conference of Social Workers was held in Montreal, with over six thousand social workers in attendance. Hospital social service was starting to grow nationally.

In her 1936 annual report, Ada Davison made the case for better facilities for the Social Service Department. She quoted from the Statement of Standards adopted by the American Association of Medical Social Workers in

1936: "Medical Social Service has been developed in the Hospital as a service to the Patient, the Physician, the Hospital, Administration, and the Community, in order to help meet the problems of the patient whose medical need may be aggravated by Social factors and who therefore may require Social treatment which is based on his medical condition and care." She went on to state that well qualified staff selection is essential and that the director must have the appropriate credentials. Thus, she advocated for "a central office ... accessible to patients and to doctors but [that would] afford privacy for interviews." She also advocated for the need for clerical assistance.[15]

In the twenty-sixth annual report in 1937, presented to J.C. MacKenzie Esq., MD, general superintendent of the hospital, the department director, Ada Davison, described the department's mission as follows: "Medical Social Work in a hospital is the searching out of social factors contributing to the physical ailments of the patient, analyzing their causes and effects, and making a plan in which as far as possible these factors may be eradicated or at least improved." The following year, Davison reported that the department served 2,268 new patients, 360 of whom were cases carried over from the year prior. She lamented the increasing volume of requests and inadequate number of staff to meet them. She detailed some of the instrumental assistance given to patients, such as, artificial eyes, spectacles, splints, and elastic stockings. She noted that, for patients unable to provide their own transportation, $495.75 was spent for taxis, railway, and car tickets. Ada Davison retired in 1939; Constance Webb was her successor.

The 1940s

The annual report for the year ending in 1940 described how the department's functioning was hampered by its inadequate quarters. Rooms on the main floor of the hospital were finally made available. Desk space was also allotted for two Montreal School of Social Work students who were doing their fieldwork at the hospital and for volunteers from the Central Volunteer Bureau. This gave the social work staff more time to work with patients.

In 1941, Constance Webb, director of the Social Service Department, noted in her annual report that the provincial Ministry of Health paid for a social worker to "bring and keep infectious patients with venereal disease under treatment.[16] Webb resigned after three years of service and was replaced by Olive L. Elmslie. The thirty-third annual report for 1944, submitted by Olive L. Elmslie, acting director, to Burnett S. Johnston, Esq.,

MD, General Superintendent, states: "The Medical Social Worker can do much to build up the morale of ... patients by frequent talks with them about their problems." These talks formed the basis of supportive counselling for patients and their families.

In 1945, Elmslie noted in her annual report the problems experienced in placing chronically ill patients, "especially those suffering with Tuberculosis, Carcinoma, and the aged sick.[17]

The shortage of beds in appropriate institutions resulted in patients staying longer at the MGH and, thereby, delaying admissions of patients waiting for treatment. She also noted that the department was encountering many cases of people suffering psychiatric problems due to the war. A year later she addressed the unmet needs of psychiatric patients by stating that a social worker needed to be hired for the new psychiatric clinic.

In her 1946 annual report Elmslie spoke about the increasing number of elderly patients: "The trend toward an older population for Canada is emphasized in the returns from the 1941 census as reported in the Canada Year Book 1943–44. We have come to realize that the increased number of old people represents a problem."

By 1947, Olive Elmslie was voicing a strong need for a chronic hospital: "Quite frequently during the past year many of our incurable patients had to be re-admitted to the ward as they were too ill." She also noted that many of the young patients seen by the department were separated from spouses either legally or as a result of the war and required a great deal of supportive help. She detailed the problem in placing Roman Catholic psychiatric patients because of the long wait for Catholic placements, thereby forcing them to languish in hospital.

Agnes Tennant replaced Elmslie but subsequently left in 1949 to be married. Mary McIlquham was therefore named as interim administrator. Her annual report for 1949 noted the many displaced persons and new Canadians who were served by the Social Service Department. "The language difficulty in many cases presents quite a handicap as the patient is at a disadvantage in trying to discuss their upset thoughts and feelings."[18] The statistics from 1 October 1948 to 30 September 1949 were reported as follows:

- 3,211 cases carried over
- 1,407 cases opened
- 1,352 cases closed
- 3,208 cases remaining
- 4,618 total number of cases served

Recognition: The 1950s

Avis Pumphrey was named director in 1950. Under her direction and in collaboration with medical chiefs of staff, ward rounds that included the social worker became established practice: "The doctor, head nurse and social worker confer together every week on the problems presented by each patient, keeping each other informed, and working as a team to help the patient to return to health as quickly as possible." She documented the expansion of services in her 1950 annual report, noting that two social workers were assigned to psychiatry. With increased recognition of the importance of social services to patients, Pumphrey was invited by the School of Nursing to lecture on emotional and social components of illness to student nurses and dieticians.

In 1951, under the direction of Pumphrey were fourteen staff members who possessed a bachelor of arts degree and a master of social work degree. The average monthly caseload of the department almost doubled from 391.3 cases in 1950 to 654.2 in 1951. In the tumour clinic the number of cases seen by the Social Service Department increased from fifty-five in March 1951 to 244 in a seven-month period. Pumphrey proudly mentioned that the value of social service was recognized by both the medical staff and the provincial health ministry with government grants for hiring social workers to work with patients with emotional disorders, glaucoma, tumours, and syphilis: "The medical or psychiatric social worker has thus been officially recognized as a member of the medical team." The social worker responsible for the syphilis casework began a social research project to identify underlying behavioural causes in order to make recommendations on community resources to meet the social recreational needs of the young Montreal population, especially those entering the city from rural areas. This social worker was seeing ten new cases per month.

In 1954, Avis Pumphrey received recognition from the American Association of Medical Social Workers in a letter stating: "Your Department of Social Service is an outstanding one … as good as we have on the North American continent."

In the spring of 1954, a subcommittee of the Medical Board, composed of Mitchell, Rowe, Alexander, and Mowry, was mandated to "study the value of Social Service in relation to the clinical treatment of the patient."[19] They noted that there had been an increase from four hundred to nine hundred cases a month since 1950. They found that forty-three percent of referrals came from doctors, 18 percent from patients and families, 17 percent from community agencies, and 15 percent from nurses. Seven percent of the referrals were from a variety of sources, such as a concerned minister or a police officer who picked up a psychotic patient.

In reviewing the departmental statistics for 1953, the subcommittee found that the major source for new referrals by service was as follows:

- 829 from medical wards and clinics
- 726 from surgical wards and clinics
- 471 from psychiatric wards and clinics
- 243 from orthopaedic wards and clinics
- 240 from gynaecological wards and clinics
- 117 from urological wards and clinics
- 343 were referred for help with resources for glasses

The subcommittee also found that, of the 5,210 new patients seen in 1953, 659 had a diagnosis of cancer.

Nursing expressed its appreciation to this subcommittee for the responsibility that the Social Service Department was taking for patients' emotional welfare and for their support in helping them return to their family and community. They congratulated the department for faithful and conscientious service: "The development of medical social service would appear to be a natural extension to clinical treatment which today considers the entire patient even though they present themselves with a specific complaint."

The Committee recommended to the Montreal General Hospital Medical Board that the Social Service Department be retained as an integral department of the MGH. In 1955, the department moved to a larger space when the MGH moved to a new building on Cedar Avenue. With the establishment of the new site, taxi transport and provision of prosthetic appliances was transferred to other departments, thereby freeing the social workers to deal with increasing numbers of referrals. At the same time, the new process of written referrals helped to eliminate inappropriate referrals. These changes helped to make the department more efficient and gave the social workers more time with patients who needed their help.

Social Service Department director Avis Pumphrey reported in 1957 that $2,500 had been donated to the department from the Women's Auxiliary of the MGH. In the 1990s, this amount was increased to $14,000 per year and continues to be of immeasurable assistance to the many patients who benefit from its use. In the form of visits and correspondence, for several years Pumphrey provided consultation to the Government of Saskatchewan regarding the establishment of medical social work. She eventually left Montreal to become director of Social Services at the Vancouver General Hospital.

In her annual reports in the late 1950, Jessie Lawrence, like her predecessors, cited the problem of a lack of facilities for chronically ill patients. She also noted the increasing number of elderly patients requiring help from the Social Service Department. In her 1959 report, Lawrence stated that more than fifty of the department's clientele required resources outside of their own home in addition to their treatment at the MGH.

The Sixtieth Anniversary, 1971

The Social Service Department celebrated its sixtieth anniversary by inviting Harvard University professor Nathan Glazer to speak. He presented a paper entitled "The Limits of Social Policy: The Case of Health Care". Glazer described North American health and social services as being in a state of crisis. He theorized that social policy had reached its limit in dealing with the breakdown of traditional societal structures. To this end, he called for the development of policies that fostered traditional social structures.[20]

Administration by the Ville Marie Social Service Centre: 1973–91

In 1973, social services in the Province of Quebec were centralized under the governance of newly created social service centres. To this end, anglophone social services, including the MGH Social Service Department staff, came under the administration of the Ville Marie Social Service Centre (VMSSC). Staff remained in the hospital but their salaries were paid by the VMSSC. The director of the Social Service Department, Jessie Lawrence, was directly accountable to the senior management of VMSSC and indirectly to the MGH senior administration.

Although services were essentially maintained in the same way, the hospital felt that it was no longer as influential in the direction of social services. Lawrence also felt that the VMSSC was too distant from the daily hospital work to effectively administer the department. However, this arrangement

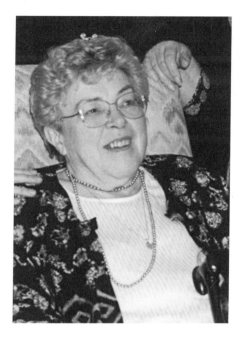

Fig. 38.1 Jessie Lawrence, director of
Social Services, 1958–83, succeeded Avis
Pumphrey in 1958. During her time as
director at the MGH, Lawrence's expertise
was also sought by the Ottawa General
Hospital. At the request of the Faculty
of Medicine at the University of Ottawa,
she helped them to establish a plan to
develop a social services department
at the Ottawa General.

continued until 1991, when, in a new reform, all social service workers were repatriated to their originating hospitals.

Jessie Lawrence served twenty-five years as department director and was succeeded by Martha Walsh following her retirement in 1983. At Walsh's untimely death Marcelle Haim assumed the responsibility of interim director. The current manager of MGH Social Services, Constance Lechman, was hired by Lawrence in 1972 to work as a social worker in the Department of Psychiatry. Lechman became the director of the department in 1991.

The McGill University Health Centre

With the merger of the MGH, the RVH, the Montreal Chest Institute, and the Montreal Neurological Hospital, Constance Lechman also assumed responsibility for these hospital social service departments. Today, social services at the MGH site are provided by twenty-six university-trained social workers who are available in all inpatient and some outpatient care areas, including the Emergency Department, and, as such, are an integral part of the interdisciplinary approach to patient care. The annual budget for the department is over $1.8 million. This is essentially for salaries, with stationary and telephones constituting a small portion of the budget.

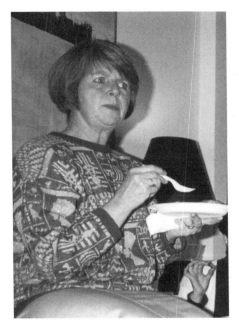 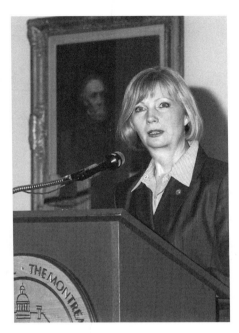

Fig. 38.2 A.M. Walsh, director of social services, 1983–91
Fig. 38.3 Constance Lechman, director of social services, 1991–

The patient population is multicultural and spans the developmental life-cycle from young adults to geriatrics. Patients present with complex medical and social problems and have a wide variety of needs, strengths, and limitations. The social service professionals help physically or mentally ill patients and their families cope with the social and psychological problems that emerge as a result of the illness or hospitalization. The range of social service interventions includes: psychosocial assessment, high social risk screening, treatment planning, counselling, discharge planning, and locating and arranging community and institutional resources. Today patients present with the same types of social problems but the response of the community is different. Today's solutions come more from governmental agencies than from churches and well intentioned volunteers.

The Social Service Department provides an educational program for social work students in collaboration with McGill University. Each year about ten students have their field training in the department. In addition to formal and informal teaching of interdisciplinary colleagues, the department engages in psychosocial research. The most recent research has found that psychosocial problem severity is a more significant predictor of length of hospital stay than is the nature of the medical problem.

It is interesting to note that the problems experienced by the department today are essentially the same as they were in the beginning years and throughout its history – namely, an insufficient number of staff, difficulty finding placements for chronically ill patients, transport problems, and scarce community resources for care of the ill elderly patients who come to the hospital's attention.

NOTES

1 "Jeanne Mance and Female Benevolent Society Respectively Founders of the Hotel Dieu and Montreal General – A Romance of Service and Charitableness," MGH Archives, MUA.
2 Helen R.Y. Reid, *Social Service and Hospital Efficiency*, pamphlet issued by the Charity Organization Society of Montreal in May 1913, MGH Archives, MUA.
3 Reverend John Lochhead, annual report of the Social Service Department, 1912, Melville Church, Westmount, MGH Achives, MUA.
4 Ibid.
5 Richard Cabot, *Social Service and the Art of Healing* (New York: Moffat, Yard and Co., 1909).
6 Avis Pumphrey, annual reports of the Social Service Department, 1950, 1951, 1954, and 1957, MGH Archives, MUA.
7 Lochhead, annual report.
8 Ibid.
9 Ibid.
10 Ibid.
11 Pumphry, annual reports.
12 Lochhead, annual report.
13 Pumphry, annual reports.
14 C.B. Webb, Report of the Social Service Department, 1941., MGH Archives, MUA.
15 Ada Davison, annual reports of the Social Service Department, 1935, 1936, 1937, 1938. MGH Archives, MUA.
16 Webb, Report.
17 Olive L. Elmslie, annual reports of the Social Service Department, 1944, 1945, 1947. MGH Archives, MUA.

18 Mary, McIlquham, annual report of the Social Service Department, 1949, MGH Archives, MUA.

19 Howard S. Mitchell, P.G. Rowe, B. Alexander, D.P. Mowry, Report of the Committee on Social Service, 1954, MGH Archives, MUA.

20 Cabot, *Social Service.*

39

Urology

Michael P. Laplante

Michael Laplante was site-director of urology at the MGH and staff urologist for over forty years.

The First Years

At the end of the nineteenth century, it was a brave surgeon who would operate on the kidney or the prostate. Surgical mortality and morbidity due to haemorrhage and sepsis were prevalent, and the science and art of surgery as we knew it even sixty years ago was unimagined to those pioneers. Lister's antiseptic techniques, in routine use in Edinburgh by 1874, were introduced and strongly promoted by Roddick at the Montreal General Hospital in 1877, but the surgical community in Montreal did not universally accept germ theory and Listerism until the turn of the century. Infection and mortality rates were high.

The practice of anaesthesia was also in its infancy and was itself hazardous. Clinical diagnosis was largely intuitive and imprecise. One can imagine the difficulties faced by a surgeon deciding to attack a kidney without imaging or biological tests to assess renal form or function. He had only his hands, eyes, knowledge of anatomy, and experience to guide him.

The development of the cystoscope by Nitze in the late nineteenth century marks the beginning of urology as a specialty. The Lowenstein modification of the cystoscope was introduced to the Montreal surgical community at the turn of the century by surgeons returning from Berlin. George Armstrong, A. Hutchison, and A.G. Garrow made efforts to learn the use of the instrument.[1] Garrow persisted and acquired status as a cystoscopist and was performing prostate resections in the early days of the twentieth century.

These early endoscopic instruments were crude by today's standards, or even by the standards of the 1950s. They were certainly a long way from the elegant fibre-optic, high definition, brilliantly illuminated video instruments in use in the first decade of the twenty-first century. Nevertheless the ability to actually see the inside of the bladder, and to catheterize the ureters, set the cystoscopist apart from his surgical colleague.

The first operation on the kidney mentioned in the annual report of the MGH was performed by Roddick in 1882. He incised a large flank abscess (presumably a pyonephrosis-dilated kidney full of pus, ór perhaps a large perinephric abscess). He drained the pus-filled cavity but the suppurating kidney was retained and the patient later died of amyloid disease.

Francis Shepherd, anatomy professor and legendary surgeon to the MGH, was reported to have performed the first successful nephrectomy in Montreal (if not Canada) in 1885, for a huge hydronephrotic kidney described by him at the time as "calculous pyelitis." The kidney was reported to have been the size of a child's head. This operation followed an unsuccessful attempt at a nephrectomy a few weeks before by William H. Hingston (later Sir) of the Hotel Dieu Hospital, a renowned surgeon with particular interest in genito-urinary surgery. Unhappily, Hingston's patient succumbed on the operating table.

Shepherd also described a difficult nephrolithotomy for a very large staghorn calculus in 1887. He was assisted in this operation by James Bell, Roddick's associate and later his successor as chief surgeon at the Royal Victoria Hospital. Shepherd did not remove the kidney as he felt it was healthy. The patient survived the operation but died three and a half months later of septic complications. Shepherd is also reported to have performed a successful operation in 1884 for imperforate anus. The subject was a three-day-old infant passing meconium from the urethra. Shepherd brought bowel out through the perineum and sutured it to the skin.

In the 1890s, surgeons did "cut boldly" for bladder stones, carrying on the tradition handed down for centuries. Shepherd, with his precise knowledge of perineal anatomy, was said to have been very skilful at the lateral lithotomy. Today's urologist cannot escape the conclusion that outcomes of this surgery were probably poor considering not only the rather crude technique used but also the fact that the surgeons of the time had no way of knowing the number of stones to be retrieved or, probably, how or why they formed in the first place.

Also a pioneer in prostate surgery, Shepherd was reported to have successfully performed a suprapubic removal in 1885 or 1886. At that time there was a very high mortality rate for this surgery, and the operation fell into disfavour for several years.

Although Urology was not recognized as a "specialty" at the end of the nineteenth century, there were certainly courageous and inventive surgeons who displayed special interest in genito-urinary surgery. Of those already mentioned, it is noteworthy that Hingston (not associated with the MGH) was one of the original members of the American Association of Genito-Urinary Surgeons (founded in 1886). Bell was elected a member in 1892, and F.S. Patch wrote in a personal account: "Dr Shepherd is rightly entitled to be numbered in this group."[2] It was not stated if he actually was.

Lists of operations performed at the MGH were published in the hospital's annual reports in the early decades of the twentieth century and indicate the scope of surgical urology at that time. In 1905, there were eight suprapubic prostate enucleations, thirteen "kidney operations," and fifty-two cystoscopies performed. There were twenty-two circumcisions, and the nature of three "other" procedures was not stated. The following year there were twenty kidney operations, eight suprapubic prostatectomies, and twenty circumcisions. Outcomes were not recorded. These numbers were more or less repeated over the next few years and indicate the limited genito-urinary surgical activity of the time.

Formation of the Montreal General Hospital Department of Genito-Urologic Surgery

Rolland Playfair Campbell was born in Montreal in 1876 and graduated in medicine from McGill in 1901. He travelled and studied in Europe for the next three years, studying with Mikulicz in Germany in 1903. He returned from Breslau in 1904 and was named medical superintendent at the MGH for two years. He was then named surgeon to the Outpatient Department and started his practice. He developed a particular interest and exceptional skill in genito-urinary surgery. His McGill appointments included demonstrator in pathology and assistant demonstrator in clinical surgery in 1907, then lecturer in genito-urinary surgery in 1912. He was appointed genito-urinary surgeon to the MGH by the Board of Management in 1911, establishing urology as a separate department.

By this time the value of cystoscopy was well recognized and was employed with increasing success. Considerable effort was made to use the instruments to catheterize the ureters and attempt to determine differential renal function by studying differences in certain characteristics of the urine samples collected from each kidney. The endoscopic image viewed by the cystoscopist was inverted, and it required significant mental exercise to convert the upside-down image to a workable perspective. There was no adjustable flow of liquid as a visual medium; the bladder had to be filled before introducing the instrument. Also contributing to the difficulties of cystoscopy was the fact that the light generated by a dry cell battery and a primitive tiny, brittle, short-lived incandescent bulb was weak and subject to frequent interruption because of encrustation by verdigris (copper carbonate) on copper contact points. One can imagine the tribulations and frustrations endured by the early urologic endoscopist.

Campbell, on being named genito-urinary surgeon, had ambitious plans for his new department, including visions of developing modern diagnostic and investigative techniques. During his all-too-brief period at the MGH prior to 1914, Campbell established himself as a dedicated and committed teacher as well as an outstanding surgeon. He formed a close working relationship with Frank S. Patch, his eventual successor, who had joined the department in 1913. It was because he wished to retain this association that he resisted recruitment by George Armstrong who had moved up the mountain to the new RVH as first chief of surgery in 1893.

Campbell was also keenly interested in clinical research and was fascinated by the demonstration of the spirochete in primary syphilis. He firmly believed that the genito-urinary specialist should follow this disease to whatever organ it eventually attacked. Unfortunately, this led to a situation in which the department's resources were almost overwhelmed by the volume of cases of neurosyphilis. Campbell was appointed officer commanding the 6th Canadian Field Ambulance in 1914 and left Montreal with his unit for France in May 1915. This unit served on the right half of the Ypres salient and, later, at the Somme as part of the 2nd Canadian Division.

Lieutenant-Colonel Campbell was killed in action near Courcellette on 16 September 1916 at age forty. His obituary in the *Montreal Star* on 29 September 1916 described him as having had no equal as a genito-urinary surgeon in Canada and as one of the best all-round physicians and surgeons in Montreal. He was remembered by his MGH colleagues as an eminent genito-urinary surgeon, pathologist, and teacher, and he was recognized for his sincerity and charm of manner. He is commemorated in a stained-glass triptych in the stairwell of the Strathcona Anatomy and Dentistry Building on the McGill campus, sharing the memorial window with John McCrae and Henry B. Yates. The tribute reads:

> To Rolland Playfair Campbell, BA, MD, CM, McGill. Lt. Col. CAMC. Surgeon, Investigator, Soldier, a man most skilled in his craft. He came here as Lecturer in Surgery in 1912 and was also Surgeon to the Montreal General Hospital an there held in affection by all. In the Great War he served with No.1 Canadian General Hospital and at the time of his death was in command of the 6th Field Ambulance. Born in 1876. Killed in Action at Thiepval, France in 1916.

The Patch Years, 1916–44

Campbell was succeeded as genito-urinary surgeon by his close associate Frank S. Patch, who had joined the department in 1913 following two years as surgeon to the Outpatient Department of the MGH. Born in Kingston, Ontario, he was a graduate of McGill (1903) and did his internship at the MGH, where he spent twelve months in the services of Shepherd and George Armstrong, during which, by his personal account, he saw only two renal operations performed by Shepherd. He did postgraduate work in Edinburgh, London, Bonn, and Vienna. He served in the Medical Corps from 1915 to 1919 and rose to the rank of Colonel.

Patch is remembered as a no-nonsense, opinionated, and assertive individual accustomed to being heard. The department practised urology by the standard of the day, a large part being venerology, and it is possible that most of the several listed members of the department in the1920s and 1930s were mainly occupied with this aspect of urologic practice. Outpatient clinics were particularly busy (second only to surgery) with a preponderance of "old" cases. In pre-antibiotic days venereal urethritis was slow to clear and treatment likely did more harm than good. Open surgery was still primitive by today's standards, the major procedures being two-stage prostatectomies, some stone surgery, and the occasional nephrectomy. Morbidity and mortality rates were high compared to the post-antibiotic and blood transfusion era following the Second World War.

Patch and his associate Ralph E. Powell were remembered as competent but unexceptional surgeons. Patch was, however, very active in medical politics. He held the post of secretary of the Board of Management of the MGH from 1933 to 1937. At the university level he was named clinical professor of urology in 1921. Later, in 1938, he succeeded A.T. Bazin as head (now called chair) of the Department of Surgery at McGill, holding that post for three years. He was elected to the Senate of McGill University in 1941. On the national scene he was elected president of the Canadian Medical Association in 1943. The same year he was elected president of the Royal College of Physicians and Surgeons of Canada.

In a personal account of the development of urology in Montreal (unpublished, circa 1946), Patch expresses regret that, during the years he was in charge of the department, he could not establish a residency system. This was largely due to the hospital policy of the time, which featured rotating internships of short duration. Only a few interns were retained for a second and occasionally a third year, and these were mainly in surgery, medicine, and Pathology. It is ironic that during the period from 1937 to 1947 Patch was engaged with the Royal College as chair of the Committee on Certification and had much to do with the establishment of certification of specialists as one of the college's principal functions.

During his years as department head at the MGH, Patch travelled extensively and gave a number of talks at meetings of the Canadian Medical Association and other scientific gatherings. He presented an elegant paper, "Pyelitis, Ureteritis and Cystitis Cystica" to the Northeastern Section of the American Urologic Association in Boston in 1938. This paper was subsequently published in the *New England Journal of Medicine*.[3] Another earlier publication, "Pyelography – Intravenous and Retrograde," offers an interesting glimpse of urologic practice and diagnostic imaging in the early 1930s.[4] He concluded that intravenous urography promised to be a valuable addition to the urologic armamentarium of the day as a supplement to the much more invasive retrograde studies. By the 1990s, intravenous urography had been highly refined, only to be gradually replaced by more precise and less invasive imaging techniques.

Patch was honoured in 1945 with an honorary MD degree from Laval University in recognition of his eminence in the medical community and his cordial collaboration with his francophone colleagues. He died in 1953, age seventy-five, nine years after retiring as head of the department.

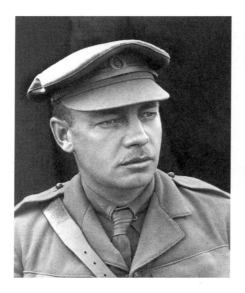
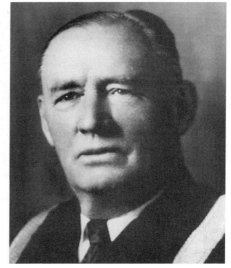

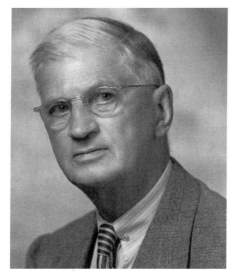

Clockwise from top left
Fig. 39.1 Rolland Playfair Campbell, first
director, Department of Urology, 1911–16
Fig. 39.2 Frank S. Patch, director,
Department of Urology, 1916–44
Fig. 39.3 Ralph Powell, director, MGH
urology, 1944–49

From 1944 to the Mid-1960s

Ralph Powell, who succeeded Patch in 1944, had the difficult task of re-establishing a war-depleted department. R. Grant Reid, who had joined the department in 1931, had been mobilized and served overseas in command of No. 6 Field Ambulance Royal Canadian Army Medical Corps from the early days of the war. K.L. Conover and A.T. Argue were also on active military service from 1940, and the surgical talent in the MGH Department of Urology was spread thin. Several other members of the department were engaged primarily in the outpatient clinics. Reid was called back from overseas in 1944 to help remedy the situation. S.A. MacDonald, returning from active service in the navy, joined the department the same year. By 1945, MacDonald was promoted to associate, along with Reid and A.M. Tanney.

In addition to demonstrating a modern approach to urologic surgery, MacDonald, who had trained at Yale and had his FRCS(C), was genuinely keen to engage in clinical research. He published articles on evolving surgical techniques and was a strong proponent of Millin's retropubic prostatectomy. His funded research focused on the development and use of haemostatic agents for control of blood loss in open renal surgery. MacDonald was respected as an excellent and enthusiastic teacher and an exceptionally skilled technical surgeon. A native Prince Edward Islander, he was a keenly competitive yachtsman and was a member of the 1960 and 1964 Canadian Olympic Sailing teams in Rome and Tokyo.[5]

In October 1949, Powell stepped down, and, as was customary at that time, by virtue of his seniority R.G. Reid was named his successor by the MGH Board of Management. Many felt that MacDonald had better qualifications. Perhaps Reid felt threatened by MacDonald, and this led to a rift not only between those two but also within the department as it limped through the next fifteen years. Reid chose not to support academic projects and disdained the Canadian Academy of Urologic Surgeons, to which MacDonald had been elected as a charter member. At a time when McGill undergraduate and postgraduate activities were rapidly evolving, Reid saw no utility either in collaborating with the "rival" teaching hospital to standardize the teaching of urology to the medical students or in integrating resident training. He resisted any move to schedule combined clinical rounds or conferences. This spirit of non-collaboration extended to relations with francophone colleagues across town at the Université de Montreal teaching hospitals. Thus, the 1950s and early 1960s were not an especially laudable period for urology at the MGH.

By 1957 Claude Moore, also ex-navy, had joined the department and brought with him expertise in transurethral prostatic surgery learned in Ottawa with Victor Berry. For unrecorded reasons, Moore and MacDonald did not get along. This did little to improve the harmony within the department.

In 1955, the MGH moved to its modern new building on Cedar Avenue on the old Cross Estate. Reid was very pleased with his new cystoscopy suite.

He recruited A.B. McLauchlin to take charge of this new facility. She had been in charge of the operating rooms at the Western Division and became a loyal and legendary figure at the MGH and the bane of their existence for many residents learning cystoscopy over the next several years. Another memorable character who moved from the old to the new MGH outpatient clinic was M. Roy, an orderly who was expert at setting up dark field preparations in the search for spirochetes in primary syphilis lesions. He was also remembered for his skills in dealing with urethral strictures and the performance of prostatic massage for patients with chronic prostatitis. It was rumoured that he also practised these skills in a "private" clinic outside the hospital on weekends.

William Lingard trained first at the MGH, then at the RVH in urology under M.B. Hawthorn. He joined the MGH staff in 1955 as assistant urologist and was soon setting records for both bed and operating room usage. He is remembered for his faithful attendance at the outdoor clinics in order to help the residents, the only member of the attending staff to do so prior to the late 1960s.

During the 1950s and early 1960s, urologic practice at the MGH was lagging behind North American standards, especially in the management of genito-urinary cancer and reconstructive surgery. S.A. MacDonald continued to perform excellent renal and prostatic surgery. He was also well ahead of his time in trying to establish databases for bladder cancer treatment. Claude Moore's health deteriorated prematurely, and, unhappily, his initial keen enthusiasm, self-confidence, and forceful surgical drive faded to the point at which he no longer enjoyed performing surgery. He retired for health reasons in 1966. Clearly a change of mission and improved personnel was required to bring the department up to the standards expected in a McGill teaching hospital. It was another, unrelated, Reid – Everett Cox Reid – who arrived on the scene in the summer of 1961 to start a residency in urology and who would ultimately be instrumental in bringing about these needed changes.

E.C. Reid, brought up in Isaac's Harbour, Nova Scotia, had graduated from Acadia University with his BSc while still in his teens and was accepted into medicine at McGill. He graduated in 1948 and interned for two years at the old MGH, where he established many valuable contacts and developed a taste for surgery. He returned to the Maritimes at the completion of his senior internship in 1950 to set up a general practice in Plaster Rock, New

Brunswick, in the upper St John River valley. Of necessity his practice included some surgery. This he had learned, in part, during his internship, some with his semi-trained colleague in Plaster Rock, and much of it self-taught, learned through his own experience and reading.

By 1960, Reid had decided he would prefer a surgical practice over a general practice, and he chose urology. This choice had been largely influenced by his exposure to the specialty during his internship, with Claude Moore, then senior resident, as his mentor. He intended to return to the US side of the upper St John valley to practise community urology, with enough leisure time to enjoy his other passions: upland game hunting, curling, and, most especially, golf.

Although the MGH residency program enjoyed a less than sterling reputation, Reid was confident his old stomping ground, now well established in its new site on Cedar Avenue, would provide him with excellent material and enthusiastic teachers in the persons of S.A. MacDonald and Claude Moore. His subsequent description of urology at the MGH in the early 1960s is revealing as it illustrates the two-tiered system of the time, when the attending staff in the teaching hospitals was largely, if not exclusively, concerned with its private practice, leaving the "public" service in the variably supervised (and variably competent) hands of the residents. A mature and surgically experienced resident (such as Reid) benefited from this very rich learning experience, as did his patients, who, under the care of a less experienced, less conscientious, and largely unsupervised resident, may not have fared as well.

Towards the end of his two clinical residency years, Reid's exceptional surgical and academic qualities were recognized by the MGH Medical Board, which realized that the Department of Urology was "not what it should be." He was vigorously encouraged to change his plans regarding a somewhat remote community practice and to pursue an academic career at the MGH. This would entail undergoing further training in urologic oncology and pathology. Despite having to leave his family behind in Montreal, he spent a year at Memorial-Sloan Kettering in New York with Willet Whitmore. He then returned to the MGH for six months of pathology with William Mathews, following which he successfully sat his Royal College Fellowship exams. His appointment as assistant urologist to the MGH in 1965 marked the beginning of a new era for the department.

The E.C. Reid Years, 1967–92

Reid brought to the department a fresh and mature approach to the practice of urology. He was soon overwhelmed with referrals, and his practice grew rapidly. He applied new modern principles of oncologic surgery to the management of genito-urinary malignancies, most especially to the treatment of invasive bladder cancer. These high standards were to apply to all urology patients, and the prevalent two-tiered public/private system underwent major changes even before the arrival of universal Medicare in 1970. All Urology patients were now to be cared for on the same ward, where specialized nursing care and equipment would be available to all. Staff supervision of residents became much tighter, and a universal standard of care became the norm.

By the end of 1966, R.G. Reid, S.A. MacDonald, and Claude Moore had all retired, leaving the department seriously understaffed. William Mathews, pathologist-in-chief, was named chair of the Search Committee for a new chief of urology. He and Fraser Gurd, surgeon-in-chief, convinced Reid to accept the position, and he was appointed in early 1967.

The first priority for Reid at the MGH was to recruit academically oriented young urologists to establish the standards of clinical excellence expected in a McGill teaching institution. This priority was clearly linked with the need to set new standards of undergraduate teaching and postgraduate training in collaboration with the other McGill teaching hospitals.

Stephen "Duke" MacIsaac, a Cape Bretoner, had trained at Dalhousie and then with Ken MacKinnon in the RVH program. With his appointment in early 1967, MacIsaac brought excellent urologic skills, memorable affability, and a very strong work ethic to the department. C.F. Douglas Ackman, Jr, and Michael P. Laplante also trained under MacKinnon and were appointed in 1968.

Ackman brought with him expertise in vascular access for renal dialysis and early experience in renal transplantation, along with exceptional enthusiasm for the rapidly evolving science of computer technology, albeit then in its infancy. He soon developed other special clinical interests in the new subspecialty now entitled andrology and was active with his gynaecology colleagues in developing assisted fertilization programs. Ever keen on innovative mechanical devises, he was somewhat of a pioneer in the use of implantable devices to correct erectile deficiency and artificial sphincters for male incontinence.

Laplante was one of the three first residents to be "charter members" of the combined McGill Urology Residency Training Program established by Ken MacKinnon with the enthusiastic collaboration of E.C. Reid. After a rotating internship and two core years of general surgery at the MGH, Laplante's urology training rotated through the RVH, Queen Mary Veterans Hospital, and the Montreal Children's Hospital, with the last six months being spent as chief resident at the MGH with E.C. Reid. A one-year McLaughlin Travelling Fellowship followed, with six months spent in at the New York Hospital with Victor Marshall (and, unofficially, with Willet Whitmore across the street) and six months in Los Angeles with Goodwin and Kaufman at UCLA, concentrating on renal transplantation.

Thus, by July 1969, a keen new team was in place, prepared to practise leading-edge urology and committed to train a new flight of residents within a fully integrated residency program. This was a source of considerable pride to Mackinnon and Reid, who had longed to see the end of inter-hospital bickering, animosity, and unhealthy competition. Weekly combined clinical rounds and other academic activities were attended by all residents and attending staff of all McGill hospitals and a true McGill training program was established, thanks to the most cordial and enthusiastic cooperation between old Maritime friends and colleagues, Ken MacKinnon and Ev Reid.

Clinical Activities: From the Late 1960s

Oncology

Reid was committed to bringing the management of urologic cancers up to modern standards, and he was especially interested in the treatment of invasive bladder cancer. This interest was enthusiastically shared by his colleagues in the department. His efforts were aimed at reducing the morbidity and the mortality associated with radical cystectomy and improving survival. Inspired by the rationale of using neo-adjuvant – that is, pre-operative – radiotherapy then being tested at Memorial-Sloan Kettering Hospital in New York by Whitmore, Reid introduced a protocol in collaboration with the MGH radiotherapists, using a short intense course of therapy immediately prior to cystectomy. This protocol was followed for several years and was the basis for several subsequent publications. At the same time, several perioperative measures were introduced to reduce wound complications and improve postoperative recovery. These included early postoperative monitoring in the intensive care unit and, with the collaboration of Hope McArdle of the MGH University Surgical Clinic basic research labs, the introduction of elemental nutritional support. New wound management techniques were developed and enterostomal care improved. All of these measures resulted in much improved outcomes for these patients, and the lessons learned are applicable to his day.

On his return to McGill and the RVH following a two-year fellowship in New York, Balfour Mount brought back invaluable experience in the management of testicular cancer. This was the first of the solid organ cancers to show remarkable response to multi-drug cytotoxic chemotherapy. Mount established a specific clinic at the RVH and soon had a rapidly growing super-specialized practice. When he decided in the mid-1970s to dedicate himself to palliative care exclusively, Laplante was asked to take over this tertiary care specialty, and the testicular tumour practice was transferred to the MGH.

In cordial collaboration with the medical and radiologic oncology departments, the MGH became essentially a centre of excellence for the management of testicular cancer and a referral centre for much of the province and beyond. With the development and use of newer and remarkably effective chemotherapeutic agents, especially Cis-Platinum, in the mid- and late 1970s, it was a good time to be at the leading edge of this segment of urologic oncology as fairly aggressive radical retroperitoneal surgery was frequently an important component of the multidisciplinary management that achieved very high cure rates.

The department also witnessed an increasingly structured and standardized approach to the management of the other urologic malignancies – that is, prostate, kidney, and non-invasive bladder tumours. Oncology was not by any means an exclusive clinical focus within the department, but it was certainly a major element of the tertiary care, along with renal transplantation.

Renal Transplantation

Ackman and Laplante had acquired considerable experience during their training at the RVH with the evolving techniques of vascular access for haemodialysis. At the MGH, these two worked closely with Michael Kaye's dialysis program to provide the same surgical services, initially with installation of external Scribner shunts (which always clotted on non-call weekends and holidays), then with the creation of A-V shunts and development of artificial A-V grafts.

The installation (and fairly frequent removal) of peritoneal catheters for patients on the chronic peritoneal dialysis program was also a part of the close collaboration with the Department of Nephrology. It was a logical extension of this collaboration that Ackman and Laplante were included as surgeons when the renal transplantation program was initiated at the MGH in October 1971. It did not take them long to learn the vascular techniques required from the vascular surgeons (Mulder, Blundell, and Scott) who participated in the earliest cases.

The transplant program directed by Roman Mangel enjoyed results comparable to those of any program in North America. L. Rosenberg, trained at the University of Michigan in renal and pancreatic transplantation, joined the program in 1988. The first combined renal and pancreas transplant recipient was operated on in October of that year and survives to the date of this account (June 2015). Unhappily for the MGH team, which was operating very smoothly, with the formation of the McGill University Health Centre, the understandable decision was made to merge the MGH and RVH transplant programs in 1997. All transplant activity was transferred to the RVH, with the ultimate exclusion of the MGH surgical component.[6]

Care of Spinal Cord Injured Patients

During his training, Laplante had developed a particular interest in the urologic care and follow-up of paraplegic and quadriplegic victims of spinal cord injuries or congenital spinal defects. In the mid- to late 1970s he became urologic consultant to l'Institut de Readaption de Montréal and conducted a weekly clinic there. This led to a large following of "paras" and "quads," with their peculiar and frequently complex urinary problems. This patient population provided much specific and challenging clinical material for the Department of Urology at the MGH.

Andrology and Information Technology

From the early 1970s, Ackman applied his keen interest and expertise to the development of computerization, not only in the Department of Urology but also, eventually, to other MGH departments. He developed early databases for the different urologic tumours, patient demographic data, and finally the very earliest trials of computer-generated clinical documentation for the medical record. These records of patient visits and some operative reports were not perfect, but they demonstrated the potential for development of the electronic medical record. In 1980, Ackman chaired a committee to advise the administration on computer use.

Ackman's particular clinical interests included male infertility and male sexual dysfunction – a subspecialty now called andrology. He was a local pioneer of mechanical incontinence and potency devices. Health problems severely curtailed his clinical activities in the late 1990s, and, later, a lung malignancy proved fatal in 2002.

Group Practice

E.C. Reid had long been convinced that the ideal organization of medical practice was entailed the involvement of a group in partnership. This seemed to him to apply especially to a group in an academic setting such as the new Department of Urology at the MGH, with four individuals with approximately equal seniority. Only the chief had the status of "geographic full time," with a salary in addition to capped clinical fee-for-service earnings. If this salary were to be included with the pooled clinical means of all the partners, and there was equitable division of the pool after all expenses were covered, then Reid felt that a very desirable, non-competitive partnership might well be possible. This indeed was agreed upon by the four, and the group was named Urobec. (Lingard's clinical activities by then were very limited and he was not included in the group.)

The chief and the three other urologists agreed to this rather simple partnership with essentially equal division of clinical income. This was an almost unheard of arrangement at the time, and it was predicated on mutual trust, long-standing friendship, and an understanding that each partner worked full time and equally. This actually led to an even closer friendship and collaboration within the department.

When GFT positions were offered in 1976 to the three partners who did not have offices in the hospital, Ackman declined. He chose instead to leave the financial arrangement of the partnership but continued to share coverage and all academic functions. MacIsaac and Laplante moved into offices in Livingston Hall with Reid, and the MGH Department of Urology had a true public/private clinic in one geographic area.

Further cooperation within the McGill faculty continued, and looked promising, under Andrew Bruce, who was named professor of surgery (urology) at McGill and chief at the RVH, replacing Ken MacKinnon. He was instrumental in acquiring McGill salaries and pension benefits for all GFTs in the McGill urology faculty. His stay in Montreal was all too brief as he was recruited away to the University of Toronto within two years.

Another collaborative McGill effort was seen in the mid-1980s under the direction of M. Elhilali, who replaced Bruce. Elhilali had been chief at Centre Hospitalier de l'Universite de Sherbrooke and was a very welcome addition to the McGill family. In the mid-1980s the entire Abitibi region was without urologic coverage. McGill urology was asked to help. Four MGH urologists and five RVH urologists shared weekly two-day rotation visits to Val d'Or to perform relatively routine surgery the first day and attend a large outpatient clinic on the second day, returning to Montreal that evening. This proved to be a bit challenging to those with limited French but, nonetheless, was a most rewarding and well appreciated experience. This itinerant coverage lasted for two years until a newly trained urologist settled in Val d'Or. Valuable contacts with the referring surgeons and physicians in the region were maintained for many years thereafter.

Evolving Technologies and Resources

The mid-1980s saw a wave of new urologic techniques and associated technologies. Minimally invasive stone management began with the development of percutaneous endoscopic techniques to fragment and remove renal stones through a nephrostomy access. This was coupled with the development of fine endoscopic instruments that were passed up the ureter, and, by the early 1990s, open surgery for stone problems was a thing of the past. These developments coincided with the construction of the new ambulatory surgery centre, which included a new cystoscopy suite on the seventh floor in space that became available after the departure of obstetrics at the end of 1982. Laser technology was well recognized by the mid 1980s as well, and a YAG laser was obtained through the generosity of Donald MacKenzie. In the new cystoscopy suite a state-of-the-art urology room was designed and equipped to perform the new minimally invasive procedures under optimal fluoroscopic control.

Meanwhile, another previously unimaginable technology for breaking up renal stones into easily passed sand and small gravel, extracorporeal shock wave lithotripsy, was introduced from Germany. Elhilali succeeded in acquiring the very expensive unit for the RVH in 1996, and this had the inevitable effect of enticing away a considerable portion of the MGH's stone clientele. Nevertheless, percutaneous nephrostomy and ureteroscopic

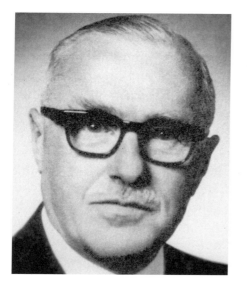
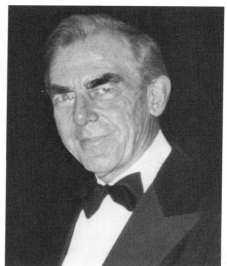
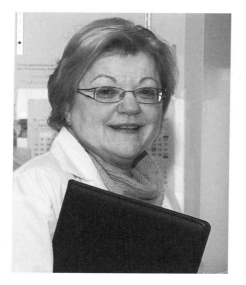
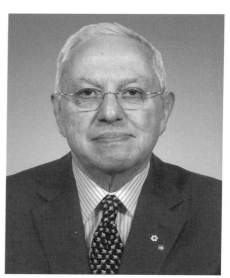

Clockwise from top left
Fig. 39.4 Grant Reid, director, Department of Urology, 1949–67
Fig. 39.5 E.C. Reid, director, MGH and Joint Department of Urology, 1967–90
Fig. 39.6 M.M. Elhilali, director, Joint Department of Urology, 1990–2000
Fig. 39.7 Simone Chevalier, director, uro-oncology research, 1990–2005

instrumentation and imaging techniques, including video cameras, continued to improve, and these activities continued at the MGH until the late 1990s, when duplication of costs and instrumentation made it impractical and non-cost-effective to perform these activities in the two hospitals. Superspecialized stone management was shifted over to the RVH.

The Elhilali Era

By the end of 1989, E.C. Reid had announced his intention to step down as chief of the department but remain in practice for another year or two. He retired completely from clinical practice in November 1992. He was succeeded as chief in 1990 by Mostafa M. Elhilali, who became the first joint chief of the MGH and RVH urology departments.

Elhilali had obtained his medical degree in Cairo in 1959 and, after completing his urology training in Egypt, came to McGill in 1965 to concentrate on basic urologic research. In 1969, he obtained both his PhD and his Royal College Fellowship and joined the staff of the Centre Hospitalier de l'Universite de Sherbrooke. In 1975, he was appointed chair of urology at the CHUS, where he developed exceptional clinical and research programs.

In 1982, he returned to McGill as professor and chair of urology at McGill and chief of urology at the RVH, replacing Bruce. He directed the ongoing refinement of the McGill Urology Residency Training Program, which came to rival any in North America.

Sharing the commitment of E.C. Reid, and before him MacKinnon and Bruce, to a group practice partnership, Elhilali succeeded in forming the McGill Urology Associates group, joining the RVH, MGH, MCH, and, later, the Jewish General Hospital McGill-appointed urologists into a very successful group practice. This group association, the first in the McGill academic sphere, was recognized by the university as an example to other McGill specialists who were urged to explore the possibility of also setting up "practice plans."

By eliminating individual financial considerations as long as all partners were committed to equal incomes and full-time workloads, this plan allowed two important principals to be implemented. First, individual partners could reserve time for academic and research activities. Second, subspecialty expertise and resources could be concentrated at the three adult sites, with liberal cross-referral between sites, without financial penalties to individuals. Thus the MGH's main focus continued to be urologic oncology, the JGH's was voiding dysfunction and female urology, and the RVH's was complex stone problems, a prostate centre, and andrology. Research activity, both clinical and basic, would be developed in each of these sites.

Thus it seemed perfectly fitting that, in 1990, Elhilali assume the joint chief position following Reid's departure. M.P. Laplante was named MGH site director and deputy chief. Elhilali's clinical activities were divided between the MGH and RVH sites, and academic activities were shared between the three adult sites.

MacIsaac had left Montreal in 1990 (to join the US Army medical corps), and, with Ackman's declining activities due to health problems, personnel at the MGH was somewhat strained. This was relieved by the transfer from the RVH of Michel Bazinet, a product of the Sherbrooke and McGill programs and a three-year oncology fellowship at Memorial. His particular interest was prostate cancer, and he distinguished himself in research and clinical activities in this field. He was joined in July 1993 by Armen Aprikian, who had also spent three years in New York, and in August 1995 by Simon Tanguay, who had spent three years at MD Anderson in Houston. Thus, a highly trained, exceptionally skilled group of uro-oncologists was soon recognized on both the national and the international scenes by virtue of their impressive clinical productivity and basic research conducted in collaboration with the teams in the research lab. Bazinet shifted his focus away from clinical practice to medical informatics in 1996 and resigned from the group to set up a private enterprise.

In 2002, the year he was named to the Order of Canada, Elhilali was appointed chair of the McGill Department of Surgery. He stepped down from the urology chair in April 2004. Later that year, Aprikian succeeded him as McGill University Health Centre chief of urology and the McGill chair in urology.

Research in Urology at the Montreal General Hospital

Prior to the mid-1970s and 1980s, publications out of the MGH Department of Urology were mainly clinically based case reports, reviews of surgical series, and essays on changes in surgical techniques and concepts. S.A. MacDonald had been funded to study the development and use of Gelfoam and Fibrin foam as haemostatic agents in renal and prostatic surgery. Results of basic histopathologic changes were published in collaboration with W.H.

Mathews of the Department of Pathology in 1948.[7] R.G. Reid had engaged one or two research fellows to work in the McGill Donner Research Labs, but no work was published.

E.C. Reid had visions of a basic research lab, but the early part of his tenure was focused on establishing high clinical and teaching standards. He nevertheless collaborated with D.M.P. Thomson in immunologic in-vitro studies of leucocyte adherence inhibition as a possible indicator of bladder cancer aggressiveness. C.F.D. Ackman and the MGH transplant team were active in a multi-institution three-year Canadian trial of anti-lymphocyte globulin as an adjuvant immunosuppressive for cadaver renal transplant recipients. Reid and Laplante had a number of significant clinical publications and presentations reporting various aspects of their work in bladder cancer, urologic care of spinal cord injured patients, and testicular cancer.

It was with the arrival of Elhilali in 1991 that plans were realized to set up a McGill urologic oncology research lab. The Molson Foundation was most generous in the establishment of the E.C. Reid Cancer Research Fund, and space was secured in the MGH Research Institute adjacent to Livingston Hall. Simone Chevalier was identified and recruited for the tenured position of scientific director. She was an FRSQ scholar and held grants from the Medical Research Council of Canada for her work on prostate cancer carried out in labs affiliated with the Université de Montreal at Hôpital Maisonneuve-Rosemont.

Elhilali's considerable effort in this project was keenly supported by Dean R. Cruess; David Mulder, chair of the Department of Surgery; Joseph Shuster, director of the MGH Research Institute; and Claude Gagnon, then McGill urology research director.

It was Chevalier's vision to work with clinical scientists to set up a uro-oncology research team working and collaborating in the subdomains of research, including biochemistry, cellular and molecular biology, and pathology. The space was set up to allow maximum collaboration and sharing of equipment, ideas, and enthusiasm by the entire research team. The lab was opened in January 1994, with Senator Hartland Molson and E.C. Reid in proud attendance. This marked the realization of Elhilali's and Reid's vision of establishing a team of clinicians and basic scientists focusing on urogenital cancer research and working together to bring bench to bedside.

Michel Bazinet was the first surgeon-scientist to set up projects with Chevalier in the new lab. He was soon followed by Aprikian and Tanguay, returning from three-year oncology fellowships in New York and Houston, respectively. Aprikian had already received awards for his work in prostate cancer, as had Tanguay for his basic research in kidney cancer. The new uro-oncology research lab was inaugurated with the first annual MGH Annual Urology Research Day, co-chaired by Aprikian and Chevalier, with the theme of prostate cancer.

Scientific and academic activities were promptly organized in the form of regular Journal Club sessions and research lab "rounds." Collaborative projects were conceived and growth was rapid. By the end of its first full year, Mario Chevrette, a molecular biologist working in the area of tumour suppressor genes with particular emphasis on prostate cancer, was recruited from the University of Ottawa and joined the team in 1995.

More space was required and secured in the Research Institute as it was felt essential to keep Chevrette geographically close to the existing team. This core of exceptional basic scientists attracted new graduate students and encouraged urology residents and research fellows to pursue projects in the new lab, often pairing basic scientists with clinical uro-oncologists. Indeed, many of the bright residents finishing their residencies had had their initial exposure to basic research in Chevalier's labs and carried their enthusiasm to their fellowships to complete their training before establishing academic careers at McGill or elsewhere.

With time, Aprikian and Tanguay shifted their attention to translational, patient-oriented, and epidemiologic-type oncologic research projects. In the early 2000s, Elhilali and Aprikian succeeded in raising substantial funds for prostate cancer research, allowing the recruitment of two additional basic scientists – Junjian Chen and Jacques Lapointe – to join Chevalier and Chevrette. Full operation of a very strong research team allowed enrolment of several students (undergraduate, graduate, and postdoctoral) as well as research fellows into projects conducted under the supervision of urology faculty members. A significant number of these students have successfully submitted masters and PhD theses and received corresponding degrees.

One of Aprikian's seminal achievements at this time (first decade of the 2000s) was to establish a provincial prostate cancer biobank, generously supported by a non-profit community organization known as Procure Alliance. This will enable concerted and collaborative efforts of urologists, basic scientists, and pathologists in all four Quebec university hospitals to address a broad spectrum of patient-oriented prostate cancer research projects. There are ambitious plans to develop similar initiatives for bladder and kidney cancers.

By 2005, Aprikian was named chair of the Department of Urology. Chevalier succeeded Claude Gagnon as scientific director of McGill urology research, and Tanguay was named director of McGill urologic oncology. A very dynamic uro-oncology research team of MGH scientists will eventually be moving to the Glen site of the McGill University Health Centre, which will be the site of the new Medical Research Institute.

By the turn of the century and the first decade of the twenty-first century the Department of Urology of the MGH should take pride in the growth it has enjoyed over the previous thirty-five years. The three missions of a university hospital department have been accomplished, with the establishment of world-class *clinical urology* focusing on oncology but practising excellent general urology as well. *Teaching* at the undergraduate level, and especially at the postgraduate residency level, is producing a new generation of extremely bright, dedicated, and energetic new urologists. Basic *urologic research* has a permanent home and an exceptional team of scientists keen to work with clinical uro-oncologists.[8] The late 1990s saw the merger of the MGH and the RVH, to be known as the McGill University Health Centre. Although construction of new physical facilities was several years away, urology was still practised at both sites.

NOTES

1 W.B. Howell, *Francis John Shepherd – Surgeon: His Life and Times, 1851–1929* (Montreal: J.M. Dent and Sons Ltd., 1934), 114–17.

2 Ibid., 178.

3 F.S. Patch, "Pyelitis, Urethritis and Cystitis Cystica," *New England Journal of Medicine* 220 (1939): 979–89.

4 F.S. Patch and W.L. Ritchie, "The Clinical and Radiologic Aspects of Pyelography, Intravenous and Retrograde," *Canadian Medical Association Journal* 26 (1932): 154–8.

5 Everett C. Reid, *The Hole Saw: An Autobiography by Dr Everett C. Reid* (Montreal: privately published, 1999).

6 In fact, with the introduction of laparoscopic living donor nephrectomy, as the equipment and expertise were initially available at the MGH, the living donor nephrectomies were done there for several years until the facilities became

available at the RVH. Maurice Anidjar, urologist, and Liane Feldman, general surgeon, were the initial laparoscopic surgeons performing living donor nephrectomies.

7 S.A. MacDonald and W.H. Mathews, "Further Studies with Gelfoam,"*Canadian Medical Association Journal* 58 (February 1948): 118–21.

8 J.S. Bennet, "The Way I See It," *Canadian Medical Association Journal* 105 (1971): 1205.

SECTION 5

Nursing Department

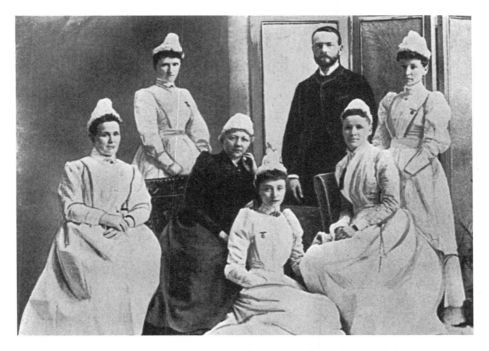

S.5 First nursing class at the MGH, 1890. Left to right: Julia English, Christina MacKay, Nora Livingston, Jean Preston, Georgina Carrol, Alicia Dunne or Ellen Chapman.

40

Mind over Matter: Early Struggles and the Livingston Era, 1821–1919

Margaret Suttie

Margaret Suttie joined MGH nursing in charge of special projects. She became responsible for nursing budgets and later chair of the Research Committee. Valerie Shannon, a former MGH director of nursing, organized five chapters on nursing written by herself and colleagues M. Suttie, M. Hooton, R. Allan-Rigby, and P. Dembeck. Margaret Suttie is the retired director of nursing at the Reddy Memorial Hospital and is involved with the MGH/MUHC heritage group.

When the doors of the Montreal General Hospital opened in 1822, Montreal was a growing port, the old city was changing shape, and the rise in the middle class was heralding political, economic, and social change. With an immediate need to grow, it had evolved from a small provincial town hidden behind fortified walls into a more open town as the fortifications were torn down. From 1800 to 1850 its population exploded from ten thousand to fifty thousand as wave after wave of English, Scottish, and Irish immigrants arrived, fleeing war and famine in search of a better life in the New World. The conditions, from which many of the immigrants came, particularly the Irish, were deplorable. They had little wealth. The ship voyage was long and insufferable so that when they arrived in Montreal, if they were not already ill, they were certainly at high risk. Diseases such as typhoid fever, typhus, and cholera were rampant. Ways to prevent the spread of infections were unknown, and medical treatments were most likely limited to bleeding, drugs, and alcoholic stimulants. Surgical interventions had not yet been developed.

It was out of the great need of these poor and ill immigrants that the women of the Female Benevolent Society opened a soup kitchen and, in 1815, with the aid of several physicians, a small hospital with four beds called the House of Recovery. The need for additional beds and outpatient services was so great that, on 19 May 1819, the MGH opened its doors on Craig Street with twenty-four beds to be followed in 1822 with a three-storey, seventy-two-bed facility on Dorchester near the river and port area.[1]

The Early Years, 1821–55

Nursing and nursing education, in the earliest days of French Canada, had their roots with the "gentle nuns [who] came from France to Canada in the seventeenth century leaving behind all they held most dear, braving hardships and death to bring religion, nursing, succour and education to the New World."[2] Behind cloistered walls institutions, founded by the Roman Catholic Church and financed partially by the state, developed to provide care to the early citizens of New France. The nursing sisters, devoted to patient care, were the mainstay of the service provided, but many lay caregivers, such as the midwives brought from France and outstanding individuals like Jeanne Mance, founder of the Hotel Dieu Hospital in Montreal, also contributed immensely to the overall network. General hospitals were also established and offered refuge for the poor, the orphans, and the mentally handicapped. For most, childbirth and sickness became the work of women in the home who were untrained and reliant on their own intuition and common sense.[3]

The earliest description of nursing indicated that it was not a discipline with any status. Nurses, considered as servants, were under the direct supervision of the Committee of Management at the MGH. In the summer of 1822, in addition to the matron, there were two nurses, a housemaid, a cook, and a manservant for seventy-two beds which, during the first six months, served 540 patients. Such activity did result in the addition of one nurse.[4]

In the first seventy years of the hospital, the recordings of the time were gloomy with regard to the women who nursed, their social status or lack thereof, the horrible working conditions, and the behaviour of the patients, to name but a few of the problems. Nursing was not an enviable or sought after profession. Some understanding of the status of nursing and the role of nurses can be gleaned from an examination of the hospital's 1822 by-laws. The matron was to visit the wards at specified times, see that nurses and patients were in their respective wards, oversee the conduct of staff and patients, and report any misconduct to the physician. In addition, she was to keep the wards clean and supplied with linens, furniture, and bedding; prevent theft; keep out unauthorized persons; and oversee the preparation of food and the adherence to dietary regimens. Little was written about the matron's working conditions or her relationship to the nurses and the provision of nursing care, but one might conclude that she was seen as "essential" to the organization as the by-laws state: "She shall not absent herself from the Hospital without the leave of the House Surgeon."[5]

Nurses were to be concerned with these responsibilities: an exact procedure for admitting the patient; what and when to report to physicians; the changing of bed linens only when ordered by the matron; the reporting of deaths; the schedule for cleaning the wards (at 8:00 AM from 1 May to 1 November, and at 9:00 AM the remainder of the year); the need for diligence in complying with orders; the need to behave with tenderness to the patients; the hydration of patients, which meant ensuring that "the vessel containing their drink [was] commodiously within their reach and ... care [taken that] they shall never be empty"; the obligation of seeing that patients take their medicines as prescribed; the necessity of controlling what is brought into the ward; the reporting of patient violations of the by-laws; and seeing that "they shall always keep themselves clean and decently clothed." Perhaps the earliest sign of concern for patient safety can be found in the fifth duty, which is: "she shall receive no medicines sent from the Apothecary's shop to the wards unless labelled and directed."[6]

There was little coherent leadership. Over a period of fifteen years, seven different women held the position of matron. However, there was an appreciation of the work of the nurses: "The management committee has also great satisfaction in being able to report the extreme neatness in which the wards have been at all times found and the great attention and humanity with which the patients have been treated by the nurses."[7]

A positive reflection on the position of nurses in the organization came to light by 1859, when "nurses" became a separate category on the pay lists and were thus differentiated from the servants. At the discretion of the matron, the nurse could receive six dollars per month. The first evidence that some standards of behaviour were in place, although not necessarily relating to quality of practice, was that the salary of an ordinary or inferior nurse would remain at five dollars.[8] Turnover of staff was a problem, so, without any other improvements in the working conditions, it was deemed expedient in 1869 to raise wages to seven dollars after one year of service.

In the meantime, nursing was evolving in other parts of the world at a much faster pace than it was at the MGH. Led by Florence Nightingale, a revolution in nursing was under way. It was a time when "compassion gave way to science as the guiding force."[9] Upon Nightingale's return from the Crimea, the British public, appreciative of her accomplishments in raising the standard of care given to the troops, donated monies leading to the inauguration of the Nightingale Fund. With this support the Nightingale School was formed in 1859 with the goal of training "competent graduates who in their turn would train student nurses."[10] Central to the program were the following beliefs: that the direction of nurses would be carried out by an intelligent nurse, that students would receive their education in a systematic manner, and that the nurse was no longer to be considered as a domestic. A nurses' home was to be provided for the comfort of the students. The medical profession, quite happy with the status quo of the nurses as assistants, was not particularly supportive of her endeavours, but, before long, her reforms were adopted and Nightingale graduates were in great demand worldwide.[11]

Although Nightingale schools did not appear in North America until some years later, recognition of the need to raise the standards of nursing surfaced at the MGH some forty-five years after the founding of the hospital in 1866 and again in 1872. On both these occasions the matron was requested to "to engage a better class of nurses than those at present in the hospital, giving them an advance on the wages now paid, their duty being to attend to patients." Also, "[to] engage charwomen to do the cleaning of the windows, washing of dishes and otherwise all the work now done by the nurses except the attendance on patients." The salary of nurses was set at seven dollars a month and a bonus of twelve dollars offered at the end of the year if they were "found worthy of it."[12] There is little evidence of any immediate change in achieving this goal.

Maria Machin, 1875–78

Not until 1874 did the MGH make a more formal effort at establishing a training school. The committee of management was coaxed by a previous matron to introduce "a system of trained hospital nurses, such as approved in England." Maria Machin, a Canadian by birth and a graduate of St. Thomas Hospital, London, arrived with several trained nurses to take up the position of "lady superintendent" on 2 October 1875.[13] During Machin's tenure, the hospital conditions were less than ideal. A local newspaper wrote an exposé on the hospital, outlining the inadequacy of the facilities for patients, the lack of windows and inadequate ventilation, the shocking accommodation for violent weak-minded patients in the basement, and the little nests of pestilence.[14] In 1877, the medical superintendent, W. McClure, reported on the inadequacy of the building with regard to overcrowding and equipment. He described attempts to isolate patients with infectious disease; however, owing to the physical conditions and the "want of nurses," patients might be admitted with one disease and contract others before discharge.[15]

Hampered by these issues and other internal dissention, Machin still had not established a training school two years after her arrival. There were two schools of thought among the decision makers – some wishing not to renew her contract and others willing to give her a further chance. Although it was deemed that the services of Machin and her nurses were laudable and their retention desirable, the overrun in costs seemed to be a major obstacle. Unlike their counterparts in England, the fact that hospitals in Canada did not have independent resources like the Nightingale Fund played a significant role in determining the direction of such schools in Canada. "Nursing schools were caught in a web of dependency with their institutional homes; the hospital relied on the inexpensive and relatively skilled labour that nursing students offered, while nursing educators were dependent on legal, administrative, and financial authority of the institution."[16] In the end, Machin resigned in 1878.[17]

Harriet Rimmer, 1878–89

Despite the desire to start a training school and improve the standard of nursing, the hospital then hired Harriet Rimmer – a woman with private means who had no formal nursing education or training but was interested in hospital work. She was authorized and did indeed proceed to hire, in 1880, Anna Caroline Maxwell, a graduate of Boston City Hospital as a "Lady Trainer of Nurses." Advertisement of the upcoming school was circulated – a two-year program, starting in January 1881, under the guidance of a competent instructor, with instruction by the medical staff and aimed at recruiting women who might either be willing to pay for the instruction or receive remuneration during the training period. The school did not succeed and, in June 1881, with no particular reasons to be found in the records and less than a year after she accepted the post, Maxwell left Montreal.[18] In 1920, she presented a paper entitled "Struggles of the Pioneers" and her reasons for leaving the MGH were revealed. "On graduation, I hastened to accept an appointment to establish a training school in a distant city." That city was Montreal. She found that the MGH had very poor physical conditions, a lack of professional practice, and little respect for the nursing staff, so she drew the conclusion that there was little inducement for women of a refined type to enter the school.[19]

Rimmer's character and high ideals attracted a better class of women into nursing.[20] What impact this had on the quality of nursing care is unknown. What *is* known is that the nurse was measured more on her appearance, her deportment, and her compliance to medical orders than on her knowledge and decision-making skills. With retention a critical issue, accommodation for these young women was a major problem. There was overcrowding, the living conditions were cold in the winter, and in the summer there was an infestations of bugs. In 1887, W. McClure and, later, in 1889, R.C. Kirkpatrick, superintendent, said that an improvement in living conditions for nurses might keep them from leaving Canada for studies in the United States and thus raise the standards at the MGH.[21]

The Livingston Era, 1890–1919

Rimmer, after some eleven years as superintendent, resigned in 1889 due to ill health.[22] The Medical Board, understanding that a trained matron was required, exerted its influence on the Committee of Management to search for a qualified nurse to replace her. A selection committee was struck to find a candidate capable of starting a training school. Even though the position was advertised in Canada, Britain, and the United States and attracted the attention of a number of applicants, none was deemed suitable or up to the challenge. The search ended in 1890, when Gertrude Elizabeth (Nora) Livingston, after some persuasion from F.J. Shepherd, a hospital surgeon, neighbour, and friend from Como, Quebec, accepted the position.[23]

Livingston, born in 1848 in Sault Ste Marie, Michigan, of English parents, moved to Como, Quebec, in 1867 along with her parents and siblings. At that time she would have been twenty, but there is little recorded as to how she occupied her time. On the 1881 census, where she can be found living in Vaudreuil with her sisters, there is no occupation listed. She entered nursing in 1889 and, at forty-one years of age, graduated from the New York Hospital Training School. After working there for a short time she returned to Canada to accept the position of superintendent of nurses at the MGH. Her conduct during the selection process demonstrated that she had a strong character and was imbued with a clear vision and plan of action, although she had little experience as a nurse and even less in the field of administration.[24]

"Frankie Shepherd must have done some impressive talking to persuade Miss Livingston to agree to come, as she only did so after laying down conditions which, although perfectly reasonable, rather startled the Committee of Management."[25] She had many questions for the selection committee about the dismaying conditions at the hospital. She also wanted to understand clearly what was expected of her and to clarify the fact she wanted nothing to do with housekeeping so that she could do her job of "directing and teaching nurses." To that end, and wishing to have people beside her who knew and understood the basic elements of nursing, she negotiated bringing trained nurses with her.

What is amazing is the speed with which she was able to make many worthwhile changes in the wards and, at the same time, within a period of two months, establish the training school. Given the conditions at the hospital when she arrived, she dealt immediately with some basic and common-sense issues: quilts and mattresses were ordered for the patients with instructions about when to change them; porters were assigned to deliver medications, a task that had previously been done by nurses; charts and medication lists were introduced and nurses taught to compute medications and write reports. Fire was an imminent danger of the times so she introduced measures for prevention and management of fires. The patients were also targets for the sweeping changes, and many of them were surprised to find they were required to take a bath. To some who had never had a bath it was their intention never ever to have one – a test of the persuasive powers of the nurse.[26]

Once the hospital was in reasonable working order Livingston turned to building a framework for training nurses. She chose applicants between twenty-five and thirty-five years of age, who possessed a good "common" school education, had positive character references, and were in sound health. Application forms were designed,[27] with a description of the regulations attached. Applicants were expected to be able to meet all the conditions or they need not apply – no exceptional cases were considered. Students lived in residence and its limited capacity restricted the number of pupil nurses that could be accepted, giving Livingston the freedom to select the cream of the crop as the number of applicants far exceeded the number that could be accepted for the spring and fall classes.

The groundwork was laid. On 11 December 1890, less than a year after the appointment of Livingston, the formal opening of the "Training School for Nurses" took place at Windsor Hall in Montreal with His Excellency the Governor General and Lady Stanley in attendance. The *Montreal Gazette* reported on the dignitaries present and the speeches given, and described the entrance of the nurses in their pink dresses, long aprons, and mobcaps as "a picture worthy of an artist's brush."[28]

The address by D.C. MacCallum gives us a glimpse into the role of women in society and in the workplace, the status of the nurse vis-à-vis the doctor, the need for a scientific program for nurses, and a genuine desire to succeed in this venture.[29] He told the nurses that they were entering an honourable profession, often fatiguing, seldom with rewards, and that the studies would not be easy: "Education and training, however, are necessary to make a nurse … to attain to a high degree of excellence, she must call into service patience, perseverance, and devotion to duty, and submit cheerfully to a thorough system of training."[30]

Although he stressed the need for a scientific education for the nurses and encouraged them "to master the principles" and "become conversant with the details of nursing," he also went on to say: "Success would be theirs if reticence and discretion were coveted but doomed for failure if inquisitive."[31] It would be many years before the culture would allow the nurse to use knowledge in a deductive or problem-solving manner and to shed the mantle of subservience.

R. Craik, representing the Committee of Management, was the final speaker of the day. He thanked the audience members for their sympathy, good will, and support, pointing out that the hospital was not well endowed and that its day-to-day running was dependent on the voluntary contributions of the citizens of Montreal. Given this constant state of chronic poverty, and leery of costly or fruitless experiments, he admitted that the MGH did seem to lag behind in providing nurses with a proper training. Whereas previously it was thought that the expenditure for a school would have been so great in proportion to the benefits that other activities would have been seriously curtailed, he believed that the cost of this program would be scarcely, if at all, greater than that of any ordinary system of unskilled nursing.[32]

The first graduation was held in April 1891 at the Natural History Society. Livingston, desperately in need of better qualified nurses, recognized the value of some of the staff already in service and offered them the opportunity to remain if they accepted a period of study of one year. Ellen Chapman, Georgina Carrol, Jean Preston, Julia English, Alicia Dunne, and Christine Mackay accepted and are recorded in the history books as the first graduates of the school.[33] According to the newspaper of the day, the nurses, in their neat and tasteful uniforms, made a picturesque scene.[34] Livingston

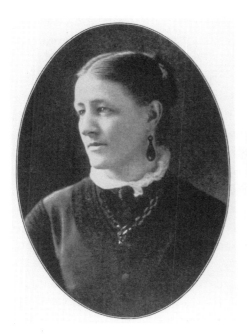

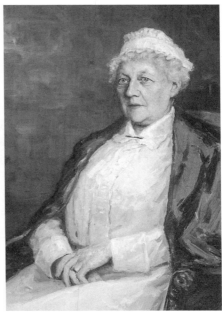

Fig. 40.1 Maria Machin, supervisor of nursing, MGH, 1875–78
Fig. 40.2 Gertrude Elizabeth (Nora) Livingston, supervisor of nursing, MGH, 1890–1919
and founder of the MGH Training School for Nurses, December 1890

agreed that "they did look lovely, red badges and pincushions." She wrote to her sisters that "it was a nice dignified ceremony with no singing or nonsense," but "the tact and finesse I have had to exercise in the affair so as to please all is a caution."[35] John Sterling, president of the board, congratulated the graduates, stressing that "the reputation of the school was to a degree in their hands and [that he] hoped they would feel the vital importance of their great work of succouring afflicted humanity." He continued, saying that "they should be very thankful for the opportunities they had had of acquiring a knowledge of their work" and, further, that "they would shed a lustre over the profession."[36]

It was left to T. Roddick to address the issue of cost in his remarks. But on this occasion there was a more positive note. After providing some statistics on the school and reviewing the curriculum, he thanked the citizens of Montreal for their sympathy and support. Despite the additional expense of three thousand dollars a year for the school, for which no provision had been made, he was quick to answer those who questioned the wisdom of this endeavour. He indicated that it was an absolute necessity and he was sure that "Montrealers' would not allow this school to suffer or degenerate into a second rate affair."[37]

The educational program used an apprenticeship model that offered training in exchange for service. Craik saw it as a decided advantage that the school was part and parcel of the hospital itself. He explained: "There is no troublesome line of demarcation between them, and what benefits the one also does good to the other. Our nurses in training, with the few necessary head nurses or instructors, do the whole nursing work of the Hospital. And they do it well."[38] The importance of this model to the institution is again stressed in the 1895–96 annual report of the hospital, in which it is noted that "the period of training has been extended to three years, an arrangement which is of decided advantage to the hospital in giving it the services of nurses for a third year."[39]

The original curriculum set out by Livingston included twenty-two hours of lectures.[40] The program evolved with regard to its content, but the main tenet of Livingston's belief system – "the patient must come first" – never disappeared.[41] Livingston's decision to lengthen the program was a landmark in nursing education as it was the first three-year course to be offered in North America and set the benchmark for other Canadian schools.[42]

Table 40.1

Lecture hours	1895[1]	1900[2]
Sciences	4	65
Pharmacology	2	25
Nursing	3	93
Hygiene	1	9
Medical/surgical	5	9
Specialties	6	3
Contagious diseases	1	6
Ethics/senior topics	1	4
Dietary	2	8
Total hours	22	287

Notes:

1 Regulations, 1890, MGH Training School for Nurses, MGH Alumnae Archive.

2 Curriculum, 1900, the MGH Training School, MGH Alumnae Archives.

Evolution of School Curriculum

Although the subjects and courses seemed appropriate, few records detailing the content exist except for the dressing of wounds, "application of blisters, fomentations, poultices, cup and leeches," the use of catheters, the administration of enemas, methods of applying friction, bandaging, making beds, moving patients, preventing bedsores, and the application of uterine devices.[43]

Probationers entered the school and if, after three months without pay, they were accepted, then they continued in the program, graduating after three years. Following the probationary period, the students were divided into three classes: junior 1st year, senior 2nd year, and head nurse 3rd year. In her third year, a nurse, if considered competent due to creditably passing an examination, would be given charge of a ward or department. The school year was from 1 October to 1 June, and the practical experience in the various branches of nursing was distributed as follows:[44] surgical and medicine – ten months each; outpatients and operating room – three months each; gynaecology – four months; private patients – one month; diet kitchen – two months.

The nurses were expected to do six months of night duty in the twenty months of the medical surgical rotation but not before they had completed one year after probation. The diet kitchen, under the watchful eye of Gracie Livingston, had little to do with learning about special diets. According to M.L. MacDermot,[45] it was hard work and, although there was a maid to wash the pots, the students did the rest. Although the hours of work were long, there was a defined vacation period of three weeks for each of the three years. In the early days of the school, Livingston, along with the doctors and head nurses, gave the lectures.

Although her annual reports were generally terse and devoid of details, Livingston wrote: "During the year [commencing 1 October 1906] a very important and progressive feature was added to the curriculum of the School in the establishment of a preliminary course for probationers; thus teaching by demonstration, etc., the simple principles of nursing before entering the wards. We already find the probationers much more valuable to the Hospital than under the old method, and there can be no doubt as to the advantage to the patients."[46] Not only did Livingston initiate the first course for preliminary students in Canada but she also assigned the first nursing instructor to the task.[47] In 1906, she wrote: "To this important post of instructor Miss M. Shaw [Flora Madeline], of the MGH Training School and Diploma, Teachers' College, Columbia University, New York" was appointed.[48]

Student life was not easy. There were long hours of work and, according to M.L. MacDermot, the students did not leave until everything was finished, which could take them beyond the usual twelve hours. Rules and regulations were strict, there were lectures to attend, studying, and then preparation for examinations at various intervals throughout the course.[49] During the first two years these exams were supervised by Livingston, but the finals were conducted by members of the Medical Board. Practical work, not defined, and deportment were included in the general average and, to receive the diploma, the nurse had to demonstrate excellence in all areas.

The rewards of a job well done could be quickly soured by one error in judgment, practice, or slip of the tongue. Punishment was meted out and could range from time added to the course to instant dismissal. Time was added if a patient was permitted to develop a bedsore or received burns from hot water bottles, mustard plasters, or overheated bedpans. Fines might have been imposed. There is a note in the minutes of the House Committee on 24 March 1893 stating that pins were being left in the sheets and sent to the laundry causing tears in the sheets. Livingston was requested to impose fines for nurses who neglected to take out the pins.[50] M.L. MacDermot reported that, prior to her time, a patient escaped from a ward while the head nurse was at supper and that three months were added to her training.[51]

M.L. MacDermot thought the nurses' quarters were comfortable. Fatigue at the end of the day left little desire for entertaining in the sitting room and, of course, dating housemen was absolutely forbidden.[52] Annie Colquoun (MGH 1892) recounted a tale in which a nurse had eloped with a medical student – an event that made the headlines: "Lovely MGH nurse elopes with medical student. Mothers fear to send their sons to McGill lest they be trapped by wily nurses."[53]

It was common practice in hospitals that the probationers did not wear uniforms. The 1890 regulations stated that the probationer's clothing was to be washable, underwear was to be plain, and that she was to bring six regulation white aprons. Once accepted as a pupil, she then wore the uniform provided by the hospital but bought at her own expense. Livingston introduced the practice of a uniform for the probationer, another first in North America.[54] The student was instructed how to purchase the plain blue uniform material and was responsible for making her own uniforms prior to her arrival at the school.[55]

Uniforms and caps gave training schools their own unique identity, and that at the MGH was no exception. Livingston first used a pink stripe for the nurses' uniform but abandoned this when a nearby hospital adopted the same pattern. She tried a pink dotted material and then finally designed a unique pattern with an MGH monogram that remained as the pattern of the school uniform until its closure in 1972. Along with their cap, it was very distinctive.[56]

Documented changes in the organizational structure were apparent in the 1898 by-laws. The superintendent of nurses "shall discharge the duties of her office subject to the general authority of the Board of Management and of the Medical Board."[57] Livingston had full control in all matters pertaining to the instruction and professional administration of the training school as well as the supervision and direction of the duties and discipline of the nurses. Mention was made of the fact that she was required to hire a house-keeper and be responsible for the female servants – tasks that, in 1890, Livingston vehemently opposed.

By 1910, the by-laws outlined that the lady superintendent would hire and discharge all graduates and undergraduates, all of whom were under her supervision. For the pupil nurses and the probationers the emphasis switched from detailed tasks to an overview of the training, affiliations outside the MGH, and responsibilities. In addition to receiving lodging and board as an equivalent for their services they were to receive a salary prorated for each of the three years. It was clear that they were under the charge of the superintendent of nurses rather than a physician. The relationship between doctor and nurse was not yet expressed as collaborative as the regulations stipulated that: "[she] shall promptly and carefully carry out all orders that may be given by the Physicians and Surgeons for the treatment, diet, and care of the patients."[58]

The functioning of a nursing unit, cost effectiveness, and the importance of nursing records were responsibilities of the head nurse who, at this time, was most likely a pupil nurse in her third year: "The Head Nurse of each ward shall be responsible for the general appearance and good order of her ward, and for the careful and proper use of everything placed in her charge; she shall see that all written orders for medicines and diet are filled and executed, that nursing records are carefully kept, and that the Night Nurses are fully instructed as to the requirements of each patient."[59]

"The Nurses on night duty shall attend to all the nursing in the Hospital between the hours of 7 p.m. and 7 a.m. They shall give special attention to patients dangerously ill, and shall report at once to the proper officer all such cases. They shall attend to the temperature and ventilation of the wards, to the proper use of the water, gas, and electricity, and shall be watchful against accidents from fire."[60] There was increasing use of the word "nursing," suggesting that there was perhaps a clearer delineation of nursing care and medical care. Events occurring inside and outside the hospital prompted changes in staffing complements and the way nursing was practised and supervised. The overall number of staff and students increased as the hospital expanded its bed capacity, but, more important, there was a gradual introduction of graduate nurses to the mix.

The following chart shows the staffing mix at three intervals during Livingston's tenure.[61]

Table 40.2

	1898	1908	1918
Superintendent	1	1	1
Day/Asst superintendents	1	1	2
Night superintendents	1	1	2
Pupil nurses and probationers	57	85	132
Graduate in-charge Operating Theatres	2	3	4
Dietician		1	1
Graduate in charge OPD		1	1
Instructor		1	1
Relief nurse			1
Graduates in charge units			9
Total students and staff	59	92	148

Adding graduate nursing staff was not without struggles between Livingston and the administration. On 27 October 1913, she responded as follows to a request to discontinue the services of an assistant and replace her with a final-year student:

> I do not think the Committee can appreciate the responsibility they have ordered me to place on the shoulders of a nurse in training. They perhaps do not know that she will be in sole charge of the public wards every Sunday night between seven and twelve; one whole night a month, and during Miss Webster's annual vacation of four weeks.

These responsibilities have always been assumed by the experienced day assistant. The continuance of vigilance heretofore observed will be impossible under the present ruling. Perhaps the Committee is right in its decision, and I may err in being over solicitous for the welfare of the patients, but the Committee, in the event of an accident, must stand between the nursing staff and the public.[62]

As the letter continued she concluded that it was in the best interest of the hospital to retain the services of a third day assistant. The hospital would never be left without an experienced graduate in charge and it would be less costly. Even in 1913 there was a "premium" for night work as the day assistant was to receive forty dollars per month and the night duty nurse sixty dollars, as "night duty is trying, unpopular, and requires great physical strength and endurance."[63]

Throughout the First World War staffing was particularly difficult given the number of nurses who were away on active duty. One hundred and five graduates of the MGH were on active duty. Hospital services were expanded and there was an increase in medical science and technology. A twenty-four-bed private ward, Ward H, slated to open in 1913, met with this response from Livingston: "I beg to inform you that I have not the nurses available for that purpose, as at the present, our Training School is taxed to its utmost capacity."[64]

We learn from the 1917 annual report that a graduate nurse was appointed to be in charge of each public ward, "thereby ensuring a continuity of service, a saving of energy, material and time, or in other words the elimination of waste."[65] The number of students in the school was increased and, as Livingston reported: "[This] makes our number per patient as it should be, and provides for our public patients the extra care needed. We no longer suffer from an inadequate supply of nurses, the lack of which so often interferes with the welfare of the patient, the education of the nurse and the reputation of the Hospital."[66]

In October 1918, there was a serious outbreak of influenza ending a year that Livingston felt "was the most trying in my experience." As many as thirty-five nurses, about one-quarter of the staff, were off duty at a time. She noted: "The constant endeavour to carry on the work so that the training of nurses should not suffer, taxed the assistants and sisters on duty very heavily, and it is entirely due to their loyalty and devotion to the interests of the hospital that we were brought through the trying ordeal. In spite of all the complications and difficulties we are able to present the record of a successful year." Without any delay and with the support of the board, just prior to Christmas the nurses were given public recognition and certificates acknowledging their "devotion to duty" during the 1918 epidemic.[67]

Throughout her tenure Livingston was always concerned for the welfare of the students. Given that students staffed the hospital, that they were required to live in residence, and that efforts to secure a higher standard of applicant were under way, it meant that the appearance and comfort of the nurses' quarters had to be appealing and suitable to the young women of the day. Shortly after the arrival of Livingston, an addition to the living quarters was completed that provided a number of comfortable rooms and a sitting room for the nurses.

In 1897, Lord Lister laid the cornerstone for the Jubilee Nurses' Home, which served as the "home away from home" for the next thirty years. Livingston recognized that a nurse required a balance in her life and that off-duty time should have a degree of comfort and security. In 1917, with an increase in staff necessitating more accommodation, she wrote: "The advantage to the hospital of a comfortable, convenient home is generally recognized, and surely in no class of women's work is there greater need for provision for rest, recreation, and hygienic surroundings, than in the Nursing profession. The present quarters at the Home are comfortable, and not unattractive, but inadequate. The nurses' quarters in the administration building are quite comfortable, but do not provide the home-like environment of a separate building."[68]

One of the risks endured by the students was the exposure to various communicable diseases and the lax application of appropriate protective measures. Although there is no direct mention of a health service for the students, Livingston acknowledged the work of one of the physicians in her 1917 report: "To Dr Tanney, the pupils are indebted for devoted personal service. By his establishing preventative measures illness has been lessened. His courtesy and skill have been much valued."[69]

Although Livingston never participated in nursing organizations at any level, she obviously saw their value and ensured that nurses went and, where possible, with financial assistance from the hospital and, later, the Alumnae Association. She was thus up to date with the developments in nursing. Moreover, she was respected by her colleagues and corresponded with Lady Stanley, founder of the Lady Stanley Institute in Ottawa, and Agnes Sniveley, superintendent of nurses at the Toronto General Hospital, on various topics.

Only three years after her arrival, and with the approval of the House Committee, she sent dolls dressed as nurses, respectively attired in their indoor and outdoor uniforms, and a unique mortuary basket to the World's Columbian Exhibition in Chicago in 1893.[70] One has to presume that the MGH collection was displayed in the Women's Building, which housed a vast array of exhibits on women's accomplishments from primitive to modern times. Although there were no MGH nurses in Chicago, Livingston seized an opportunity to display her creativity and take credit for some of her innovations.[71]

The exhibition served as a gathering place for nursing leaders and saw the birth of many nursing organizations, including the Nurses' Associated Alumnae of the United States and Canada. Mathewson credits these alumnae associations and their members with the foresight to realize that uniting at various levels would serve to enhance the standard of nursing education and promote nursing as an honourable profession.[72]

In 1905, encouraged by Livingston, the Alumnae Association of the Montreal General Hospital School of Nursing, as it is known today, took root.[73] It set as its goal "the maintenance of the honour and character of the nursing profession, the promotion of good feeling and loyalty among members."[74] From the very beginning it demonstrated clearly the devotion and commitment of the members to the advancement of the nursing profession, to the welfare of its members, and to the community at large through its involvement in social, educational, political, and charitable ventures.

In 1909, with the movement to organize a national association for nurses, the alumnae sent three delegates to Ottawa. Flora Madeleine Shaw (MGH 1896) was elected secretary-treasurer of the new group, later to become the Canadian Nurses Association. Similarly, in 1914, the alumnae responded to a request and sent two nurses to sit on a committee for provincial registration leading to the formation of the Registered Nurses Association of the Province of Quebec. It was the beginning of a long tradition in which alumnae members were involved in nursing organizations, often in a leadership role, and in policy making at the local, national, and international level.[75] Education for the alumnae members was addressed at each meeting, where lectures could be of a professional nature or relating to the current issues of the day, literature, or politics. For example, a lecture in 1913 was given on "the rights of children born and unborn," while in 1914 the topic chosen was Kingsley's *Water-Babies*.[76]

Long before the days of collective agreements with guarantees of job security and social benefits, the alumnae established a sick benefit fund for the nurses. It was spearheaded by Nora Tedford (MGH 1895), raised funds to support the benefits, and served its members at home and in the hospital until it closed in 1996. In addition, the alumnae raised money to support nurses at conferences and in continuing education. From the outset, the Alumnae reached beyond the boundaries of nursing to become involved in movements of importance to women. In 1909, it joined the Council of Women and through it was implicated in the suffrage movement. It extended its hand to the community with many initiatives, among which, in the early days, related to First World War efforts such as contributing to the prisoner-of-war fund of the Imperial Order Daughters of the Empire (IODE), knitting, and preparing care packages for the troops.

No less important was keeping in touch with the graduates of the school. In her 1907–08 annual report Shaw writes: "Our absent members appreciated keenly the letters of the corresponding secretary, being grateful for any news of their old acquaintances and the Montreal General Hospital."[77] Annual dinners were started to honour the graduates and to give members a chance to meet and socialize. Today, over one hundred years later, the tradition of the dinner and the newsletter still unite the members living here and abroad.

Nora Livingston's "firsts" are well documented. To accomplish what she did took great determination against overwhelming odds. But what of the personal side of her nature? Julia English, the second official graduate of the school, shared her recollections. At eighty-two years of age and dressed in her black satin and lace dress with her medal proudly pinned on her dress, she described life at MGH in 1891. Of Livingston she said: "[She was a] "disciplinarian but had a heart of gold, and was always doing things to make the nurses comfortable."[78] Mary A. Samuel, a graduate of the New York Hospital and a school visitor in Quebec for many years, wrote after her friend's death: "Two outstanding characteristics seem to me the keys of her great achievement: her remarkable ability as executive and administrator and her delightfully keen sense of humour."[79]

Livingston's letters to her sisters in the early 1890s while they were in Europe offer some insight into the challenges she faced, how she handled certain situations, and what interests she had outside of the hospital. They offer a keen, humorous yet often cutting description of her administrative counterparts, the doctors, and the nursing staff. She spoke of her long days with frequent meetings with various individuals followed by teaching classes in the evenings. She was not afraid to get into the fray, intervening in a rather dangerous fire situation in one account and filling in the gaps in service in others. On one occasion, after organizing work in the operating room in Dunne's absence, she wrote: "The nurses are all very nice to me; I can get them to do anything. Of course, they would have to, but is much pleasanter to have willing service."[80]

One individual who figured highly in her letters was Kirkpatrick, the medical director when she arrived at MGH. Her comments speak of her relationship with him as well as giving a glimpse of her own self-image. Just prior to the end of his term of office she wrote: "Poor Dr K., he reminds me so much of myself in every way; gets heaps of praise, no brains, all luck and diplomacy, liked and popular, everyone, seemingly, getting their own way, but in the end he does just as he pleases. We work well together, and I always felt I could go to him with anything. I hate myself sometimes for being so civil-silky to people."[81] She obviously missed him as, at a later date when he was ill, she again wrote in her letters that his successor could not compare and that Kirkpatrick, something like herself, "would sympathize almost to tears, but he held his own, and bowed them out [i.e., out of office] pleased with themselves. It is training, this institutional life."[82]

At other times the letters seem frivolous and superficial, seemingly out of character with the picture of a highly efficient and effective administrator. They centre on material for dresses, the latest fashion, and light-hearted gossip about their circle of friends. She did not suffer fools lightly and showed those who did not meet her standards quickly out the door. Following the dismissal of one young woman whom she dubbed a "beauty probationer," she commented to her sisters: "The funny idea of nursing and hospital life that some women have is rich, more poetical than practical."[83]

On 20 February 1915, the alumnae held a reception in honour of Nora Livingston's twenty-fifth anniversary as lady superintendent of the training school. Graduates, doctors, and their wives and members of the Committee of Management gathered as Henrietta Dunlop (MGH 1893) made "a very appropriate speech" and presented her with a platinum and diamond watch in appreciation of her years of invaluable service. Sir Montague Allan, president of the board, then presented her with a very handsome silver tea tray and hot water kettle, and the Medical Board presented her with a basket of lovely American Beauty roses.[84]

Livingston was not invited on a regular basis to meetings of the Board of Governors, the House Committee, or the Committee of Management, yet she commanded their respect and she worked in harmony with the medical directors. At her side in nursing she had, among others, Jennie Webster

(MGH 1895), night superintendent; Nora Tedford (MGH 1895), head nurse in the operating room; Flora Madeleine Shaw (MGH 1896); and Sara E. Young (MGH 1900), her assistant and successor. These nurses receive more attention later in this book.

An individual, who stayed on the home front, and perhaps did not get the same public attention, is Flora Strumm (MGH 1900). She appears, from all accounts, to have been a very quiet yet devoted and respected member of the staff. After graduation and some private duty work, she worked in the operating room and then as an instructor for five years before becoming an assistant to Livingston in 1915. When she retired in 1941, after working with three directors, there were 545 signatures on the gift from the Alumnae Association of the MGH School of Nurses and accolades from the Association of Registered Nurses of the Province of Quebec, the doctors, and her peers. Francis Upton, representing the ARNPQ, said her record of service had no parallel in Canadian nursing history. She praised her loyalty, her steadfastness of purpose, her gentleness, her devotion, her ability to hold fast to those good things of former years and to weave them seamlessly into the work and thought of later and present times, and, finally, for her cheerful laugh.[85]

By 1919 Nora Livingston, then seventy-one, continued to attack her job with vim and vigour. Nurses and other personnel were returning from war, and there was renewed activity and expansion at the hospital. Unfortunately, she suffered a stroke and was forced to retire on 20 August. She went to live in Como with her sister Gracie and a pension of $1,425 a year from the hospital. A marble slab, erected by the alumnae at her burial place in Como, marks her death on 24 July 1927.

A biography of Livingston states that she "must be considered *the* pioneer of nursing education in the province of Quebec."[86] No higher praise could be given. American nursing leaders Nutting and Dock wrote: "To Miss Livingston is due, not only the efficiency of the nursing department of the Montreal General Hospital, but the high tone and standard of nursing today in many parts of Canada." Maxwell wrote: "The pioneers of nursing had to have had courage, patience, and perseverance of rare quality."[87] Livingston, with her forceful character and forward thinking, took nursing out of the dark ages and ensured that the status of nursing "was raised from that of an untrained domestic worker to one of the most honoured callings available to women."[88]

NOTES

1 F.J. Shepherd, *Origin and History of the Montreal General Hospital* (Montreal: Gazette Printing Co., Ltd.,1925), 3–6.

2 Jean Bannerman, *Leading Ladies, 1639–1967* (Dundas, ON: Carswood, 1967), xii.

3 C. Bates, D. Dodd, and N. Rousseau, *On All Frontiers: Four Centuries of Canadian Nursing* (Ottawa: University of Ottawa Press, 2005).

4 Minutes, 1 May–1 August 1822, MGH Committee of Management, in H.E. MacDermot, *A History of the Montreal General Hospital* (Montreal: Montreal General Hospital, 1950), 23.

5 Montreal General Hospital by-laws, McGill University Archives (hereafter MUA) RG 96, 1822, 431–779.

6 Ibid., duty no. 5.

7 MacDermot, *History* (MGH), 25.

8 Minutes, 1859, MGH Committee of Management, in MacDermot, *History* (MGH), 29–30.

9 E. Desjardins, E.C. Flanagan, and S. Giroux, *Heritage History of the Nursing Profession in the Province of Quebec* (Montreal: Association of Nurses of the Province of Quebec, 1971), 48.

10 Ibid., 98.

11 Ibid., 99.

12 Minutes, 1866, MGH Committee of Management, in MacDermot, *History* (MGH), 31.

13 H.E. MacDermot, *History of the School of Nursing of the Montreal General Hospital* (Montreal: Southam Printing, 1961), 17.

14 Newspaper report, 1877, in MacDermot, *History* (MGH), 78.

15 McClure's report, 1887, in MacDermot, *History* (MGH), 79–80.

16 K. MacPherson, "The Nightingale Influence and the Rise of the Modern Hospital," in Bates et al., *Frontiers*, 77.

17 MacDermot, *History* (School), 26.

18 Ibid., 29.

19 Anna C. Maxwell, "Struggles of Pioneers," paper read at a meeting of the New York State Nurses' Association, Albany, 1920, 5.

20 MacDermot, *History* (School), 32.

21 Ibid., 33–5.

22 Ibid., 35.

23 H.E. MacDermot, "Nora Livingston and Maude Abbot," address delivered at the fiftieth reunion of the 1907 McGill Class of Medicine, 1957, MUA, RG 96, 422-662, 228.

24 MacDermot, *History* (School), 36.

25 MacDermot, "Livingston and Abbott," 229.

26 E.A. Collard, "Getting Patients to Come Clean Was Daunting," *Montreal Gazette*, 1999.

27 Form of Application, 1890, MGH Alumnae Archives.

28 "Formal Opening, Training School for Nurses," MGH (Montreal: Gazette Printing Co., 1890).

29 Ibid., 9.

30 Ibid., 11.

31 Ibid., 18–20.

32 Ibid., 25–30.

33 MacDermot, *History* (School), 45.

34 Newspaper clipping, 1891, "Trained Nurses," MUA, RG 96, 422-647.

35 Nora Livingston, *Some Letters Written to Her Sisters, 1890–1891* (Made for the Archives of the MGH by F. Wise, Montreal, 1942).

36 Newspaper Clipping, 1891, MUA, RG 96, 422-647.

37 Ibid.

38 "Formal Opening," 29.

39 Annual reports, MGH, 1895–96, MUA, RG 96.

40 MacDermot, *History* (School), 46.

41 Ibid., 74.

42 Ibis., 46.

43 Ibid.

44 MacDermot, *History* (School), 53.

45 M.L. MacDermot, "Nursing Training 45 years Ago," *MGH Bulletin* 2, 6 (1954): 15–17.

46 Department of Nursing, annual report, 1906, MGH, MGH Alumnae Archives.

47 Maxwell, "Pioneers," 25.

48 MacDermot, *History* (School), 54–5.

49 MacDermot, "Nursing Training," 15–17.

50 Minutes, 24 March 1893, Committee of Management, MGH, MUA, RG 96.

51 MacDermot, "Nursing Training," 15–17.

52 Ibid

53 MacDermot, *History* (School), 116–17. Annie Colquhoun's entire speech may be found in MGH School of Nursing, MGH Alumnae Archives.

54 Maxwell, "Pioneers," 25.

55 Regulations, 1890, 40.

56 History of uniforms, MGH Alumnae Archives.

57 Montreal General Hospital by-laws, 1898.

58 Charter and by-Laws, 1910, MGH, MUA, RG 96, 432-779, chap. 20, 43.

59 Ibid., chap. 21, 44–5.

60 Ibid.

61 Department of Nursing, annual reports, 1898, 1908, and 1918, MGH Alumnae Archives.

62 Livingston to the Committee of Management, 27 October 1913, MGH, MUA RG 431-765.

63 Ibid.

64 Ibid.

65 Department of Nursing, annual report, 1917, MGH Alumnae Archives.

66 Ibid.

67 Department of Nursing, annual report, 1918, MGH Alumnae Archives.

68 Ibid., 1917.

69 Ibid.

70 Minutes, 6 March 1893, Committee of Management, MGH, MUA, RG 96, 45.

71 Website: www.nursingworld.org, American Nurses Association, formerly Nurses' Associated Alumnae of the United States and Canada, search Women's Building, 1893 Worlds Exposition.

72 J.M. Murray and M.S. Mathewson, *Three Centuries of Canadian Nursing* (Toronto: Macmillan, 1947), 355.

73 Letter to graduates, 1905, MUA, RG 96, box 421, file 643.

74 Constitution and by-laws, 1983, the Alumnae Association of the MGH School of Nursing, MGH Alumnae Archives.

75 Minutes, 18 May 1914, Alumnae Association of the MGH School of Nursing. MGH Alumnae Archives, 51.

76 Annual reports of the Alumnae, 1905–2005, MGH Alumnae Archives.

77 Ibid.

78 C. Birkenhead, 1939, interview of Julia English, MUA, RG 96, 429-691.

79 M.A. Samuel, circa 1927, "The Late Miss Livingston," *Alumnae News*, NY Hospital Training School, MUA, RG 96, 422-662.

80 Livingston, *Letters*, 53.

81 Ibid., 82.

82 Ibid., 120.

83 Ibid., 32–3.

84 Newspaper clipping, 1941, *Montreal Gazette* vol. 152, no. 142.

85 Desjardins, *Heritage*, 180.

86 Newspaper clipping, "Miss Livingston Set High Standard," Montreal *Gazette*, 26 July 1927, MGH Nursing Archives.

87 Maxwell, "Pioneers," 5.

88 MacDermot, *History* (School), 116–17.

41

Building for the Future under Young, Holt, and Mathewson, 1919–53

Valerie Parker Shannon

Shannon became director of nursing at the MGH in 1984. With the formation of the MUHC she was the last director of MGH nursing and the first director of MUHC nursing. She held a joint appointment at the McGill School of Nursing.

During this time, nurses both provincially and nationally created organizations to represent their issues and protect their interests. The first serious nursing shortages began after the First World War and continued intermittently throughout this thirty-three-year period. In this tumultuous yet energizing context, three directors of nursing at the MGH made their mark not only anticipating and responding to the changes required but also dealing thoughtfully with the challenges of the day.

The Sarah Edith Young Years, 1919–27

The first to take on these challenges, Sarah Edith Young, had also to contend with Livingston's formidable reputation. Young was born in Quebec City in 1877 and received her education there. She came to the MGH in 1897 to study nursing, graduating at the head of her class in 1900 and, like many others, did private duty nursing. She returned to the MGH as the second assistant superintendent and then became assistant superintendent to Livingston. In 1916, Young joined the No. 1 Canadian General Hospital as matron and was sent to England and France, where she received the Royal Red Cross for distinguished service. She was recalled to Canada in 1917 and appointed matron of the Tuxedo Military Hospital in Winnipeg, where she was responsible for the military nursing district in Manitoba. On 2 November

1919, Young was appointed to the position of lady superintendent of nurses and principal of the School for Nurses at the MGH.

Nursing Training

One of Young's first actions was to hire Edith C. Reside and Mabel K. Holt (MGH 1919) as instructors, a role that had lapsed during the war.[1] The existing curriculum allocated 25 percent of the student's time to studying natural sciences, 4 percent to studying social sciences and ethics, and 71 percent to studying nursing.[2] As infectious diseases were rampant in Montreal, the medical sciences that most influenced the curriculum continued to be principles of asepsis and antisepsis. Reading materials consisted of textbooks on anatomy and physiology, nursing techniques, and a hospital procedure manual for standards of nursing care. Visits were made to the anatomy and pathology museum at McGill and lectures in public health and social conditions were given at the McGill School for Graduate Nurses. It is interesting to note that nursing ethics consisted of rules governing hospital etiquette, principles of student government, and the social and moral obligations of a nurse. Good moral conduct implied not being concerned about economic matters.[3] The development of the character of the nurse was a powerful theme at the MGH throughout its history. Physicians continued to play a dominant role in the instruction of nurses, but they did not concern themselves with the organization of the teaching programs or the management of the school and nursing services.

Rayside described the intent of the curriculum, stating: "It is now conceded that the nurse is no longer a bedside attendant who is expected to perform a few practical duties; nor, indeed, is she called upon to merely serve the needs of a single institution – she must be prepared to serve the whole community … and meet the conditions as she finds them."

The model of education continued to be the apprenticeship method, whereby students were given some formal instruction but fundamentally learned through watching others and through repetitive supervised practice. Students were assigned to the public wards only and were guided by the head nurse who was always a senior student or an MGH graduate. In 1921, the students worked sixty hour weeks and twelve hour days. They had one day a week off starting at 10:00 AM and five hours off on Sunday when it was strongly suggested that they worship at a place of their choice. They were paid ten dollars a month. They provided their own uniforms and, in exchange, received room, board, and instruction. They worked four to six months of night duty over the course of their three-year training program and had three weeks of annual vacation.

Always concerned with the quality of residence life, on 15 October 1923, Young introduced student government. The first president was Grace Tanner (MGH 1924). Young also began a big sister program for the probationers in 1923 to ease their transition into the role of student nurse.[4] A staff health service was soon established that looked after the students and graduates.

An ongoing concern for Young was the overcrowding in the nurses' residence as the total staff increased in number. New space had to be found and, in 1921, the hospital rented a house on Sherbrooke Street to accommodate eighteen nurses. This proved to be insufficient, and Young continued to be preoccupied with the need to deal with the lack of space in the nursing residence to accommodate the expanding hospital needs. She was persuasive and persistent, finally convincing the Board of Management that a new nurses' home was needed. The monies for the building were obtained from the government of Quebec ($200,000), which was not customary, and from individual members of the hospital's Board of Governors ($270,000). Many of the furnishings were given as gifts from the governors. On 20 December 1926, the new nurses' residence and teaching unit was officially opened by the Honourable L.A. Taschereau, premier of Quebec, and Colonel Herbert Molson, president of the MGH Board of Governors. The new building, located on the north side of Dorchester Street, faced the front of the hospital and was connected to it by an underground tunnel. Above the entrance were two stone cameos of Jeanne Mance and Florence Nightingale.

Young made the graduation ceremony and its accompanying activities an important social occasion, which was well publicized in the newspapers in recognition of the value and contributions of the students to the hospital. There were three main events – the graduation exercises, the alumnae dinner, at which the new graduates were invited to join the Alumnae Association of the MGH School for Nurses, and a graduation ball. Between 1919 and 1927, an average of thirty-eight nurses graduated each year, with the number ranging from thirty to forty three.[5] Young noted that, as of 1926, a total of 902 nurses had graduated from the MGH.[6]

In the early 1920s, there were very few graduate nurses on staff at the MGH. If they were hired, it would usually be into a head nurse position either on the wards, in the operating rooms, or in the outpatient department.

They worked twelve-hour days, and the hospital provided them with room, board, and uniforms. In 1920, the head nurse of the ward made nine hundred dollars a year, while the nurse in the outpatient department and the nurse anaesthetist made twelve hundred dollars a year.[7] In comparison, the average annual income for a nurse in Canada aged twenty-five to forty-nine in 1921 was $735 a year.[8] Although the cost of living was low, it was difficult for nurses earning these salaries to save enough for the annuities they would need to be self-sufficient in retirement. To compensate for lack of finances, an MGH graduate who became ill and was a member of the Alumnae Association Graduate Nurses Benevolent Fund had her medical expenses paid for. If she was not a member, she received a 50 percent discount on medical fees. The MGH Alumnae Association also subsidized and made arrangements with the MGH to have graduates looked after on a private ward at the cost of $1.50 a day.

In spite of educational and some professional developments, opportunities for graduate nurses in general were limited. As mentioned previously, wages were low and the working conditions were difficult. To address some of the nurses' concerns, the Catholic nurses in Quebec formed the first nursing union, called L'association des gardes-malades catholiques licenciées de la province de Québec in 1928.[9] Quebec led the way in Canada in terms of organizing nurses into unions, but the English nurses did not join these unions or form their own because the boards of the anglophone hospitals, like those of the MGH, generally followed the guidelines for salary and working conditions issued by the Association of Registered Nurses in the Province of Quebec. It also established the Shepherd Convalescent Fund in 1922 to augment the other funds that were established by the MGH Alumnae Association to look after ailing MGH graduate nurses.[10] In addition, some senior nurses upon retirement received a lifetime annuity.

Medical specialization was on the increase, and MGH physicians led the way in Montreal. This influenced the development of new roles for graduate nurses. In 1920, Haywood, the superintendent, authorized the hiring of the earliest recorded specialized nursing role – a nurse anaesthetist.[11] In addition, a graduate nurse was hired in 1921 by the nursing office to provide discharge planning to reduce length of stay as a way to give more access to patient's needing specialized care.[12] Similarly, new nursing roles were developed in the outpatient department. Young sent head nurses to New York and Boston to observe the role of nurses in well developed ambulatory care settings. Consequently, the graduate nurse in the early MGH clinics attended to patient flow, assisted the physicians, and provided specialized nursing care ensuring that the clinics operated efficiently. Specialized clinics expanded and physicians frequently requested that graduate nurses be hired.

With changes in societal values and conditions and the effects of the First World War, the demand for graduate nurses increased across the country, creating the first sustained nursing shortages, and solutions had to be found. In the United States, the Rockefeller Report on Nursing commented on the need for auxiliary workers. In Canada, Marie Louisa Parker (MGH 1903), acting on this report, started the earliest school for trained attendants.[13] Parker had worked with voluntary aid detachments in military hospitals in Canada during the war, and, though the attendants were poorly prepared, she felt they could be taught to offer greater help. After demobilization in 1921, she established a three-month training school at the Montreal YWCA. In 1923, under the patronage of many notable MGH physicians, she established the Parker School for Trained Attendants.[14] It was not clear if the MGH employed these trained attendants during Young's tenure.

In 1924, the MGH merged with the Western Hospital to provide more specialized care, to increase the teaching facilities, to improve the surroundings for private patients, and to gain economies in overhead by combining management positions. Nursing took the lead in making the merger work. Under the tactful and sensitive leadership of Young, the school for nurses at the Western and its graduate staff gradually became part of the MGH. Jane Craig, a graduate of St Luke's Hospital in Chicago, remained the lady superintendent of the Western Division until her resignation in 1932.

Another important development for graduate nurses was access to postgraduate university education. In 1919, the University of British Columbia offered the first post graduate courses, and in 1920 McGill followed suit with Flora Madeline Shaw as its first director.[15] The McGill School for Graduate Nurses offered diplomas in teaching, supervision, and public health.

Young was also very involved professionally and was one of eight nursing leaders in Quebec who spearheaded the formation of the ARNPQ. On 14 February 1920, an act recognized the existence of the ARNPQ despite opposition from physicians, hospitals, and other public agencies for economic, religious, and emotional reasons.

Not long after the new residence and teaching facilities were becoming well established, Young's health deteriorated. She died on 4 December 1927 at fifty years of age and was given a full military funeral at the Cathedral of the Holy Trinity in Quebec City. In 1927, two other outstanding MGH nurses died: Nora

Livingston (24 July) and Flora Madeline Shaw (27 August). To fill the leadership vacuum, Mabel Kathleen Holt was invited to return to the MGH.

The Mabel Kathleen Holt Years, 1928–45

Mabel Kathleen Holt became the lady superintendent of nurses and the principal of the MGH School for Nurses in 1928. Born in 1893 in England and educated there, Holt was a tall, distinguished-looking woman who was viewed as very approachable and warm. As evident in her formal portrait, she always wore a blue, military-like dress with a white collar and cap, despite the fact that she never served in the war. Holt graduated from the MGH in 1919 and immediately became Young's second assistant. She taught at the MGH School for Nurses from 1920 to 1922 and graduated from McGill in 1924. Holt subsequently accepted a position of assistant superintendent of nurses at the Hamilton General Hospital. From 1928 to 1932, she was the president of the ARNPQ and, in that capacity, presided over the first congress of the International Council of Nurses (ICN) held in Canada in 1929. She went on to give the ARNPQ nineteen years of exemplary, continuous voluntary service.

Nursing Training

Like Young, Holt was already an experienced administrator when she began her tenure at the MGH. She knew the importance of the training program and moved quickly to appoint Martha Batson (MGH 1921) as the first named director of education, a position that she held from 1928 to 1946. To better understand what it was like to be a student during this era, retired assistant director of nursing Phyllis Snow Read (MGH 1934) wrote an account of her student days circa 1931.[16]

> A gong got us out of bed at 6 AM. We were sent to the wards at 7 AM until 8:45 AM to make all the beds … rushed to diet kitchen for a glass of milk and a slice of buttered bread before going to classes until noon. At noon we were given two hours … [for]… our lunch. As the dining room was on the top of the hospital and we had to wait until everybody senior to you entered the elevator before we could set foot on one, it took us a long time to get [there] … At 2 PM, we returned to class until 4 PM … [then] went to the wards to help with suppers, pile linen from the carriers on to the linen cupboards … so that everything was absolutely straight – if one sheet or towel was out of line the head nurse

would make us re-do the whole thing. Another gong was sounded at 10:30 PM for us to be in bed. Nurses were not permitted to smoke in the residence ... [Those] who disobeyed were sent home for six months as punishment ... they would have to come back and finish their training six months after their own class had graduated.

Despite this regimentation and punitive attitude, Read states: "We were proud and strutted accordingly ... we felt like a breed apart. Every year one of our graduates obtained the highest marks on the RN examinations. We were fiercely loyal and loved our institution." Graduation continued to be an important occasion on which the addresses mirrored the current thinking or key issues affecting nursing. The personal qualities and altruistic virtues of the nurse as well as the loyalty to and confidentiality of the doctor-nurse relationship were repeatedly stressed.

The Weir Report and the MGH School for Nurses

Low wages, poor working conditions, and questionable educational standards across Canada led to a major study called the Weir Report (1932) sponsored by the Canadian Nurses Association and the Canadian Medical Association. It was a historic milestone in nursing education and made many important recommendations. It also commented on the hotly debated issue as to whether nurses even needed to be educated. Weir clearly felt that they did and was very concerned about the overemphasis on disposition.[17]

Weir characterized the "good old days" of nursing education as driven by apprenticeship learning and rule-of-thumb standards and said that the twentieth-century world would have "more exacting and specialized demands on intelligence, knowledge, ingenuity, resourcefulness and social adaptability."[18] The report noted that, "sooner or later, the university, in affiliation with the well-equipped hospital, must face the problem of educating the nurse. Evolutionary trends point in this direction ... The field of nursing ... presents sufficient scope and wealth of content to warrant the establishment of degree courses."[19]

Weir also noted that recent specialized advances in medical treatment had greatly increased the cost of illness and hospitalization. He stated: "Science[,] in a word, has outstripped economics."[20] With great insight and forethought, Weir insisted that some form of national insurance would be required in the future.[21]

In the end, the report issued many recommendations, of which the key ones are: (1) there is a need for a standardized curriculum for nursing in Canada that allows for new knowledge and emerging fields of practice; (2) nurses' homes must be improved; (3) science courses must be part of the curriculum; (4) the hours of work for students should be decreased; (5) texts must be available; (6) a history of nursing in Canada should be written; (7) housemaid's work, after the first six months, should be eliminated from the curriculum; (8) as soon as possible, the training school for nurses should be established primarily as an educational institution, closely affiliated with a hospital but enjoying financial independence, as do other educational institutions that perform a national service; and (9) higher salaries should be available for those in teaching or administrative positions.[22]

Having already implemented many of the suggested changes, the MGH School for Nurses led the way in educational reform. It had already met or actually surpassed the requirements that the Canadian Nurses Association had developed in response to the Weir Report. In 1936, the school hired a public health nurse to teach all aspects of health and to look after the health of the students in collaboration with MGH physicians. In 1939–40, 18 percent of the courses and labs were in the natural sciences, down from 25 percent, social sciences and ethics increased from 4 percent to 17 percent, and nursing courses were decreased from 71 percent to 65 percent. Yet, the number of hours of study increased overall from 454 in 1921–22 to 850 in 1939–40. In 1941, the work week of the students was reduced from sixty hours to fifty hours, which meant that they provided service 88 percent of the time rather than 95 percent. The teaching and administrative staff of the school earned more than the general duty nurses and, at the time of the writing of the Weir Report, nurses in Quebec had the highest salaries in Canada, perhaps because the majority of them were unionized.[23]

Nursing Service

The first ten years of Holt's leadership were influenced by consequences of the Great Depression of 1929. The MGH struggled to balance its growing debts compounded by the expansion of treatment possibilities. Revenues from the government were limited and inconsistent. In 1932, the Board of Management established a permanent committee on nursing services, with Holt as an active member, to study and consider all matters pertaining to the nursing staff and training school. Their initial and ongoing principal focus was that of cost control. After consultation with the committee, the board decided to cut wages temporarily because of the prevailing conditions. In addition, fewer nurses were sent on affiliation, with the result that fewer graduate nurses were needed to replace them. The student allowance of ten dollars per month was cut, and they were provided with books and uniforms instead. Later on, the board also decided to decrease the number of graduate nurses at the Western Division and replace them with students.[24]

Given these rather draconian measures, it was surprising that the Board of Management agreed to sponsor Holt's initiative of an internship course for newly graduated MGH nurses. It was her way of assisting nurses who were having difficulty finding employment due to the economic conditions. No doubt the medical staff welcomed better prepared nurses to work with the new techniques and treatments associated with increasing medical specialization.

At the Western Division, Holt appointed Blanche Herman (MGH 1925) to serve as nursing superintendent. She held that position from 1933 to 1955, with the exception of the time she was oversees during the Second World War. Blanche G. Herman was an MGH legend, who, upon her graduation, chose the following quotation for her yearbook: "Like Alexander I will reign and I will reign alone." She said that her ambition was "speed, accuracy and neatness" and her hobby was "tidying up."[25] This glimpse into her character foretells a strong, determined, and fastidious woman who had high standards and ruled the Western Division like a four-star general – with an iron fist and booming voice. She was a native of Lunenburg, Nova Scotia, graduated from the School for Nurses of the MGH in 1925 and from McGill University with a diploma in teaching and administration in 1930. From 1933 to 1955 she was the superintendent of the Western Division of the MGH , and, in 1940, she joined the army nursing service and went overseas in 1941 as matron of the twelve-hundred-bed No. 14 Canadian General Hospital. Posted to the Mediterranean as principal matron of the Canadian nurses in 1942, she was on board the SS *St Helena* when it was torpedoed two days out of Gibraltar. To honour their good work, one Italian made each sister a plate "denoting the landmarks of their wartime experience."[26] In recognition of her wartime service, Herman was decorated with the Royal Red Cross, First Class, and was mentioned in despatches for her courageous work. On her return to Canada, she resumed her position of superintendent at the Western Division.

In the midst of the educational turmoil associated with the Weir Report and with a view to the future, Holt began to make her case in 1931 for a stable staff of graduate nurses. Several earlier decisions facilitated this change. First, the internship course had been a great success resulting in a corps of well prepared graduate nurses. Also, Herman had introduced the eight-hour day at the Western Division, which improved the quality of life of the graduate nurse. Last, the reopening of the private pavilion at the Western Division provided an opportunity to showcase the value of an all-graduate staff to a largely paying clientele.

The Second World War, the need for nurses in industry, the eight-hour day, and improved economic conditions that permitted marriage at an earlier age all made staffing the hospital a major challenge. By 1943, 170 MGH graduates were serving overseas. In order to compensate for the shortages, she hired one hundred Volunteer Aid Detachment staff to serve in the Central Division along with practical nurses. That year the federal government offered financial assistance to increase student nurse enrolment, enabling the MGH to add thirteen more students and a clinical instructor. At the provincial level, the age of admission to nursing schools was lowered to eighteen. This was designed to attract women into nursing rather than losing them to other careers or university, but Holt was hesitant about the younger applicants as she felt a certain maturity was necessary.

To cope with the nursing shortage, functional nursing was introduced. This structural change divided tasks among the staff according to the care required and their level of skill. The MGH version of functional nursing required that medications and vital signs be checked by a nurse, that some beds be made by ward aide staff, and that the other nurses give complete care to their patients. This approach required greater vigilance and responsibility on the part of the head nurse or ward sister, who was considered to be the nursing expert. A former head nurse from the MGH said: "It was much more autocratic [in the early days] ... It was the head nurse that put all the pieces together ... she took care of seeing that procedures and examinations were done; she met with the families and oversaw the discharge of patients. She had control of everything. The graduate nurses worked under her direction."

As nursing at the MGH and elsewhere was acquiring more influence, another crisis arose. In 1932, the McGill School for Graduate Nurses experienced grave financial difficulty. Francis Upton (MGH 1908), a teacher at

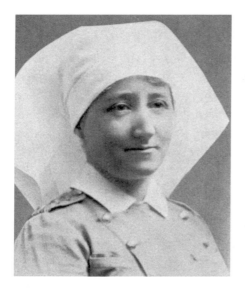

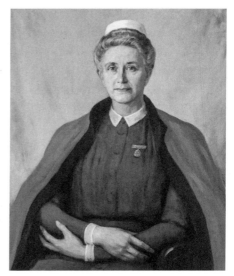

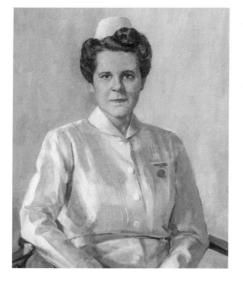

Clockwise from top left
Fig. 41.1 Sarah Young, director, MGH
Nursing, 1919–27
Fig. 41.2 Mabel Kathleen Holt, director,
MGH Nursing, 1928–46
Fig. 41.3 Mary Seabury Mathewson,
director, MGH Nursing, 1946–53

McGill, solicited the MGH Board of Management for financial assistance.
The matter was referred to the committee on nursing, but it concluded that,
"due to the financial state of the hospital, nothing could be given." Loyalty
to the MGH was the top priority, and the profession's aspiration for higher
education was not shared by all, as the committee's decision demonstrated.
In support of its stance, the Board of Management, in 1934, tabled a copy of
a letter from J.C. Meakins sent to Upton indicating that he "deprecated the

present tendency of nurses' training schools to insist upon the higher education of nurses."[27] Despite the disappointment Holt must have felt, she was unfazed and proceeded to challenge the view of the board by asserting that three years was not enough time in which to accomplish the real process of education and that postgraduate study was essential. In support of her viewpoint, she pointed out that all seven MGH graduates who had done postgraduate work at McGill had obtained positions of responsibility across Canada and that it was a requirement of the MGH School for Nurses that the instructors have a university certificate in teaching and administration. Seemingly at odds with its own position, the MGH Board continued to give generous scholarships for higher education. The MGH nurses, though, did not rely solely on the board to support them in their educational aims as they also received generous help from the MGH Alumnae Association. To keep pace with the demand for qualified nurses to assume leadership positions in all areas of nursing, Holt managed to increase the number of bursaries provided by both the board and the alumnae association. In 1944, the McGill School for Graduate Nurses began offering a two-year course for graduate nurses, leading to a bachelor of nursing rather than a diploma. According to Keith Gordon, Holt played an important role in making this happen. Holt noted that two MGH graduates were enrolled in the new program and proudly pointed out that eleven MGH graduates were doing postgraduate work at McGill and that one was at Columbia University working on a master of arts.

With such successes, and after eighteen years of illustrious service as superintendent of nurses and principal of the School for Nurses and a total of thirty years at the MGH, Mabel Holt retired in September 1946. Holt's chief contribution, which changed the way the hospital functioned forever, was to employ graduate nurses in increasing numbers. Not only did this improve the quality of care but it also enabled the students more often to be primarily learners. In retirement, Holt led an active life as a volunteer until her death on 15 August 1967 in Charlottetown, Prince Edward Island.

On 21 August 1946, Mary Seabury Mathewson succeeded Holt as the director of nursing. Mathewson's appointment maintained the tradition of the director of nursing being an MGH graduate with considerable educational and leadership experience. She was born in Montreal on 25 June 1898, graduated from the MGH in 1925, and did postgraduate work at both McGill (1929) and at Teacher's College, Columbia University in New York, where she obtained a bachelor of science. She was the first director to have a degree as well as a diploma in nursing and the first to use the title of director of nursing. Mathewson practised in the public health field, where she gained a reputation for her work on child welfare issues. In 1934, she was appointed assistant director of the McGill School for Graduate Nurses, where she worked for twelve years and was in charge of its public health nursing course. Continuing the close connection between McGill and the MGH, Mathewson served as the president of the MGH Alumnae Association from 1936 to 1940 and was a member of the executive of the Mutual Benefits Association within the alumnae for many years. At the time of her appointment to the MGH, she was active in the Association of Nurses in the Province of Quebec as first vice-president and was chair of its board of examiners for many years. One of her earlier accomplishments was the publication of the first book about the history of Canadian nursing, entitled *Three Centuries of Canadian Nursing*, which she co-authored with John Murray Gibbon.[28]

Nursing Education

Mathewson, like her predecessors, was very involved in the education of students. In 1947, she appointed Norena Mackenzie as the director of nursing education, a position she held until 1955. Mackenzie came from Ontario to study at the MGH, from which she graduated in 1926. She taught in the MGH School for Nurses and then spent a year doing postgraduate study at the McGill School for Graduate Nurses in 1928. Her teaching skills were recognized early on, and, in 1932, she was one of two Canadian nurses sponsored by the Florence Nightingale Fund to study in Great Britain. She gained international recognition for her knowledge of teaching, and, in 1951, she was appointed nursing consultant to the World Health Organization's expert commission on nursing. She was also an outstanding administrator. She was a head nurse at the MGH for five months in 1933, the educational director at the Hospital for Sick Children in Toronto in 1936, and the director of nursing at the Jeffery Hale Hospital in Quebec City before returning to the MGH.[29]

Mackenzie and Mathewson faced numerous challenges, but they were a strong team with great determination and a strong professional orientation. In 1947, they changed the MGH School Pledge, which all student nurses repeated at their graduation ceremony, in several ways. First, the name of the school was changed from "School for Nurses" to the "School of Nursing," thereby putting more emphasis on the substance and developing discipline of nursing rather than on the nurses themselves. Second, in addition to pledging their loyalty to the school, they added "to promote the welfare of my patient and to uphold the honour of my profession," thereby acknowledging nursing's expanded responsibilities to patients and society.

In 1949, Mackenzie made major revisions in the curriculum to better integrate theory and practice. A link was made between the basic sciences, the welfare of human beings, and their relationship to the environment. Growth and development and community organization were subjects added to the curriculum followed by a clinical experience in the field of public health. Given the rise of the public health movement, more emphasis was placed on the social sciences and the emerging field of psychiatric nursing. In 1951, twelve graduate nurses and eleven selected students were given a two-month course in psychiatric nursing. Also, during the affiliation to infectious disease hospitals, students were introduced to the concept of chronic illness through the study of tuberculosis. There was less use of mannequins for simulated learning and more time spent at the bedside with greater emphasis on experiential learning and the identification and use of scientific principles underlying care practices. These curriculum changes laid the groundwork for future nursing practice developments.

An objective of Mathewson from the start was to decrease the weekly working hours of students. In 1948, this was not possible due to a significant drop in student enrolment at the MGH as well as nationally, which emphasized the nursing shortage and illustrated the continuous challenges with which the directors of nursing had to contend. Mathewson worked closely with Mackenzie to adopt other means of improving the students' work life. Drawing on Mackenzie's experiences in Great Britain, a "study day plan" was implemented that permitted students one day a week in a sixteen-week rotation to study or work in the library. If they were working nights, they were not wakened for classes, or, if they were on affiliation at another hospital, they were not required to return for lectures. Although the working hours for the students were not shortened, they were freed from attending classes on their day off. This was considered to be a major change. In 1948, the MGH Alumnae Association, which had given bursaries for graduate nurses only, now offered bursaries to student nurses. Also, the Brainerd Bursary was established in 1952 to provide for needy students.[30]

A student nurse association was also created and funded books and records to be used in leisure time. Vacation time was increased from three to four weeks in 1948, and, in 1950, the students were given one whole day off each week. Adequate space in the nurses' residence was an ongoing problem, as was the location of the school in the seedy part of downtown Montreal, which some parents considered to be a deterrent to their daughters studying at the MGH.

On 19 February 1947, Mathewson was asked to respond at the Board of Management meeting to the proposition from the Canadian Nurses Association to experiment with a new system to train nurses. This new approach, which had funds attached to it, would make the schools independent of the hospitals. She informed the board that she did not favour divorcing the nurses' training schools from larger general hospitals as the "spirit and atmosphere of the wards was conducive to better training."[31] She listed all the barriers that the hospitals would have to overcome if a change like this were to happen. Given her years of teaching at McGill, her academic preparation, the close working relationship with the university, and her awareness of the Weir Report, it was surprising that she was not willing to explore what could have been a major innovation.

So, the apprenticeship model of training continued to flourish. It relied now not only on the instructors in the classroom but also on the expertise of graduate nurses and head nurses on the wards. An ongoing concern was having enough experienced head nurses to give the students sound teaching at the bedside and to be role models for good nursing care. For example, when new services were developed, like neurology and neuro-surgery, the graduate nurses visited hospitals like the Montreal Neurological Hospital so that they could learn to care appropriately for this new patient population and help in teaching the students. Early in 1953, new MGH graduates were offered a year's rotation with salary through a series of clinical services according to the individual nurse's interest. This provided additional specialized education for the young graduate through ward conferences, readings, and a planned experience at the bedside along with some administrative work.

Nursing Service

Mathewson's first priority in 1946 was to continue to ensure the highest possible standards of patient care. To accomplish this, she developed personnel policies that would encourage a more permanent nursing staff, and she recruited more capable ward helpers who were supervised closely. In 1946–47, she increased the number of ward helpers, had the students and the graduate nursing staff temporarily work longer hours, hired married nurses on a part-time basis, and hired forty more nurses. This resulted in putting the students in bunk beds in the larger rooms. Mathewson, with board approval, increased nurses' salaries, closed whole wards in the summer months, adjusted the work space, and replaced aging equipment as best she could considering the shortage of supplies and equipment after the Second World War.[32] Since the Parker School for Trained Attendants had closed, Mathewson sought support from the directors of nursing from the other English hospitals and financial help from the MGH Board of Management to open a nurses' aide school at the Montreal Convalescent Hospital. She hired its graduates to do work that did not have to be done by nurses. It is interesting to note how systematic and contemporary her solutions were.

The number of graduate nurses doing general duty on 20 January 1947 was seventy-nine. To assist them there were 129 support staff who worked as nurses' aides, ward helpers, ward maids, and orderlies. On that same day, there were 151 students on general duty.[33] These numbers indicate that the hospital still depended heavily on the students to provide care. This was very common in the early 1950s, when it was noted that 60 percent to 80 percent of the care in hospitals in Quebec was provided by student nurses.

The ever-increasing need for space for patients, nurses, physicians, and other related facilities was great, and managing two hospital sites was increasingly problematic. Consequently, the Board of Management took the momentous decision to build a new hospital on Cedar Avenue. Planned innovations in the new hospital included wards of thirty-two to thirty-six beds in single-, double-, and four-bed combinations. This change was met with some scepticism by members of the nursing staff as they felt more confident being able to see all their patients at a glance and were concerned that this arrangement would require more nurses. A central supply department was also envisioned, which pleased the nurses greatly. When it came time to name the new nurses' residence, the nurses were consulted. The committee on nursing, after consultation with the MGH Alumnae Association and the nursing administration, recommended to the board that it be called Livingston Hall after the school's legendary founder. This decision was accepted on 17 February 1954. The original plan for Livingston Hall was reduced by one hundred rooms in 1952 due to escalating costs, but the building was erected to accommodate additional floors, which would serve the hospital well in the future.[34]

An Abrupt End ...

The health of Mathewson was never robust. In 1949, it was mentioned in her annual report that she had been off most of the year. On 13 March 1953, Mathewson died suddenly at the age of fifty-five. The hospital community and nursing staff were shocked and anxious as many changes were about to occur and her steady and decisive leadership would be missed. The former executive director of the MGH, Burnett S. Johnston, said Mathewson was "a distinguished and brilliant member of the nursing profession, a loyal and selfless women of great integrity and an educator of vision whose single purpose was the high standards of the nursing profession."

NOTES

1 H.E. MacDermot, *History of the School For Nurses of the Montreal General Hospital* (Montreal: Alumnae Association, 1940), 63.
2 A. Petite, *Les infirmières: De la vocation a la profession* (Montreal: Boreal, 1989), 193.
3 Edouard Desjardins, Suzanne Giroux, and Eileen C. Flanagan: *Heritage: History of the Nursing Profession in the Province of Quebec* (Montreal: Association of Nurses of the Province of Quebec, 1971), 86.
4 Department of Nursing, annual report, 1923, MGH Alumnae Archives.
5 Ibid., 1919–27.
6 Ibid., 1926.
7 Board of Management, minutes, 1 September 1920, MGH Archives.
8 Desjardins et al., *Heritage*, 93.
9 Ibid., 87.
10 Board of Management, minutes, 23 August 1922, MGH Archives.
11 Ibid., 5 August 1920, MGH Archives.
12 House Committee, minutes, 23 November 1921, MGH Archives.
13 Marie L. Parker, "Training Auxiliary Workers," *Canadian Nurse* (1946): 563–6.
14 Ibid.
15 Barbara L. Tunis, *In Caps and Gowns* (Montreal: McGill University Press, 1966).
16 Phyllis Read and Margaret MacLeod, "Nurses' Training at the Montreal General Hospital Forty Years Ago," an account written for the 150th Anniversary of the Hospital in 1971, MGH Alumnae Archives.

17 G.M. Weir, *Survey of Nursing Education in Canada* (Toronto: University of Toronto Press, 1932), 385–6. An extraordinarily comprehensive survey of nursing education in Canada written more than eighty years ago. Prophetic and changed nursing teaching.

18 Ibid., 380.

19 Ibid., 392.

20 Ibid. 474, 495–6, 504–6.

21 Ibid., 299–301.

22 I compared the hours per course in the curriculum at the MGH after 1941 (available through the MGH Alumnae Archives) with the standard curriculum proposed by the Canadian Nurses Association, which was published in J.M. Murray and M.S. Mathewson, *Three Centuries of Canadian Nursing* (Toronto: Macmillan, 1947), 947.

23 Committee on Nursing, minutes, 5 April 1932, MGH Alumnae Archives.

24 MGH Alumnae Association of the School of Nursing website: http://www3.sympatico.ca/mmsut.mtl.

25 Ibid.

26 Ibid.

27 Letter from Francis Upton to Mabel Holt, 19 September 1946, MGH Alumnae Archives.

28 Gibbon and Mathewson, *Three Centuries of Canadian Nursing*.

29 H.E. MacDermot, *History of the School of Nursing of the Montreal General Hospital*, rev. ed. (Montreal: Southam, 1961), 85.

30 Department of Nursing, annual report, 1952, MGH Alumnae Archives.

31 Board of Management, minutes, 19 February 1947, MGH Archives.

32 Department of Nursing, annual reports, 1946 and 1947, MGH Alumnae Archives.

33 Canadian Nurses Association Spot Survey on Nurse Patient Ratios for Bedside Care, 20 January 1947, MGH Alumnae Archives.

34 Committee of nurses, 17 February 1954, MGH Alumnae Archives.

42

Nursing Comes of Age: The MacLeod Years, 1953–74

Margaret Hooton

Hooton, a McGill nursing graduate, has been involved with the McGill School of Nursing, awarded a Distinguished Teaching Award from her alma mater, and named Grande Infirmière by the Ordre des Infirmières et Infirmiers du Québec.

As the 1950s took shape, Canada was recovering from the shock and turmoil wrought by the Second World War. The society was maturing into an industrial nation with the accompanying values and attitudes. Quebec nationalism was on the rise, with individual rights attaining more prominence, and unionism was emerging as a social force.[1] The responsibility for meeting these challenges and leading nursing through the myriad of changes at the MGH was assumed by Isobel Black MacLeod.

Isobel Black MacLeod Years, 1953–

MacLeod accepted the position of director of nursing and principal of the School of Nursing in 1953 amid some controversy. Born in Sturgeon Falls, Ontario, and after living and working in many different Canadian cities, she came to Montreal to be the director of the Victorian Order of Nurses. Her appointment as director broke a long and valued tradition as she was neither an MGH graduate nor a hospital graduate, having acquired her basic nursing education at the University of Alberta. But, like Matheson, her professional practice was in public health. As part of her conditions for accepting the position, she negotiated a leave to acquire a master's degree in nursing administration (Columbia University, 1954). Then she took the unprecedented step of getting married in 1954. Her credentials, although championed by the Board of Governors, were not unanimously endorsed by the nurses, and her appointment was met with some dismay and a degree of resistance.

Student Life, Entry to the School, and the Curriculum

Not only did the MGH acquire a new director but also, in 1954, the hospital moved into a new building on Cedar Avenue with a new residence for students. Known as Livingston Hall, the new student quarters with the accompanying amenities certainly enhanced the quality of students' living arrangements. It was fitting that the president of the MGH nursing alumnae association, Norena Mackenzie, laid the cornerstone as the alumnae had always been interested in and committed to students. Such things as the length of uniforms, make-up, jewellery, and nail polish were all scrutinized. Infractions of the codes continued to result in reprimands and, frequently, punishments. Other aspects of the student's life also monitored included curfews, study time, and conduct in the "beau" rooms. Given the responsibility students assumed for patient welfare, it was ironic that they were perceived to lack the judgement to control personal aspects of their own behaviour. Blanch Herman became associate director of nursing in charge of the residence, which meant she had the responsibility for overseeing students. Known for her strict supervision, in today's language she would probably characterize her behaviour towards students as "tough love," MacLeod's focus with students was similar to that of all the directors who preceded her. She wanted them to learn how to govern themselves. Student government had waned since the Young era, but MacLeod reenergized it and renamed it the student council. This body was responsible for addressing student issues, and, from their experience students, learned how to govern their peers. As a standing member of the "house committee," MacLeod encouraged the students to gain a perspective on each issue brought before it and assisted them in arriving at a reasonable decision. But she did become the decision maker if she deemed the issue or student behaviour to be at odds with her standards.

Ever attentive to the health of the students, MacLeod and the MGH Board of Management became concerned when several suicides occurred within the student group. In 1958, she moved quickly to address the situation with the appointment of a mental health counsellor for the students and with the formation of the MGH School Associates.[2] This latter group was a representative mix of parents of the students and administrators in the School of Nursing. Not only were the parents exposed to the aims of the educational program but they also informed the school administrators of the numerous social changes that affected their daughters' lives. The dialogue between the two groups was designed to help young women develop into responsible members of a professional community.[3]

As always, there was no lack of applicants as women continued to have limited career opportunities, but residence facilities restricted the number of admissions. Such a drawback was bothersome to hospital administrators because the number of graduates available for hire was directly linked to the number of students admitted. Whereas previous applicants had to be eighteen to be eligible for admission, seventeen and one-half became the minimum age for entry. They had to pass a physical examination, meet the academic requirements of junior matriculation with ten papers, and be interviewed by the principal of the school of nursing.[4] MacLeod considered this personal contact with the students an important way for them to meet the leader of their school and for her to glean an impression of the applicants as young women. In 1953, there were 163 students enrolled in the MGH School of Nursing, fifty-nine of whom graduated that year. In previous years two classes were admitted each year, but, beginning in 1959, admission to the school was limited to one class a year. By 1964, 133 students were admitted, resulting in a total of 340 in the program, with 109 ready for graduation.[5]

As with most curricula, revisions were made in tandem with changes in the society or the nature of health services. For many years, selected student learning experiences in neighbouring hospitals were needed. But changes in disease patterns and an increase in relevant services at the MGH altered those arrangements in such areas as infectious diseases, obstetrics, and psychiatry.[6] Within the curriculum, "social sciences and human growth and development" received more emphasis than had previously been the case.

As for nursing sciences, research was just beginning and the knowledge generated was minimal. In his analysis of the change of content in nursing curricula, Petitat mentioned that social sciences, between 1921 and 1971, had increased from 4 percent of the MGH curriculum offerings to 21 percent. During that same period the natural sciences (biological) decreased from 25 percent to 8 percent. He argued that the latter decrease was not due to an actual reduction in the biological content but, rather, to its shifting to the nursing courses. With no increase in the proportion of nursing courses in the curriculum, as they remained at 71 percent, nursing content changed to incorporate the new biomedical knowledge and treatment modalities.[7] In her overview of the school of nursing curriculum from 1956 to 1971, MacKenzie concurred with Petitat's analysis but emphasized: "it [i.e., the curriculum] did take on a more community oriented approach, began to stress the social context within which patients lived and to emphasize an individual orientation towards patients and their families.

Although head nurses had previously exercised control over the students' ward experiences, clinical teachers gradually assumed that responsibility so congruency between curriculum content, learner needs, and learning experiences was enhanced. Marilyn McQueen Dewis and Jackie Hall Shrive were two people who assumed such a role and have credited MacKenzie for their success. They also attributed much of their enjoyment on the clinical units to head nurses Joy Hackwell (MGH 1955) and Molly O'Donovan. In 1957, there were three part-time clinical instructors, but their numbers had surged to nineteen full-time equivalents by 1967, and when the school closed in 1972 there were thirty-one teachers in total.[8]

Setting the Stage for Educational Reform

Throughout the 1960s, major strides were made in reducing the amount of nursing service provided by students, and the nursing approach to patient care became more congruent with the orientation of the curriculum. Even with these changes, MacKenzie acknowledged that problems persisted when student clinical learning experiences were at odds with the demands of nursing service in the hospital. The continuing conflicts prompted her to write a letter to MacLeod complaining that the functional method of assignment for students continued on some wards. She contended that "passing linen, washing all the patients by an assigned time, taking all the patient's temperatures etc. did not reflect the concept of total patient care. Moreover, opportunities to engage in problem solving were thwarted and the extent to which independent thinking and planning could be done was restricted."[9] Much earlier in his 1954 address to the graduating class, Preston Robb had voiced his reservations regarding educational practices. He saw tension existing between demands for service and the time students require for reading, thinking, and studying.[10]

It has been mentioned that, in Quebec, students gave 60 to 80 percent of the care to patients in the 1950s. Although the MGH required less patient care from students, in 1962 it attempted to address the education/service dilemma. A proposal was made to offer most of the students academic study in two years so that they could have an internship in their third year that would focus mainly on service. In the existing curriculum, third-year students already had a "ward training" experience from which their contributions to service were costed as twenty-five graduate nurse positions at a saving of $35,920 to the hospital.[11] While the MGH was in the midst of studying this proposal, many external bodies continued to express dissatisfaction with hospital involvement in nursing education and advocated the separation of nursing schools from hospitals.

Cognizant of the dissensions and disagreements emanating from those with vested interests in nursing, the CNA launched a study to determine the educational adequacy of Canadian hospital schools of nursing. The association was interested in discovering the number of schools able to satisfy its criteria for program approval, which were stipulated in the study. The results, presented at its 1960 annual meeting, evoked an outcry both inside and outside nursing. Of the schools studied, 84 percent were deemed inadequate.[12] The MGH School of Nursing participated in the study and was one of the few to receive a favourable report. This assessment was rendered despite the criticism of the allocation of student hours on the wards, which was divided equally among days, evenings, and nights. Moreover, the report noted that the MGH had limited control over course content offered to the students during the time they spent at other institutions.[13] Given the CNA's negative report versus the MGH's favourable assessment, many more studies were undertaken before the fate of hospital schools was resolved.

Three studies by the Canadian Nurses Association in support of moving hospital programs into the mainstream of education were: the Royal Commission on Health Services, *Nursing Education in Canada*, and *A Path to Quality*. Two prominent nurse leaders had previously shared their ideas on the subject. In 1951, the dean of the Faculty of Nursing at the University of Toronto, Kathleen Russell, had said: "Nursing schools should be divorced from hospital administration and re-established as educational institutions." And the director of the McGill School for Graduate Nurses, Rae Chittick, had stated in 1960: "We cannot educate nurses the way we have in the past." She cited Cyril James, principal of McGill, as telling nursing students that "we need a different kind of nurse for the society which is emerging."[14] By 1964, it was clear that the cumulative recommendations and position statements, if adopted, would affect nursing education and service in a significant way. MacLeod asked for a summary of the main thrust of the proposals to determine the Department of Nursing's response. Essentially the studies recommended having both diploma and university basic education. Diploma education was not to be financed by hospitals. Students were to pay for their education and receive financial support through a bursary system

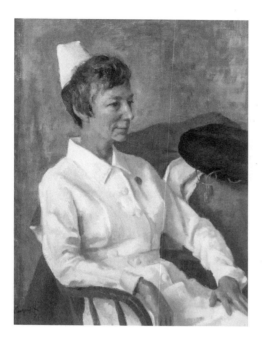

Fig. 42.1 Isobel Black MacLeod, director
of nursing and principal, MGH School
of Nursing, 1953–75

and not by the provision of service. Commenting on the summary, MacLeod
stated: "The department of nursing would study them with great delibera-
tion and would decide its own course of action based on the best interests
of the MGH."[15]

Concurrently, the Quebec government released the Parent Report, which
became the cornerstone of extensive reform in education in the province. It
endorsed a relocation of "vocational" education into a new institution for
all postsecondary school education – called College d'enseignement general
et professionnel. The authors argued that technical education was inadequately coordinated with general education and that more cultural and advanced content needed to be introduced into the program.[16]

Faced with a potentially volatile situation due to these proposals, Joan
Gilchrist, then director of nursing at the Jewish General Hospital, said action was urgently needed. Through her presidency of the CNA, MacLeod
had learned that Canadian hospital schools were not all of the same calibre
as that of the MGH and that, for the good of the profession, the status quo
was not acceptable.

Given the momentum to transform nursing education, the outcome was
inevitable. The final chapter was written when the president of the MGH
Board of Management received a telegram on 16 March 1970 from Gelinas,

deputy minister of health (Quebec), stating: "The cabinet has decided to further its policy to include nursing in the programs of the CEGEP's by extending it to Dawson and Vanier ... Consequently your school of nursing shall accept no more applicants for the first year of training in 1970/71."[17] Whereupon the president conceded that "this appears to finalize the future of our nursing school and the last graduates will leave August 1972 at which time the school will close." After eighty-two years of outstanding accomplishments, and with 4,275 graduates, the venerable school ceased to exist. Not surprisingly, unanimous approval for the decision did not exist. Even though most leaders in nursing expressed strong agreement, reaction among other interested partners was mixed. Barbara Whitley, the first female member of the MGH Board of Governors, sadly opposed the decision and said, "If a similar situation arose today I would be as opposed as ever."[18] Hospital administrators were sceptical, and MGH graduates were dismayed, saddened, and even angry. In his address to the 1967 graduates, John Hinchey admonished nursing leaders for supporting the closure of hospital schools of nursing. He contended that the same kind of nurse with which he was familiar and whose skills he had come to value would not come from the new systems.[19]

Certainly there was support for Hinchey's view that the MGH graduate was a quality nurse. Over the years they had demonstrated this as they became leaders in many different professional arenas and assumed the presidency of many professional organizations. In recognition of her many accomplishments, the only chair in nursing at McGill, the Flora Madeline Shaw Chair of Nursing, was created in her honour in 1957. As the executive director of the Association of Registered Nurses of the Province of Quebec from 1929 to 1949, E. Francis Upton (MGH 1908) strove to improve the standards for nursing education. Jennie Webster, OBE (MGH 1895), and Laura Holland, CBE, RRC, LLD (MGH 1913), were recognized by King George V in 1934. Webster was honoured for her devoted, long-standing service and her reputation as the "ideal nurse." Holland was awarded her medal for her work as a pubic health nurse in child welfare in British Columbia. F. Moyra Allen (MGH 1943), an educational expert and innovator, led the way in the development of nursing curricula and establishment of accreditation criteria at the international, national, and provincial levels. She was named an Officer of the Order of Canada in 1986. Other graduates chose to contribute at the local level. Margaret MacLeod (MGH 1930), Audrey MacKenzie Scott (MGH 1947), and Florence MacKenzie (MGH 1947) were each recognized

by the MGH with an Award of Merit and each earned her respective reputation in a different sphere of service. MacLeod, as a head nurse, worked
tirelessly to promote patient care; MacKenzie concentrated her efforts in
educational and Scott gave generously of her time and talents through her
volunteer efforts.[20] Although incomplete, this snapshot presents a picture
of the scope and nature of nursing influenced by MGH graduates. McGill
University recognized this reputation when it conferred on Isobel MacLeod
an honorary doctor of law degree in 1971. William Storrar cited that it was a
way of "honouring the Montreal General Hospital School of Nursing and its
prominence in nursing in Canada and the world."[21] Thus ended a vital era
in the history of the MGH.

Education for Nurses at the Montreal General Hospital and Links with McGill University School of Nursing

Events leading up to the educational milestone had monopolized the nursing agenda for many years, but practice issues gradually thrust themselves
into the foreground. The preparation and qualifications of head nurses
needed to be reviewed. In 1954, only 10 percent had the level of education
warranted by such an illustrious institution.[22] Moreover, more and better
prepared teachers were needed to deal with curriculum demands and the increasing number of students in the school. Emphasizing study in the fields
of teaching, supervision, and administration, MacLeod capitalized on existing bursary systems sponsored by the alumnae association and the hospital
to encourage nurses to seek advanced preparation. Between 1954 and 1968,
sixty-eight nurses each received a thousand-dollar bursary. The amount
actually increased to $1,250 per bursary in 1963. Each recipient was required
to reciprocate with one year of service. As of 1967, twenty-three of the
awardees were still on staff.[23]

As a member of the advisory committee at McGill's School for Graduate
Nurses, MacLeod established consultative links within and between the university faculty and the hospital nursing staff. Prior collaborative efforts with
Chittick had facilitated the opening of the McGill Bachelor of Science (nursing) program in 1957.[24] MacLeod provided facilities and material resources
for the students in that program and seconded them to the MGH for their
clinical learning experiences. By 1969, there were 143 university students (not
all from McGill) onsite at the MGH.[25] McGill students, in particular, were
not always received or perceived in a positive light by the MGH nurses.

McGill nursing students did acquire more legitimacy when the MGH was declared a McGill teaching institution in 1969.[26]

The MGH-McGill connection had begun with the appointment of Flora Madeline Shaw as director at McGill and strengthened over the years with many more MGH graduates joining the faculty. In 1969, McGill appointed two MGH nurses – Jane Mitchell Henderson (MGH 1957) and Marilyn McQueen, University of Toronto – as part-time lecturers to help with the clinical teaching of the McGill students.[27] From the MGH perspective, involvement with students and the university served to entice graduates to become future staff members, which many McGill graduates did.

Nurses and Unionism

But no matter how well prepared and connected nurses became, their working conditions remained an important factor in determining their performance. As MacLeod said, nurses in 1953 were usually single, lived in residence, and accepted long hours of work, split shifts, and low salaries.[28] Even the preparation of the nursing budget was the jurisdiction of the hospital administration, a condition that changed only much later in her tenure.[29] But the ANPQ forced change with its 1953 recommendation of an eight-hour a day, five-day work week. It even proposed nurses' salaries be increased by ten dollars a month, resulting in a $215-a-month salary, about which the MGH Board of Management was less than enthusiastic. If adopted, it calculated, thirty thousand dollars would be added to the year's expenses. Even though the board eventually acquiesced to the proposal, there was no ensuing rapid rise in salaries.[30] As of 1964, staff nurses still only received $325 a month and head nurses $590 a month.[31] In 1961, the Department of Nursing had grave concerns about the workload issue due to the fact that nurses worked fewer hours per week. Also, there was increased bed occupancy, longer patient stays, and more complex patient conditions. Adding to the problem was a stipulation of the Hospital and Insurance Diagnostic Services Act, 1957, that there be a professional nurse on all shifts.[32]

To cope with such demands nurses wanted to exercise more control over their professional work and its conditions. They arrived at the conclusion that unionization was the way to attain that goal. An additional impetus for unionization, other than the nurses' agenda, was the government's refusal to engage in salary discussions with other than a certified union, a condition already in existence for their francophone colleagues. Supported by the directors of the English hospitals of Montreal and the McGill School for Graduate Nurses, the nurses initiated a series of meetings, information sessions, lobbying activities, and consultations with many different people. As a result of all their efforts the United Nurses of Montreal was formed, and it was granted certification with the Quebec Labour Relations Board in 1966. This was the first step of many that led to the nurses in each anglophone hospital voting to accept the United Nurses as their bargaining unit. Next, there needed to be agreement on the issues to include in a contract proposal. Each of these steps took time and was compounded by the 1966 strike of support staff in the anglophone hospitals.[33] Therefore, it is not surprising that the first contract was not ready until 1973. Implementation of its many clauses would require several more years of negotiation.

The staff orientation clause did become problematic when the MGH School of Nursing closed. Its graduates had great familiarity with the many regulations, protocols, daily activities, and routines of the hospital and nursing department, so they required a minimum orientation when joining the staff. Margaret Suttie (MGH 1963) said that new CEGEP graduates and those from the university did not possess the same information, so a longer and more extensive orientation program was needed. Unfortunately, the hospital did not provide funding for an expanded program. With insufficient funding, it was a struggle to support the new graduates in the development of the skills and knowledge needed to adjust quickly to the hospital milieu.[34]

Although there were gains with unionization, workload and number of staff were not addressed. Perhaps that is why nurses resisted being "floated" from one unit to another in time of need. MacLeod felt that unionization may have contributed to a lack of cohesiveness in the nursing team and a diminished sense of obligation to the MGH, to one's peers, and to the patients. Suttie added that nursing administration lost some control over the allocation of its human resources as the union contract stipulated vacation time, shift assignments, and rotations. Equally problematic was the failure of the government to provide sufficient funds to meet requirements of the non-monetary clauses in the contract.[35]

Simultaneously, the Quebec Hospital Insurance Services (QHIS) was setting quotas for nursing staff in each institution and funding accordingly.[36] For instance, in 1970, the QHIS authorized a budget for 735 nurse positions at the MGH, but it already had 748 on staff. This anomaly put the MGH into deficit and exemplified the financial conflicts between hospital institutions and provincial health and welfare services.

Obviously, government incursions into the operations of nursing departments was steadily increasing and the composition of the nursing group was changing. In 1969, of the 712 on staff, 397 came from Quebec, 101 from other Canadian provinces, and 214 from other countries.[37] Diversity within the nursing group challenged traditional ways of doing things as many nurses held values different from those found among the MGH graduates. Adaptation to the changes proved to be difficult.

Shortage of Nurses and Their Effective Use

In an attempt to address the nurses' concern over "staff shortage," a refresher course was started in 1957 at the MGH to encourage nurses who had stopped working to return to their profession.[38] When the ANPQ and the Quebec Ministry of Education became involved in continuing education in 1971, the program changed and became an eight-week course with sixteen nurses in the first class at Dawson College (CEGEP). In addition, massive recruitment campaigns were conducted in other provinces, other countries, and throughout Quebec. Publicity materials were produced and distributed in an effort to attract staff.[39] Also, when the nursing assistant program at the Queen Mary Veterans Hospital closed, the ANPQ asked the MGH to start one. In 1962, a program began with Elizabeth Chalmers (MGH 1948) as its director, but later it was relocated to Rosemount High School in accordance with the 1967 Parent Report recommendations. Nurses at the MGH had welcomed the 1962 program as they felt the new assistants could provide routine care while freeing the nurse to provide more specialized aspects of care. Although feasible in theory, the rapid development of specialized medical care interfered with the nursing assistants becoming fully integrated members of the team as they did not have the knowledge to make a significant contribution to patient care.[40]

No matter how many proposals were implemented the chronic shortage of nurses persisted. In 1970, with the inception of the CEGEP program, MacLeod felt the shortage problem would be exacerbated because the hospital no longer had a graduating class each year of about 110 nurses whose preference was to remain at the MGH on staff and to stay for extended periods of time. In 1971. she said that recruitment efforts were compounded by the Quebec government's stipulation that nurses coming from outside Canada needed a working knowledge of the French language to receive a permanent licence to practise. The situation worsened as fewer nurses were graduating from the English CEGEPs than had graduated previously from all English hospitals. In 1973, there were only 269 of these graduates to supply all the English hospitals. This number did not even meet the MGH requirement of 385 new staff. In an attempt to redress this situation, the directors of nursing of the English hospitals petitioned the ANPQ to pressure the government into increasing enrolments in the CEGEPs.[41] Concurrently, the Quebec Nurses' Act was amended to legally admit men to the profession, a condition that had the potential to also augment enrolment.

Meanwhile, ways were sought to use nurses more effectively and efficiently in delivering nursing care. Earlier the Department of Nursing, when faced with a limited number of nurses, had adopted a system called "team nursing."[42] The system incorporated all of the ward staff under the rubric of a team. Nurses, students, nursing assistants, and orderlies all participated in determining care for a group of patients. Responsibility for the delivery of care was allocated to the caregiver with the skill and knowledge needed for the situation. The nurse assumed a more supervisory and leadership role. However, lack of continuity occurred because team leaders had to work on a rotational basis. Therefore, there was considerable time spent preparing nurses to assume the role of team leader and, at times, the stability of the team's functioning was absent.

Much earlier, in 1955, Mills alluded to the issue of making better use of nurses when she mentioned that secretaries, an inter-room phone system, a centralized sterilization unit, and a linen delivery system were part of the modernization processes that came with the new MGH building.[43] With nurses divested of many housekeeping chores, MacLeod continued to search for ways to make better use of the ever-increasing nursing knowledge and skill. To assist her in these endeavours she mobilized a capable and selected group of MGH graduates whom she had developed and nurtured. Cruikshank became associate director (service) with responsibility for staff. It was within this definition of her role that she became involved in the unionization process.Mary Buzzell became associate director in-service. Viola Aboud was a special assistant to the director and made the clinical arrangements for university students, while J. Henderson was assigned to special projects. Joy Hackwell resigned her position as a head nurse and became a supervisor. With the closure of the school, Margaret Suttie joined the Department of Nursing. Initially, she was responsible for special projects related to staffing and recruitment. Later she also became the first nurse to assume responsibility for the nursing budget, its development, and management.[44] That all of these assistants were "home grown" helped alleviate the suspicions and tensions that accompanied the change process. They also provided MacLeod with the inside knowledge of institutional values, culture, and vested interests to which she as an "outsider" might not be privy and which would be so important in implementing any initiatives. MacLeod consulted with Elizabeth Logan, director of nursing at McGill, and asked her to provide faculty to conduct studies on staffing patterns that could enhance nursing care. Logan concurred with MacLeod that the whole question of the utilization of nursing personnel was urgent due to the persistent shortage of nurses and, especially, of qualified nurses.[45]

To free the nurse to do nursing, more changes were made at the MGH. A six month postgraduate program in operating room nursing, led by Barbara Robinson Young (MGH 1954), was offered from 1957 to 1972. In 1968, it became a course to prepare operating room technicians who assumed many roles previously held by nurses. Also in 1968 admission of patients was centralized and delivery of narcotic drugs to the units was done on a routine basis by the pharmacy department. Other actions to further liberate the nurse included the use of audiotapes as a way of sharing patient information with their colleagues at the change of each shift, and a study was undertaken to explore the feasibility of work reorganization.[46]

MacLeod was particularly interested in the work of the head nurse and her staff. Head nurses were caught between clerical, clinical, and management demands. Assigned to examine this dilemma, J. Henderson did a preliminary study in 1966 and found the head nurse spent less than one-quarter of her day with patients but spent over one-third of it concerned with ward maintenance and procurement of supplies. Based on these findings a pilot called "Project 16" was designed to assess the potential benefits of a position of "ward manager." The study aimed to find ways to provide relief for all nurses from the overwhelming amount of clerical work. As part of the design, nursing and non-nursing functions were separated. Non-nursing activities were assigned to the ward manager, who liaised with all hospital departments, and unit secretaries who answered the telephone, filed reports, and noted when patient tests had been carried out. The site chosen for the project was 16 West, and the ward manager position was budgeted within the hospital administration system. The Donner Foundation agreed to fund the implementation phase of the project. Results of the study showed that the head nurse became more engaged in nursing care, teaching of staff increased, discussions of patient care with doctors occurred on a more consistent basis, and patient care improved.[47] Despite the outcomes, funding was not continued. Convinced the new arrangements made a positive difference in patient care, MacLeod and the Department of Nursing found a way to finance it, and eventually the ward manager position came under its jurisdiction and budget.

New Trends in Health Care and Nursing Practice

As has been mentioned, tremendous and astonishing discoveries in curative medicine and the related sciences had been made and have continued unabated. In 1971, Castonguay and Lalonde released their reports, which questioned the exclusive attention on disease and proposed a stronger health promotion orientation within a family and community context. This approach needed hospital and community cooperation.[48] Isobel MacLeod had long agreed with this focus, as demonstrated by the liaison program between VON and the MGH, which she introduced in 1954. This program, a first in Canada, helped ease the transition of patients from the hospital to the community. MacLeod maintained that the efficacy of such a program required a multidisciplinary team and active family and patient participation in planning care. The MGH program was so successful it eventually became a home care program that operated across the city. According to the recommendations of the Castonguay Report, this VON home care program was to be incorporated into the Department of Community Health, but, until that occurred, Gail Tedstone (MGH 1964) said the program came under the jurisdiction of the MGH Family Medicine Unit.[49]

Although the themes of health promotion, patient participation, and multidisciplinary collaboration began to appear in nursing practice, the continued dominance of an illness focus in hospital care made the introduction of these components a challenge. In the 1960s, the intensive care units for cardiac surgery, neurology, and general surgery were in the early stages of their development. Patient care in these units, and to a large extent on the general hospital units, focused on disease treatment and required many new technologies that nurses needed to operate and monitor in support of patient care. For these reasons nurses could easily become preoccupied with and immersed in the use of the equipment and the medical prescriptions. Despite these pressures, M. Buzzell and J. Hezekiah maintained: "Nursing in the 60's was becoming more patient centered with a focus on patient nursing needs. There were also attempts to have patients and families participate in their care. Nurses were beginning to rely less on doctor's directives as they increased their own knowledge base and nursing care plans began to have health teaching as a central component."[50]

Mildred McCann: An MGH Icon

Every era has its icons, and one remarkable person known to all personnel during this period had to be Mildred McCann (MGH 1938). A decorated Second World War veteran, she returned to the MGH and became a head nurse on 9 East in the new building. No doubt her war experiences were as important in shaping her as were her experiences as a student in the MGH School of Nursing. Known as "Miss" McCann, she ruled her domain. A strict adherent to regulations, she had an authoritarian style and rigorously monitored the "comings and goings" on her unit so that entering her territory was done with considerable trepidation. Students remember almost every word she ever spoke to them. Tedstone recalls the day she received her nursing medal, which recognized her as a nurse. When she returned to the ward with her new status, she gave her patient a narcotic for pain and he went into shock. McCann admonished her for failure to question the doctor's orders. That she deserved the reprimand Tedstone accepted, but did it have to be done on such an important day? It made her question whether she was deserving of the title "nurse." Jennifer Dymond Martin (MGH 1972) recalls the severe scolding she received from this strict "disciplinarian" for arriving on the ward without her "cap" and for daring to presume that privileges granted to graduates would apply to her. Marcia Beaulieu, a student in a graduate nursing program at McGill that did not require any prior nursing studies, said that "scepticism" was an inadequate descriptor to attach to McCann's reaction to the program and its students. Research in nursing was viewed not only with some suspicion but also with a degree of curiosity, as were the students who engaged in the process. Unable to find a title for them, she simply said, "Oh, it's you!" Regardless, she treated everyone in the same way. When patients played their radios too loudly during the compulsory afternoon rest period, she confiscated the radios. When a ward manager tried to enter her ward unnoticed, she yelled: "Why are you sneaking around, Sidel?" When new medical students arrived on her ward they were indoctrinated into the required and acceptable rules of conduct. And when she disagreed with a medical prescription for a patient, she was just as likely to have it modified or changed. Dr Hanaway recalls McCann calling him into *her* office for his indoctrination in 1960 and also telling him that the nurses were for the patients and not the doctors. However, this same woman had a humane side, as is shown by a soft, gentle smile on her face, which Tedstone observed when she found McCann standing in front of the nursery window and gazing down on the newborns. Arguably, the strict control she maintained over events and personnel on her ward were in aid of good patient care. That she accepted all kinds of students on her ward and was willing to expose the patients and herself to their behaviour had to attest to her commitment to learning. Unable to pigeonhole this formidable and dedicated woman, one can only say she was a loyal MGH graduate who devoted her entire professional life to the hospital – to our benefit.

Expanded Role of the Nurse

Cognizant of all the changes in health care and no longer preoccupied with educational responsibilities, Isobel MacLeod was prepared for Ian Henderson when he approached her for help. He wanted to replicate the multidisciplinary team approach in oncology, which had been so successful during his time at Harvard. He identified the nurse as a key member, so he needed MacLeod's help to find one for his team. Prepared to meet resistance, she amazed him when she immediately said it was what she had always wanted to develop and agreed, on the spot, to fully fund a nurse.[51]

Nancy McCormick Cunningham (MGH 1957), head nurse of the postpartum unit, and Dorothy Scott Stoutjesdyk (MGH 1959), head nurse of the nursery, said the change to integrated family maternity care was driven by families wishing to be involved in the birthing process and their newborns' care, by the changes in the nursing curriculum, and by the skill of the nurse clinicians. Implemented to help patients and families adapt the dialysis regimen to their daily patterns of living, the dialysis home care program was the second of its kind in Canada.[52] Arlene Thompson, head nurse of the unit, and Glenda Oscar, liaison nurse, were adept in helping the families learn how to work with the complex technology, measure its effectiveness in care, and make adjustments as needed.[53] Carol McCone, in the preadmission surgical clinic, helped the patients learn about their surgeries, post-operative expectations, and hospital protocols and procedures. Valerie Shannon, head nurse in the cardiac monitoring unit, developed a two-pronged rehabilitative program for patients who had experienced a major cardiac event. In addition to patients and families learning about their illness, she used her mobilization protocol in care.[54]

In the three remaining programs the nurse functioned within an interdisciplinary team. Evelyn Malowany, the nursing coordinator for psychiatry, appointed two nurses to two different teams.[55] Diane Moreau Hemmings (MGH 1966) became a member of the psychiatric consultation service and functioned in a similar way to the nurse on the oncology team. Sandra Chidoda became a member of the team in the community mental health clinic. Finally, the program in the Family Medicine Unit was a collaborative venture between the MGH Department of Nursing and the McGill School of Nursing. It was supported by research funds from the National Health Research and Development Program, with principal investigator M. Allen stipulating the approach to nursing. The nurse focused on the health status of the patient/family and complemented the physician's role in the delivery of care.[56]

MacLeod then shifted her focus to the role of the staff nurse. She formed a committee to examine the feasibility of changing the way the staff nurse practised in the hospital units. She argued that nurses had come to rely on their own judgment and creativity in determining nursing care and less on hospital policies and regulations. She maintained their role should reflect that reality and be "expanded."[57]

Finally, John Briscoe, business manager, was asked to propose a reorganization of the Department of Nursing. He recommended the creation of a business and recruitment manager. Similar to the ward manager position in Project 16, this new position divested the nurse administrators of many clerical and management activities not directly related to their professional responsibilities.

Sceptical in the beginning, nurses came to value MacLeod and her expertise. On the occasion of her resignation in 1974, Cruikshank said: "Dr MacLeod's qualities of warmth, sensitivity to human need, reliability and a deep confidence in nurses' worth, made her an example to which all could strive. MacLeod attached importance to working collaboratively with her nursing colleagues and with other members of the health team."

NOTES

1 S. Lee, *Quebec Health System: A Decade of Change in Quebec, 1967–77* (Ottawa: Canada: Institute of Public Administration of Canada, 1979), 1–5; K. Russell, "A Half Century of Progress in Nursing," *New England Journal of Medicine* 244 (1951): 1155–60; R. Chittick, "A New Nursing Program at McGill," *Nursing Alumnae Letter* 1958, 3–4, Montreal, McGill University Archives, RG 96, Montreal General Hospital (hereafter cited as McGill University Archives (MUA), RG 96); F. MacKenzie, "The Hospital School of Nursing in Canada," *Plenary Session: Education for To-day and To-morrow: Basic Programs-ICN Quadrennial Congress*, 6 June 1969, 5, MUA, RG 96.

2 Montreal General Hospital Nursing Service Committee Minutes, 24 September 1958, 92, Montreal, Alumnae Association of the Montreal General Hospital School of Nursing Archives (hereafter cited as MGH Nursing Minutes).

3 MGH Nursing Minutes, 11 February 1960, 98.

4 The Montreal General Hospital School of Nursing Calendar, 1957–59, 1-27 Montreal, Alumnae Association MGH School of Nursing Archives.

5 MGH Nursing Minutes (1953), 67; (1959), 100; (1964), 117

6 I. MacLeod, annual reports for the Montreal General Hospital Department of Nursing (1964) 57, (1969) 53, Montreal, Montreal General Hospital Archives (hereafter cited as Annual MGH Nursing Report).

7 A. Petitat, *Les infirmières: De la vocation a la profession* (Montreal: Boreal, 1989), table 5.1, 192–3.

8 Mackenzie, "Hospital School of Nursing," 7.

9 Letter from Norena MacKenzie to Isobel MacLeod, director of nursing, 27 January 1970, McGill Archives, RG 96.

10 P. Robb, "Address to Graduating Class: MGH School of Nursing," 2 June 1954, McGill Archives, RG 96.

11 MGH Nursing Minutes, 28 February 1962, 110–11.

12 Canadian Press, "Education Stressed at CNA Convention," *Montreal Star*, 27 June 1960, D2, McGill Archives, RG 96.

13 Canadian Nurses' Association, Report of Survey of Educational Programs in Nursing *ESN2051*, Canadian Nurses' Association, Ottawa, 24–29 November 1958, McGill Archives, RG 96.

14 Russell, "Half Century of Progress," 7; R. Chittick, "Inventing the Future," address to the 40th Annual Meeting of the Association of the Province of Quebec, 1960, 13, McGill Archives, RG 96.

15 Annual MGH Nursing Report, 1964, 1–2.

16 Education in Quebec before and after the Parent reform. http://www.mccord-museum.qc.ca/scripts/explore.php?lang. An excellent review of the subject.

17 Montreal General Hospital Board of Management Minutes, 15 April 1970, 62, MGH (hereafter cited as MGH Board of Management Minutes).

18 Personal communication with Barbara Whitley, 7 July 2006.

19 J. Hinchey, "A Surgeons View on Nursing Education," *Montreal General NEWS* 6, 3 (1967): 17–19

20 M. Suttie, "The Alumnae Association of the Montreal General Hospital School of Nursing 1905–2005," Alumnae Association of the MGH School of Nursing Archives, 3, 9–10.

21 W. Storrar, "Citation: Mrs. Isobel MacLeod, Honorary Doctor of Law Degree," Special Sesquicentennial Convocation, Montreal, McGill University, 1971.

22 MGH Nursing Minutes, 1954, 65.

23 Annual MGH Nursing Report, 1967, 65

24 Chittick, A new nursing program at McGill, MUA, RG 96.

25 MGH Board of Management Minutes, 8 October 1969, 34

26 Nursing Calendar, McGill University School for Graduate Nurses, 1969, 6–7.

27 Ibid., 1969–95.

28 H. Bercovitz, two interviews with Isobel MacLeod, director of nursing, MGH, 1989–90, Alumnae Association, MGH School of Nursing Archives.

29 Ibid., 8.

30 MGH Nursing Minutes, 30 January 1957, 83–4.

31 Annual MGH Nursing Report, 1969, 3.

32 Hospital Insurance and Diagnostic Services Act and Regulations, 1957, at http://en.wikipedia.org/wiki/health__insurance_diagnostic_services_act

33 J. Turner, "The Strike and the Montreal General Hospital," *Montreal General News* 6, 1 (1966): 11–12.

34 Personal communication from M. Suttie, 15 September 2006

35 Ibid.

36 Annual MGH Nursing Report," 1970, 76.

37 Ibid., 1969, 70.

38 MGH Nursing Minutes, 24 September 1958, 80.

39 Annual MGH Nursing Report, 1971, 80.

40 E. Chalmers, "The Transfer of the Hospital Schools of Nursing Assistants into the General Education System," 150th Anniversary: The MGH Department of Nursing, 1821–1971." 1971, 31-14, McGill Archives, RG 96.

41 Annual MGH Nursing Report, (1970) 78, (1971) 80, and (1973) 89.

42 E. Lambertson, Nursing Team Organization and Functioning, New York: New York Teacher's College Columbia, (1953), 12.

43 N. Mills, "A Nurse Comments," *Canadian Hospital* 32 (October 1955): 59–60.

44 Personal communication from M. Suttie, 15 September 2006.

45 E. Logan, Annual Report McGill School for Graduate Nurses, Montreal: McGill University, (1968–69), 18.

46 Annual MGH Nursing Report, 1948, 56.

47 J. Henderson, "Research in Nursing: Project 16," *Montreal General News* 8, 2 (1969): 5–7.

48 M. Lalond, Report of Royal Commission of Inquiry on health and Social Welfare: A New Perspective on the Health of Canadians, Ottawa: Government of Canada Publications, (1974).

49 G. Tedstone, "The Family Medicine Perspective," in *Recollections: A Retrospective View of Nursing Achievements at the Montreal General Hospital, 1971–96.* Montreal: Alumnae Association of the MGH School of Nursing, (1977), 60–2.

50 Personal communication from M. Buzzell and J. Hezekiah, 17 July 2006.

51 Personal communication from I. Henderson, 8 August 2006.

52 M. Lewis, *Recollections: A Retrospective View of Nursing, at the MGH, 1971–1996* (Montreal: Alumnae Association of the MGH School of Nursing, 1996), 126–9.

53 Personal communication from A. Thompson and G. Oscar, 15 August 2006.

54 V. Shannon, "The Transfer Process: An Area of Concern for the CCU Nurse," *Heart and Lung* 2, 3 (1973): 364–7.

55 Personal communication from E. Malowany, 15 December 2006.

56 M. Allen, "Nursing in the Family Practice Unit of the Montreal General Hospital," unpublished report, Montreal: McGill University School of Nursing, 1973.

57 Annual MGH Nursing Report, 1970, 76.

43

Delineating the Parameters of Professional Practice: The Taylor Years, 1975–83

Ruth Allan-Rigby

Ruth Allan-Rigby established the research unit in nursing and health care at McGill in 1976. She was a prominent nurse-educator at the MGH.

Helen Taylor, 1975–83

When Helen Taylor was appointed as director of nursing in June 1975, tradition was restored as she was an MGH graduate of 1953. She was born in Montreal and had a good command of the French language. Taylor received a diploma in teaching and supervision (1961), a bachelor of nursing (1962), and an MSc (applied) (1975), all from McGill University. Prior to her appointment, she had been a head nurse and then the director of nursing at the Sir Mortimer B. Davis-Jewish General Hospital in Montreal.

Taylor did inherit a better prepared nursing staff thanks, in part, to her predecessor, Isobel MacLeod and her colleagues, who established a generous bursary system, thus encouraging nurses to continue their studies. However, there remained debate and little consensus about what exactly constituted adequate education preparation, particularly for nursing management and clinical nursing positions. As the School of Nursing had been closed prior to Taylor's appointment, she had more time to focus on developing hospital nursing practice and fulfilling a significant role in provincial- and national-level health care organizations.

Clinical Developments

Taylor's goal for nursing practice was to maintain excellence in nursing care in spite of the complex and turbulent times. She envisioned developing the role of the nurse within the health team and encouraging a more decentralized approach to decision making. Taylor inherited the recent structural change in the Department of Nursing, as suggested by the findings of John Briscoe. The position of assistant director of nursing was continued and the daytime supervisors were replaced with three divisional nursing directors for medicine, surgery, and special services, respectively (see photo). Madeleine Cargeege replaced John Briscoe as the recruitment and business manager. The role of evening and night supervisors remained unchanged, with Barbara Zinck as assistant director (evenings) and Amelie Huber as assistant director (nights).

The senior nursing management team and Taylor held formal weekly meetings at which a range of issues were discussed, including primary nursing, various patient classification systems, and methods to evaluate the quality and consistency of nursing care.[1] These discussions resulted in a statement of nursing philosophy and major objectives for the department. The head nurses, in turn, using these departmental objectives as guidelines, set their own unit goals annually. They were used as standards of care for their units and formed the basis for staff evaluations. Similarly standard care plans were also developed for each specialty in order to facilitate the consistency and quality of care as patients were often transferred between units. Gradually these collective changes built an atmosphere of collaborative and consultative relationships as opposed to the previous supervisory ones.

Concurrently, the Department of Nursing reviewed the system of organizing patient care. Team nursing and total patient care had been practised for many years. However, many staff members and management nurses were dissatisfied with this approach since it tended to result in fragmented care, indirect communication, and lack of accountability. The primary nursing model, first implemented by Marie Manthey, had been discussed in the literature for some time.[2] This model created a system in which the primary nurses accepted responsibility and accountability for planning and managing the care of a small caseload of patients from admission to discharge. When the primary nurse was off duty, an associate primary nurse replaced her. Such a system focused on clients' needs, increased the opportunity for the development of rapport between the nurse and the patient/family, and increased continuity through their being fewer nurses, each guided by a detailed plan of care, responsible for each individual patient. This method of care delivery facilitated the decentralization of decision making to the level of the staff nurse, and, thus, one crucial component of professional practice, accountability, became an expectation for the individual nurse at the bedside.

Primary nursing was initially implemented on four units. In 1983, Helen Beath, nurse clinician medicine, conducted a comparative study on these four units to evaluate the impact of primary nursing on job satisfaction, patient satisfaction, and documentation of the nursing process in to compare the results to units without this model. Kathy Randall (interim director of nursing, 1983–85) canvassed for funds, which were finally obtained from the MGH Foundation. Two years later, Sara Frisch, the first director of the nursing research department at the MGH, analyzed the data. She concluded that primary nursing seemed to produce greater job satisfaction among the MGH nurses and to improve nursing documentation but that it had no effect on patient satisfaction.[3]

Although this new approach did support and encourage greater collaborative and decentralized decision making, it required considerable education and clarification of roles, especially in the short term. At the unit level, the medical staff had to learn to go to the primary nurse with their queries about care rather than to the head nurse. Measures were also required to support the autonomy of the primary nurse in terms of delegation and appropriate decision making. This encouraged the staff nurse to be accountable for patient care decisions as ell as more peer review. As a result, the head nurses' practice evolved to include more coaching and consultation.

Communicating this new approach to the hospital community was a major challenge and was addressed in various ways, including through articles in the *MGH News*. Marketing and communication were important areas of interest. In March 1983, the focus of the Isobel MacLeod Lecture was "marketing in the nursing profession." The public image versus the reality of nursing was explored and marketing strategies useful to nursing were discussed.[4]

One important aspect of professional practice became the ability to measure the quality of care. In 1978, Taylor employed a part-time clinician/researcher, Shirley Sultan, to implement and establish a quality assurance (QA) audit program. Sultan had graduated with a master's degree from Boston University and had acquired considerable nursing research skills. As part of her mandate she held discussions with all levels of nursing staff about the concept of quality assessment, seeking their interest and participation. Topics for the individual audits varied as the head nurses determined what was most pertinent to the improvement of nursing on their units. According to Sultan: "The goal of the nursing audit program is simply to study nursing care throughout the hospital. It is not a panacea – it is merely a tool to be used by nursing managers to provide the best possible nursing care. Looking into the future the nursing audit encourages nursing study and research"[5]

In 1973, l'Ordre des infirmiers et infirmières du Quebec (OIIQ) were required to respond to new legislation enacting a professional code that mandated the establishment of a peer review process to assure competence and quality. By 1976, professional inspection regulations were established defining the four elements of competency as knowledge, skills, attitudes, and judgment, but it would be several years before the OIIQ developed the necessary tools to carry out this evaluation. The first visit to the MGH Department of Nursing from the OIIQ was in October 1984.

The mandate for the MGH was historically the care of acutely ill patients. However, from the mid-1970s the number of elderly patients visiting the emergency department increased. Some required short-term admission but many stayed for long periods of time as no other accommodation was available. Bill 65 further reinforced this change as the government mandated that 10 percent of the bed capacity be reserved for chronically ill, long-stay patients, the majority of whom were elderly. A multidisciplinary committee was struck and a federal grant obtained to develop a motivational and recreational program for long-term institutionalized persons. With a strong impetus from nursing and the inspired direction of the head nurse, Ann Smith, an active rehabilitation unit was established.

The numerous technological advances in medicine, introduced in the 1970s, challenged and shaped the practice of nursing. The MGH Oncology Centre opened in 1975, employing three full-time nurses. Likewise a bone marrow transplantation service began in 1979, and a special isolation unit needed for this procedure was established on 17 West in 1983. This unit provided care for patients from all parts of eastern Canada. Open-heart surgery was performed more frequently, as was renal transplantation, and the home dialysis program was expanded. All these advances created a further impetus for the expanding of additional intensive care units. These appointments included a diabetes nurse consultant and an enterostomal therapy nurse consultant. This trend would evolve and develop over the next two decades.

The move towards greater ambulatory care affected bed utilization. In 1955, the bed capacity of the new hospital had been 910. By 1981, the rated number of beds had decreased to 822, with a daily average of 687.[6]

Livingston Hall, the former nurses' residence, became a centre for ambulatory care. The shift to ambulatory care provided many new nursing opportunities. Still the recruitment of nurses with the appropriate knowledge and experience was a challenge.

In response to this demand for an expanding knowledge base, nurses began to lobby for specialty certification. The CNA viewed certification as a voluntary process that confirmed that a registered nurse had demonstrated competence in a medical specialty by having met predetermined standards. Although proposed during Taylor's presidency, it was not until 1986 that the CAN designed and approved a certification program.

Problems in the recruitment of nurses was made even more challenging when legislation passed by two consecutive Quebec governments, Bill 22 (1974) under Robert Bourassa and Bill 101 (1977) under René Lévesque, required nurses to be sufficiently fluent in French to pass the professional examinations. These language rulings did alter the sources of potential nursing candidates. Subsequently, most nurses were recruited from within Quebec. The MGH, as an institution, had to obtain a certificate of francization to prove it could function in French with its employees and with outside institutions.[7] Furthermore, recruitment was negatively affected by wide differences in salaries between provinces. Taylor recalled that the average nursing salary in Quebec at that time was about half the average in Ontario. After a full-scale withdrawal of nursing services in mid-October 1975, Taylor indicated that the nurses received a retroactive settlement that many considered to be their first ever acceptable salary.

At this time there were several new trends in health care that influenced the MGH. In the area of community health, Bill 65, a product of the Castonguay-Nepveu inquiry into the organization of health and social services in Quebec,[8] resulted in the MGH being classified as a "centre for highly specialized care."

Yet the government, cognizant of the collaborative ventures undertaken at the MGH (see chapter 42), together with the onsite expertise in research and epidemiology, requested, in 1974, that the MGH develop a Départment de santé commuautaire (DSC). This would become a prototype for the government's vision of community-based primary care. Taylor and the director of the Department of Community Health, Alexander Macpherson, together hired a nursing coordinator, Lorna Davis, who participated in the planning of this new department. She was also appointed a joint faculty member at the McGill School of Nursing. All the nurses employed in the community and schools became employees of this new department. They formed the early community health outreach program as the province developed a system of local community health centres under the auspices of each DSC. This necessitated a new collaborative partnership between the hospital and the community to achieve the objectives of health promotion and disease prevention as well as to supply some primary care services. This was one of many examples of external legislation affecting the mandate of the MGH, and this shift in focus continued to evolve over the following decades.

In 1978, the MGH agreed to accept "temporary" responsibilities for providing services to the Inuit and Cree populations in northern Quebec. The Module du Nord Québécois (MNQ) was established to assure ongoing accessibility to specialized and ultra-specialized care in the south. The MNQ was requested to "provide transport, interpreters and lodging for patients and their escorts," according to Nancy Anderson, the nursing coordinator.[9] Over time, they were an important link with the northern populations, whose culture and health behaviours were well understood and actively embraced by the nurses.

A trend of increasing amounts of paperwork and over 600, 000 patient records necessitated the establishment of the computer advisory committee in 1978. This paperwork and records accounted for 10 to 15 percent of the annual budget of the MGH.[10] The committee had representation from all sections of the MGH to examine the feasibility of considering a central patient registry. The MGH and International Business Machines (IBM) implemented the first patient information system, referred to as health care systems. The system underwent evaluation and cost analysis for a period of six months. The hospital then decided to implement a new computerized registration, discharge, and transfer system for patients. According to Tom Harrison, assistant director of hospital services at that time, this system was to be the basic building block for the future expansion of computerized systems into radiology, laboratories, nursing units, hospital information systems, admission after registration, and dietary and pharmacy services.

In-Service Education

As the move towards professional practice involved life-long learning, an even greater emphasis was placed on continuing education. Taylor undertook several projects to achieve this goal. A more comprehensive central orientation program was implemented to acquaint new recruits with primary

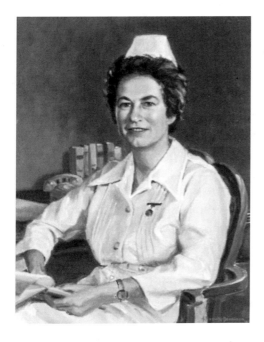

Fig. 43.1 Helen Taylor, director, MGH
Nursing, 1975–83

nursing and the expectations for practice at the MGH. The nurse clinicians
also assisted with the unit-specific orientation. In-service education was also
instrumental in developing a variety of professional programs and tools to
assist the staff nurses with practice issues. These included workshops, unit-
based programs, manuals, and standardized nursing care plans for complex
cases. Nurses were also funded to attend conferences locally and nationally and to report back to their colleagues on new developments. Through
peer education, this encouraged the application of ideas and new knowledge
to practice.

The in-service education department also coordinated the clinical experiences for nursing students from CEGEP and university programs at the
MGH. On any given day, there were between sixty and one hundred students
located on the clinical units. Several nurses in the master's program at McGill
University used data from their clinical experience at the MGH for papers
and research. A close working relationship with the various faculty members
enabled the MGH to understand more fully what the students needed and to
provide them with an enriching milieu. Furthermore, as Taylor held a joint
appointment with the McGill School of Nursing as an associate professor, and
participated in a course for nurses in the baccalaureate program, there was
close collaboration between the hospital and the university.

Meanwhile, the Isobel MacLeod Lecture, underwritten by the MGH Alumnae Association, developed into an annual event at which important nursing issues of the day were discussed. The first of these lectures addressed a very complex but highly relevant nursing challenge, that of pain management. An American nurse with much authority, Margo McCaffrey, gave the keynote address. The topic of pain management was chosen as the hospital had recently established a multidisciplinary pain clinic staffed by Ronald Melzack, Joseph Stratford, Richard Monk, and Mary-Ellen Jeans.[11] World renowned Ron Melzack participated in the successful launch of the MacLeod Lecture.

In addition, monthly grand rounds were established in 1978 to enable the discussion of professional issues and complex nursing cases. This was a useful forum in which nurses could exchange knowledge and keep up to date on the practice of nursing.

Taylor lobbied intensely for maintaining a separate nursing library, as had existed in the MGH School of Nursing under the watchful guidance of Mary C. McRae (MGH 1944). Upon McRae's retirement, Barbara Covington, a nurse who was qualified in library sciences, was appointed librarian in 1981. After the closure of the nursing school, the population using the library changed from principally student nurses to graduate nurses, educators, staff nurses, and administrators.[12] In keeping with the alumnae's tradition of supporting nurse's education, it contributed financial support to the library.

The Beginning of Nursing Research

In the early 1970s, nurses were beginning to systematically study their practice, as evidenced by their behaviour in the seven clinics during the MacLeod era. More formal studies were undertaken by Jane Henderson and M. Allen in the Family Medicine Unit, which was a collaborative effort between the MGH and McGill. These ad hoc arrangements became more formalized after Allen (MGH 1943) established the research unit in nursing and health care at McGill in 1976.[13] Nurses were asking important questions about the most effective practice on their clinical units. When the research committee was established, Mary-Ellen Jeans, administrative director of the pain centre at the MGH, became the first chair. When she resigned to become associate dean (nursing) at McGill in 1984, Margaret Suttie (MGH 1963), then nursing director for special services, became the chair.

Fiscal Restraint

According to Taylor's recollections, the ever-present cloud of fiscal restraint was a constant challenge of this era. She recalls that 10 percent, or $2 million, was removed from the budget of the Department of Nursing between 1981 and 1983. The Ministry of Health and Social Affairs notified the teaching hospitals in Quebec, half way through the fiscal year, of the requirement to cut approximately 7 percent of their budget while, as much as possible, maintaining both the volume and quality of services rendered to patients. As the Department of Nursing budget represented a large segment of the overall hospital budget, the impact was profound. The director of nursing, like her predecessor, was a member of the hospital's Board of Directors, the Budget Control Committee, the Management Committee, and the Medical Advisory Committee. As such, she had a key voice in the affairs of the hospital. All these venues were critical for the Department of Nursing operations, and Taylor took advantage of her membership to convey the impact that this cost cutting would have on the quality and organization of patient care.

This required that the hospital make difficult decisions. One decision was the closure of the obstetrical department. By 1982, it did not have a sufficient number of admissions and births to justify keeping the service. This closure displaced seventy-one staff members, many of whom had much seniority. They were able to "bump" less senior members according to the procedures outlined in the collective agreement. The resulting displacements led to many discussions among the nurses about the place and role of competency versus seniority in a changing world of specialization and the mandate of the organization to guarantee patient safety. The significant costs of retraining had not been considered in making this change. This same year a summer closure on four units was undertaken to reduce expenditures. It provided some cost savings without compromising nursing's strong and enduring stance that the established ratio of registered nurses to other nursing staff and patients must be maintained.

Influencing Nursing Nationally and Internationally

Because of her major contributions at the provincial, national and international levels, Helen Taylor was instrumental in enhancing the profession of nursing. She became president of the Association of Nurses of the Province of Quebec in 1969. She was appointed president of the Canadian Nurses' Foundation from 1973 to 1975. Taylor was the first nurse to be chair of the board of the Canadian Council on Hospital Accreditation from 1977 to 1978, and she was a respected surveyor of hospitals in that organization for over twenty years. On the international stage, from 1980 to 1984, Taylor was the first and only Canadian to head the Commonwealth Nurses Federation. This prestigious federation was founded in 1973, and it exists to influence health policy throughout the commonwealth, enhance nursing education, improve nursing standards, and strengthen nursing leadership.

From 1978 to 1980, Taylor was appointed president of the Canadian Nurses Association, a personal honour and one that gave the MGH a direct view on national nursing issues and the process of influencing health policy. The most significant priorities under review during her tenure were nursing standards, quality of nursing practice, accreditation of nursing education programs, and the development of a code of ethics.[14]

In 2003, Helen Taylor was one of twenty nurses the CNA nominated to receive the Jubilee Medal to commemorate the fiftieth anniversary of the reign of Queen Elizabeth II. All the recipients had made a significant contribution to their fellow citizens, their community, and to Canada. Taylor's tenure came to an end in 1983 when she moved to Toronto following her marriage to Malcolm Taylor, a scholar in the field of Canadian public policy.

Katherine Randall: An Influential and Respected Leader, 1983–84

Given her depth and breath of knowledge about the running of the former school and the Department of Nursing and her positive working relationships with others, it was no surprise that Katherine Randall was invited to hold the position of interim director of nursing from 1983 to 1984 after Taylor resigned. Katherine Randall was born in Ottawa in 1938 and graduated from the MGH in 1959. She obtained a diploma in public health and then completed her bachelor of science in nursing in 1967 at the University of Western Ontario. On her return to the MGH, she was clinical coordinator in the School of Nursing responsible for a group of clinical instructors. She also held a joint appointment with the McGill School of Nursing as a lecturer. Randall was well respected among nurses for her strong nursing knowledge base and people skills together with her collaborative relationships with the medical staff. She made two major decisions that would have long-term implications for the Department of Nursing. She established a committee on primary nursing to coordinate the implementation of this care delivery system throughout the nursing department. She renamed the in-service education department the staff development department and appointed Peggy Sangster, hired by Taylor in 1982, as its first director. This renaming was prompted by the changing demographics of the nursing personnel, changes in the workplace, and emerging new trends in staff development. There was also a belief that centralizing the clinicians was a more effective way of using scarce resources.

In 1981, a hospital strategic planning committee had been established. Randall, Margaret Donaldson, Margaret McNicoll, and Margaret Suttie sat on this important committee. Three years later the MGH capital campaign raised $30 million from the private sector. The fundraising was necessitated by the government's reduction and reallocation of health dollars, and it required tremendous efforts by the executives and many senior nursing managers to establish a priority list of potential hospital projects. The first phase of the implementation of priorities comprised the ambulatory care project, including outpatient services for gastro-intestinal diagnosis, a pulmonary laboratory, and a tropical disease unit. The second project of this period was major funding to the Research Institute.

After her untimely death in 1990, the main nursing conference room on the sixth floor of the hospital was renamed the Katherine Randall Conference Room in recognition of her many years of service and the high esteem in which she was held by the MGH nursing community.

Conclusion

From 1975 to 1983, the health care system was affected by the government priorities of fiscal balance, the desire to develop a system of community-based care, and technological advances. In light of this, it is remarkable that so many changes were embarked upon during Helen Taylor's tenure. The move towards primary nursing, the continued decentralization of the nursing structure, the beginning of hospital nursing research, and further specialization were her major contributions to the MGH.

NOTES

1 Personal communication with Helen Taylor, May 2006

2 M. Manthey, *The Practice of Primary Nursing*, Boston: Blackwell Scientific Publications, (1980), 1

3 S. Frisch, "Research News," *En Avant Nursing Onward* 1, 2 (1985): 3.

4 Isobel Macleod Lecture, *MGH News*, Summer 1983, 5.

5 S. Sultan, "The Nursing Audit," *Canadian Nurse* 76 (1980): 33.

6 Montreal General Hospital, annual reports, 1981–82, 9, MUA.

7 P. Boyer et al., *From Subjects to Citizens* (Ottawa: University of Ottawa Press, 2004), 168.

8 G. Blain, "The Impact of Bill 65 on Quebec Hospitals," *Canadian Hospital* 50, 1 (1973): 12–15.

9 N. Anderson, "MNQ: Fifteen Years of Change," *En Avant Nursing Onward* 11, 3 (1996): 9.

10 D. Ackman, "Computer and the Montreal General Hospital," *MGH News*, Winter 1996, 6.

11 M.E. Jeans, Joseph Stratford, P. Taenzer, Sandra LeFort, and Kitty Rowat, "The MGH Pain Centre, 1974–2000: The Contributions of Ronald Melzack," *Pain Research and Management* 5, 3 (2000): 223–7.

12 M. Lewis, *Reflections: A Retrospective View of Nursing Achievements at the MGH, 1971–1996* (Montreal: The Alumnae Association of the Montreal General Hospital School of Nursing, 1997), 126–9.

13 School of Nursing, annual report, 1977, McGill University, MGH Alumnae Archives.

14 Ibid., 1978, 12.

44

The Shannon Years, 1984–98: The Evolution of the Discipline of Nursing in a University Teaching Hospital

Paula (Urch) Dembeck

Dembeck is a long-time staff member and one-time director of MGH Nursing.

Valerie Shannon was appointed director of nursing in 1984. Like Isobel MacLeod, she was not an MGH graduate, but, like Helen Taylor, she had extensive hospital experience. She obtained a BSc(N) from McGill (1970) and a master's of science in Nursing (MSN) from the University of British Columbia (1976). In addition, during her years as director at the MGH, she became a fellow in the Johnson and Johnson/Wharton Program for Nurse Executives at the University of Pennsylvania. Prior to her appointment, Shannon had experience in England as a staff nurse and in Canada as a staff nurse, head nurse, and director of surgical nursing. She also held a joint appointment in the McGill School of Nursing.

Nursing Practice

Although the search for efficiency was a factor in fuelling many changes, providing a supportive context for the evolution of nursing practice was the primary goal. Leadership required not only choosing the right thing to do but also choosing the right time to do it.[1] The timing of each of these changes was critical, and Shannon wisely spread them over time as staff knowledge, skills, and confidence grew. For these practice and role changes to be fully realized, legislative as well as system orientation changes were required.

Shannon continued the development of primary nursing begun by Helen Taylor and her colleagues. During the 1980s, nursing directors Margaret Donaldson (MGH), Linda Stephens, Paula (Urch) Dembeck (MGH), and Katherine Randall (MGH) worked with the nurse managers to consolidate this delivery system on all the nursing units. To facilitate the process, a primary nursing advisory committee was appointed to define the key concepts, clarify roles and responsibilities, and provide the required support.[2] Nurses became more independent in clinical decision making and accepted accountability for planning and evaluating care for a group of patients. Nurse managers stepped back from their role as primary clinical decision makers. To support the changing roles, relationships, and care processes, new documentation tools were developed, which incorporated elements of functional assessment, charting by exception, and focused charting. Implemented in 1994, these changes required legal advice, interdepartmental collaboration, and hours of training, but they proved to be an efficient way to communicate.[3]

The next step in the process was the closure of the remaining nursing supervisor positions and the creation of a nursing resource manager position on evenings, nights, and around the clock on weekends. The emphasis changed from supervising care to providing staff support, coordinating overall activity in the hospital, and collaborating with medical staff over placement of patients admitted from the emergency room. In addition, in 1994, the patient attendants, previously managed centrally, were allocated to individual nursing units.

An outgrowth of primary nursing was the introduction of case management. This approach, implemented with selected types of patients, built on the vision of ambulatory care outlined in the Rochon Report and Bill 120.[4] The first group of patients selected for case management required complex care, numerous caregivers, and an array of support services. A case manager coordinated care across settings and ensured collaboration among members of the care team, which now included the patient and family. Two patient groups who benefited from this approach were elderly patients with fractured hips who subsequently required fewer days in hospital, and patients with addictions who expressed greater satisfaction with care.[5]

As part of ongoing quality assurance activities begun by Taylor, staff developed new indicators, measured, and made improvements. These processes provided a foundation for the introduction of total quality management (TQM), which was implemented as a hospital-wide program. TQM was based on several assumptions: that organizational complexity requires collaborative problem solving by those who do the work, that quality is everyone's responsibility, and that organizational units must serve customers.[6] As time evolved, quality assurance activities became integrated with clinical program planning, development, and evaluation.

Bill 120 mandated another quality initiative that required all health care institutions to create a council of nurses. This new body was accountable to the Board of Directors for assessing the quality of nursing care and making recommendations about nursing policies and resources. It also advised the executive director on both the scientific and technical organization of the institution and ways to maintain standards of care.[7] When the legislation for Bill 120 was tabled, Shannon and her directors used this opportunity to explore the philosophy of shared governance. Subsequently, the department adopted a framework for the council of nurses that enabled it to proceed with fulfilling its mandate.[8] With more independence in decision making nurses gained confidence in raising and resolving their own issues and embraced their new roles in the council.

During her time, Taylor had introduced nurse consultants who worked in specialty clinics or who provided specialized nursing care or advice across the hospital. In the 1980s and 1990s, some of these consultants played important roles nationally and internationally. As nursing care and its evaluation became more complex, in 1990 Shannon introduced the clinical nurse specialist (CNS), who was a master prepared in nursing and had specialized knowledge and expertise. The nursing literature was beginning to show the impact of this role on clinical outcomes such as length of stay, complications, and the patient's ability to manage her or his illness.[9] The CNS delivered care to patients and families in select situations, provided education and consultation at the request of the primary nurse, and had defined responsibilities for research. CNS positions were created in areas or programs where nursing expertise could clearly make a difference. Margaret Eades (MGH 1967), the first MGH CNS, used her skills with patients with cancer. Later, specialists were hired to work with the elderly, those requiring palliative and critical care, victims of trauma, and those with mental health problems. With decreased time in hospital, patients and families needed support to manage their care at home. Staff nurses' took it upon themselves to help patients and families with this challenge.

As nursing knowledge grew, and staff nurses became more interested in evidence-based practice, changes were made in approaches to care. The development, testing, and use of new tools allowed nurses to better measure, manage, and control pain. Common clinical problems such as delirium and confusion were explored, resulting in improved approaches and treatment. The vision and concept of rehabilitation was expanded and incorporated into the care of those with cancer.[10] Increased knowledge of family needs and dynamics facilitated a deeper commitment and ability to include patients and families in the care process.

As patients and families became more knowledgeable and assertive about their expectations, nurses sought feedback on how care could be improved. Questionnaires and the Listen to Learn Program, which explored how elderly patients and families experienced care in hospital, helped caregivers examine their approaches.[11]

As in previous eras, the MGH Department of Nursing continued its close relationship with McGill University. Gradually, the number of MGH joint appointments with the McGill School of Nursing increased. The university also modified its structure to address the linkages between the practice and educational settings.

Addressing Challenges in Delivering Care

The shortage of nursing staff was a persistent and intractable theme throughout the history of the MGH and continued to be so through the 1980s and 1990s. Now, however, it took on a different dimension as the number of available graduates decreased due to the demographic shift to fewer young people and because nursing was less frequently chosen as a career. Also, provincial language requirements were strictly enforced and many non-Quebec graduates unable to progress sufficiently in learning French were forced to leave the province. Finally, more nurses left the profession early, driven by stress or searching for new careers, convinced that rotations and shifts were incompatible with healthy family life. To address the shortage, all members of the nursing department became actively involved. In 1987, work groups were created to discuss, question, or confirm the department's direction and to generate ideas and solutions. Recruitment efforts were once again extended to looking abroad. In an innovative approach, the Department of Nursing entered into a partnership with Concordia University to develop an English language program for francophone nurses. Ninon Yale, reporting on its success, stated that, since the inception of the program in 1988, sixty-six new nurses had joined the staff by 1992, and, of these, 77 percent were still working at the MGH. This retention rate was comparable with other graduates hired at the MGH in the same time period.[12]

From these work groups two recommendations focused on retention were implemented: the creation of a career counselling service and the development of the awards of excellence. The career counsellor helped nurses already at the MGH discuss continuing career options. Expert nurses were offered the opportunity to become prepared to work in more than one setting, which provided them with challenging and diversified experiences and at the same time increased staffing flexibility. In another staff-led initiative, awards of excellence were created to recognize nurses whose contributions to practice, education, research, and leadership were noteworthy.

Charged with the delivery of increased complex care, it became evident that nurses spent valuable time supervising the care of nursing assistants and delivering care that the nursing assistants could not legally provide themselves. On staff were approximately 150 nursing assistants, many whom were graduates from the disbanded MGH School for Nursing Assistants. Capitalizing on the experience of other hospitals that had demonstrated the positive financial and clinical impact of reducing the number of nursing assistants, Shannon received government approval to close ten positions. The remaining nursing assistants were reassigned to areas where care was less acute and more predictable. Over time, nursing assistants were replaced by nurses through a gradual process of attrition. Therese Wallace, nurse manager in psychiatry, spearheaded a project in which nursing assistants were deployed to assist in the integration of psychiatric patients into the community.

Nurturing professional practice in a unionized environment was difficult in Quebec, where relationships between the nursing unions and the provincial government had historically been antagonistic. A strike in 1975 during Taylor's period, with no provision for essential services, left nursing staff with valid concerns about the withdrawal of patient services. In 1982–83, the government bypassed the collective bargaining process in the entire health and social services sector and unilaterally rolled salaries back by twenty percent. The subsequent contract in 1986–87 failed to address the rollback, and when negotiations stalled in 1989, nurses staged an illegal five-day provincewide strike. The strike came to a sudden close with the application of Bill 160, which imposed heavy fines and loss of seniority for the union executive and those nurses who had participated in the strike. This very punitive piece of legislation generated feelings of vulnerability and anger among the nurses. Salaries continued to be a major concern, although they improved slowly but steadily. As previously mentioned, they increased from under one hundred dollars per year in the late 1800s to under nine hundred dollars in the early 1900s. The last information available in 2006 cites the salary of a beginning diploma graduate as $33,542 per year and $49,995 after twelve years and that of a beginning BSc(N) graduate as $34,450 per year and $63,459 after twelve years.[13]

Staff Development

At the MGH, nursing leaders always believed that the development of staff would advance nursing practice and improve the quality of patient and family care. Peggy Sangster, the director of staff development, and her team of nurse clinician educators (NCEs) systematically planned, implemented, and evaluated educational activities in response to identified learning needs. Using adult learning principles, they facilitated professional competency through role modelling and problem solving. Since there were only eight NCEs for nine hundred staff and thirty-two nursing units, they had to plan strategically to be available and visible. Adopting an approach pioneered by Dorothy Del Bueno at the University of Pennsylvania, they used her competency-based framework for their programs and activities.[14] They also introduced a number of educational strategies to reach staff at the MGH and, later, in the McGill hospital network by means of self-instructional learning modules, tele-medicine conferences, and journal clubs.

On the nursing units, the NCEs helped staff master technologies, carry out complex tasks, and deal with demanding interpersonal situations. Given that each NCE was responsible for more than one patient care unit, the role of the unit-based preceptor, an experienced staff nurse, was developed and introduced on many nursing units.

The nursing shortage made it difficult for staff to attend educational programs. In 1994, a learning centre close to the nursing units was created, increasing accessibility to computers and providing a quiet space for learning. Innovative methodologies such as a twenty-four-hour one-week blitz to meet CPR recertification standards reached 85 percent of the staff.

Departmental education funds, including legacies from the MGH School of Nursing, provided opportunities for nurses to attend professional meetings or to further their studies. In the early 1990s, the government provided funds for baccalaureate study and continuing education through the new collective agreements. Representatives of the nurses' union and nursing management decided jointly how the funds were to be used, a function later assumed by the nursing council. Support was also given to nurse managers. Educational sessions helped them develop and manage their budgets, understand organizational effectiveness, and develop their management and leadership skills. They were also expected to keep abreast of the knowledge in their clinical field, and many were active in the professional associations related to their clinical specialties. This expectation was modelled by Shannon, who, as nurse manager of the MGH Coronary Care Unit, was the founding chair and first president of the Canadian Coronary Care Nurses Association in 1973–74 and the first nurse named to the Board of Directors of the Canadian Heart Foundation in 1974.

The MGH continued to support the development of nursing students, making them feel welcomed and valued. Each year more than three hundred nursing students from three English CEGEPS and two universities, studying at the diploma, baccalaureate, master's, and doctoral levels, were present in the clinical setting.

From the creation of the division of staff development in 1984 until 1990, Professor Florence MacKenzie from the McGill School of Nursing acted as a consultant. As the last associate director of nursing in charge of education at the MGH School of Nursing, MacKenzie maintained her links with the hospital.

The Challenge of a Changing Health Care System

A new day surgery unit opened in 1989 and selected surgical inpatient beds were closed.[15] Similar clinical services were relocated and regrouped to streamline care, more ICU beds were created, and care for the elderly was consolidated on one large unit with a modified environment that reflected their needs. Nurses staffed a newly created preoperative test centre in expanded roles. They prepared patients and families for the surgical experience and organized for or carried out diagnostic testing and preoperative procedures. Surgical patients requiring hospitalization were admitted the same day as their surgery. By September of 1989, day surgeries had increased by 50 percent, and 43 percent of all surgeries were day procedures.[16]

The realignment affected all areas of practice, including medicine and psychiatry. Chemotherapy was administered in ambulatory clinics or in the patient's home.[17] Day treatments in other specialties were also expanded. Patients with mental health problems were quickly reintroduced to the community in programs such as the award-winning Community Link Service, a first in Montreal. Nurses provided care for this group in the community wherever these patients would meet them, thereby reducing the frequency and length of their hospitalization and improving their quality of life.

The closure of nursing units and the realignment and relocation of patients from 1990 to 1998 was a difficult feat to accomplish in a highly unionized environment. In 1990–91 alone, one hundred nurses in the surgical division were affected by what is known as the bumping process.[18] During this period, Shannon and her directors worked closely with the union to ensure safe care. Management's concern was to have patients receive knowledgeable care from nurses who had expertise, while the union's mandate was to ensure that senior nurses had the priority to choose a position wherever it existed based on their seniority and not their expertise. Much of the success in managing these opposing positions was due to the skilful work of Phyllis (James) Havercroft (MGH 1963). The process resulted in some nurses working with unfamiliar patients in different environments, and unit-based teams were disrupted. The lack of expertise and team cohesion interfered with patient care and increased the nurses' workload. Nurses felt vulnerable, frustrated, and in conflict with their professional values as their contract required them to submit to a set of rules that neither valued nor respected their expertise

The CLSCs, created in the early 1970s to deliver primary care in the community, struggled with their mandate. Concern grew throughout the province as patients continued to gain access to primary care through doctors' offices and emergency rooms rather than the CLSCs. This resulted in long waiting times, crowded conditions, and more patients staying overnight in the ERs, particularly the vulnerable elderly. In 1989, to address the situation with the elderly, the province provided funds for an assessment team at the MGH to work with this group of patients. Nurses played a pivotal role as leaders and coordinators of this team. They provided support to patients in the ER, worked with families, and mobilized community resources to support home care. In 1985, a provincial study group, La Groupe tactique d'intervention pour les problématique des urgences, was created to study and make recommendations about the deteriorating conditions in all provincial ERs. Carmen Millar of the MGH was one of its members. After the group visited the MGH in the early 1990s, measures such as an improved nurse triage process and protocols for patients presenting with common conditions were introduced to streamline care. When the MGH was designated a Level 1 trauma centre in 1992, assessment tools and guidelines for care were

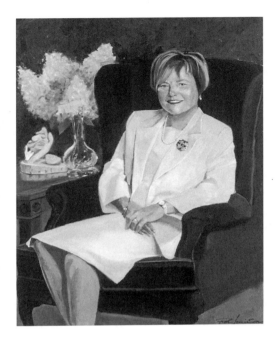

Fig. 44.1 Valerie Shannon, director
of MGH/MUHC nursing, 1984–98

created for these patients, and some of these were subsequently used in emergency rooms in other Quebec hospitals.[19]

In the MNQ, practice patterns were changing as the Inuit and Cree took charge of their health and social services in the 1990s. Physicians frequently went north to perform screening and minor procedures, although patients continued to come south for specialized care. By adopting a case management approach with the Inuit, the length of stay in the south was reduced from sixteen to twelve days, and with the Cree from thirteen to ten days. These were important accomplishments as both groups were uncomfortable away from their northern homes and care in the south was costly. In April 1995, the Cree services were completely repatriated, followed by the Inuit in January 1996.

Research

The establishment of new systems and protocols is not sufficient to improve care, and research has been acknowledged as a necessary condition for the development of knowledge. Initially, nursing projects had been carried out by researchers from other disciplines, but nurse researchers gradually assumed this responsibility. This was fuelled by the creation in 1983 of the first

Canadian ad hoc doctoral nursing program at the McGill School of Nursing and, in 1993, the funded joint doctoral nursing program between McGill and l'Université de Montréal.[20] Gradually, the number of nurses with the credentials to carry out systematic study of the discipline emerged, as did the number of clinical and academic faculty at the MGH and McGill.

With the aim of moving the research agenda forward, Valerie Shannon hired Linda Groom (MGH 1970) as a research consultant and asked her to examine how research was addressed by nursing in health institutions across Canada and on the eastern seaboard of the United States. Based on Groom's report, Shannon approached Harvey Barkun, the MGH executive director, with a proposal to establish a nursing research department and hire a recognized researcher as its director. In agreement with the proposal, Barkun acquired an annual grant of $150,000 from the MGH Foundation to fund the operations of the department. Sara Frisch, PhD, an educational psychologist with a research background in education and program evaluation, was hired as the first director. To have access to collegial support, she and Groom were both appointed as joint faculty at the McGill School of Nursing.

One of the first studies emerged from nurses' observations in the operating room. Recognizing that patients had to lie for long periods of time in one position, they questioned the effect of this practice on skin integrity. In 1989, DuPont funded a "Clinical trial on the prevalence of pressure sores among hospitalized patients." Initially, this study was conducted within the MGH and was led by Frisch, Cathy Foster, Marlene Elliott, and D. Fleiszer. In 1994, it became an external multi-site study conducted in Montreal, Hamilton, and Ottawa. The results of the study led both to changes in practice and the purchase of new equipment.

During the period between 1980 and 1996, the research committee assessed 125 nursing research proposals for ethics, scientific merit, and feasibility. The majority of proposals dealt with patient care issues such as pain management, coping, and social support. Nurse issues such as job satisfaction, worklife, and turnover were the subject of 20 percent of the proposals.[21] As Frisch said: "It is outstanding how much we got done given that we did not have PhD prepared people carrying out the activities of these roles." The number of research studies actually undertaken, as opposed to those reviewed, increased from nine in 1986 to twenty-seven in 1994. Approximately $3 million in external funds came from the Social Sciences and Humanities Research Council, the National Health and Research Program, the Conseil québécoise de la recherche social, and the DuPont Company. Internal funding came from the MGH Foundation and "seed" money from the research department itself.[22]

Many more research-related initiatives followed. The Pfizer Lectures continued but now included other activities, such as research-based clinically focused workshops and poster sessions illustrating the use of research in practice. Mary Grossman, having completed her doctoral research at the MGH, became the first nurse scientist in the Department of Nursing. MGH nurses with joint appointments attended research colloquia held at the McGill School of Nursing with others from the McGill network. And, in 1991, the MGH Nursing Research Committee published a booklet entitled *Guide to Nursing Research: The Friendly Manual for the Inquiring Mind*, a resource that was of such high quality that the CNA asked to reproduce it for its members.[23]

Frisch also continued to support and facilitate the participation of nursing staff in research activities. She scheduled workshops with nurse managers and staff nurses to help them understand the significance of research findings, their use, and their impact on care. By focusing on the study of a particular clinical issue such as the syndrome of confusion, she helped nurses examine, analyze, and discuss the relevant research studies. In addition, journal clubs and articles in *En Avant* were used to increase understanding of the research process and to discuss and disseminate research findings. As Frisch said in 1994, "The growth in formal research projects is paralleled by a growth in nurses' use of research findings, methods and approaches to enhance their daily practice."[24]

Additional evidence of the increasing credibility and importance attached to research was demonstrated by the Department of Nursing when it revised all job descriptions to include behaviours reflective of research mindedness and mandated that all new and revised policies, procedures, and patient education materials, where appropriate, reflect and document evidence from research. Nursing research continued to made great strides. Not only were studies conceived and developed by a team of researchers within the MGH, but many collaborative efforts took place with the university and its extended network.

Like Isobel MacLeod before her, Valerie Shannon was committed to the value of life-long learning. She modelled the behaviour she expected in others, continuing her own learning in administration, carrying out nursing research with her peers, writing in peer-reviewed journals, and presenting papers at provincial, national, and international conferences. She continued the tradition of linking the hospital with McGill so that nurses at the MGH and faculty at the university had new and different opportunities to learn, grow, and develop. The significance of Shannon's contribution to the MGH, McGill, and the provincial nursing network was recognized in 2005 when she was awarded the MGH Award of Merit and in 1997 when she received the Insigne de mérite from the OIIQ, the highest honour a nurse can achieve in Quebec.

Two key areas of significant progress marked the Shannon era: increased professionalization of nursing and the establishment of knowledge-based practice through research. During this period, nurses took on more independent roles in clinical decision making and developed expanded roles.

The McGill University Health Centre

The nursing community applauded the 1992 proposal for the McGill University Health Centre, and the directors of nursing from each site were involved in all steps of the process both in the hospitals and at the university. In August 1998, the hospitals were merged to create the MUHC, and, a year later, a process was put in place to select the first director of nursing, Valerie Shannon. This was a bittersweet moment as it meant that she was the last director of nursing at the MGH.

NOTES

1 Rudolph W. Giuliani, *Leadership* (New York: Miramax Books, 2002), 123.

2 Department of Nursing, annual report, 1984–85, MGH Alumnae Archives, 219.

3 Ibid., 1993–94, 284–5.

4 Quebec, Bill 120, An Act Respecting Health Services and Social Services, 1991. http://www.mss.gouv.qc.ca/sujets/organisation/sss.

5 Personal communication from Valerie Shannon, 3 February 2007.

6 Valerie Shannon, "From the Director's Desk," *En Avant Nursing Onward* 7, 4 (1992): 3.

7 K. Kenny, "The Council of Nurses," *En Avant Nursing Onward* 9, 2 (1994): 6.

8 T. Porter-O'Grady, N.D. Como, and B. Pocta, eds., *Implementing Shared Governance* (St. Louis: Mosby Year Book, 1992).

9 D. Brooten and M.D. Naylor, "Nurses Effect on Changing Patient Outcomes," *IMAGE: Journal of Nursing Scholarship* 27, 2 (1995): 95–9.

10 M. Eades, "Rehabilitation Is an Important Part of Cancer Care," *En Avant Nursing Onward* 9, 1 (1994): 9.

11 D. Mosher-Trattford, "Choosing to Listen ... the Valuable Lessons Learned," *En Avant Nursing Onward* 10, 1 (1995): 11.

12 N. Yale, "The Education Project," *En Avant Nursing Onward* 7, 1 (1992): 5.

13 The United Health Care Professionals, *History Is There to Recall What the Memory Fails to Remember*, 2006, 2. Available at www.pssu.qc.ca/pages-en/historique.php.

14 D.J. Del Bueno, F. Barker, and Christmyer, "Implementing a Competency-Based Orientation Program," *Journal of Nursing Administration* (February 1981): 24.

15 Department of Nursing, annual report, 1989–90, 278.

16 Ibid.

17 J. Constantin, "17 East Innovation Ambulatory Infusion Pump Program," *En Avant Nursing Onward* 11, 4 (1996): 2.

18 Department of Nursing, annual report, 1990–91, 276.

19 M. Antoniazzi, "A Decade of Progress in Emergency at the MGH," *En Avant Nursing Onward* 10, 2 (1995): 11.

20 Seventy-fifth anniversary of the McGill School of Nursing, "Government Funding for a Joint PhD Nursing Program between McGill University and L'Université de Montréal," 1993; *McGill School of Nursing Newsletter*, Fall 1995, 4.

21 S. Frisch, "Nursing Research: A Retrospective," in *Recollections: A Retrospective View of Nursing Achievements at the Montreal General Hospital 1971–1996*, ed. M. Lewis, 116–22 (Montreal: Alumnae Association of the MGH School of Nursing, 1997).

22 S. Frisch, "Facts and Figures: Nursing Research Projects at the MGH," *En Avant Nursing Onward* 11, 3 (1996): 17.

23 Department of Nursing, annual report, 1990–91, 310.

24 S. Frisch, "Nursing Research and Clinical Practice," *En Avant Nursing Onward* 3, 4 (1998): 1–2.

45

The Alumnae Association of the Montreal General Hospital School of Nursing

Margaret Suttie

Margaret Suttie joined MGH nursing in charge of special projects. She became responsible for nursing budgets and later chair of the Research Committee.

The Founding of the Alumnae Association

E.H. Bensley, speaking at the Alumnae Association of the Montreal General Hospital School of Nursing dinner in 1955, said: "The records of the meetings of fifty years ago clearly reveal that your founders were exceptional in their ability, their energy and their vision."[1] Clearly, the action of those few laid a solid foundation for what today is still a vibrant and active organization that continues to uphold as its object "the maintenance of the honour and character of the nursing profession, the promotion of unity, good feeling and loyalty among the members."

Since its inauguration in 1905, the players have changed, the backdrop in which the alumnae operates has varied as the decades have rolled by, and the faces of nursing and nursing education has evolved. Yet, on reading the minutes and annual reports, one can trace the thread of continuity over these one hundred plus years. Demonstrated clearly is the devotion and commitment of the members to the advancement of the nursing profession, to the welfare of the members, and to the community at large through its involvement in social, educational, political, and charitable ventures.

Inspired by the initiative of Louisa Parker (MGH 1903) and under the guidance of Nora Livingston, Louise Parker, Nora Tedford, Ina McCutcheon, Jennie Webster, Sara Young, Flora Strumm,[2] May Young, and others gathered in the boardroom to lay the foundation of what was to become known as the Alumnae Association of the Montreal General Hospital School of

Nursing. Parker became the first president and, on 17 April 1905, a letter was sent out to the graduates of the training school inviting them to join the Montreal General Hospital Nurses' Club. She had been unable to convince Livingston to have the club named after her.

Parker rented a house at 59 Park Avenue, where fourteen to sixteen nurses could be accommodated. The clubrooms were large and at the disposal of members for lectures, teas, and occasionally to entertain their friends or to enjoy the privilege of reading and writing. In addition, a sewing machine and a nursing registry were included in the five-dollar fee.[3] The club house, handsomely furnished, thanks to the good taste of Livingston and the generosity of four friends, was opened with an informal "at home" on 22 June. By 1913, however, the clubrooms were abandoned and all subsequent alumnae activities took place in the original nurses' home, the Jubilee nurses' home since 1955, in Livingston Hall.

At the fiftieth anniversary celebrations in 1955, Louise Parker spoke of her dream for the "Nurses' Club" and the early days as it evolved into the Alumnae Association. She christened the gavel, still in use today, made from the original handrail of the stairway in the 1822 building. At that time she was conferred with the title of "honorary president," a title that she held until her death in 1961.[4]

In the first few years of operation the alumnae underwent a number of changes, and finally, in January 1909, under the presidency of Flora Madeleine Shaw (MGH 1896), it adopted the name of the Alumnae Association of the Montreal General Hospital Training School for Nurses. Although some have questioned the date of origin, Norena Mackenzie (MGH 1926) put the issue to rest in 1953 when she said:

It was on the seventeenth of April 1905 that the Alumnae Association was given birth. Although a new constitution and a new name did not occur until 1907 the minutes of the meetings held between the years 1905 and 1907, reveal that, consciously or unconsciously, the object of the Nurses' Club, proclaimed in their constitution, and the efforts directed toward its realization, were those of a body of professional women with a great sense of responsibility for the future of nursing. If we accept that birthday, it is a pleasure to remind members – and the reminder implies an obligation – that the Association will celebrate its fiftieth anniversary in 1955. It is an anniversary that must receive the attention worthy of its age.[5]

And indeed, from all accounts, it was a memorable occasion.

In *Three Centuries of Canadian Nursing*, Mathewson writes: "Organization among nurses on the American continent began with the grouping of individual Training Schools in alumnae associations."[6] She credits these alumnae associations and their members with the foresight to realize that uniting together at various levels would serve to enhance the standard of nursing education and promote nursing as an honourable profession. Although the MGH alumnae was not the earliest in Canada, when it did emerge on the scene it played a significant role. In 1907, Flora Shaw, who was president, sowed the seeds for what was to be a very long and dedicated involvement of alumnae members in the formation, shaping, and evolution of nursing associations at all levels. She wrote:

> The second matter, to which I ask you to give a full measure of thought, is the question of how we may best develop in and through our Association the spirit of Professional Responsibility. That spirit which is essential to any true advancement of the profession of nursing, the promotion of which is one of the objects of this Society. That spirit whereby we realize our duties to the whole nursing body – to the state, to humanity, not merely to our own Association and School.[7]

In 1924, the Western Hospital of Montreal became the Western Division of the MGH, and the following year the School for Nurses and the Western were closed. It was believed that there would be greater strength to accomplish projects, to achieve mutual protection from adverse conditions, and to mould ideals if the two alumnae associations merged. So, in 1933, at the reception in the nurses' residence at MGH, the alumnae members of the Western were welcomed into the fold of the MGH Alumnae, with many already being fast friends as a result of their mutual experiences of the Great War.

Links to Nursing Organizations and the Community at Large

With the movement to organize a national association and in response to a request from Agnes Snively, president of the Canadian Society of Superintendents of Training Schools, the alumnae sent three delegates to Ottawa in 1909. The election of Flora Shaw as secretary treasurer of the newly formed group assured, that as an association, we were in on the early development

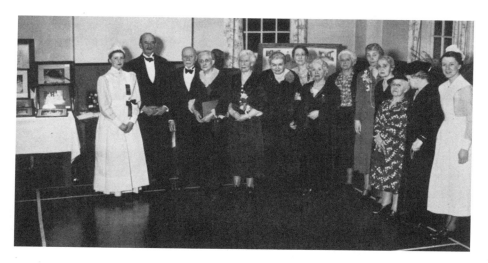

Fig. 45.1 Nursing group on the 50th anniversary of the MGH School of Nursing

of what was to later become the Canadian Nurses Association. It was the beginning of the alumnae's long involvement in nursing beyond the local scene as members, supported in part by funds from the association, then travelled across Canada and around the world to attend meetings at such organizations as the CNA and the International Council of Nursing (ICN).

In 1909, Norah Tedford (MGH 1895), chosen from the Alumnae Association and then delegated as the secretary for Canada, went to England to the Congress of the ICN. In the archives of the CNA one can find her graphic written account of the proceedings.[8] This experience was obviously something that she cherished very much. In a letter of congratulations to Mabel Holt (circa 1944) on her appearance at an international meeting, Tedford spoke of her own pride at the ICN in London in 1909. In addition to her duties as secretary she was chosen to present a bouquet of orchids and lilies-of-the-valley to Agnes Snively, president of the Canadian National Association of Trained Nurses, at the final session.[9]

Flora Madeline Shaw (MGH 1896), third president of the Alumnae Association, played a major role in the early evolution of the association and its link to the profession at large. A glimpse into her remarkable career shows that, in 1905, Nora Livingston appointed her as the instructor for probationers, the first in Canada, and that, in 1920, she became the first director of the School for Graduate Nurses at McGill. She played an active role in

provincial, national, and international nursing organizations.[10] It is no wonder that, in 1934, the Alumnae Association erected a memorial to her with
these words from the president, Frances Upton: "We trust that no nurse will
ever be permitted to graduate from this school without having learned of
Miss Shaw's contribution to the education of Canadian nurses and of her
life and leadership in this community." Today, this memorial hangs in the
entrance of Livingston Hall.

Evidence of the links previously mentioned by Mathewson between alumnae associations and developing nursing organizations can be found in the
minutes of 8 May 1914,[11] in which Georgina Colley (MGH 1895), president,
reads a request from the CNA asking the alumnae to appoint two members
to act with its committee on provincial registration. Without hesitation,
Birch and Lottie Fraser were proposed and were willing to act. Over the next
few years members of the alumnae were encouraged to support the fledgling organization then known as the Association of Registered Nurses of the
Province of Quebec ARNPQ). It is with pride that we can say that many presidents came from our ranks: Flora Madeline Shaw, Caroline V. Barrett (MGH
1915), Mabel K. Holt (MGH 1919), Margaret Wheeler (MGH 1940), and Helen
Taylor (MGH 1953), as well as countless others who served on various committees of the organization.

E. Francis Upton, AARC (MGH 1908) and eighteenth president of the
Alumnae Association (1932–35), further demonstrates the involvement and
influence that MGH graduates had on the nursing world. Upton was key in
organizing the ICN to be held in Montreal in 1929. Working with Mabel
Hersey, president of the CNA, her organizational abilities became evident,
and, in September, she assumed the office of executive secretary and official
school visitor for the ARNPQ, a post she held until her retirement in 1949.
She focused her efforts on the all-important work of raising standards of
nursing through better administration of nursing schools and more effective educational programs. As an alumnus of the School for Graduate Nurses
at McGill she also worked tirelessly to ensure the survival of the school. In
recognition of Upton, the Association of Nurses of the Province of Quebec
(ANPQ) established a relief fund for nurses in 1955. Also, to perpetuate her
memory, and that of Hersey, the alumnae associations of the MGH and the
RVH schools of nursing donated sufficient funds to equip the ANPQ library,
which opened in 1969.

From early on, the Alumnae Association reached out beyond the boundaries of nursing to become closely allied with movements of importance to

women. One of the first organizations joined by the alumnae was the Council of Women in 1909.[12] Through this association, the Alumnae Association and its members were deeply involved with the suffrage movement. In 1935, Martha Batson (MGH 1921), president, reiterated the importance of that link as "it has brought us in to close contact with movements of importance to women – useful work which is being accomplished by women for the good of society."[13] This valuable link continues into the twenty-first century.

Benefits of the Alumnae Association

Long before the days of hospital insurance, permanent nursing positions, and fringe benefits, the Alumnae Association made it a priority to provide for its members if ill or disabled. The formation of the Sick Benefit Fund, which later became the Mutual Benefit Association, owes much to the creativity and hard work of Nora Tedford, one of the original founders of the association and the first graduate in charge of the operating room. She established the Sick Benefit Fund and, with Henrietta Dunlop (Class 1893), the first treasurer, saw that funds were raised and that the early terms were negotiated, laying the foundation of an association that served the members at home and in the hospital until it was closed in 1996.

In addition to the monetary benefits and assistance that a member could acquire through the mutual benefits, a sick visiting committee was also in operation. In 1923 it was reported that flowers were sent to seventeen nurses and that ninety-one visits were made.[14] An interesting note in 1931, without explanation, that flowers would be sent only after the member had been in hospital for one week – a sign perhaps of the economic depression. Today, members who are shut in, ill in hospital, or at home are visited by alumnae members, with special recognition of birthdays and festive events.

Educational Programs

The programs run in conjunction with the regular meetings of the Alumnae Association were not always limited to professional issues but, indeed, broadened to include literature as well as social and political issues. From *Rights of Children Born and Unborn* (1913) to *The Canadian Patriotic Society* (1919), from Charles Kingsley's *Water Babies* (1914) to *Mussollni* (1927), and from *Mr. Punch and His Merry Men* (1923) to *Preservation of Quilts* (2003),[15] the planning committee ensured that the members had a broad spectrum of current issues to digest as well as the latest trends in medicine and nursing.

In the early days, most of the meetings seemed to be held in the comfortable rooms of the nurses' residence, where, after a pleasant evening, tea was served. On 11 May 1915, thirty-two members attended the meeting held in the surgical theatre of the MGH, where, prior to observing E.M. Eberts perform two surgeries, they approved the minutes of the last meeting and passed a resolution to send a note of sympathy to the president of the board, Sir Montogue Allan on the loss of his daughters aboard the *Lusitania*. Eberts then operated under local anaesthesia an excision of rib for drainage of empyema.

His second patient was a chronic tuberculosis case on whom he produced an artificial pneumothorax by injecting nitrogen gas into the pleural cavity, thus putting the lung at rest and giving it a chance to heal. Eberts also demonstrated the apparatus for intravenous anaesthesia, for intratracheal anaesthesia and the thermos bottle with attachments used for subcutaneous saline injections.[16] The secretary, not named, ends the meeting with "Tea was served afterwards in the Nurses' home with the meeting adjourned."

One gets the feeling that "the show must go on" was a motto by which the alumnae lived and died. However, in September 1916, educational programs at the meetings were suspended. According to the members: "It was an imposition to ask the doctors who are already overworked to address the meetings during this time of war. Miss Dunlop moved that instead of addresses the meetings that year should take up Red Cross work."[17] This motion was passed with hearty approval, and so for many months to come the click of knitting needles could be heard.

Support for the Education of Nurses

Bazaars and bridge parties gave way to a "weighing party" in 1925 as means to raising funds. And a success it was, as $650 was raised to send Winnifred Cooke (MGH 1924) off to McGill, inaugurating the first scholarship of many given by the alumnae for postgraduates studies.[18] Through fundraising activities, endowments, and wise investments, the Alumnae Association has supported the education of countless undergraduates and graduates.

Following the closure of the school in 1972, the tradition of supporting nurses' education carried on, as did financial support for nursing research and the nursing library. Today, funds continue to be made available for continuing education and studies at the postgraduate level for MGH alumnae members, and the same is true regarding assistance to the sons and daughters of those members who are pursuing careers in nursing. On a broader scale, the association offers scholarships to nursing students enrolled at McGill and in the CEGEPs. In 2004, it named one of the scholarships given to the School of Nursing at McGill in honour of Florence MacKenzie (MGH 1947), recognizing her contribution as the associate director of nursing education in the School of Nursing at the MGH prior to its closure, her subsequent appointment to the faculty of the School of Nursing at McGill, her dedicated work as chair of the Bursary Fund of the Alumnae, and her untiring support of the Alumnae Association and its work.[19]

The Alumnae Dinners

Entertaining the new graduates was a tradition that began early in the history of the Alumnae Association. Beginning in 1908, the new graduates were entertained in the Governors Hall,[20] then, in 1912, they were given a Valentine's party.[21] Shortly thereafter, a dinner to honour the graduates became an annual event. Prior to the closing of the school in 1972, many illustrious guest speakers graced the dais at the Ritz Carleton. And, although it was an event for MGH graduates, tradition was put aside when it came time to honour or recognize others: all the head nurses were invited in 1973 in recognition of their important contribution to the education of the students over the years, and, in 1982, on the tenth anniversary of the closing of the school, teachers who had by then scattered across the country gathered for a reunion. What a delight in 2003, when Edith Boyd Crawford and Isabel Tanner Bell, both from the Class of 1933 and celebrating their seventieth reunion, came to the annual dinner. The applause was overwhelming when they accepted bouquets of flowers, signifying an outstanding occasion.[22]

Although there are no new graduates today, the dinner lives on and serves to strengthen the bond established over those three years of living in almost convent-like conditions. A visit on the first Friday in May to the lounge in Livingston Hall or to the evening dinner will require earplugs. Screams and screeches of joy and surprise fill the air: "Mary, is that really you?" or "Janie, you haven't changed one little bit!" can be heard over the babble. Time does not seem to diminish the camaraderie and friendship that was established so many years ago, despite the various paths that each has taken from that glorious day when a medal was pinned onto the graduate uniform and the register was signed in the presence of the director of nursing. A nurse at last!

Welcomed into the fold of the Alumnae Association were nurses, although not graduates of the School of Nursing, who worked with and embraced the association's values. The first honorary president was Nora Livingston, and, among those who were conferred the title of "honorary member," were the three more recent MGH directors of nursing – Isobel MacLeod, Valerie Shannon, and Ann Lynch.

Recognition of Accomplishments

To this day, the Alumnae Association supports the Awards of Excellence in the Department of Nursing. Since its inauguration in May 1989, the recipients of these awards have been invited to the annual dinner as guests of honour. The winners, most of whom graduated after 1972 and have never experienced the "joy" of living in a residential setting for three years, are so incredibly amazed at the obvious display of warmth and pleasure at meeting old friends as well as the loyalty demonstrated to the school and the Alumnae Association.[23]

Just as the fiftieth anniversary of the founding of the Alumnae Association was feted in 1955, so the one hundredth anniversary was recognized in May 2005. The past presidents were invited as guests, and, as a means of sharing our history, we commissioned the building of a display cabinet that stands proudly in the sixth-floor corridor of Livingston Hall, sometimes known as Peacock Alley. Sharing our past with today we exhibit, on a rotating basis, the uniforms of yesteryear, books written by alumnae members, quilts made of the pink and blue monogram uniform material, as well as many other precious pieces of memorabilia.

The sense of loyalty to the school and the alumnae as well as a desire to recognize the accomplishments of the association's members has been illustrated many times over the years. Various funds were established in recognition of outstanding alumnae and were most often used to assist in the education of nurses. Endowments such as that from the estate of Helen McMurrich, Croix de Guerre (MGH 1908), contributed greatly to the work that the Mutual Benefit Association was able to do for sick and disabled nurses.[24] The alumnae contributed towards the building of a memorial to nursing sisters who lost their lives in the Great War, which was unveiled in 1925 in the National Hall of Fame in the Parliament buildings in Ottawa.

For some, such as Jennie Webster, OBE (MGH 1895), and Laura Holland, CBE, RRC, LLD (MGH 1913), recognition came from King George in 1934. Webster's fame as the "ideal nurse" had spread around the world, and Holland was recognized for her work as a public health nurse in child welfare in British Columbia.[25]

Closer to home, Margaret MacLeod (MGH 1930), Audrey MacKenzie Scott (MGH 1947), and Florence MacKenzie (MGH 1947), all active members of the Alumnae Association, were recognized for their contributions to the MGH with the hospital Award of Merit.

Following the completion of her doctorate at Stanford University, Moyra Allen (MGH 1943) made a name for herself in the field of nursing education. As a professor at McGill, her work and research centred primarily around curriculum development in nursing education and, in later years, the study of how nurses could practise in an expanded role. According to Marie-France Thibadeau, dean of nursing at the University of Montreal, she was a "visionary" who not only had an impact on nursing here in Canada but also around the world. To name but a few of her accomplishments, she initiated *Nursing Papers*, Canada's only nursing research journal; played a significant role in the development of the research unit in nursing and health care at the School of Nursing at McGill; was the first president of United Nurses of Montreal; developed a model for the "evaluation of education programs in nursing," and co-chaired a committee to establish a PhD program co-jointly with the University of Montreal. The scope of her influence can be measured in the many awards that were accorded her during her illustrious career: L'insigne du Merite, from the Order of Nurses of the Province of Quebec; honorary doctorates from both the University of Montreal and McMaster; the Order of Canada; the Canadian Nurses Association Award; and professor emeritus at McGill University.[26]

Keeping in Touch

The monthly meetings held in Montreal and the annual dinners were only two of the ways in which the members of this elite group kept in touch. Little is recorded of early communications, but it was evident that graduates who had moved away from Montreal or who were not actively nursing paid dues to the Alumnae Association and received news from home. Shaw writes in the 1907-08 Annual Report: "Our absent members appreciate keenly the letters of the Corresponding Secretary being very grateful for any news of their old acquaintances and The Montreal General Hospital." By 1959, there is mention of an Ottawa branch that was two years old, and it was the first of many to come in various parts of the country. A need for news and information that did not belong in the annual report sparked the first newsletter to members in 1959. For a time, alumnae news was incorporated into the *Hospital Bulletin*, but today members, who are spread far and wide, can look forward to the newsletter – "a thread of continuity" published every spring – or they can tune into the alumnae's own website.

Helping Others

One of the things that stands out when reading the annual reports is the generosity, not only in terms of time but also in terms of financial support, that members of the alumnae directed towards a variety of worthwhile causes in the community. It is of particular significance in the first fifty years of the organization when one considers the long hours that the early nurses worked and the less than generous salaries that they earned. The list is endless. Among these many notable projects are: the prisoners of war fund of the IODE in the First World War; support, over many years, for a bed and cot for a mother and child in Canada Hospital in Nasak, India, in memory of Sarah Young; Indian missions, the Spitfire fund, and mobile canteens in the Second World War; a fifteen-thousand-dollar contribution to the joint hospital fund in 1950; and monies for the countless number of socks and scarves knitted by members during wartime. More recently, the association has supported the following endeavours: a hospital bed for Fulford House, a senior's residence; the creation and printing of brochures advising oncology patients on exercise as well as posters relating to hand washing; support for educational conferences on a palliative care unit and the purchase of a "physicians pack" for a community in Kenya. And these only scratch the surface of the contributions made by the Alumnae Association.[27]

Ties with the Past

Our history lives on in many ways. Thanks to the work of Blanche Herman, RRC, MID (MGH 1925), Betty Chalmers (MGH 1948), Phyllis Macdonald (MGH 1951), and countless others, some of our early photographs and memorabilia were catalogued and given to the McGill University Archives for safekeeping. In 1940, at the fiftieth anniversary of the founding of the School of

Nursing, H.E. MacDermot was commissioned to write *History of the School of Nursing of the Montreal General Hospital*,[28] or "the pink book," as it is more affectionately known. It offers a lively account of the early challenges of nurses at the MGH throughout the years, with many amusing and interesting anecdotes about our founders as well as the letters from Livingston to her sisters Gracie and Alice, while travelling on the continent. Updated in 1972, following the closure of the school, there is a complete listing of all 4,225 nurses who graduated between 1891 and 1972.[29]

We have much in our past to cherish, and luckily people like to share their memories. Recently, the Ottawa branch of the Alumnae Association published a booklet called *MGH Memories, a Collection*, with many interesting and amusing anecdotes from members.[30] Members and their families continue to send us memorabilia, photographs, and trinkets relating to their special days at the MGH. Each one helps to piece together a small part of our history. Some early photographs, those taken by the Notman Studio, are housed at the McCord Museum, while other memorabilia can be found at the Museum of Civilization in Hull. Recently, we were asked to participate in a project undertaken by Christina Bates of the Museum of Civilization regarding the history of nursing uniforms, giving us an opportunity to showcase our collection.

Walking the halls of the MGH, particularly Livingston Hall, is a trip down memory lane. The name itself conjures up the very beginning of the School of Nursing. With plans under way for the "new" MGH in 1954, the board had decided that the custom of naming wings after distinguished individuals would be discontinued. However, the nurses had recommended that the residence and school be named after Nora Livingston. Arthur Westbury, executive director of the hospital, consulted with the alumnae, and, in the 17 February 1954 minutes of the Executive Committee, we find the following statement by Norena Mackenzie: "the Committee agreed that the name Livingston Hall was quite appropriate. There would never be any doubt as to the Livingston we are immortalizing."[31] On 29 May 1954, Mackenzie, president of the Alumnae, laid the cornerstone for the new nurses' residence – Livingston Hall.

Proudly hanging on the walls entering Livingston Hall are two memorials erected by the Alumnae Association to pay tribute to the MGH graduates who served in both world wars. On the invitation to the unveiling of the Second World War memorial on 3 March 1958, guests were invited to an evening affair and were asked to wear afternoon dress and medals.[32] The alumnae also saw fit to erect a tablet commemorating the loss of Margaret Jane Fortescue (MGH 1905) and Gladys Irene Sare (MGH 1913), who, along with twelve other nursing sisters, lost their lives when the *Llandovery Castle* was torpedoed on 22 June 1918.

In more recent times, on the occasion of the one hundredth anniversary of the founding of the School of Nursing, the Alumnae Association, in partnership with the Department of Nursing, mounted a collage of photos depicting the early days at the MGH. Following the death of Katherine Randall (MGH 1959), a former acting director of nursing (1983–84), and under the auspices of the association and the Department of Nursing, a conference room was named in her memory. On the walls hang photographs of graduates over the years, from the first class in 1891 to the grand finale, the graduation exercises at Place des Arts for the Class of 1972.

Conclusion

Membership in the alumnae has had its peaks and valleys. From the early tightly knit group mainly centred in Montreal, through the times when nurses were very mobile, to the closure of the school, there have been great fluctuations in the number of members. The focus of the organization has never changed or wavered, but the ways in which these goals are realized today have altered. The home base in Montreal, small in numbers, keeps the home fires burning, along with the branches across the country. Numbers may be small but enthusiasm is still very evident.

The accomplishments and the impact of the Alumnae Association cannot be summed up in a few words. Some outcomes and benefits are more obvious than others. Less evident are the skills that nurses acquired, whether officers of the association or not – skills that were valuable at work, at home, or in the community while caring for patients and leading and educating others. Within its framework the association provided many opportunities to gain familiarity with parliamentary procedures, skill at minute taking and report writing, the ability to manage of finances as well as to develop organizational skills, an understanding of and a chance to help those less fortunate, and opportunities for expressing ideas in many different fora.

More obvious accomplishments of the Alumnae Association of the MGH School of Nursing might include its promotion of collegiality, its continued commitment to life-long learning, its concern for its members, and its involvement in the issues of the day as well as its considerable contribution to individuals and charitable organizations.

But the association is a lot more than that. It was and is the collective work of many creative and dedicated individuals – too many to name here. Some have received public recognition for their achievements. But most have been quietly acknowledged by colleagues, friends, and themselves for a job well done. This chapter only touches the surface of such a rich history, and it salutes all members of the Alumnae Association of MGH School of Nursing, who, from 1905 to the present day, have indeed made an immeasurable contribution to nursing and society at home and abroad.

NOTES

1 E.H. Bensley, "The Alumnae Association of the Montreal General Hospital," *Montreal General Hospital Bulletin* 2, 7 (1955): 25.

2 H.E. MacDermot, *History of the School of Nursing of the Montreal General Hospital* (Montreal: Southern Printing Co., 1961), 56–8, 122–4.

3 Letter to graduates, 1905, MUA, RG 96, box 421, file 643.

4 Louise Parker, "Address to 50th anniversary dinner," 1955, AAMGHSN, MUA, RG 96, box 429, file 727.

5 AAMGHSN, annual reports, 1905–2005, MGH Alumnae Archives.

6 J.M. Murray and M.S. Mathewson, *Three Centuries of Canadian Nursing* (Toronto: Macmillan, 1947), 355.

7 Ibid.

8 Norah Tedford, *A Brief History of Canadian Nurses Association* (Winnipeg: Saturday Post printers, 1929).

9 Letter, 1945, MUA, RG 96, box 423, file 681.

10 M. Batson, I. Welling, and A. Slattery, *Pioneers of Nursing in Canada* (Montreal: Gazette Printing Company Ltd., 1929).

11 AAMGHSN, minutes, 8 May 1914, 51, MGH Alumnae Archives.

12 AAMGHSN, annual reports, 1905–2005.

13 Ibid.

14 Ibid.

15 AAMGHSN, minutes, 11 May 1915, 107, MGH Alumnae Archives.

16 Ibid., 8 September 1916, 139.

17 AAMGHSN, Annual Reports, 1905–2005.

18 Ibid.

19 Ibid.

20 Ibid.

21 AAMGHSN, newsletter, 2004, MGH Alumnae Archives.

22 Helen Beath, "Awards of Excellence," *En Avant Nursing Onward* 7, 3 (1992): 8.

23 AAMGHSN, Annual reports, 1905–2005.

24 Ibid.

25 Marie-France Thibadeau, presentation for honorary doctorate, 1990, University of Montreal.

26 AAMGHSN, Annual Reports, 1905–2005.

27 H.E. MacDermot, *History of the School of Nursing of the Montreal General Hospital* (Montreal: Southam Printing Co., 1961).

28 MacDermot, *School of Nursing* (update, 1972).

29 Ottawa Branch of the MGH Alumnae Association, *MGH Memories: A Collection* (Ottawa: MGH Alumnae Association, 2005).

30 AAMGHSN, minutes, Executive Committee, 1954, MGH Alumnae Archives.

31 AAMGHSN, invitation, 1958, MGH Alumnae Archives.

SECTION 6

Additional MGH Items

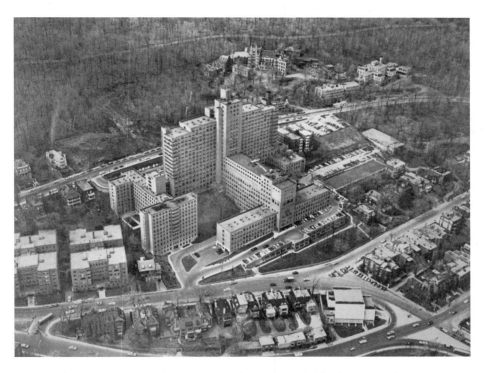

S.6 1955 MGH from Pine Ave. showing the Children's Memorial
and Shriners in the background

46

The MGH Foundation

Ronald W. Collett

Ron Collett is the first president of the MGH Foundation. He has overseen its development as the major fund-raiser for the hospital from its inception to the present day.

This is the story of the Montreal General Hospital Foundation told from the
perspective of the president who arrived on the scene on 1 January 1990. The
story of the MGH Foundation is one of foresight, perseverance, and fundraising success in a changing environment for medical care, research, and
fundraising, with an emphasis on governance.

The MGH Foundation was established in 1973 with the foresight and leadership of Melvyn G. Angus and his confreres, F.S. Capon, C.F. Carsley, T.M.
Galt, Hon. G.M. Hyde, Peter Kilburn, Campbell W. Leach, A.D. Nesbitt, C.H.
Peters, J.W. Tait, C.W. Webster, and H. Rocke Robertson. While Canada benefits from a publicly financed health care system, these leaders recognized
that the MGH and its patients could benefit from private-sector support that
would allow the hospital to be on the cutting edge of medical care teaching
and research.

The MGH Foundation undertook a successful capital campaign, but it
was not until 1989, under the chairship of the late Don Wells, that the determination was made to build a full-fledged, modern, professionally led foundation. Three visionary board members – Chair Don Wells, Chair elect Eric
Molson, and senior board member Robert Swidler – took on the responsibility to recruit a president to lead the foundation. Bob Swidler found a
prospect for president in Halifax, a Winnipeg lad, Ronald William Collett,
who had helped establish and was at the helm of the IWK Children's Hospital Foundation. Bob Swidler, a leader in his field of executive search, then

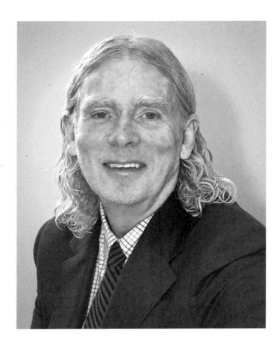

Fig. 46.1 Ron Collett, president,
MGH Foundation, 1990–2014

as today, sensed how well the aspirations of the MGH Foundation and the
future president, Ronald Collett, could meld.

Don Wells, in meetings both in Halifax and Montreal, was a strong
advocate for the MGH Foundation and its potential. However, it was Eric
Molson, the chair elect, with his modesty, love for "the General," and quiet
determination, who convinced the future president to join him, Don, Bob,
and other members of the board to build the best possible health care
foundation. Today the MGH Foundation is proud to have as a Director Eric's
son, Andrew Molson, the seventh generation of Molsons to be associated
with and serve the MGH. Indeed, through the Molson family, the MGH
Foundation is connected to the founding of the MGH in 1821.

Arriving on 1 January 1990, priorities and challenges for the president and
foundation were many, but it was decided to tackle governance and fundraising in tandem. For many years, governors of the foundation, who comprise
its membership, were committed donors who contributed twenty-five dollars per year to it. In consultation with existing governors, and to meet the
fundraising needs of a leading academic health care institution, it was determined that the governors of the MGH Foundation would be those contributing $250 per year or more annually. Existing governors and new donors

responded with enthusiasm and support. Today, the MGH Foundation benefits from the annual support of three thousand governors.

It was determined from the outset that the board (then twenty-four members) would be responsible for policy and the president for executive and administrative decisions. The president is the chief executive officer and signing officer for the foundation. The Board of Directors meets quarterly, and the president is a full-fledged voting member of the board. Further, it was determined that the Foundation would concentrate on gifts from individuals, corporations, and foundations rather than on events.

The mission of the MGH Foundation, a founding partner of the McGill University Health Centre, is to raise funds in support of excellence in patient care, education, and research, primarily at the MGH. These funds are applied to the priority needs of the hospital and its patients, in accordance with the wishes of donors.

Over the past twenty-two years, the foundation has made possible the reconstruction to world standards of several units at the MGH, including intensive care, cardiac care, mental health care, palliative care, gastroenterology, and orthopaedics. Acquisition of advanced major equipment in these and other disciplines, such as ophthalmology, would not have been possible without the leadership support of the MGH Foundation.

In 2006, under the leadership of Jean-René Halde, the chair of the Governance and Nominating Committee, the Board of Directors embarked on a full review to ensure best governance practices. It was recommended by the Governance Committee, and adopted unanimously by the board, that board membership be reduced to twenty-one. Quorum was established at seven members. To ensure renewal, directors may serve a maximum of ten consecutive years, commencing in 2007.

The Foundation is fortunate to have had as chairs the leaders listed in table 46.1. The Governance and Nominating Committee is one of six committees of the Board of Directors, the others being fundraising, grants review, audit, investment, and human resources.

Building strong professional relationships with donors and strong stewardship of gifts are components of good governance. The funds entrusted to the MGH Foundation for endowment are managed by professional managers, with oversight by the board's Investment Committee. The Investment Committee, comprised of seven members of the board, sets investment policy and supervises the investment of the foundation's endowed funds by

Table 46.1

Melvyn G. Angus	1973–83	Brian P. Drummond	1998–2001
Herbert K. McLean	1983–84	Gail Marilees Jarislowsky	2001–03
Alexander D. Hamilton	1984–86	J. Robert Swidler	2003–05
Donald S. Wells	1986–89	Bertin F. Nadeau	2005–08
Eric H. Molson	1989–91	Michel Vennat	2008–10
Douglas T. Bourke	1991–93	Peter Coughlin	2010–12
Derek A. Price	1993–95	David L. McAusland	2012–
Peter R. O'Brien	1995–98		

seven professional investment managers. Funds are managed on a conservative basis, and the committee reviews the performance of the investment managers on a quarterly basis.

The Fundraising Committee under the leadership of long-serving board member Jonathan Birks concentrates on expanding the very successful Governor Program and on soliciting support for the Single Patient Room Sponsorship Program. Donors with a gift of seventy-five thousand dollars may sponsor rooms providing for single patient care in the redeveloped MGH. Already rooms have been converted to single patient care in palliative care, cardiac care, and the Melvyn G. Angus and the Honourable W. David Angus QC, AdE, mental health care units.

On an annual basis, the Grants Review Committee asks the Hospital for support on priority projects, equipment, and research, and makes recommendation to the Board of Directors. As part of good governance, it was determined that the Audit Committee, comprised fully of external directors, would meet twice per annum: (1) mid-fiscal year to plan the annual audit in advance of (2) meeting annually with external auditors to assess financial statements and to make recommendation for approval to the board.

The Governance Committee determined that there would be no Executive Committee, based on the belief that board members participate more fully when decisions are not taken in advance by an executive committee. The Board of Directors reports annually to the members within six months of the fiscal year end, which is 31 March. New directors are elected at this annual meeting, upon recommendation of the Governance and Nominating Committee. A concerted effort is made to renew the board with leaders from the "next generation." Governors who have supported the MGH Foundation for fifty years are designated honorary life governors and are honoured at the annual meeting. To date we have designated eighty-three honorary life governors.

The Board of Directors of the MGH Foundation is comprised of senior community leaders. Building on its formal mission, the board also assumed the mandate of leading advocate for redeveloping the MGH on it current site to ensure its continued leadership as a level 1 trauma centre.

Good governance combined with a strong board and a small dedicated team of professionals has allowed the foundation to grow and innovate. In 1989, it raised $3.7 million; in 2001, it raised $15.7 million. The foundation is extremely proud that its total annual fundraising costs are less than 8 percent, making it the leader for foundations in Canada – another important example of good governance.

The MGH Foundation is comprised of eight dedicated team members with in excess of seventy-five years of service to the foundation. With leadership from the president, the first McGill University/MGH Foundation chairs were established in 2009. These chairs greatly facilitate the ability to recruit the best and the brightest to Montreal and the MUHC. The chair and president of the foundation have a strong working relationship with the chair and director general of the MUHC, and, while the foundation is autonomous, its president and the director general of the hospital meet regularly to ensure optimum cooperation and the advancement of hospital projects.

The president also collaborates closely with the director of the Research Institute of the MUHC. Each year in October the MGH Foundation, in collaboration with the Research Institute, hosts the Annual Awards Dinner to honour and recognize the best and brightest young clinician/researcher and to present awards to assist them embark upon or advance their research careers. Good governance dictates that the awardees be selected by a scientific scholarships committee chaired by Joseph Shuster and comprised of the chiefs of most major departments. Over eighty awards, valued at more than $2.8 million, were presented in October 2012. These awards cover a wide range of clinical/research disciplines.

In 2012, Wael Hanna received the Astral Media Award. Hanna's research focuses on the improvement of the efficiency and quality of the delivery of surgical care. Valerie Panet-Raymond, who received one of the Simone and Morris Fast Awards for Oncology, has been evaluating different methods of radiation delivery to minimize toxicity in patients with central nervous system traumas. Anne Choquette, who was awarded the Eureka! Fellowship in Nursing Research, is studying how adolescents respond to returning to school after cancer treatment.

Awards amount to as much as $70,000 renewable on performance for up to three years. The average annual award is for $30,000. Benefactors who have provided endowed funding to support awards attend as special guests and are seated with the recipients. This allows donors to receive personal appreciation from the recipients of their awards and to be briefed on the awardees research.

The MGH Foundation is proud of its role in helping to establish, within itself, the Saku Koivu Foundation and the Max Pacioretty Foundation. Saku and his foundation, in partnership with the MGH Foundation, helped raise over $3 million to acquire the first PET/CT in Montreal. Saku shares the following message with potential donors:

> I am proud and honoured to be a partner, personally and through the Saku Koivu Foundation, in contributing to the greatness of the Montreal General Hospital, particularly in the areas of cancer and trauma care. Like you, I know very well what a special place the MGH is and how great are its doctors, nurses and support personnel. I invite and encourage you to join with me in giving your support to the Montreal General Hospital Foundation. With thanks and best wishes, Saku Koivu.

On 10 March 2011, near centre ice at the Bell Centre, Montreal Canadiens star forward Max Pacioretty suffered a devastating concussion. Attended to immediately by team physician David Mulder, he was transported to the MGH. During his hospitalization, in appreciation for his superb care, Max committed to the president of the MGH Foundation to give back in order to benefit others.

On 7 November 2011, at a press conference chaired by Geoff Molson, president of Les Canadiens, Max, together with his wife Katia, committed to help raise $3.5 million to make possible the acquisition of an advanced functional MRI, which will ensure the MUHC's continued leadership in the research and treatment of concussions and other traumatic brain injuries. "I received great care at the Montreal General Hospital and now that I have fully recovered I want to do my share and give back," said Pacioretty. "The fact that this new MRI unit has several applications not only for athletes but for concussion patients of all ages, adult and children, is really important.

Also, members of the Canadian Armed Forces suffering Post Traumatic Stress Syndrome (PTSS), will benefit from this new equipment."

Fundraising in 2013 presents a greater challenge then it did in 1990. For example, when we undertook the Critical Needs Canvass in 1990 to support new trauma and intensive care facilities at the MGH, we were able to meet with the CEOs of most major Canadian corporations. Today companies have donations committees that are often several decision levels removed from the CEO, with many more restrictions relating to donations. Nevertheless with a dedicated fundraising team, with a strong board, and with good governance, the MGH Foundation continues to thrive as a leader in its field.

47

MGH and Les Canadiens

Douglas G. Kinnear and David S. Mulder

Doug Kinnear was team physician for Les Canadiens for thirty-five years. He was succeeded by David Mulder. Both have been on a first-name basis with a succession of players and owners.

The first Canadien hockey player who hobbled across Cabot Square to be treated at the Western Division of the MGH started a relationship with the hospital that has grown over the years. Many physicians at the MGH have participated, up to Doug Kinnear (1962–98) and Dave Mulder, who assisted the former for years was named team physician 1998. The relationship has opened all specialty care for the team at the MGH, including the Sports Medicine Department at McGill.

Many have asked how and when the current relationship between the Montreal Canadiens and the MGH developed. One must examine the history of these two great Quebec organizations for an explanation, and there are many books which chronicle both.[1] We make no attempt to duplicate this colourful history but, rather, present the salient points to supply the background for today's partnership. Pivotal to this relationship has been the influence of seven generations of the Molson family and their impact on both the Canadiens and the MGH.[2]

Who could imagine that the festive occasions of the laying of the cornerstone, 6 June 1821 and the opening date, 3 May 1822, in the rapidly growing trading centre on the St Lawrence would someday be related to the medical care of the Montreal Canadiens Hockey Club, which was to come into existence nearly one hundred years later (see chapter 2 for the early development of the MGH, the Montreal Medical Institution, and McGill's Faculty of Medicine).[3]

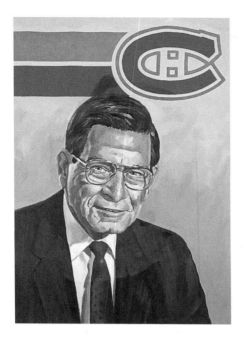
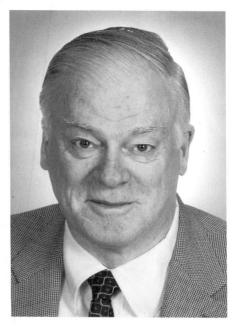

Fig. 47.1 Doug Kinnear, team physician for Les Canadiens, 1962–98
Fig. 47.2 Dave Mulder, team physician for Les Canadiens, 1998

Turning to the development of the Montreal Canadiens organization, the Montreal Forum has served as the home of the Montreal Canadiens dating back to November 1924 and extending to its closure on 11 March 1996.[4] The original forum was built in record time by the Canadian Arena Company on a city block bounded by Atwater and St Catherine Streets (previously the locale for a roller skating arena called the Forum. The original investors included Herbert (father of Hartland Molson) and William Molson, Sir Herbert Holt (Royal Bank), Sir Charles Gordon (Bank of Montreal), and numerous Montreal business leaders. The architect (also an investor) was John S. Archibald. The pressure to build the forum was related to the size (i.e., seating capacity) and lack of consistent artificial ice-making facilities of the previous arenas.

Prior to 1924, the Montreal Canadiens commenced playing hockey at the Jubilee Rink on St Catherine Street (1909–10 season). This arena was originally built by Patrick J. Doran, who was the owner of the Montreal Wanderers, and could seat thirty-five hundred spectators. The team then located to the Westmount Arena on St Catherine and Wood. This was a more modern building with appropriate dressing rooms and a seating capacity of seven thousand. Unfortunately, it was destroyed by fire on 2 January 1918, and this necessitated a move to the Mount Royal Arena for a short period of time. There is no question that the Montreal Forum became the mystical hockey shrine for all Quebecers. For over seventy years, the "ghosts of the Forum" became a factor at virtually every game – and certainly during Stanley Cup playoffs.

The opening of the Western Division of the MGH in October 1924 was a major factor with regard to establishing "geographical proximity" key to the MGH and Montreal Canadiens relationship.[5] The hospital emergency room was now just a short walk across Cabot Square from the Montreal Forum medical clinic. Elmer Lach describes many occasions when he put on his skate guards and walked across Cabot Square during a game for treatment in the emergency room of the Western. One of these occasions involved the insertion of a posterior nasal pack for a broken nose – following which he returned to play. Harry Scott, a retired MGH surgeon, describes attending games in his "whites" while being on call as a surgical resident at the Western Division. The residents in training were allowed to stand behind the glass in close proximity to the Montreal Forum medical clinic ("a mutually beneficial arrangement"). L.G. Hampson explains that Egbert McKay recruited members of the hospital staff to provide medical coverage for Forum games. This geographic proximity was clearly the basis for the early close relationship between MGH physicians and the Montreal Canadiens.

Despite the global increase in hospital beds with the addition of St Mary's, the Jewish General Hospital, and the Montreal Neurological Institute in the 1930s, overcrowding and functioning on two separate sites became problematic. The lack of land around the Dorchester site and the distance from the McGill University campus, along with the continued demand for services, led to a desperate search for a new location to consolidate and enlarge the MGH. This came to fruition on 13 May 1948, when the hospital board purchased the land on Cedar Avenue, the current site of the MGH.[6] The persistence and vision of Thomas and Hartland Molson made construction of the current MGH a reality by 1955. Hartland Molson was the prime fundraiser for the new construction, and Tom Molson, who was a long-term governor of the MGH, played a lead role in the construction of the current hospital. He worked with the same architects and consulting engineers (MacDougall) for the hospital construction as he used for the brewery's expansion and renovation in Montreal and the new brewery in Toronto. This clearly explains the many similarities in basic construction details between the hospital and the brewery.

The newly opened MGH resulted in a transfer of all patients from the Central and Western Divisions to the new Cedar Avenue location in May 1955. This newly constructed hospital was now closer to McGill University and continued, along with the Royal Victoria Hospital and the Montreal Children's Hospital, to be a major teaching institute for McGill's Faculty of Medicine. The hospital's long interest in trauma care, spearheaded by Fraser B. Gurd, H. Rocke Robertson, and Fraser N. Gurd, led to the development of a level 1 trauma centre at the MGH in 1993. The newly located MGH continued to be associated with the Montreal Canadiens Hockey Club and, indeed, served as the major emergency room for several life-threatening emergencies that took place at the Montreal Forum and the newly built Molson Bell Centre.

It appears that the Molson family/brewery first became involved with the Montreal Canadiens when Herbert and William Molson formed the Canadian Arena Company while building the original Montreal Forum (1924). Hartland and Tom Molson became owners of the hockey club in September 1957. They sold it to a trio of younger cousins (David, Peter, and William Molson) on 15 May 1964 for approximately $5 million. Edward and Peter Bronfman purchased the Montreal Canadiens in December 1971 and sold the team to Molson Breweries in August 1978. This was under the terms of an agreement with Carena Bancorp and included purchase of the hockey team and a long-term lease on the Montreal Forum, covering operation of the team as well as the entertainment division. It was during this tenure that Eric Molson and Ronald Corey built the Molson Centre near the old CPR Station (Windsor) on La Gauchietere Street – opening in March 1996. The official ground-breaking for the Molson Centre took place west of Windsor Station on 23 June1993. It was attended by Eric, Steve, Senator Hartland Molson, and Ronald Corey. On that day, Eric Molson stated: "It is very special that C.P. and the Molson Companies could once again collaborate on a project destined to become the city's number one sports and entertainment centre."[7]

Molson Brewery sold the arena and a majority of the hockey club to George Gillett's group in January 2001. Molson Inc. retained a 19.9 percent share of the hockey team, and the arena was renamed the Bell Centre. Once again, the concept of geographic proximity to the MGH. and its Level 1

Trauma Centre was important in several life-threatening injuries at the Bell Centre (McCleary, Audette, Zednick, etc.). The Molson family entered the scene again in June of 2009, when Geoff, Andrew, Jason, and their group purchased the Montreal Canadiens Hockey Club, the Bell Centre, and Gillett Entertainment from the Gillett family group.

During the 2009–10 NHL season, the Montreal Canadiens celebrated its one hundred years of existence in many special ways. Readers are referred to Jenish's historical description of the franchise for further details.[8] We had hoped to document all the medical personnel for the one hundred years of the Montreal Canadiens franchise, but, for many reasons, this proved to be too difficult. The initial medical coverage for the Montreal Canadiens appeared to be informal and conducted by players' personal physicians or physicians working with team ownership or management. There are several well documented episodes of key players needing sophisticated medical care. Perhaps the first occurred in 1926, when I.E. Dube, who was the personal physician of George Vezina, diagnosed the prominent goalie with pulmonary tuberculosis. He was sent to the Hotel Dieu in Chicoutimi for sanatorium care (which was traditional for the time), and it was there that he died of his disease.[9] In 1937, Howie Morenz suffered a fracture of his left tibia and fibula and was treated in St Luc's Hospital by I.A. Hector Forges. He died of complications (probable pulmonary embolism) related to this fracture, and his funeral was celebrated at the Montreal Forum.[10] After speaking with senior alumni of the Montreal Canadiens Hockey Club and examining historical documents, it appears that Egbert MacKay was one of the earliest recognized team physicians.

J. Gordon Young was the team physician in 1951 when Maurice "Rocket" Richard suffered a major head laceration and concussion after a hit by Leo Labine.[11] He was taken off the ice and sutured by Young and then returned to the ice, probably in a concussed state, to score an important goal. L.G. Hampson served as team physician along with J.D. Palmer, providing surgical support for Young for ten years (1952–62).

From D'Arcy Jenish we learn that, in 1959, Ian Milne was recruited by Larry Hampson as the team internist and played an important role in helping to create Jacques Plante's first goalkeeper's mask.[12] Milne worked with Bill Birchmore (Fiberglass Canada) and Mary Gzowski (an MGH medical artist) to create a mould that would serve as the prototype for the first Jacques Plante mask. Mary Gzowski had worked with plastic surgeons Jack

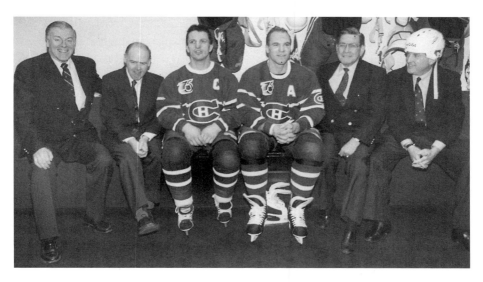

Fig. 47.3 Doctors for Les Canadians (*left to right*) David Mulder, John Little,
players Guy Carbonneau and Brian Skrudland.

Gerrie and Fred Woolhouse to produce moulds to guide complex facial re-
constructions following facial trauma.

Ian Milne's illness required Doug Kinnear to replace him and, in 1962,
Doug took over as team physician, a position he held from 1962 to 1998. He
was one of the longest serving-team physicians (often single-handed) in the
NHL. David Mulder, W. Keon, and Tony Popieraitis were recruited to provide medical coverage of the Montreal Junior Canadiens in September 1963.
Mulder later cared for the American League team (Montreal Voyageurs) and,
in 1970–71, formally began as a surgical assistant to Kinnear. In 1998, he and
assumed the role of team physician for the Montreal Canadiens.

A list of team physicians, associate team physicians, and orthopaedic
consultants is appended. In addition, however, virtually every department
and division within the MGH and McGill University have been utilized
to provide optimal care to the Montreal Canadiens and its family, including alumni.

In addition to the importance of geographic proximity, the MGH/Cana-
diens' relationship provides the hockey team with immediate access to quaternary health care practised by a complete array of health care professionals.
All levels of care are included, from paediatrics to geriatrics. The access to

McGill's Department of Sports Medicine and residency programs has provided mutually beneficial educational programs. Important research programs at McGill address the frontiers of medical care for the elite athlete. These included improved bio-physiological assessment (pre-season), concussion studies, airway management, the role of hyperbaric oxygen for sports injury, abdominal wall injuries (causation and surgical repair), and minimally invasive arthroscopic treatments – to name just a few. The McGill students of sports medicine and orthopaedics have benefitted from the focus on the care of the injured elite athlete.

The Montreal Canadiens medical team has taken a lead role in many NHL activities. The NHL Team Physicians Association, designed to optimize the health care of all athletes, focuses on the development of an electronic health record, concussion studies, optimal emergency standards for the arena clinics, and so on.

Concluding Remarks

The MGH and the Montreal Canadiens are both prestigious Quebec organizations. The hospital has been in existence since 1819 and played an important role in the establishment of McGill University. The Montreal Canadiens began their storied franchise in 1909. The opening of the Western Division of the MGH in 1934 brought the two institutions into geographic proximity, which was critical to their relationship. It was key to the MGH physicians assuming a role in the care of injured players, and it led to the first team physicians to be hired specifically for the hockey club. Prior to this, players were cared for by their own doctors or by physicians known to management.

A common thread in this relationship was the Molson family. The MGH was opened on the strength of John Molson's 1821 petition to government for additional hospital beds for the rapidly growing city of Montreal. The Molson family is now in its seventh generation of being involved with the MGH at all levels. Current ownership represents the fifth generation of the Molson family's involvement with the Montreal Canadiens.

Table 47.1
Montreal Canadiens Medical Staff

Team MD	Associates	Ortho consultant
E. MacKay (1950–59)		
G. Young (1952–62)		
J.D. Palmer (1952–62)	L.G. Hampson	J. Shannon
I. Milne (1959)		
L.G. Hampson (1954–64)	D.G. Kinnear	T. Percy
	J.D.Palmer	F. Greenwood
D.G. Kinnear (1962–98)	D.S. Mulder	E. Lenczner
	C.Clement	T. Percy
		F. Greenwood
		C.E. Brook
		D. Burke
D.S. Mulder (1998–present)	T. Razek	E. Harvey
	K. Khwaja	P. Martineau
	V.J. Lacroix	G. Berry
		R. Reindl
		E. Lenczner

NOTES

1 H.E. MacDermot, *A History of the Montreal General Hospital* (Montreal: Montreal General Hospital, 1950); H.E. MacDermot, *The Years of Change, 1945–70* (Montreal: Sesquicentennial Committee for the 150th Anniversary, MGH Publication, 1971); Darcy Jenish, *The Montreal Canadiens: 100 Years of Glory* (Toronto: Double Day Canada, 2008).

2 S. Woods, "The Molsons and the MGH," chap. 1, this volume.

3 J. Hanaway, "The Early Years, 1819–85," chap. 2, this volume.

4 Jenish, *Montreal Canadians*, 285.

5 MacDermot, *History*, 101.

6 Ibid., 122–4.

7 Jenish, *Montreal Canadians*, 287.

8 Ibid., 68–70.

9 Ibid., 87–89.

10 Ibid., 134.

11 Ibid., 159–61.

12 Ibid., 160.

48

Governance

Joseph Hanaway

Introduction

There are three sections to this chapter. Section 1 deals with the governance of the MGH as it evolved from 1819 up through the McGill University Health Centre/Centre Universitaire Sante McGill (MUHC/CUSM – cited as MUHC). Section 2 deals with the government control of health care in Quebec and Canada and its effect on the governance of the MGH. It is not my intention to cover government health care in Canada and Quebec in depth but, rather, to give the reader enough information to appreciate the extraordinary challenges it presented to the MGH administration. Section 3 presents a brief history and chronology of events leading to the creation, planning, and construction of the MUHC and discusses how MGH independence and governance changed as it joined the super-hospital.

Governance of the MGH, 1819–1961

Written in 1823, the original administrative structure establishing the governance of the MGH was a twenty-page, folio- sized document in a Board of Governors' minute book. A blueprint for the management of one of the first public hospitals in Canada "The Statutes, Rules and Regulations of the Montreal General Hospital" carefully outlined the composition and responsibilities of the Board of Governors, the Committee of Management, and the Medical Board (the only boards) as well as the duties of all the personnel.[1]

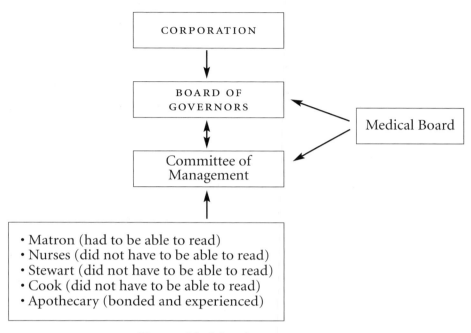

Fig. 48.1 Administrative structure, 1823

To be a member of the MGH Corporation in the first half of the 1800s required a contribution of two to five pounds per year, and a life governor had to contribute ten to fifteen pounds per year. Starting with about thirty-five members in the 1820s, the corporation grew to more than one thousand members by 1890. The Corporation owns the property for which it responsible. Elected by the Corporation annually, thirteen volunteer business executives and professionals and an additional thirteen from life governors were appointed to the Board of Governors, making a board of twenty-six, which met four to six times per year to make broad decisions for the hospital. The Board of Governors is the corporation's ultimate governing body, and it makes broad policy decisions. Appointed annually by the Board of Governors were the members of the Committee of Management, who run the hospital directly day to day. Responsible for all hospital affairs and business, the Committee of Management met weekly. The Medical Board, a board of all the medical staff, controlled the patient diets and set standards for house physician and staff appointments to the hospital. It reported to the Committee of Management and its responsibilities increased over the decades.[2]

The volunteer members of the board had management experience, but none of them had experience running a public institution like the MGH. Learning on the job, the Committee of Management struggled with inadequate funding from local churches, the city, the province, and from silent benefactors like John Richardson. To keep the hospital running, these dedicated men had to contend with real challenges. Uneducated and illiterate attendants; food, coal, ice, milk, and spirit vendors; oil lamp and gas lighting that led to fear of fire; poor heating and plumbing; rats and roaches; straw mattresses full of insects and hospital finances – all were committee fare.[3]

Two random examples of the Committee of Management's concerns were: (1) the laundry and (2) frequent staff turnover. With regard to (1), all helped with hand washing. Sheets and other bedding were boiled and washed in large utility sinks. Because there was no space for drying, bedding had to be hung anywhere it could be draped over something – in the lobby, on stair railings, in the wards and basement. With regard to (2), only the matron had to be able to read: the remainder of the staff were usually illiterate and came and went frequently. Poor salaries, no incentives, poor supervision, and poor working conditions were the reasons for this, and, without enough income, little could be done about it.

Welcomed capitol expansions (given by donors – the Richardson Wing 1832, and the Reid Wing 1848) managed by the Board of Governors in fact created problems. The need for more attendants to care for the increased number of patients put a greater strain on tenuous hospital finances, which were so bad that, at times, the Committee of Management had to close wards, furlough staff, and slow admissions to control the budget. Paying the attendants as well as paying for the food and apothecary needs became absolute priorities. Maintenance repairs to the plumbing and building could only be done with extra money, which meant that bathroom plumbing at times didn't work, that holes in the floors never got repaired, and that the dingy walls did not get painted.

Despite all these challenges, the men on the Committee of Management never let the hospital close. Because of the increasing number of daily problems, by 1880 the committee convinced the Board of Governors to appoint a medical superintendent who would deal with daily problems that were taking too much committee time. James Bell, MD, CM, Holmes Gold medalist of 1877 and a brilliant physician was chosen the first superintendent. He served in this position for three years before becoming a great surgeon under Roddick at McGill.[4]

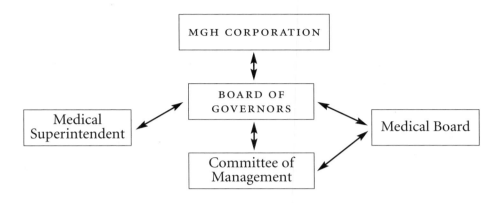

Fig. 48.2 Administrative structure, 1881

His successors, all outstanding medical graduates with no experience in administration, performed remarkably well and eventually became indispensable in dealing with daily problems. But, by 1910, it was clear that the (now) general superintendent had to have administrative and business experience. James Fyshe was hired as the general superintendent while the board was looking for someone to meet these requirements and, in 1917, found A.K. Haywood, MD, whose primary interest was not medicine but hospital administration and management. Haywood found the MGH deficit approaching $5000,000 and began to organize the administration to ensure better financial management. He created new positions in the business office, but budget constraints and inexperience limited his plans between 1918 and 1930.[5] The new financial management under Haywood, however, could not reduce the creeping debt caused by expansion of services, advancing technology, and inadequate funding.

The hospital coped for decades, gradually changing after Arthur H. Westbury, a trained accountant, came on the scene in 1930. He started as secretary to the Board of Management, learning how to manage the hospital and its financial problems, and in two years became chief accountant.

During the Second World War General Superintendent John MacKenzie and his assistant Burnett Johnston went overseas. William Statkoff directed the hospital until Johnston returned as the general superintendent. He retired in 1952, when Westbury took his place.[6] Despite his accounting background, Westbury decided to centralize financial management at the MGH.

He would not delegate authority or establish budgets, satisfied to manage the business of the hospital himself. The definitive micromanager, Westbury insisted on an austere and Spartan operation and signed most of the purchase orders himself. The Board of Governors tolerated his management style because it was a great improvement over the past. The deficit continued to increase.

Government Health Care and Its Influence on the MGH Governance, 1961–97

The first bill to improve medical care in Quebec and in all of Canada, the jointly funded, federally proposed Hospital Insurance and Diagnostic Services Act (HIDS), 1957, covered all hospitalization and ER visits, to which the province subscribed in 1961 with its own bill (Quebec Hospital Insurance Plan).[7] The government supplied the money while the province designed its own health care program.

The bill mandated better financial management at the MGH, and Westbury assigned increasing responsibilities to his assistants until he retired in 1966. An unexpected result of the Quebec hospitalization plan was flooding of the ER at the MGH, which was open 24/7 and where the medical care was free. This spilled over into the hospital, and, when there was no inpatient room, patients, at times, remained in the ER for days.

Starting in 1960, the MGH administration began to be influenced by political, social, and economic forces that had not been seen before. Under Liberal premier Jean Lesage (1960–66), the province, which had been under the non-progressive and reactionary government of Maurice Duplessiss and the control of the Roman Catholic Church for years, began a period of intense modernization. Lesage rapidly secularized Quebec society and took public education out of the hands of the church to establish a modern educational system. The province that had so vigorously opposed change before 1960 now welcomed it. With the expropriation of church-owned hospital and school properties, and other bold business takeovers, the province resuscitated its economy and created the historic "Quiet Revolution" that changed Quebec society forever, was a high point in its history, and kindled the smouldering fire of provincial nationalism.[8]

Fortunately for the MGH, the man who succeeded Westbury, the very able William Storrar, MD, had had considerable medical administrative experience during the Second World War and postwar years as Saskatchewan's assistant minister of health. He came to the MGH in the early 1950s as an assistant to Westbury and made his reputation as an organizer with the 1955 hospital move from the Central and Western Divisions to the new hospital on Cedar Avenue. On Sunday, 14 May, 180 student nurses moved; on Sunday, 22 May, seventy patients from the Western Division moved; and, on the following Sunday, 103 patients from the Central Division did so. It took three weeks of frantic ambulance and van trips back and forth with no serious incident – all carefully orchestrated by Bill Storrar.

Storrar immediately decentralized the financial administration of the MGH to cope with HIDS and other mandates and surrounded himself with professional hospital administrators. W. Atchison and George Jackson were kept on from the previous administration, and he hired Tudor Roberts, Christian Primavese, and Jacques Nolet, all of whom had master's degrees in health care administration and accounting. Storrar also hired a director of finance, Richard Criddle, to complete his team. He introduced departmental budgets and greater accountability as he began to form a professional administration to manage the evolving hospital business.[9]

During the 1960s, the Board of Governors became the Board of Directors, still comprised of business and professional leaders who volunteered their time to manage the hospital. Now, with the rising professionalism of the administration, the board, once autonomous, shared the responsibility of running the MGH more than ever before. On the one hand, board members were chosen for their proven management experience and ability to make policy decisions; on the other hand, financial and management professionals in the administration dealt with the details of running hospital business. Both groups worked closely to maintain the mission of the MGH.

In 1964, the federally funded Hall Commission Report on the state of health care in Canada was released. It not only recommended universal health care in Canada but also revealed that the Québécois did not have the same level of medical services and access to GPs and specialists as did people elsewhere in the country. Hospitalization had been taken care of with the HIDS, but doctors' bills and outpatient tests were not covered.[10] To this end, in 1965, Lesage asked Claude Castonguay to head a commission to evaluate health care and social services in Quebec – a survey he expected would take a few years. The Castonguay-Nepveu Report of 1967 confirmed the Hall Commission's report:[11] the Québécois did not have the level of health care found in other provinces. Hard on the heels of this, a 1968 federal opinion poll asked Canadians whether or not they would accept an increase in taxes to pay for a federally supported, provincially run medicare program. Sixty-four percent of Quebec responders voted "yes" to the proposal, the highest percentage in the country.

On the federal scene, one year before in 1966, Prime Minister Pearson introduced the Medical Care Act (Canadian Medicare),[12] with the government paying 50 percent of the cost of hospital and doctor bills. This extended the 1957 HIDS Act's cost-sharing, allowing each province to develop a universal health care plan. Again the government did not want to direct Medicare, only to supply the money for the provinces to develop their own plans.

Lesage definitely wanted to develop a separate provincial-directed health care plan that was within the province's jurisdiction. By the time of the 1967 Castonguay-Nepveu Report, the liberals had been voted out by Union Nationale candidates from 1966 to 1970, and the Liberal health care plan was put on hold. In March 1970, at the eleventh hours, Jean Bertrand, Union Nationale premier (1968–70), submitted his own health plan but was voted out of office one month later by the Liberals, who were led by Robert Bourassa.

In retrospect, 1970 may be remembered as the most tumultuous year in modern Quebec history. It started with Liberal Party leader Robert Bourassa winning the provincial election in April 1970 and appointing Claude Castonguay minister of health (he had left the commission, at Bourassa's request, to run for office – a proviso being that he could submit his report to the legislature). The final form of the Castonguay-Nepveu Report was submitted to the legislature as a bill, to be debated and voted upon in mid-October. Named the Quebec Medical Insurance Act, or Bill 65,[13] it called for sweeping changes in the administration of Quebec hospitals and in medical practice as well as for complete government take-over of health care in the province.

The province took over management of all the hospitals, democratizing the boards and committees, making them more representative of the people. Also, and more controversial, the bill challenged the dominance of the Anglo/French specialists in the hospitals, the medical schools, and the Quebec College of Physicians and Surgeons. It set fees for specialty care, allowed no added billing, prohibited private insurance for covered services, and allowed no opting-out of the plan (something that had been promised). These and other issues threatened the specialists' hold over medicine in Quebec and, according to them, represented a "socialist-communist" attempt to dictate medical practice. Not surprisingly, they vehemently opposed the bill.[14]

Sentiments were so high that, at a meeting of forty-five hundred medical personnel in Montreal's Maurice Richard Arena, 27 August 1970, the specialists, acting through their union (Federation des Médecins Spécialistes du Quebec), voted to strike as of 1 October. Their timing could not have been worse, and, in addition, they misread the importance of their claims, which had not gained much public support or sympathy.

Unfortunately, the specialists' strike and the government's effort to get Bill 65 passed in October coincided with the 1970 October Crisis created by the separatist terrorist Front de Libération du Québec (FLQ). It had been bombing sites in Quebec for years (approximately two hundred bombs placed, one of which was on the McGill campus, with no injuries) but now resorted to kidnapping and murder to promote its separatist fervour.[15] MGH business was apparently not nearly so affected by the turmoil surrounding the FLQ as it was by Bill 65, which was going to change the governance and the administration dramatically over the next few years.

The beleaguered Bourassa government, refusing to give in to FLQ demands to release popular jailed separatists, feared widespread civil disobedience. To prevent this, Mayor Drapeau of Montreal and Premier Bourassa asked Prime Minister Trudeau to send in the army, invoke the War Measures Act (15 October 1970), declare the FLQ a criminal element, and arrest its leaders, all of which was done, putting an end to the crisis.[16] On the same day the Quebec legislature, in a twelve-hour marathon session, passed Bill 65, the Quebec Medical Insurance Act.

Regarding the specialists' walkout on 1 October , they were legislated back to work. It was simple: those who wanted to continue practising in Quebec either returned to practice by 1 November or lost their licences and were fined daily. With the Liberals back in power in April 1970, the full force of Bill 65, Quebec's version of Medicare, was beginning to be felt and to worry people. The hospital was going to suffer from too much change in too short a time. Frankly, neither the hospital nor the government had the personnel or expertise to manage the unfolding of Bill 65. As Quebec began to enforce its regulations, for a few years it was a one-sided situation, with the hospital trying to catch up.

The immediate problems presented to the MGH at the end of 1970 were:

1 The suspension and cancellation of all building projects, including the MGH Research Institute, which had been planned for years.
2 The failure of the Regie d'Assurance Maladie du Quebec to reimburse the MGH for medical care services and for the mandated salary increases for employees negotiated before Bill 65 but not enforced until

1970. The MGH was forced to borrow large sums of money from the banks to meet its agreement, and Quebec refused to pay the bank interest rates for a problem it created.

3 The abrupt way in which Bill 65 was implemented, right in the middle of the October Crisis, which had everyone's attention.

4 Worry about the impending reorganization of the MGH administration from top to bottom and job security. Bill 65 created such an unpredictable and indefinite political and economic climate, as well as mistrust of Quebec City's socialistic policies, that many physicians fled the province (about fifteen from the MGH). "What are they going to do next?" was the question everyone was hearing and reading.

Unrest did not start with Bill 65: interns and residents had walked off in the spring because of salary disputes, and the specialists had walked off in October because of the perceived stranglehold Quebec now had on medical practice. In 1971, the Quebec Health Services and Social Services Act (HSSS) had a major effect on MGH governance by mandating specific personnel changes in the hospital administration and management.[17] Updated in 1973 (Quebec was unhappy with the slow response to HSSS), the boards were abolished and reconstructed. This involved determining who and how many people were designated to be on each board, committee, and council, what their charges were, and how often they were to meet. This attempt at democratizing the administration meant that a lot of inexperienced people found themselves in unfamiliar positions, and this slowed down hospital business for months to years.[18]

Despite the administrative nightmare, MGH president Melvyn Angus and executive director William Storrar began to work with Regie d'Assurance Maladie du Quebec to establish budget stability, both sides reiterating that they still did not have the personnel to speed up negotiations. Bill Storrar resigned in 1972 after twenty years, and Harvey Barkun, MD, the French-educated and able administrator, took his place. Barkun was comfortable in each culture. The money for the Research Institute, to be built on the Pine Avenue side of the MGH, was granted in 1972, and, more important, the chronic budgetary delays and difficulties were regularized by Quebec ending decades of uncertainty and delays. (Keep in mind that the government had to deal with two hundred hospitals in the province, all of which were clamouring for attention.)

Table 48.1
Required membership of the Board of Directors of a hospital centre and
the mode of selection

Constituency	No. of representatives	Mode of selection
Users of the hospital (patients)	2	Elected by a meeting of constituents
Major "socioeconomic groups" in the community	2	Proposed by local civic groups; final choices, made by the government
Hospital corporation (including former board)	4	Elected at annual meeting of the corporation
Hospital professionals (e.g., nurses, social workers)	1	Elected by constituents
Physicians and dentists in the hospital	1	Elected by constituents
Hospital non-professional staff (housekeeping, orderlies)	1	Elected by constituents
Local community clinics with referral contracts to the hospital	1	Appointed by clinics
University (if hospital is a teaching unit) of the	1	Appointed by board university
Interns and residents	1	Elected by constituents

Source: J.M. Eakin, "Survival of the Fittest? The Democractization of Hospital
Aministration in Quebec," *International Journal of Health Services* 14, 3 (1984):
397–411.

It appears that Quebec underestimated the uncertainty and threat to job security and the problem of the transition of MGH management from the small board of experienced executives to a large mandated board of inexperienced people who had little to no preparation for governing an enterprise as large as the MGH.[19]

Fortunately, the existing board members in 1970, recognizing this, continued to serve, working closely with the administration for three to four years while the mandated board members learned on the job. The tempo of change had quickened with the mandates of the early 1970s, and there was no slowing down once the bills began to come out of Quebec City updating the original health care acts. New board members had to learn how to function as an effective body, learning from the older members, who also had to teach sessions on board protocol. Meetings were long with much discussion.[20]

At the same time, at the MGH, issues had to be decided, and the older board members continued to do this, frequently outside the boardroom in order to avoid excess discussion. As the takeover gradually occurred, the mandated board members assumed more responsibility and the governance structure became very complex, with subcommittees, councils, and other advisory bodies. As this happened, the senior board members retired. Younger leaders, whose experience and advice was still part of the overall executive control of the MGH, replaced them. There were constant delays in renovation plans because Quebec insisted that any change had to be approved, even if paid for with private funds.

In 1974, Quebec requested that the MGH establish a department of community health (DSC) to develop a community-based health care system for the greater Montreal area. Under the DSCs, local community health centres (centres local de services communautaires [CLSCs]) were created (about 147 or more in the province at this writing) to be the main entry point into the health care system in Quebec. Staffed by a variety of professionals – MDs, RNs, therapists, and social workers – this comprehensive concept failed because of physicians' objections to the salaried positions. Less than 20 percent of primary physicians have elected to join the CLSCs, and the public has not been sold on them because they cannot see their own physicians in these centres. Also, the CLSCs operate on a nine-to-five schedule, not the 24/7 schedule of the private doctor family medicine groups that have successfully competed with them.[21]

Legislation to strengthen the French language in Quebec over the years has passed, but none of these pieces of legislation has affected the MGH administration as much as Bill 22 (Bourassa, 1974),[22] which declared French the only language in Quebec and created a constitutional storm over bilingualism. Bill 101, Lévesque's 1977 Charter on the French Language,[23] mandated that all business in the province be conducted in French, including that performed in Anglo hospitals. Anglo hospital personnel were even required to take French competency exams. This sparked a flame of resentment in the Anglo community, resulting in well organized resistance at different professional levels. Seeking "acquired rights" from the province, the organized groups successfully appealed to the government to modify the policy and to allow the Anglo hospitals to carry on business in English and/or French whenever needed. Barkun, with his French background, greatly helped the MGH administration adopt the language changes that were ultimately imposed.

In 1977, the Established Program Financing Bill shifted the funding sources for the HDIS and the MCA federal cost-sharing programs to the province, thus decreasing federal control over provincial health care. It did this by shifting taxes that formerly would have gone to Ottawa directly to the provinces.[24]

By 1978, a major internal problem for the MGH concerned paper records generated by the hospital that had reached a staggering number and had consumed about 10 to 15 percent of the annual budget. Under CEO Barkun, a computer advisory committee recommended that an IBM system be installed on a trial basis for registrations, discharges, and transfers. A uniquely Canadian program had to be developed centred around patient records (unlike the US system, which is centred around billing and accounting). The MGH hired Thomas Harrison to work with IBM to expand the program. By 1991, eighteen systems had been established related to patient care, plus systems for medical records, nursing, radiology, the pharmacy, personnel, financial management, and accounting. This can be considered Barkun's greatest legacy to the MGH.[25] There was no significant budgetary problem in 1978, and a fire in the laundry required a major renovation that was long overdue.

In 1980, a major budget cut of 7 percent across the board, reflecting a national recession, was mandated and occupied one year of endless hours and meetings of work. On a positive note, additional space for psychiatry was provided when the McConnel family presented its indoor tennis court facility to the MGH for clinical use, thus relieving a chronic space problem for psychiatry without having to spend money for renovations. There were now strict quotas on the numbers of residents. Initially, there was concern about patient care being compromised, but this did not happen even though the resident staff had been reduced.

Since 1960, financing of the hospitals in Quebec has been based on historical data. Global budgets have been allocated by the provincial government, rarely taking into account activity levels within the institutions. Hospital boards have been able to launch capital campaigns for bricks and mortar, and fundraising initiatives by auxiliaries and foundations have raised money for new state-of-the-art equipment. Staffing of the hospitals has remained confined within historical global budget allocations. Deficits have mounted. From time to time, these have been partially addressed by the provincial government.

The Ministry of Health did not like hospital deficits and was very unhappy with the anticipated 1981–82 MGH deficit of $8,039,539, mostly due to the cost of maintaining the seventh floor OBS unit. Quebec offered $2.5 million to help cover the deficit and required a plan to reduce that amount by 50 percent by the end of 1982. Trusteeship, the obvious threat, galvanized the MGH into action.[26]

The Board of Directors appointed a special committee of priorities to propose a solution to the problem of the rising deficit. The first, which was to close the pregnancy termination unit (PTU), was rejected; the second, which was to close the entire OBS unit, was not. The board referred the second proposal to the Executive Committee of the Council of Physicians and Dentists, which didn't like the idea of closing the OBS unit but saw no alternative if it was to meet Quebec's requirements.

So important was this decision that an information session called for the entire hospital staff (150 attended) to come and hear the decision of the board: among the invitees were the president of the board, the director general, and Dean Richard Cruess of the Medical School. The president of the board reviewed the problem and reluctantly approved the decision to close the OBS unit as of 30 June 1982.[27] One year later, the annual report for 1982–83 stated that the $8,039,539 debt had been reduced by $8,019,000 by closing the OBS Unit.[28]

The Canada Health Act, 1984 (CHA),[29] reaffirmed the 1957 HIDS Act, 1957, and the Medical Care Act, 1966 (MCA), which established Medicare. It stated the five criteria of health care – public administration, comprehensiveness, universality, portability, and accessibility – that the provinces had to follow to get federal funds and that, on the federal level, prohibited user fees and extra billing for covered services. The CHA did not affect the MGH administration, but the Quebec Prescription Drug Insurance Plan, 1997,[30] did, mandating that all Québécois have private (through employment) or public drug coverage. The main impact was on the MGH pharmacy, which had to expand its inventory and its delivery service.

In 1988, the MGH was running smoothly considering the proposed budgets cuts. Renovation projects were being undertaken in pathology and radiology, and the parking garage was enlarged, as was the "Day Centre" in psychiatry.

In 1997, with the MUHC, the governance of the MGH changed. The MGH surrendered its independence to the MUHC but had an on-site director, an associate deputy general of professional services (doctors, dentists, and pharmacists), and an associate deputy general of nursing services. They manage MGH business independently, adhering to MUHC policies, guidelines, and budgets, and they seek aid from the MUHC administration only when needed.

The MUHC and the Change in the MGH Governance, 1997–2013

Contemporary history is a challenge for any author because details and facts not currently known about events that are constantly evolving always affect and alter the perspective on what has been written. Recognizing this, I write the history of the MUHC from what is presently known, knowing that new information in the future will no doubt change the story.

By the 1980s, it became apparent that, to maintain two full-service, large, general hospitals (i.e., the RVH and the MGH) just over a kilometre apart was too costly and impractical. Merger was investigated and found, in a questionable study, to save so little as not to be worth it. Also, the staffs at both hospitals had little interest in merger plans.

In 1992, Nicholas Steinmetz, CEO of the Montreal Children's Hospital approached Quebec City and Richard Cruess, dean of medicine, with a proposal that McGill combine all its hospitals (the MGH, the RVH, the MCH, the MNI, and the Montreal Chest Hospital) into one super-hospital in the Montreal region. Contingent on a number of issues, Quebec City as well as the dean and McGill principal David Johnston generally agreed with the plan.[31]

In 1994, the board chairs of the hospitals met to discuss the proposal for a McGill University Hospital centre. Enthusiastic about the project, The RVH, with its time-limited one-hundred-year-old buildings (opened 1893), which posed serious problems transporting patients and installing new equipment, had ninety-centimetre granite walls that were impossible to modernize. The annual accreditation visits praised the RVH staff but frankly decried the outdated buildings, stating the need for a new facility.[32]

The MNI/MNH, a McGill property, vigorously resisted the idea of moving, even in the face of losing the RVH, with its support services (e.g., kitchens, dining room, general labs, consult services, etc.), proposed counter-plans that delayed the ultimate decision to move to the Glen site. A decision has now been made to move, but the ultimate date remains uncertain due to questions about financing.[33]

Initially, the MGH also resisted moving but was saved in 2003 when the province wanted to have a level 1 adult trauma centre in the downtown area and designated it to be in that hospital (which had already been designated a level 1 centre in 1989). Also, because of the long delay (six years up to 2003) in getting the MUHC project started (it would take until 17 June 2010 to break ground), the cost of moving the MGH had become a concern. The MGH therefore was to remain on Cedar Avenue, its other functions to be decided.[34]

The MCH, like the RVH an outdated structure that there was reluctance to renovate and with research facilities in rented space blocks away, was ready for a new facility. Finally, the tiny Montreal Chest Hospital decided to move with the RVH.

The Sir Mortimer Davis Jewish General Hospital (JGH) had declined to join the MUHC from the outset, fearing losing its image in the MUHC and potentially losing funding from the wealthy Jewish community. It remains associated with McGill and is a well endowed clinical research centre.

In 1995, the Quebec government formally agreed to the merger plans to form the MUHC. In 1997, after three years of legal negotiations, the MUHC, officially established now controlled all the hospitals with onsite managers until the final move. Sites for the super-hospital (about seven) were evaluated over a few years, and, in 2001, the old CPR Glen switching yards in NDG met provincial approval but needed a major environmental cleanup.[35]

Progress beyond the planning stage in the MUHC was stalled because of Quebec red tape and because the province did not want to spend a lot of

money on an anglo hospital without spending the same amount on the similar French Centre Hospitalier de Université de Montreal. Unfortunately, the
hospitals associated with the University of Montreal engaged in prolonged
planning, which held up the entire project for a few years.[36]

In late 2004, Quebec appointed Brian Mulroney and Daniel Johnson
(prominent political leaders) to form a commission to investigate the stalled
hospital projects.[46] They were to report on public opinion and support for
establishing the Anglo (McGill) and French (University of Montreal) super-
hospitals in Montreal, to be paid for by taxes. The report, released in March
2005, endorsed the Anglo/French plans for modern hospitals that would benefit the Montreal and Quebec communities and gave the go ahead to start
the projects. It agreed with the Glen site for the MUHC and suggested a better site for the CHUM than the one that had been proposed. Of particular
note, in the strongest terms, it recommended the public-private partnership
(PPP) management model for both projects.

Regarding the MUHC now that construction was approved, a multi-
million-dollar Glen site cleanup of Dioxin and other contaminants, referred
to as an "environmental remediation," had to be carried out before any idea
of foundation work was considered.[37] Frustrated by the lack of progress since
1997, in 2004 the MUHC appointed a selection committee to recruit a
decisive leader who could cut through the morass of Quebec red tape and get
the MUHC built. A headhunting firm recommended Arthur Porter, MD,
who had been working in Detroit on a hospital project and who was ready
to move on. Unfortunately, the firm failed either to uncover lawsuits filed
against him ($5 million in one case and $137,000 in another) for not repaying
business loans and or to find out that members of the board of the Detroit
hospital had resigned in protest over Porter's irregular financial activities.
With insufficient knowledge of his character, the firm's recommendation
was accepted and he was appointed CEO of the MUHC project. Deftly
working his way through the political and social networks of Montreal,
Porter convinced everyone of his ability and even secured outside positions
on the Board of Air Canada (2006) and the headship of a committee in
Prime Minister Harper's government (2008).[38] Porter set out to kick start
the MUHC and, with his remarkable ability to get people to do what he
wanted, gets the credit for getting a stalled project started. In 2006, with the
Glen site cleanup finished, Quebec started the selection process for a PPP
model for the MUHC, recommended by the Mulroney-Johnson Commission in 2005.[39]

In 2008, the Lachine Hospital joined as the only French-language hospital in the MUHC. It has been modernized by the province, and its Pavilion Camille-Lefebvre has been renovated for chronic respiratory care. It is the only such hospital unit in the Quebec. The Montreal Chest Hospital at the Glen site will care for acute respiratory problems and cancer.

An ultramodern, $280 million clinical and basic research institute has also been added to the Glen site adjacent to the hospitals. It is the intention to have this facility available for clinical research, just as the McGill-RVH University Clinic was in 1924.[40]

On 17 June 2010, ground was finally broken at the Glen site thirteen years after the creation of the MUHC in 1997. In the same year, Quebec selected a public-private partner, the Groupe Immobilier Santé McGill, to manage the project to its completion and beyond.[41]

Modernization of the MGH proposed in 2008 was too costly and disruptive. Revised in 2010, it has, to date, led to a new cardiology investigative and treatment centre, renovations on the mental health unit, and upgrades on the gastroenterology unit.[42] A preliminary distribution of services to the MGH (subject to change) included the following: some general medicine and surgery, the emergency department, trauma service, orthopaedics, plastic surgery, geriatrics, and neuroscience research. Clinics for these services will be at the MGH and relocations can be expected. By 2011, the MUHC foundations were poured and finished and the project emerged from the ground ready for the superstructure.

After a few years, two elements of Porter's management style began to surface. First, he dominated his associates, keeping the activities of the MUHC board a secret. All meetings were closed, members were bound legally to keep all board activities confidential, none of the oversight committees mandated by Quebec were invited, and he controlled the board that was supposed to control him. Second, as time went on, Porter's outside business interests became more and more important and he spent less time in Montreal. In 2012, he managed the MUHC on his Blackberry, and between January and April he was in town only eight times.[43]

Fraud, corruption, and an alleged lack of oversight and transparency in MUHC business was revealed by a Quebec government audit released in December 2012. It found that the anticipated $12 million running cost of the multiple aspects of the project had ballooned to $115 million. In addition, a Quebec anti-corruption task force uncovered major fraud in a separate MUHC budget (one contractor, to get the $1.3 billion project award, allegedly paid CEO Porter and some associates, $22.5 million in consulting fees), and this was also released in December 2012. However, the building project, which was on a separate budget, never lost time.[44]

The government reacted by appointing a senior medical administrator to "accompany" the hospital as it attempted to put its finances in order. McGill and the MUHC moved quickly to restore faith in the project, with able people coming to the rescue and with strict oversight within a year. The overall project was on time – in fact, it was ahead of the scheduled 2015 opening. As for Arthur Porter, who had left the country at the end of 2011 (he popped in and out of Canada a few times on MUHC business) was found by Interpol and presently resides in a Panamanian prison awaiting extradition.

The MUHC's Glen site, completed in the summer of 2014, replaced the existing facilities of the RVH, the MCH, and the Montreal Chest Hospital and provides a research institute and a cancer centre.[45] It will also be the new home for the Montreal Shriners Hospital for Children, which was saved from moving to London, Ontario, by a goal-line stand on the part of 250 committed Montreal professionals, doctors, politicians, and business leaders who went to Baltimore, Maryland, on a chartered flight on 4 July 2005, all wearing T-shirts emblazoned with "Please Don't Close Our Montreal Hospital." At the meeting, the group, including Quebec premier Charest, Mayor Tremblay, Health Minister Couillard, two McGill medical deans, Alex Paterson, MUHC CEO Porter, and many others sang a special song to the tune of "My Bonnie Lies over the Ocean" to the Shriners to plead their case, and they prevailed by fewer than five votes. The hospital is part of the MUHC campus but will operate independently.[46]

After 1997, the MUHC Board of Directors rotated meetings between the RVH and the MGH for a few years, then it rented space in a building on Guy above de Maisonneuve. Now that the board meetings are mostly public, they are held in the old Air Canada Building, owned by the MUHC, on the Glen site. The elaborate structure of nine to ten associate deputy generals, fourteen committees, and six councils, all part of MUHC governance, meet at many locations to get regular space.

Regarding the clinical departments, there is an MUHC chief for each department somewhere in the system and an onsite departmental director for the same specialty at the other hospitals. When the Glen site opens, it will include medicine, surgery, and paediatrics. The location of the public clinics for each clinical discipline is now a concern. The MUHC was built as a tertiary and quaternary care centre and, for budget reasons, a clinic system was not planned. As for now, the clinics will be located wherever the principal activity of the specialty is located. Orthopaedics and plastics will have clinics at the MGH, and cardiology and other specialties such as dermatology and nephrology, located at the Glen site, will rent space in nearby buildings. Information on the elaborate administrative structure of the MUHC in 2013 – the Board of Directors, the CEO and director general of the MUHC, the assistant DG of medical affairs, its fifteen committees, six councils, and nine associate DGs can be found at http://muhc.ca/homepage/page/.

The Legacy Committee held its opening meeting and dinner and awarded two honorary degrees in a special ceremony at the end of March 2015. Patients moved into the Glen MUHC at the end of April and the Grand Opening and ribbon cutting was held in warm weather in the middle of June 2015.

Otherwise, the problems of who is in charge of patient care (the physicians or the bureaucrats), the distribution of the clinical services (which will still be duplicated) among the hospitals; the location of the multitude of clinics throughout the MUHC system; the current fate of the MNI/MNH now that the RVH and its services have closed (e.g., dining room, laboratories, and consult services); the need for an airport-like transport system to get visitors around the vast institution; the inadequate accommodations for the professorial staff; the fate of the combined auxiliaries, which have donated millions to the hospitals and have no place in the Glen MUHC to continue their essential work and donations; who is going to qualify for admission to the Glen MUHC and its billion-dollar facilities; what to do with orthopaedic, plastic surgery, or psychiatric emergencies who arrive at the Glen ERs when the services are at the MGH; and how it is going to be paid for in light of the present provincial austerity policies covering the costs of two superhospital systems are to be settled in the future.

NOTES

1 Rules and Regulations of the Montreal General Hospital, June 1823, Register of Proceedings, vol. 1, 1822–32, MUA.
2 Ibid.
3 J. Hanaway, "The Early Years," chap. 2, this volume.
4 H. Berkovitz, "A History of the Montreal General Hospital," unpublished ms, 1992, 104–7. Presented by Berkovitz to Joseph Hanaway and John Burgess for their files.
5 Ibid.

6 Ibid.

7 Hospital Insurance and Diagnostic Services Act, 1957, available at http://en. wikipedia.org/wiki/ health_insurance_diagnostic _services_act. Excellent review of this landmark health legislation (five pages, eight references); Health Care in Canada, available at. http://en.wikipedia.org/wiki/health_care_in_ canada. A comprehensive nineteen-page review of the subject (ninety-three references); and .J.G. Turner, "The Hospital Insurance and Diagnostic Services Act: Its Impact on Hospital Administration," *Canadian Medical Association Journal* 78 (1958): 768–70.

8 Claude Belanger, "The Quiet Revolution," 1960, available at http://faculty. marianopolis.edu/ca. Belanger/quebechistory/events/quiet.htm, 2000; "Quiet Revolution," available at http://en.wikipedia.org/wiki/quiet_revolution. This is a comprehensive history of the historic secularization and modernization of Quebec led by Liberal premier Jean Lesage (thirty-one references, 2014); and "Quebec's Quiet Revolution: Summary and Significance," available at http://schoolworkhelper.net/quebec_quiet_ (slanted toward Quebec nationalism).

9 Berkovitz, "History," 104–7.

10 Hall Commission Report, 1961–64 (Royal Commission on Health Services in Canada), available at http://www.hc-sc.qc.ca/hcs.sss/com/fed/hall-eng.php. This report proposed universal health care in Canada but also revealed the relatively poor access to health care professionals in Quebec compared to other provinces.

11 Castonguay-Nepveu Report, 1967 on Health Care and Social Services in Quebec, available at www.historymuseum.ca/cmc/exhibitions/hist/medicare/medic.

12 Medical Care Act, 1966, available at http://en.wikipedia.org/wiki/medicare (Canada). This bill established Medicare in Canada, introducing the concept of universal health care (eight pages, sixty references); Michael Rachlis, "Medicare Made Easy," *Globe and Mail*, 26 April 2006; and Alex Patterson, "History of Medicare in Canada," speech given October 2012 at the Canadian Club in Yamaska, Quebec. This is a good review of the history of health care legislation in Canada from someone who had been on various boards at McGill and its hospitals during this period.

13 Medical Insurance Act, 15 October 1970, "Bill 65," available at http://www. mastermyhealth.com/html/quebec-health-insurance act.html.

14 Quebec and Medicare, available at http://www.historymuseum.ca/cmc/ exhibitions/hist/medicare/medic-6h03e_shtml. This the best account of the specialists strike, the reasons for it, and its consequences. Short and sweet.

15 Gerard Pelletier, *The October Crisis* (Toronto: McClelland and Stewart, 1971). Pelletier was a member of Bourassa's cabinet, and he wrote this book one year after the event.

16 William Tetley, *The October Crisis, 1970: An Insiders View* (Montreal and Kingston: McGill-Queen's University Press, 2007). A comprehensive chronology of the events leading up to October 1970 and after.

17 Quebec Health Serves and Social Services Act, 1971, available at http://www.mss.gouv.gc.ca/sujets/organisatin/ssss.

18 J.M. Eakin, "Survival of the Fittest? The Democratization of Hospital Administration in Quebec," *International Journal of Health Services* 14, 3, (1984): 397–411.

19 Ibid.

20 Ibid.

21 M. Breton, R. J.-F. Pineault, and W. Hogg, "Primary Care Reform: Can Quebec's Family Medicine Group (FMG) Model Benefit from the Experience of Ontario's Family Health Teams?" Available at Longwoods. Com. Health Care Policy, 7 October 2011. This is a comparison of the CLSCs and FMGs in Quebec

22 1974 Official Language Act (Bill 22) in Quebec, available at http://en.wikipedia.org/wiki/official_languag_act, Bourassa's Bill 22 declared French the only official language in Quebec, which met major legal opposition from constitutional scholars at McGill (two pages, six references, including the infamous sign legislation and the language test for non-French children). This ill-conceived and unpopular bill backfired on Bourassa, who resigned as party leader.

23 1977 Charter on the French Language (Bill 101), available at http://en.wqikipedia.org/wiki/charter_of_the_French language. Lévesque's Bill 101 declared that French was to be the language of work, instruction, communication, commerce, and business. Lévesque wanted all business, even hospital business with patients, to be in French (fourteen pages, forty-two notes, twelve references).

24 History of Health and Social Transfers, available at http://www.fin.gc.ca/fedprov/his-eng.asp.

25 Bercovitz, "History," 104–7; and D. Ackman, "The Computer and the MGH," *MGH News* 6–7 (Winter 1996).

26 J.E. Coffey, chapter 27, this volume. See also MGH, annual reports, 1981–82 and 1982–83, MUA, which provide the actual tax deficits.

27 Ibid.

28 Ibid.

29 Canada Health Act (CHA), 1984, available at

http://en.wikipedia.org/wiki/canada_health_act. A ten-page comprehensive review of the CHA (sixteen references).

30 Public Prescription Drug Plan (1997 in Quebec), available at http://www.ramq. gouv.qc.ca/en/citizens/prescription-drug-insurance

31 McGill University Health Centre (MUHC), Project's History, available at http://muhc.ca/new-muhc/page/redevelopment-project's history, 1–2. This offers a brief list of events, by year, from 1997 to 2011, leading to the building of the MUHC.

32 Ibid.

33 Ibid.

34 Ibid.

35 Ibid.

36 Personal conversations and e-mails between November 2013 and June 2014 with Richard and Sylvia Cruess, ex-dean of medicine Abe Fuks, Alex Paterson, and Barry Cappel about the MGH and MUHC. These communications confirmed and clarified information already obtained and gave me insight.

37 Daniel Johnson and Brian Mulroney, Executive Summary of Commissions Report (Commission to Analyze the Implementation of the Projects for the Hospital Centre of the University of Montreal [CHUM] and the McGill University Health Centre [MUHC]), April 2005. Available at : http://www.premier. gouv.gc.ca.collections.banq.gc.ca/ark:/52327/bs47247; and MUHC, Project's History, 1.

38 Ibid.

39 G. MacArthur and D. Montero, "Meet Arthur T. Porter, the Man at the Centre of One of Canada's Biggest Health Care Scandals," *Globe and Mail* 22 December 2012. This is a detailed account of Porter's career in the MUHC; D. Seglins and John Nicol, "Who's Who? McGill University Hospital $22.5 M Bribery Case, 'Targets of the Biggest Fraud and Corruption Investigation in Canadian History,' Says Sureté du Quebec," BCB News, 3 September 2014. This program names six others involved in the contract scandal of the MUHC and is available at http://www.cbc.ca/news/who-s-who-mcgill-univeristy-hospital-22-5m-bribery-case.

40 MUHC, Project's History, 2.

41 Ibid.

42 Ibid.

43 MacArthur and Montero, "Meet Arthur Porter"; Seglins and Nicol, "Who's Who."

44 Ibid.

45 Progress at the Glen Site, 2012, available at
http://muhc.ca/new.muhc/article/progress-glen-site; B. Wurst, "MUHC Super-
hospital: A New Horizon," *Montreal Times*, 12 January 2014, available at
http://mtltimes.ca/social-life/muhc-Superhospital-newhorizon. This is the best
short account of the MUHC project.

46 A.K. Paterson, *My Life at the Bar and Beyond* (Montreal and Kingston: McGill-
Queen's University Press, 2005), 179–81. An excellent first-hand account of the
Save the Shriners Hospital campaign by a remarkable group of academics and
politicians written by one of the great names associated with McGill in the last
four decades. Because of this effort, the Shriners made one of the best hospital
location decisions in its history by placing its new facility in the Glen along
with, but independent of, the MUHC/CUSM.

General Works regarding MGH Governance

These include H.E. MacDermot, *History of the Montreal General Hospital*
(Montreal: Montreal General Hospital, 1950); H.E. MacDermot, *History of
the School of Nursing of the Montreal General Hospital* (Montreal: Alumnae
Association of the MGH, 1940); and H.E. MacDermot, *The Years of Change,
1945–70* (Montreal: MGH, 1970). The latter was published by the MGH for
its 150th anniversary in 1970, this is MacDermot's excellent update on his
1950 history of the institution.

Also of interest is F.J. Shepherd's *Origin and History of the Montreal General Hospital* (Montreal: self-published, 1925). Published privately by the author, this little book is hard to find and is written by a man who lived
through MGH history from 1872 to 1929. H.E. MacDermot, A.T. Bazin, E.H.
Bensley, G. Fisk, P. Edgell, and A.H. Westbury's *The Montreal General Hospital, 1821–1956: A Pictorial Review* is a special *MGH Bulletin* (vol. 2, no. 8
1956) offers many pictures of past presidents, board chairs, medical directors, and directors of nursing plus many scenes of the hospital's history. E.
Bensley, R.R. Forsey, and J. Grout's *The Montreal General Hospital since 1821*
(Montreal: MGH, 1971) was published by the 150th Anniversary Committee of the MGH in May 1971. This little known book, which is full of pictures of MGH life, is a complement to H.E. MacDermot's 1970 paperback
update on MGH history.

Editors' Final Note

The editors and authors have written an historic account of the MGH from a multi-specialty point of view covering the 178 years (1819–1997) of its existence. The various specialty histories are about the MGH as we have known it, an independent institution, up to 1997, when the McGill University Health Centre was officially established. Now, having been integrated into the MUHC, the MGH, dubbed the MUHC Mountainside Campus, will gradually lose its identity, the preservation of which is one of the purposes of this volume.

The editors wish to praise the extraordinary people who have directed and managed the course of the MGH up to 1997. For 178 years of unprecedented political and social change, they have never failed to meet the challenges and never forgotten the mission statement located in the lobby on Cedar Avenue, taken from the building on Dorchester Street. (Please note that "178 years" refers to the MGH founded on Craig Street in 1819 and not the Dorchester Building opened 1822.)

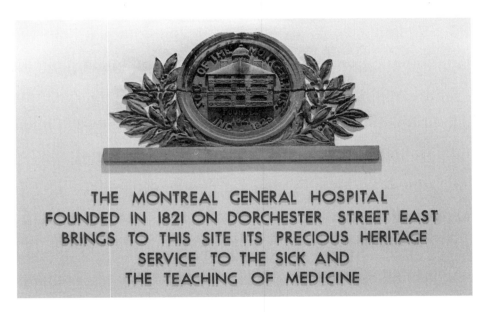

THE MONTREAL GENERAL HOSPITAL
FOUNDED IN 1821 ON DORCHESTER STREET EAST
BRINGS TO THIS SITE ITS PRECIOUS HERITAGE
SERVICE TO THE SICK AND
THE TEACHING OF MEDICINE

Fig 48.3 This is the mission statement of the MGH found in the lobby
in the Cedar Avenue building.

Contributors

Ruth Allan-Rigby, BN, CIC, former director of MGH research unit in nursing and health care.

Donald W. Baxter, OC, MD, FRCPC, former director, Division of Neurology, MGH, and Montreal Neurological Institute emeritus professor neurology and neurosurgery, and of medicine, McGill University.

James D. Baxter, MD, CM, FRCSC, former chair of otolaryngology, McGill University professor of otololaryngology (retired), McGill University.

Garth M. Bray, MD, FRCPC former director, Division of Neurology, MGH, emeritus professor neurology and neurosurgery, and of medicine, McGill University.

C. Emerson Brooks, MD, CM, FRCSC, former chief, Department of Orthopaedic Surgery, MGH, associate professor of surgery (retired), McGill University.

John H. Burgess, CM, MD, CM, MACP, FRCPC, emeritus cardiologist, MUHC, professor of medicine, McGill University.

C.J. (Ray) Chiu, MD, FRCSC, former director, Division of Cardiovascular and Thoracic Surgery, MGH professor of surgery, McGill University.

Michael Churchill-Smith, MD, CM, FRCPC, former director, Emergency Room, MGH, associate professor of medicine.

J. Edwin Coffey, MD, CM, FRCSC, obstetrician and gynaecologist, MUHC, associate professor of obstetrics and gynaecology (retired) McGill University.

Ron Collett, president and CEO, MGH Foundation.

Neil Colman, MD, CM, FRCPC, former director, Division of Respirology, MGH, professor of medicine, McGill University.

Larry Conochie, MD, CM, FRCSC, former orthopaedic surgeon, MGH, assistant professor of surgery (retired), McGill University.

Duncan Cowie, BA, MA.

Paula U. Dembeck, RN, BN, MEd, former associate director of nursing.

Donald Douglas, PhD, clinical chemist, MGH, associate professor of medicine, McGill University.

John Esdaile, MD, CM, FRCPC, former director, Division of Rheumatology, MGH, former associate professor of medicine, McGill University.

R. Roy Forsey, MD, FRCPC, former chief, Department of Dermatology, MGH, professor of medicine (retired), McGill University.

Samuel O. Freedman, OC, MD, CM, FRCPC, emeritus professor of medicine, former dean of medicine and vice-principal (academic) McGill University.

Carolyn Freeman, MD, FRCPC, chief of radiation oncology, MUHC, professor of radiology, McGill University.

Abraham Fuks, MD, CM, FRCPC, professor of medicine and former dean of medicine, McGill University.

William Gerstein, MD, FRCPC, former director, Division of Dermatology, MGH, associate professor of medicine, McGill University.

John Gibson, MD, FRCPC, former radiologist, MGH, assistant professor of radiology (retired), McGill University.

Lyson Haccoun, former pharmacist, MUHC.

Joseph Hanaway, MD, CM, FAAN, associate professor of neurology (retired), University of Missouri School of Medicine, Columbia, MO.

Jacqueline Harvey, MPhys Ed, former physiotherapist, MUHC.

David Hawkins, MD, FRCPC, former director, Division of Rheumatology, MGH professor of medicine (retired), McGill University.

Margaret Hooton, RN, BScN, MSc(A), former staff member of MGH nursing.

Lois Hutchison, past-president, MGH Auxiliary.

Guy Joron, MD, CM, former director of toxicology, MGH, associate professor of medicine, McGill University.

Michael Kaye, MD, FRCPC, former director, Division of Nephrology, MGH, professor of medicine (retired), McGill University.

Douglas G. Kinnear, MD, CM, FRCPC, former director, Division of Gastroenterology, MGH, associate professor of medicine, McGill University.

Michael Laplante, MD, CM, FRCSC, associate professor of surgery, urology, McGill University.

Constance Lechman, MSW, MBA, former director of social service, MUHC.

Eric Lenczner, MD, CM, FRCSC, orthopaedic surgeon, MGH, associate professor of orthopaedic surgery, McGill University.

Michael Libman, MD, FRCPC, director, Division of Infectious Disease, MUHC, associate professor of medicine, McGill University.

J. Dick MacLean, MD, CM, FRCPC, former director, McGill Centre for Tropical Diseases professor of medicine, McGill University.

Alan Mann, MD, CM, FRCPC, former psychiatrist-in-chief, MGH, professor of psychiatry, McGill University.

Jacqueline McClaran, MD, CM, former director, Division of Geriatrics, MGH, assistant professor of family medicine, McGill University.

Ian Metcalf, MD, FRCPC, former chief of anaesthesiology, MGH, associate professor of anaesthesiology, McGill University.

David S. Mulder, CM, MD, FRCSC, former chair, Department of Surgery, McGill University professor of surgery, McGill University.

Ross Murphy, MD, CM, FRCSC, former orthopaedic surgeon, MGH, assistant professor of surgery (retired), McGill University.

Sean Murphy, OC, MD, CM, FRCPC, former chair, Department of Ophthalmology, McGill University professor of ophthalmology, McGill University.

Edwin Podgorsak, PhD, radiation physicist, MUHC.

John Richardson, MD, FRCPC, former chair, Department of Pathology, McGill University professor of pathology, McGill University.

Sandra Richardson, MD, CM, former director, Division of Geriatrics, MGH, associate professor of family medicine, McGill University.

Richard Robinson, MD, FRCPC, anaesthesiologist, MUHC, assistant professor of anaesthesiology, McGill University.

David Rosenblatt, MD, CM, FRCPC, director, Division of Clinical Epidemiology, MUHC professor of medicine, McGill University.

Leonard Rosenthall, MD, CM, FRCPC, former director of nuclear medicine, MGH professor of radiology, McGill University.

Valerie P. Shannon, BScN, MSN, former director of nursing, MUHC, former director McGill School of Nursing.

Joe Stratford, MD, FRCSC, former director, Division of Neurosurgery, MGH, professor of neurosurgery, McGill University.

Margaret Suttie, BScN, former chair of MGH nursing research committee.

Michael P. Thirlwell, MD, FRCPC, director, Division of Medical Oncology, MGH, associate professor of medicine, McGill University.

H. Bruce Williams, former director, Division of Plastic Surgery, MGH, professor of surgery, McGill University.

Shirley E. Woods, Jr., author.

Figures

The names in this list, starting with chapter 3, are the chairs of MGH departments and divisions up to 1997, although in some cases into the 2000s. These represent the pictures that could be found with extensive searching.

Index

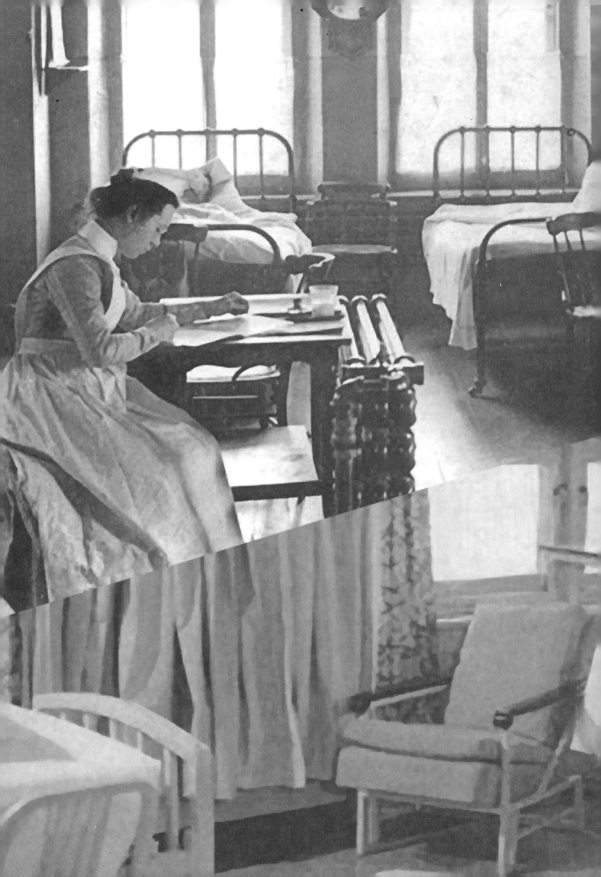